SELECTED WRITINGS OF
JOHN HUGHLINGS JACKSON

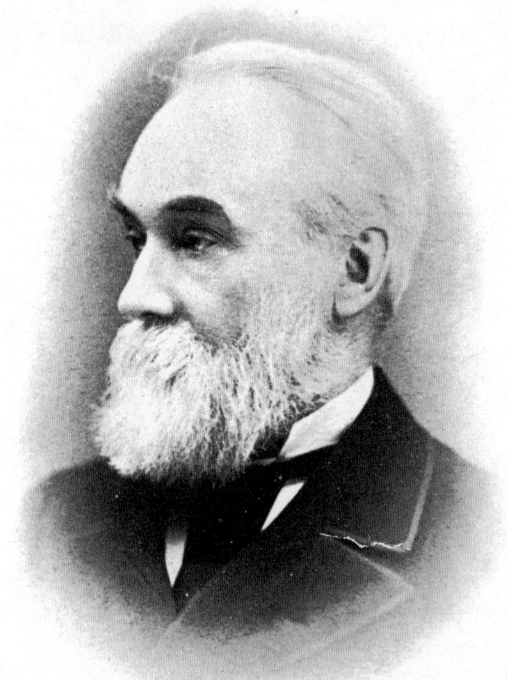

J Hughlings Jackson

[*Frontispiece*

# SELECTED WRITINGS

OF

# JOHN HUGHLINGS JACKSON

## VOLUME ONE

## ON EPILEPSY AND EPILEPTIFORM CONVULSIONS

EDITED
FOR THE GUARANTORS OF "BRAIN"
BY

JAMES TAYLOR
M.D., F.R.C.P.

WITH THE ADVICE AND ASSISTANCE OF

GORDON HOLMES
M.D., F.R.C.P.
AND
F. M. R. WALSHE
M.D., F.R.C.P.

BASIC BOOKS, INC.
New York

First printing, 1958
PRINTED IN THE UNITED STATES OF AMERICA

# PREFACE

It has always been a matter for regret that Dr. Hughlings Jackson himself was never able to make a selection from his writings which he would have regarded as adequately illustrative of his views and theories. A request that he should make such a selection was conveyed to him in 1901 in a letter from Dr. Osler, who wrote on behalf of himself and Dr. Weir Mitchell and Dr. Putnam. To this Jackson replied that he was so highly stimulated by a request from three such men that he would " endeavour a kind of reproduction," and that he hoped to make a volume which would contain in a methodical way most of what he had done in neurology, and another volume of minor contributions. Unfortunately he was never able to carry out his intention.

The question of republishing some of Jackson's papers has been discussed at various times among neurologists, and last year the Guarantors of " Brain " decided that such a republication was desirable, and they decided to undertake it. On offering to put at their disposal the collection of his papers which I had made, I was asked to undertake the work of editing the necessary volumes. I consented to do this, only stipulating that I should have access to Dr. Gordon Holmes and Dr. Walshe for any advice or assistance I might find necessary. I need only say that I am deeply grateful for the help they have most willingly given me.

It was considered that two volumes of about 500 pages each would be necessary, and satisfactory arrangements for publication were first made with Hodder and Stoughton Ltd. It was decided that the first volume should contain the papers dealing with Epilepsy and Epileptiform Convulsions, while the second volume should contain the more philosophical papers together with several lectures and addresses.

I am much indebted to the Editors and Proprietors of the various publications in which the articles originally appeared for their permission to reproduce them. Sir James Crichton-Browne, in giving his most cordial consent to the inclusion of articles from the West Riding Asylum Reports, expressed his pleasure in the publication of these volumes, which, he says, " will be the payment of a debt long overdue to Jackson's memory, and to medical science." I have to thank Messrs. Churchill for permission to reprint articles from the *Medical Times and Gazette*, and the Editors of *The Lancet*, *British Medical Journal*, *Medical Press and Circular*, *Medical Times*, and the *Journal of Medical Science* for so willingly giving their consent to the inclusion of articles which appeared in their journals. I am greatly indebted to Mr. W. R. B. Prideaux for the care and skill with which he has prepared the index.

JAMES TAYLOR.

*April*, 1931.

## PUBLISHER'S NOTE

The present publisher wishes to express his gratitude to the Guarantors of "Brain" for their kind permission to reprint this neurological classic, which will, it is hoped, be of value to this generation of students and to the future.

# TABLE OF CONTENTS

PAGE

Introduction . . . . . . . . . . . . ix

Unilateral Epileptiform Seizures attended by Temporary Defect of Sight . . . . . . . . . . . . 1

Epileptiform Seizures—Aura from the Thumb, Attacks of Coloured Vision . . . . . . . . . . . 1

Blow on Left Side of Head, Loss of Speech and Hemiplegia on the Right Side: subsequently Unilateral Epileptiform Seizures, beginning in Side Paralysed . . . . . . 2

Loss of Speech with Hemiplegia of the Left Side, Valvular Disease, Epileptiform Convulsions affecting the Side Paralysed . 3

A Digression on Epilepsy . . . . . . . . . . 4

Extract from an Article, " Note on the Comparison and Contrast of Regional Palsy and Spasm " . . . . . . . . 5

Case of Convulsive Attacks arrested by stopping the Aura . 6

A Study of Convulsions . . . . . . . . . . 8

On the Anatomical and Physiological Localisation of Movements in the Brain . . . . . . . . . . . 37

Observations on the Localisation of Movements in the Cerebral Hemisphere, as revealed in Cases of Convulsion, Chorea, and " Aphasia " . . . . . . . . . . . . 77

On the Anatomical, Physiological, and Pathological Investigations of Epilepsies . . . . . . . . . 90

On the Anatomical Investigation of Epilepsy and Epileptiform Convulsions . . . . . . . . . . . . 112

Remarks on Systemic Sensations in Epilepsies . . . . . 118

On Temporary Mental Disorders after Epileptic Paroxysms . 119

On Epilepsies and on the After-effects of Epileptic Discharges (Todd and Robertson's Hypothesis) . . . . . . 135

On the Scientific and Empirical Investigation of Epilepsies . 162

PAGE

Intellectual Warnings of Epileptic Seizures . . . . . 274

Lectures on the Diagnosis of Epilepsy (Harveian Society) . . 276

On Right- or Left-sided Spasm at the Onset of Epileptic Paroxysms and on Crude Sensation Warnings and Elaborate Mental States . . . . . . . . . . . 308

On Temporary Paralysis after Epileptiform and Epileptic Seizures: a Contribution to the Study of Dissolution of the Nervous System . . . . . . . . . . . 318

Epileptiform Convulsions from Cerebral Disease . . . 330

Localised Convulsions from Tumour of the Brain . . . 341

A Contribution to the Comparative Study of Convulsions . 348

On a Case of Fits resembling those artificially produced in Guinea-pigs . . . . . . . . . . 362

On Post-epileptic States: a Contribution to the Comparative Study of Insanities . . . . . . . . 366

On a Particular Variety of Epilepsy ("Intellectual Aura"), one Case with Symptoms of Organic Brain Disease . . . 385

Case of Tumour of the Right Temporo-sphenoidal Lobe, bearing on the Localisation of the Sense of Smell and on the Interpretation of a Particular Variety of Epilepsy (with Dr. C. E. Beevor) . . . . . . . . . . 406

On Convulsive Seizures (Lumleian Lectures) . . . . 412

Case of Epilepsy with Tasting Movements and "Dreamy State"—very Small Patch of Softening in the Left Uncinate Gyrus (with Dr. W. S. Colman) . . . . . . . . 458

Epileptic Attacks with a Warning of a Crude Sensation of Smell and with the Intellectual Aura (Dreamy State) in a Patient who had Symptoms pointing to Gross Organic Disease of Right Temporo-sphenoidal Lobe (with Dr. Purves Stewart) . . 464

Observations of a Case of Convulsions (Trunk Fit or Lowest Level Fit) (with Dr. Douglas Singer) . . . . . 474

Further Observations on a Case of Convulsions (Trunk Fit or Lowest Level Fit?) (with Dr. Stanley Barnes) . . . . 482

Index . . . . . . . . . . . . . 487

# INTRODUCTION

It is not an easy task to make such a selection from the writings of Hughlings Jackson as will give an adequate idea of the extent of his work or explain its influence on neurological thought and research since his time. His contributions are so numerous, scattered through the pages of so many periodicals over many years, that it has been found impossible to make a small selection illustrative of his methods and doctrine. One has been forced to select generously, and the reader will find that there is much repetition. He will also find, however, that although the same idea is enunciated in different places it is often arrived at by different routes, so that the repetition is so far justified.

There were always the two sides to his teaching, the clinical and the philosophical, but these two sides are in such intimate combination that there is no corresponding division of his papers which would enable one to devote a volume to each. The plan adopted has been to reserve the first volume for articles dealing with "Epilepsy and Epileptiform Convulsions," the subject apparently of his earliest interest. The papers which are included in this volume are arranged chronologically, as it is hoped that by this means, the reader will be able to trace the gradual development of Jackson's views on the subject under discussion. Although the clinical interest is naturally predominant in this volume, the philosophic side is by no means absent. In the second volume many lectures and philosophical addresses will be included, but here, on the other hand, the clinical side will be found frequently obtruding itself.

Jackson came to London in 1859, then aged 24. His medical education had been conducted in York, and he returned there, after he qualified, to take office at the local dispensary. There he was associated with Laycock, who afterwards became Professor of Medicine in Edinburgh University. Laycock had in 1841 enunciated the doctrine that the brain was subject to the laws of reflex action and was therefore in this respect not different from the other ganglia of the nervous system. Jackson at the beginning of one of his papers (p. 37) quotes this doctrine of Laycock's, and in the first volume of the *London Hospital Reports* one of the published cases—hemiplegia of the right side with loss of speech—is from the records of cases under his care at the York Dispensary. So I think we are justified in inferring that when Jackson came to London he was already interested in the functions of the nervous system and its disturbance as a result of disease. We know he was interested is Psychology, for Jonathan Hutchinson tells us that Jackson at this time had fully resolved to give up medicine and devote himself to philosophy. Hutchinson was able to persuade him to continue his medical career, and neurologists at least must always be grateful to him for this service.

Soon after his arrival in London he was associated with Hutchinson in reporting for the *Medical Times and Gazette* cases from Hospital practice and from the proceedings of medical societies. He thus became well known to members of the Staffs of the chief London hospitals and had opportunities of seeing many cases. It is not difficult to identify the contributions of the two men, and it is soon evident that Jackson's interests were overwhelmingly neurological. These interests were confirmed by his early appointment as Assistant Physician to the National Hospital, Queen Square, an appointment which he received the year before he joined the staff of the London Hospital. At this time Brown-Séquard was one of the physicians at Queen Square, and there is no doubt that Jackson was stimulated and encouraged in his neurological work by this brilliant physician and physiologist.

Jackson's early writings are much concerned with convulsive seizures of limited range and of deliberate onset, attacks which were first described by Bravais in 1824, but are now universally known as Jacksonian. A study of his writings reveals not only his interest in these conditions, but also indicates their significance in determining the lines in which his researches and speculations developed. He first pointed out, for instance, that these attacks begin mostly in the face, hand or foot—the parts which suffer most in the ordinary form of hemiplegia—and he contrasted the conditions found in local convulsions with those occurring in hemiplegia. He recognised that these limited attacks, although commencing locally, do not always remain local, but sometimes spread so as to affect the whole of one side of the body or even the whole body, and that when this occurred consciousness was lost, while in the limited seizure consciousness might be retained throughout the attack. If the attack were severe it was not unusual to find after the attack weakness of the side affected, and this he identified with the epileptic hemiplegia previously described by Todd. He also pointed out what had previously been observed, that an attack could often be aborted by pulling or pressing on the part in which the convulsion began.

In many of these cases of local attacks he found evidence, sometimes confirmed by post-mortem examination, of " coarse " disease of the brain—glioma, syphiloma, abscess—and when such a condition was diagnosed and confirmed in a case in which a seizure commencing locally had been present, *e.g.* in the hand or in the foot, the seat of the minute changes associated with the convulsion could be inferred. He claims that in thus observing local convulsions and their underlying causes he is studying convulsions generally, and that by such a method of approach he is more likely to arrive at definite ideas as to the nature of the much more complex condition—idiopathic or genuine epilepsy. Such observations also are useful in helping to determine the region of the brain from which movements are initiated and controlled.

Such ideas were of course revolutionary, for it has to be remembered that at this time the prevalent view as to the cause of epilepsy was that it depended upon disturbance of the Medulla oblongata. The objections raised by the defenders of the old doctrine were that these cases of localised convulsion with which Jackson was concerned were not epileptic at all !

These early observations were summarised and analysed, and his views enunciated more fully in " A Study of Convulsions," a paper published in the *Transactions of the St. Andrews Medical Graduates Association*, and afterwards reprinted in pamphlet form (see p. 8), and it was then evident that Jackson was advocating a completely new outlook on the nature and cause of epilepsy. He was no longer concerned to know whether there was loss of consciousness, or tongue-biting, or relaxation of sphincters. What he was concerned with was the nature of the convulsion, the mode of its onset, the march of the spasm and the subsequent condition of the patient, whether paralysed or otherwise affected, so that he might by means of such observations discover not only the significance of the convulsion but also the region of the nervous system in which the unstable focus was situated, the nature of the disturbance and its pathological cause.

Another disease of analogous nature which he studied in connection with local convulsions and paralysis was chorea, and he classed all three together as dependent upon vascular disturbance in the " region of the middle cerebral artery." Chorea he regarded as due to changes occurring in the terminal branches of this artery in the " region of the corpus striatum " and alluding to the then prevalent idea that it was often the result of fright, he said that while it might be permissible to regard chorea as the result of mental shock, such a cause could hardly be invoked logically to account for the condition in a case of hemi-chorea. Although his views on the pathology of chorea are no longer accepted, his arguments on the nature of its anatomical basis are still of interest, more particularly as he placed this in the corpus striatum, where, according to recent experiences, the essential lesion probably exists.

In 1873 Jackson received what must have been to him most welcome confirmation of his views from the researches and experiments of Ferrier, who wrote [1]: " The objects I had in view in undertaking the present research were twofold: first to put to experimental proof the views entertained by Dr. Hughlings Jackson on the pathology of epilepsy, chorea and hemiplegia by imitating artificially the destroying and discharging lesions of disease which his writings have defined and differentiated—and secondly to follow up the path which the researches of Fritsch and Hitzig (who have shown the brain to be susceptible to galvanic stimulation) indicated to me as likely to lead to results of great value in the elucidation of the functions of the cerebral hemispheres, and in the more exact localisation and diagnosis of cerebral disease."

At the conclusion of his article he writes: " The pathology of epileptiform convulsions, chorea and epileptic hemiplegia receives much light from the foregoing experiments. I regard them as an experimental confirmation of the views expressed by Dr. Hughlings Jackson. They are, as it were, an artificial reproduction of the clinical experiments performed by disease, and the clinical conclusions which Dr. Jackson has arrived at from his observations of disease are in all essential particulars confirmed by the above experiments."

This almost dramatic confirmation, from the experimental side, of his clinical observations and conclusions must have been very gratifying to Jackson, yet in the next year he writes: " In spite of the encouragement I have received from these researches I feel that it requires more skill than I possess to make my subject clear to those who have long worked at epilepsy from a totally different point of view."

It would seem as if Jackson's early interest in and study of these local convulsions were the starting-point of all his subsequent work. Among his earlier observations was one on the affection of speech after some of these local convulsions, usually of the right side of the body, and he knew that there was often permanent defect of this faculty with decided hemiplegia. His attitude to Broca's claim that speech is localised in the third left frontal convolution is shown by his statement in 1864 that while " viewing with great respect and deference the evidence adduced by M. Broca," he neither accepted the old view that the brain is a double organ, nor the new one that the faculty of

[1] *West Riding Asylum Reports*, vol. iii, p. 30.

language resides in the left hemisphere only. He claimed that there were advantages in remaining neutral, and pointed out that there were other paths of investigation, especially the investigation of the temporary interferences with speech which occurred after some local convulsions. Jackson's work on speech, valuable as it is, is only touched on in some of the papers in this volume. It has been so exhaustively investigated by Sir Henry Head [1] that it has not been considered necessary to reproduce any of the papers specially devoted to its study.

Local convulsions are of course often associated with intracranial growths, and Jackson's interests were early invoked in the symptomatology of these, and some of his most interesting communications and lectures dealt with this subject. The introduction of the ophthalmoscope was a great stimulus in the observation of these cases, and Jackson was never tired of insisting upon the necessity of repeated and persistent use of this instrument, in the use of which he himself was proficient. He was among the first to point out how necessary such examination was, even in cases with no evidence of impaired vision, as he recognised that often vision may be perfect even in the presence of intense optic neuritis. This aspect of Jackson's work has been dealt with in considerable detail elsewhere.[2] That many of the local fits were syphilitic in origin naturally resulted in a close study of syphilitic conditions, both hereditary and acquired, and he published many papers on syphilitic affections of the nervous system.

Another subject which engaged Jackson's attention was vertigo. So-called epileptic vertigo he recognised early, *i.e.* attacks of giddiness and reeling with momentary or longer loss of consciousness. He himself was subject to attacks of auditory or labyrinthine vertigo, and his interest naturally led him to investigate the whole subject. He regarded the vertigo associated with ocular paralysis as a link connecting various varieties of vertigo, and his investigations into its manifestations and pathology are most instructive.

An aspect of epilepsy which early excited Jackson's interest was the relation of subjective sensations to attacks of unconsciousness. In a paper published in 1866 he mentions that the first symptom in certain epileptiform seizures is a subjective sensation of smell, generally a disagreeable one, and he refers to sensation of colours, etc., in connection with these seizures. He regards these sensations as psychical states attending nervous discharges, and warns us against regarding them as nervous discharges. Sometimes these sensations are crude, sometimes they seem to merge into an elaborate state, as when coloured vision—a crude sensation—is followed by "seeing faces." Similarly a crude sensation of smell is sometimes followed by a voluminous psychical state—the "dreamy state"—but he insisted that such a psychical state cannot be regarded as an elaboration of a sensation of smell, although it is not without significance that in normal persons certain scents or smells do develop very voluminous reminiscences.

The nature and significance of these psychical states, which had been named "intellectual auræ," were dealt with in a later series of papers. He rather deprecates the term "intellectual aura," preferring the term "dreamy state," for this "dreamy state" is not an aura in the sense that the crude sensations of smell, etc., so often associated with it, are auræ. The crude

[1] *Brain*, vol. xxxviii, 1915, p. 1, and vol. xlvi, 1923, p. 355.
[2] *Brain*, vol. xxxviii, 1915, p. 391.

sensations, he pointed out, occur during epileptic discharges, the elaborate "dreamy state" arises during slightly raised activities of healthy nervous arrangements. "Dreamy states" with or without olfactory or gustatory phenomena were later found to be associated with tumours or other lesions of the uncinate region, and Jackson therefore proposed for the variety of epilepsy characterised by these auræ the now generally accepted term "uncinate epilepsy."

Even the most philosophical of Jackson's writings, those concerned with evolution and dissolution of the nervous system, seem to be related to his early work on local convulsions. Destructive lesions of different levels of the nervous system produce symptoms, as paralysis of movement, that differ in kind as well as degree, and the same fact applies to convulsive phenomena, whether local or general. Arguing from these facts, Jackson came to the conclusion that not only had the nervous system evolved from the simple nervous system of the lower vertebrates by the addition of new parts, but that these new levels were organised differently, to use the words of Spencer, his favourite author among the philosophers. He was almost forced to a consideration of evolution in comparing and contrasting the facts of convulsion and palsy. Palsy results from destruction of fibres, so that a lesion low down in the nervous system, *e.g.* in the corpus striatum or lower, results in marked paralysis. But as we ascend to the cortex the condition becomes much more complex, the fibres more numerous, so that a destructive lesion of the same extent at this level is not nearly so paralysing as one lower down in the nervous system. And conversely as the increasing complexity of fibres necessitates more ganglion cells—the supposed explosive material—discharge here produces severe convulsion. In other words, destruction of those parts, irritation of which produces the most severe convulsion, may result in little or no palsy.

This view of the nervous system implies that the most lately developed level controls and inhibits the lower levels. Destruction of it—dissolution—a negative condition, cannot by itself produce active symptoms. The symptoms which follow such a condition are the result of the now uncontrolled action of the lower healthy levels, and in this fact is sought the explanation of such widely different conditions as the increased knee-jerk after a destructive lesion in the internal capsule and the violence of epileptic mania. "Theoretically," Jackson says, "we should expect that the epileptic patients most likely to become insane would be those who have discharging lesions in the very highest nervous arrangements. In such cases the disturbance initiating the attack would be in an area in which there exists the most complex and elaborate arrangements for the representation of movements. The attack would be sudden, the convulsion almost immediately universal, and occurring as it did in such a complex area there would be no warning." Such cases are of the most severe type, and it is of no little significance in reference to the absence of aura in these that Sir James Crichton-Browne has stated, with all the authority of wide experience, that in asylum practice an aura is of rare occurrence in cases of epilepsy.

The implications of this view of the evolution of the nervous system and its application to the explanation of nervous disease, although alluded to in parts of this volume, are much more fully set out in papers which will appear in the second volume.

Between 1893 and 1909 Jackson published a series of short papers under the title of *Neurological Fragments*. They excited much interest at the time, as they dealt with many interesting neurological questions. They are not included in either volume, as they were published separately a few years ago with a short biographical memoir.[1]

I should like before concluding this introduction to give two short quotations from an early lecture of Jackson's illustrative of methods which only those were familiar with who knew him by the bedside. Former house-physicians will be able to recall similar short disquisitions. " How foolish," he says, " we should look if we diagnosed brain disease in a case like this. A young man supposed to be quite healthy falls down in convulsions. He soon regains consciousness, but his urine is found to be bloody and albuminous, and it is ascertained that several of his brothers and sisters are then suffering from scarlet fever. Here, obviously, the condition was disorder of the functions of the brain, but the organ anatomically changed was one remote—the kidney." The other quotation is a piece of advice, remarkable as it was, given at a time when attention was largely focused on the auscultatory phenomena of heart disease: " Never treat a patient on stethoscopic evidence only. The heart may be a bad musical instrument and yet a good force-pump. However noisy the first sound may be at the base of the heart, if the apex be in the right place, if there be no signs of hypertrophy, no anæmia, if the pulse be good, and, above all, if the patient does his work well, we have nothing to treat. To treat such a case would be to treat a sound. It would be just as great a mistake as the drunken captain made who tried to navigate his vessel round a speck of dirt on his chart which he mistook for an island."

These quotations are illustrative of the more practical side of his teaching. His writings have been called theoretical and obscure, and it is true that they are sometimes not easy to follow, and they are frequently overloaded with footnotes. Yet with persistent study they become clear, and in places really luminous, displaying the incisive analytical mind of the philosopher, while quotations like those I have just given show the sound practical common sense of the physician.

[1] *Neurological Fragments*, Oxford Medical Publication, 1925.

# EPILEPSY AND EPILEPTIFORM CONVULSIONS

These few papers which serve to introduce this volume are selected from a very large number which were published between 1861 and 1870 by Dr. Hughlings Jackson on Epilepsy and Epileptiform Convulsions. They are included merely as examples of his early contributions to various Medical Journals and to the London Hospital Reports, on which he founded much of his later systematic work. These papers were very numerous, and naturally include many repetitions, so that it would be impossible and unnecessary to publish all of them. They were really the raw material out of which developed the paper, *A Study of Convulsions* (see p. 8).

## Unilateral Epileptiform Seizures Attended by Temporary Defect of Sight [1]

In the following case there was, as well as the epilepsy, some temporary defect of sight. As a clinical fact, this is common in cases of epilepsy in which the attacks are unilateral. Sometimes in such cases the temporary defect of sight passes into a permanent one, but more frequently epileptiform seizures follow amaurosis. Such is, we repeat, the clinical fact, but the causes of the temporary loss of sight are very various, being due in some merely to a passing defect of the accessory apparatus of the eye, and in others to defects in the circulation of the retina itself. In a case of epileptiform convulsion in a patient who had recently suffered from syphilitic rash recorded in this Journal, January 31, 1863, the slight defect of sight appeared to be due to want of parallelism of the eye from convulsive action of the external rectus muscle on the side of the body affected, as this muscle was afterwards paralysed in the hemiplegia which followed a severe attack. In other cases there appears to be evidence that the defect of sight is due to some change in the circulation of the retina itself, and these are more likely to be followed by amaurosis.

A young robust-looking man consulted Dr. Hughlings Jackson November 1862 for epileptiform convulsion of the left side. He had then had only one complete attack. In this case the sight failed at the beginning of the paroxysm. A few months after, he lost the sight of both eyes. In a case now under the care of Dr. Brown-Séquard, at the hospital, there has been complete amaurosis for twelve months, followed by epileptiform convulsions of one side.

## Epileptiform Seizures—Aura from the Thumb—Attacks of Coloured Vision [2]

Alice F., a married woman, æt. 49, was admitted as out-patient under the care of Dr. Hughlings Jackson on November 28, 1862. Until about seven or eight months ago she had had good health and indeed looked in fair health and was very intelligent. She had not menstruated for twelve months, and complained a good deal of "sinking," of faintness, weakness, etc., symptoms so common at the change of life. Until the attack to be described she had

[1] *Medical Times and Gazette*, vol. i, 1863,p. 588. [2] *Ibid.*, p. 589.

had no definite ill-health, except a pain in the right arm of no very special character, so far as could be ascertained.

Five weeks before, she had a tingling sensation in the right thumb. It began under the nail and extended about as high as the styloid process of the radius and then " went to the face." The part of the face first attacked was the upper lip on the right side ; next the whole of that side of the face and the tongue also ; " it took her speech away for five minutes." She was not at all insensible. She had great pain in the arm, but the leg was not affected in any way. She had had about 20 of these attacks before admission.

It is interesting to note that, before any question was asked, she said that catching the shuttle with the thumb and finger would sometimes bring on a fit. She gave a circumstantial account of this. She had also attacks in which there was coloured vision, which were distinct from the seizures just described. The first was about four days before the seizure described above.

This patient took iodide of potassium. At her next visit she was better and had only had one attack. It was now ascertained that she had had tape-worms three years ago. December 19.—She had had no fit, but " had had the colours dreadful." It affected the right eye only, as she shut each eye in turn, in order to ascertain. The coloured vision was attended by pain in the right superciliary region. Both the pain and the colour came and went suddenly, lasting each time about ten minutes. She could see things, in spite of this peculiarity, but rather dimly. The colours were violet, white, and orange, and seemed about three yards distant. At other times the sight was good, and she had no pains. She had not at any time during these attacks any vertigo or insensibility, but numbness of the right leg. She had considerable pain still from the elbow to the fingers, but this was constant. A dose of the oil of male fern was prescribed.

Case 37.[1]—*Blow on the left side of the head, loss of speech and hemiplegia on the right side : subsequently unilateral epileptiform seizures, beginning in the side paralysed.*

The patient, a man 34 years of age, received a blow from a handspike November 1861 on the left side of the head. (When I saw him July 4, 1863, there was a depression of the skull about a square inch on the left side of the middle line about the anterior 1/3rd of the parietal bone.) He said that for ten hours after the blow he had been insensible, and that when he came to himself, he found that his speech was gone except to say " yes " and " no " and that he was paralysed on the right side. He could not get out of bed for four months.

After he had got rid of the paralysis, he became subject to convulsions affecting the side previously paralysed. The first seizure began by a tingling in the right hand, five months after the accident, but it was incomplete and was not followed by insensibility. Of these he had had 18, all beginning in the same way. But for nine months before I saw him the fits had been complete. He had had, of these, 5 or 6. I most unfortunately did not inquire whether speech was temporarily affected after the fits or not. I noted that he spoke " thickly," and that he said he could not write from slight weakness of the right hand.

In this case there can be no doubt the injury was near the left 3rd frontal

[1] *London Hospital Reports*, vol. i, 1864, p. 469.

convolution. By way of contrast I may mention that I now have under my care a patient who has extensive injury to the skull, including the part depressed in the case just related and much more. He has partial hemiplegia on the left side and left unilateral convulsions. The attacks began in the same way, but in the left instead of the right hand. He never lost speech, for his injury was on the right side, but he had double amaurosis.

## Loss of Speech with Hemiplegia of the Left Side, Valvular Disease, Epileptiform Convulsions Affecting the Side Paralysed [1]

The following is the only case I have ever seen of hemiplegia of the left side with loss of speech. Indeed, when I saw him he could talk almost as well as ever, but it is perfectly clear that speech was lost after the attack. Mr. Corner, under whose care the patient was at first, kindly sent him to me, and gave me much of the following information.

I first saw the patient on March 19, 1864. He was a healthy-looking man 49 years of age. On February 5, 1863, at 11 a.m. he complained of severe headache and left work. At 7 p.m. after a walk he sat down and became speechless, and by the time he was got to bed, lost the use of the left arm and leg. He did not speak at all for six weeks, except to say " yes " and " no," and then asked what time it was. He was not insensible, but simply unable to talk. He put out his tongue when Mr. Corner asked him. For two months there was considerable paralysis of the arm and leg, and he never got well enough to go to work ; on July 19 the same year he had a second attack, but this was not followed by any notable paralysis. It was a convulsive seizure and affected but one side, the side previously paralysed. It began in the left side of the tongue and next the arm and leg were convulsed, and he became insensible. He has had 4 attacks since, May 27, October 17, January 10, and again in July of this year. They all began in the same way, viz. by an " aura " in the tongue on the left side, and the left side of the body was convulsed in each.

It may look like special pleading, but I must record the fact that in the first attack, the face was, Mr. Corner tells me, paralysed on the right side and the limbs on the left, so that probably the left side of the brain was affected as well as the right.

This patient had when I saw him, what appeared at first to be simply difficulty in articulation, but on referring to Mr. Corner's account, and on again questioning the patient's wife, there is the clearest evidence that he was speechless for some time. On his first visit he could put out his tongue, and said he could eat and swallow well. Then the difficulty in talking was not a thickness, but rather a clumsiness, a kind of talking which is found in patients recovering from loss of the faculty of articulate language—the aphasia of Broca.

The case has great interest in several ways,—first as being an exceptional case, secondly as being complicated with unilateral epileptiform seizures, and thirdly as presenting a valvular lesion. There was a loud diastolic murmur heard best below the ensiform cartilage.

One chief point of interest is, that there were periodical convulsive seizures, not distinguishable from what would, by most medical men, be called epilepsy.

[1] *Medical Times and Gazette*, vol. ii, 1864, p. 166.

These affected the left side, and were no doubt the result of softening from imperfect supply of blood to the brain in the region of the right middle cerebral artery. I have seen several cases of epilepsy of this kind with valvular disease. In each there was more or less hemiplegia, and, in those in which the right side was affected, more or less defect of speech. Cases of unilateral epileptiform convulsions coming on suddenly in very healthy-looking young men suggest the inquiry whether some quasi-accidental cause, like embolus, be not more frequently the origin of epilepsy than is generally supposed. This is the more likely when it can be pointed out that the muscles first affected by spasm in those cases are the same as are paralysed in plugging of the middle cerebral artery: and again that the hemiplegia which sometimes follows the unilateral convulsion (epileptic hemiplegia) is also of the same kind as that which follows plugging. In the next case [1] the patient was not young, and had no valvular disease, yet the fact that she had temporary aphasia with the hemiplegia is enough to render it certain that she had disease in the range of the middle cerebral artery, even if the vessel itself was not primarily diseased.

Such cases seem to me to prove beyond doubt the truth of Dr. Radcliffe's views, that the convulsions depend on enfeebled power of the nervous centres, or diminution of blood supply, rather than on increased irritability or on congestion. Now and then convulsions usher in hemiplegia from embolism. Here it is inconceivable that the condition of the motor tract, the corpus striatum, can be any other than one of anæmia. It may be said that the medulla oblongata and not the corpus striatum is concerned in convulsion. Whatever the medulla oblongata may have to do in some links of the seizure, it is a fact that unilateral convulsions do follow from affections of the corpus striatum, as in the instance of embolism, and that they do follow disease on the surface of the hemisphere. The medulla oblongata may be diseased as well, but post-mortem examination shows that in unilateral convulsions the middle cerebral artery itself, or some part of the brain in its range, is diseased too.

## A Digression on Epilepsy [2]

(The following occurs in a paper on a case of loss of power of expression, inability to talk, to write, and to read correctly after convulsive attacks.)

I think, as I have elsewhere suggested, that the term (epilepsy) should be degraded to stand for our knowledge, or rather for our ignorance of the various permanent and temporary conditions of nerve tissue in functional divisions, or perhaps in nutritive regions, which conditions cause or prevent temporary failures or losses of functions. Thus epilepsy would not, in this sense, convey the idea of convulsions, but of temporary disorders of functions of many kinds, sensory as well as motor and mental as well as physical. For instance, epileptic loss of speech might mean failure of any part of the "circle" by which mind outside lives in words. But to give a more simple instance, and in more general terms, and with but indirect reference to speech, I would study convulsions according to (1) tissues affected or the nature of local damage which affects those tissues, (2) organs injured, (3) functions disordered. The first (1) might be many things betwixt, let us say, health and cerebral hæmorrhage.

[1] The case referred to is one described in the same paper, which it has not been thought necessary to include.

[2] *British Medical Journal*, vol. ii, 1866, p. 328.

And the standard of value in each (in one convulsion in cerebral hæmorrhage as well as in the most common chronic seizure) would not be any supposed types such as idiopathic epilepsy. The grouping of one's thoughts would be about health of (1) tissues, (2) organs, and (3) functions, so far as we know or can get to know about their healthy states. I have spoken of convulsions in preference to temporary failures of speech, but the principle is the same in each instance. For our point of departure in cases of defect of speech should be from what we know of healthy mind, language and movement—an imperfect knowledge it is true, but one with most of the elements of progress in it. In this way of looking at them temporary defects of speech are very important, although unfortunately they are very difficult to study.

I hope shortly as a plan of work to attempt the comparison and contrasts of (1) unilateral irregular movements, (2) unilateral attacks of spasm, and (3) unilateral paralysis. I would work at these, as if we had forgotten the terms chorea, epilepsy and hemiplegia, according to (1) the tissues affected, (2) the organs damaged, and (3) the functions disordered.

There are at least two chief views on the periodicity or intermission of convulsive paroxysms and other temporary disorders of functions, to both of which views I would pay attention as equally as I could. One is that the nutritive changes in the enfeebled region itself are the causes of the occasional attacks of spasms ; the other that the injured part fails in some general change in the organism—a change possibly starting from the medulla oblongata or beginning in the vaso-motor system. . . . The convulsion of cerebral hæmorrhage (ground currents from decomposition of nerve tissue around the clot ?) and possibly convulsions from plugging of vessels, seem to be instances of the first, and the fits which depend on the secondary changes of foreign bodies, *e.g.* tumours of the hemisphere, of the second.

## Extract from an Article, "Note on the Comparison and Contrast of Regional Palsy and Spasm" [1]

Such cases suggest a more positive method of inquiry than we usually adopt—*viz.* an examination in many differing cases of the whole of the states of muscles in the various parts—face, arm and leg—of the region the corpus striatum governs and of their conditions in time—from health, through nearly continuous irregular movements and occasional spasm to permanent palsy. I fear we too frequently arrange our thoughts on cases according as the symptoms approach supposed types—such as genuine epilepsy, real chorea, etc. Then we hear it discussed whether genuine epilepsy is always attended by loss of consciousness or necessarily implies spasm of muscles, whether epilepsy ever proves fatal, whether apoplexy causes an epileptic fit or an epileptic fit causes apoplexy, if the convulsions of children are true epilepsy or not, if epilepsy be hereditary, if epilepsy causes insanity, and frequently, of a particular case, whether it be a case of genuine epilepsy or not. Indeed I fear the student—it was so in my early medical career,—imagines there is some entity of which epilepsy is the proper name. When we see a man in a fit we cannot from the paroxysm itself tell whether there is a cerebral hæmorrhage or not, or uræmia, or whether the case be one in which there is no obvious change in the nervous system at all. Above all, when we see a man in a first severe convulsion we cannot

[1] *Lancet*, vol. i, 1867, pp. 205, 295.

tell from what we see whether he will die or not. I submit it is better to state what occurs in many striking cases of convulsion, and, when opportunity occurs, what we see after death—whether it be a large clot in the brain, or merely a little extra blood in the veins,—rather than study what causes the clinical entity genuine epilepsy, and what genuine epilepsy causes. We should still have further work to do to settle—What is the slight alteration in nervous matter which permits occasional spasm of muscles or other signs of disorder or failure of function ?

I trust that working in the narrow field I have mentioned we may study cases of palsy, spasm, irregular movements and tremors, as departures from what we can learn of the healthy condition of a region of the nervous system, and the outward parts this region governs, without undue adhesion to the views the words "epilepsy," "chorea" and "paralysis agitans" are supposed to convey.

## Case of Convulsive Attacks Arrested by Stopping the Aura[1]

Cases of epileptiform seizures, in which the "aura" is stopped by the application of a ligature, or by extension of the muscles first affected, are not very uncommon. This is sometimes so even when the fit manifestly depends (indirectly) on gross organic disease of one cerebral hemisphere. The following is not a common case, although it belongs to a common class. For the best account of cases of this sort it is scarcely necessary to say that Dr. Brown-Séquard's work *On Epilepsy* is to be consulted. It may occur to the reader that possibly the partial fits would not go on to a full fit in the case now to be related if nothing were done. It would not, however, be justifiable to make the experiment ; and the whole tenor of the case is in favour of the real value of the procedure adopted.

The patient, C., a man 52 years of age, was first under the care of Dr. Brown-Séquard in 1861, and then Dr. Hughlings Jackson saw him ; the notes, of which what follows is a partial abstract, were taken at that time. The account is purposely given nearly in the man's own words, so that the opinions expressed and the theoretical terms used are the patient's and not the physician's. Only so much is abstracted as appertains to the peculiarities the case exhibits as one of particular fits stopped by a definite procedure.

1861. He (the patient) rarely has genuine fits ; but he has sensations which would go on to fits if they were not prevented. Before he knew how to stop them, each sensation invariably resulted in a full fit ; and it would now if he had not timely assistance.

*Description of the full fits.*—He used to have them once a fortnight, and had never had two together. The left leg would begin to draw up and "the nerve worked," and it went up and up the spine ; and then he became insensible. The first shock was from the base of the great toe ; it next passed to the inner side of the foot. After he became insensible, or about that time, his son said that the arms and legs were violently worked ; the face also worked, it became of a *dark pale*, and the tongue was generally bitten. He remained insensible about half an hour—once two hours ; but even after the lapse of that time he was not quite himself, and wandered. However, he shortly went into a deep sleep for two or three hours.

[1] *Lancet*, May 10, 1868, p. 618.

*Description of the partial fits.*—About three years ago he tried to stop the fits by tying a string round the toe, and that would sometimes, though rarely, stop them. Afterwards he tied a string round the ankle, but he never applied anything higher. One morning he asked to have his leg rubbed, and has since been able to stop the fits. When a fit begins, he falls if there is nothing to catch hold of. He is, however, raised, and the leg, which becomes flexed, is rubbed. The following is copied, with a few verbal alterations, from Dr. Hughlings Jackson's case-book : " His son tells me, partly by words, but chiefly by demonstrations, how he proceeds when the attack comes on. His father being standing, and holding by something, the son kneels in front of the leg, pushes his head against the knee, and holds the heel to the ground, and rubs the calf violently. When he gets the leg straight, it is all right. He occasionally asks someone to help him to get the heel down. The muscles of the calf sometimes stand out quite hard and stiff, and the leg works and twists all manner of ways. The patient says he has a pain like a cramp from the middle third of the leg behind, and it goes higher, but how much higher he cannot say. If the leg can be kept down, there is, the son says, no working about the knee. Whilst all this is going on, the patient feels very ill, and his nerves are all at work. He feels as if shaken to pieces. Occasionally he is jerked all over, and especially when the fit is leaving ; it gives then several jerks, and goes away. He often has a slight jerk in the leg without anything further."

At one visit he remarked to the effect that by touching the foot at or about the crossing of the tibialis anticus tendon, the jerking and the seizures can be brought on ; but touching that spot on this occasion produced only a " feeling of something like an electric shock to the little toe." The following extract from Dr. Hughlings Jackson's notes is also of much interest : " He is quite clear that when the fits used to be severe (he means the fits described above as full fits), he did not lose power in any of his limbs ; but now that the fits are stopped, the left leg is ' paralysed ' after each attack. He can, he says, bear no weight on it after the seizure, and on getting along by help he drags the foot with the toe on the ground. The leg gets well gradually in about an hour."

May 1865. Dr. Bathurst Woodman, then resident medical officer of the London Hospital, was a witness at the Old Bailey on a trial on which the patient C. was a witness too. Dr. Woodman on that occasion saw an attack which was so strange that he would have suspected malingering had it occurred in an out-patient. C. cried out suddenly " Rub my leg." His son (C. always goes about with his son, so that skilled assistance may be had promptly when a fit begins) knelt down and began to rub it violently, the father urging him on. Dr. Woodman felt the lower part of the thigh, the muscles of which were lax ; he then felt the calf, and found the muscles firm. From the first the leg was in continual agitation. Soon C. said, " Rub away, it's getting higher " ; and now, on feeling, Dr. Woodman found that the previously lax muscles of the thigh were firm and rigid. After some time the man said, with a sigh of relief, " It's all gone now." He was shortly called into one of the offices, and as he walked away, Dr. Woodman noticed that the left leg was dragged with a slight swing. He told Dr. Woodman that it was always so after a fit, and he complained that the hand and the arm of the same side were numb and weak, although he could make almost any movement with the limb.

## A STUDY OF CONVULSIONS[1]

A CONVULSION is but a symptom, and implies only that there is an occasional, an excessive, and a disorderly discharge of nerve tissue on muscles. This discharge occurs in all degrees; it occurs with all sorts of conditions of ill health, at all ages, and under innumerable circumstances. But in this article I shall narrow my task to the description of one class of *chronic* convulsive seizures. The great majority of chronic convulsions may be arranged in two classes.

1. Those in which the spasm affects both sides of the body almost contemporaneously. In these cases there is either no warning, or a very general one such as a sensation at or about the epigastrium, or an indescribable feeling in the head. These cases are usually called epileptic, and sometimes cases of "genuine" or "idiopathic" epilepsy.

2. Those in which the fit begins by deliberate spasm on one side of the body, and in which parts of the body are affected, one after another.

It is with the second class only that I intend to deal in this article.

But although I thus limit myself to one class of cases, I contend that the title of my article is correct.[2] I trust I am studying the general subject of convulsion methodically when I work at the simplest varieties of occasional spasm I can find. Cases of unilateral convulsions are unquestionably the simplest. We can, when we are luckily present at a paroxysm, watch the march of the spasm. I have known a fit of this kind last ten minutes. (Case 5.) For instance, we may first see movement of the index finger, then of the hand, then of the whole arm, then of the face, leg, etc. Besides, patients can describe the onset and much of the march of such seizures. We can therefore compare and contrast these convulsions with hemiplegia—which form of palsy the convulsion not unfrequently leaves. In some of these cases we find *gross* disease of the brain (see Case 7, syphilitic nodules) post-mortem, and thus we can infer the seat of the minute changes on which the discharge producing the spasm was dependent. This done, we have, as in Case 7, on the one hand a record of the events occurring in a certain kind of convulsion, and on the other hand, a knowledge of the internal part diseased. We are free, therefore, from the great vagueness of the word "epilepsy." We do not care to say that a tumour of the brain (or minute changes near it) had "caused epilepsy," but that changes in a particular region of the nervous system—say

[1] *Transactions St. Andrews Medical Graduates' Association*, vol. iii, 1870.

[2] Those who say that the two classes differ "only in degree" make a remark the truth of which is admitted. In both there are occasional, excessive, and disorderly expenditures of force on muscles, the discharge depending on instability of nervous tissue. But in what kind of degree do they differ? Not merely in degree of more or less spasm—more or less instability of nervous tissue—but also in degree of evolution of the nervous processes which are unstable. A convulsion which is general, and in which the muscular regions affected are affected nearly contemporaneously, must depend on discharge of parts in which the nervous processes represent a more intricate co-ordination of muscles in Space and in Time than those parts represent, which, when discharged, produce a convulsion which begins in one limb and has a deliberate march. My speculation is that the first class differs from the second in that convolutions at a greater distance from the motor tract are discharged.

in the region of the left middle cerebral artery—led to convulsions, in which the spasm began in the right hand, spread to the arm, attacked next the face, then the leg, etc.

I chiefly wish to show in this article that the most common variety of hemispasm is a symptom of disease of the same region of the brain as is the symptom hemiplegia ; *viz.* the " region of the corpus striatum." The loose term " region of the corpus striatum " is advisedly used. Hemiplegia shows damage (equivalent to destruction) of the motor tract, hemispasm shows damage (equivalent to changes of instability) of the convolutions which discharge through it. Palsy depends on destruction [1] of *fibres*, and convulsion on instability of *grey matter*. As the convolutions are rich in grey matter I suppose them to be to blame, in *severe* convulsions at all events ; but as the corpus striatum also contains much grey matter I cannot deny that it may be sometimes the part to blame in slighter convulsions. Indeed, if the discharge does begin in convolutions, no doubt the grey matter of lower motor centres, even if these centres be healthy, will be discharged secondarily by the violent impulse received from the primary discharge. Now both these parts—the corpus striatum and many convolutions—are supplied by one artery, the middle cerebral or Sylvian, and this artery circumscribes the region I speak of.

By hemiplegia in this article is meant the common form of hemiplegia, the result of destruction of part of the corpus striatum or of part of the optic thalamus. I shall, however, illustrate by hemiplegia due to disease of the corpus striatum. As we usually see hemiplegia there is partial paralysis of the face (scarcely more than a little weakening of the cheek), a trifling turning of the tongue on protrusion to the side paralysed, and weakness of the arm and leg of the same side as that on which the face is paralysed. But in *complete* hemiplegia, say of the right side—complete in range I mean—there is turning of *both* eyes to the left, turning of the head to the left, turning of the face to the left (and some weakness of the right orbicularis palpebrarum), weakness of the right side of the tongue, palsy of the right arm and leg. In large lesions the muscles passing from the trunk to the limbs are paralysed also.

The muscles which suffer most are those which can act independently of their fellows of the opposite side. Those which must act along with their fellows of the other side—for instance the intercostals—do not suffer at all ; and those which are, so to speak, half-way in their action—*e.g.* muscles which turn the two eyes and the head to one side—suffer only in very large lesions, and then but for a short time, a few hours or days. It is but putting these facts in another way to say that parts suffer directly as the actions they engage in are voluntary, and inversely as the actions they engage in are automatic. This is seen in the order of recovery. The muscles serving in the more automatic actions recover first. Now just the same principle applies to cases of hemispasm, so far as this at least, that the fit begins most frequently in those parts which suffer most in hemiplegia. This point is now to be considered in some detail.

[1] The word " destruction " is scarcely the correct word to use. By it is not meant that the nerve fibres are necessarily broken up, although they often are in palsy, but simply that there is a change in them which *destroys their function*. Thus, see pp. 13 and 25, palsy is supposed to follow a convulsion because the axis cylinder of the nerve fibre has temporarily lost its function, from the effects of the excessive quantity of nerve force it has had to " carry." Here the nerve fibres are not physically destroyed, since the palsy quickly passes off. With this qualification the word " destruction " may be conveniently used.

Fits beginning unilaterally may doubtless begin by movement in any part of the region which is paralysed in hemiplegia, *i.e.* in the face, in the arm, or in the leg. But I know few cases of fits of this class which begin other than in the side of the face (usually the cheek), in the hand, or in the foot. They very rarely begin in the upper arm, or in the calf. The fit usually begins, it is to be observed, in that part of the face, of the arm and of the leg which has *the most varied uses*. (I use the term *varied*, instead of voluntary, non-automatic, and the like, as it carries fewer special implications.) Moreover, taking numbers of cases of convulsions which begin unilaterally, the same law, if I may so call it, is exemplified. Fits beginning in the hand are common, fits beginning in the cheek and tongue are less frequent, fits beginning in the foot are rare. The law is to be exemplified in details. For again taking numbers of cases, the fits which begin in the hand begin usually in the index finger and thumb ; fits which begin in the foot begin usually in the great toe.

The above-mentioned facts are obviously very significant in regard to what is under different aspects variously named " co-ordination," " grouping," " localisation," " plan of structure of nervous organs," etc. ; although it may be that the order of frequency mentioned points merely to an order of frequency in liability of parts to become diseased. I have considered such cases from this point of view (*Medical Times and Gazette*, December 14 and 21, 1867, August 15, 1868), but now I have to speak of the bearing of the facts in the study of convulsions.

Parts which have the most varied uses will be represented in the central nervous system by most ganglion [1] cells. I say most *varied* movements, as it is not only a question of number of movements, but also of number of *different* movements.

We shall speak of three varieties of convulsions beginning unilaterally :

1. Those beginning in the hand.
2. Those beginning in the face and tongue.
3. Those beginning in the foot.

The seizures occur in all degrees. There may be, for instance, twitching limited to the thumb and index finger, or the whole body may be convulsed. In the same patient we find all degrees. The fit may stop, so to speak, at almost any stage, and indeed (as in Case 4) it may be artificially stopped by a ligature in its earliest stage. Admitting that the fits occur in all degrees, we may conveniently take three degrees for consideration.

1st. The spasm attacks only the unilateral muscles of the side in which it begins, say the right.

2nd. It passes on to the bilateral muscles of both sides.

3rd. It goes still further, and attacks the unilateral muscles of the other side—the left—and probably the bilateral muscles of both sides a second time.

To say that the seizures " occur in all degrees " is not a vague statement when qualified as above. There are not merely degrees of more or less *quantity* of spasm. The point of significance is that the spasmodic movements are not contemporaneous, but follow a distinct march, and a different march according as the spasm begins in the hand or in the foot. The sequence is, however, not simple. The spasm does not affect the arm, then cease, next affect the face,

[1] Although both the nerve fibre (axis cylinder) and the ganglion cell " store up force," it is the latter which stores it up in large quantity, and to instability of grey matter, therefore, will be chiefly owing the excessive discharges in convulsions.

etc. It is a *compound* sequence. For instance, the face begins to be affected before the spasm of the arm ceases.

When observing the paroxysms we have therefore to note two things.

First, the region affected ; for instance, we say the face, arm and leg of one side are in spasm.

Secondly, the order in which parts are involved ; for instance, we say the spasm began in the hand, passed up the arm, then attacked the face and lastly went down the leg—" out at the toes," one of my patients said.

It will be best now to give clinical illustrations, and I shall add to each case remarks on such subjects as tongue biting, loss of consciousness and hemiplegia. These digressions are necessary for the main argument, but are most conveniently placed near the reports of the cases.

*Case* I.—*Occasional spasm in the right arm beginning in the index finger and thumb.*

A married woman, 43 years of age, but looking ten years younger, consulted me at the London Hospital, December 13, 1864. I use largely in the following the patient's own expressions. Exactly a week before, at 9 or 10 a.m., her right forefinger and thumb began to work, and the working continued up to the elbow, and then all the fingers worked. (She imitated the movements by alternately shutting and opening the hand.) There was no other attendant sensation. I inquired carefully for giddiness, temporary defect of sight, for abnormal feelings in the face, leg, etc. The fit was strictly localised as above described. She had had three attacks, and after each the hand felt " heavy and dead," and for some time she could not use it well. For instance, she could not " feel " the needle on the day of her visit (the third fit having been the night before).

She was healthy-looking, and had had good health, but said she was nervous. At the next visit I found no albumen in the urine. I have no note of any examination of the heart. There were two circumstances which may be supposed to have had an influence in the development of the fit. She had weaned a baby, aged 11 months, three days before the first fit. She had suffered from ascarides several years. My object at present is, however, to give illustrations of varieties of hemispasm, and the question as to the causation of the fits will be discussed later.

On her visit December 20 she had had another attack, beginning in the whole of the fingers of the right hand at once, and after this to February 20, when I lost sight of her, she had had no more attacks.

Now the most utilitarian question we can put about such a case is—Will a patient suffering so little have more fits, and will they be severe, *i.e.* general ? [1]

[1] After this was in type I sought the patient out. She still looks in very good health and feels quite well. There is no cardiac murmur. Since I saw her she has had *severe* fits. These began a year or two after I saw her, and she had three or four a year, but none for the last eighteen months. She describes their onset just as the onset of the slighter ones is described in my notes taken six years ago. In these severe attacks the arm " drew up " so strongly that no one could hold it down—her husband tried " with all his strength." When the arm was much drawn up she became insensible. She did not bite her tongue, and her speech was not affected before she lost consciousness, nor when she came to herself. The arm was weak after the attacks, but there seems to have been no considerable loss of power. She was evidently anxious, and I did not like to make her uneasy by questions which might increase her dread that she should become paralysed. All the severe attacks have been in the night. She says she has had no slight attacks such as she had when attending at the hospital, but it seems she really has, for she is occasionally awakened at night by " starting " of the *right* arm, and sometimes of the right index finger only—that finger in which the fits, slight and severe, have invariably begun.

I never saw the patient again, and therefore I can only speculate as to what would become of her. My impression is that she would have fits extending to the whole of the side, and possibly general convulsions. I think so because we sometimes see patients the subjects of severe convulsions, who for a time had had slight seizures such as Mrs. R. had. I have recorded such a case (*Medical Times and Gazette*, January 31, 1863). In that case the fit began in the index finger of the left hand, and I remember the patient told me that before the attacks were severe, he thought so little of the twitching of the hand that he used to show it to his fellow workmen as a curiosity. In the same journal, June 6, 1863, I have noted another case in which a severe fit occurred one month after a warning of movement of the first two fingers of one hand. But I cannot be sure Mrs. R. will have more fits. It may be that many people have such local twitchings, and that they remain " a curiosity " only, and do not show them to a doctor. I therefore ask those in family practice, who can watch patients longer than a physician can, if they can give records of cases in which such attacks of spasm have continued thus local, and therefore comparatively unimportant, for some years ? I may say, however, that I should never declare a patient to be safe who had attacks, even so slight as this woman had. I am not referring to cases where there is what is called " live blood," nor to the fidgety movements of the limbs which occur in weak, and especially in aged, people. Nor do I speak of cases where, without spasm, the patient becomes occasionally numb on one side—as he may say, " dead." These last-named cases are not cases of spasm at all ; they are probably cases of very slight palsy, and have a different clinical significance. Such symptoms occur in patients who have valvular disease of the heart, in patients who have renal cachexia, and occasionally in people who seem to be quite healthy. They point, I believe, not to instability of ganglion cells, but to destruction—slight in amount—of nerve fibres.

*Case 2.—Fits beginning in the right hand. Loss of power after a seizure.*

William G., aged 11, a healthy-looking boy. July 1, 1864. Yesterday, his mother said, a shaking began in his right hand, first in the fingers, and then it went up to the eye (orbicularis doubtless). It lasted for five or ten minutes. In the night the boy was awakened by another attack of the shaking, and his mother, who saw him when it was over, found that he could not speak. How long he remained speechless is not known, but next morning he could speak, and had two or three more trifling attacks in the hand.

Whilst I was taking these notes a fit came on. There was only a little twitching of the right hand for about two minutes. He stood through it, and talked when questioned. I saw nothing wrong with the face, but he felt " it " in the right side of the face and in the region of the orbicularis palpebrarum. The leg was, as in the other fits, not affected. The arm was weak when the fit was over, and he could not by any effort pick up a pin with his hand.

Four years before he had had attacks on the right side for several weeks, but his speech was then in no way affected.

He spoke a little thickly, but this was always so with him, but his mother fancied he spoke a little worse than he had done the day before.

I heard of him again in February 1867. He had had one fit in the interval betwixt February 1865 and May 1866. He was in service.

This boy seemed to be in good general health, and I could arrive at no conclusion as to the cause of his seizures.

### Remarks on Epileptic Hemiplegia

The cases I am describing are those cases of chronic convulsions which are so often followed by hemiplegia. It is the epileptic hemiplegia of Dr. Todd. I do not know how it is that some patients have no palsy after these seizures, and some have. The same patient is hemiplegic after some of his seizures, and not after others. The presumption is that the degree of palsy depends on the severity of the convulsions, *i.e.* on the *quantity* of discharge. When the convulsion is limited in range, the palsy left by it is limited in range. This is seen in Cases 1, 2 and 5. I have recorded a case (*Medical Mirror*, September 1869) in which palsy of the arm only followed a convulsive seizure—the spasm, according to the patient, being limited to that limb. In this case there was a new growth in the hemisphere in the hinder part of the superior frontal convolution. (Compare with Case 5.) When the fit is severe, there may be hemiplegia complete in range, except perhaps for deviation of the head and eyes. But the hemiplegia, however complete in range, and however decided in degree, is transitory, and we may very safely tell our patient that it will pass off in a few days or weeks, and we may usually say so when we feel certain that the fits are the result of organic disease in the head. The palsy does not depend directly on the organic disease (see p. 24), but is doubtless the result of " overwork " of the nerve fibres which pass from the part discharged to the muscles convulsed. The nerves and the muscles require time to recover from the effects of the sudden and excessive discharge.

But although we can assure our patient that his palsy will pass off, we shall be obliged to confess that both his fits and the palsy will *probably* return again and again.

It is not said that hemiplegia after a convulsion is transitory, but that hemiplegia after a convulsion deliberately beginning unilaterally is transitory. Hemiplegia after a convulsion may signify large cerebral hæmorrhage destroying the motor tract, and then the palsy is permanent, or it may signify plugging of the middle cerebral artery.

*Case 3.—Fits beginning in the left hand. Some fits arrested by pressure on the limb.*

A healthy-looking lad, 17 years of age, came under my care July 8, 1868. Six months before, he had been struck on the buttock, but he suffered next to nothing from the blow, and went on with his work. Probably the blow had nothing to do with the symptoms he afterwards had. He had " not been well since," but he looked well and could give no definite statements as to the nature of his supposed ill health. Six months later—a few days before I saw him—on a Thursday, when helping to kill a bullock and after being at work about half an hour, the left hand " began to work " ; there was, he remarked, " gentle movement of the fingers." He showed it to his mother but did not stay with her. Soon he had to call to his brother to catch him. He became insensible, and bit his tongue. In a quarter of an hour he was seemingly well, having no headache. On the Friday, about 7 a.m., the arm began " to work " again, but his brother " touched him on the wrist," and then the " working " stopped. He went on with his work and kept well until about half-past five, when a similar movement occurred ; he called his brother, who caught him. He had a severe fit, but in an hour could walk about again.

I gave him a dose of oil of male fern, but he passed no worms.

July 15. He had had a single movement of the hand, but it was stopped by pressure. I saw him no more after August 5. He had had no further seizures.

In this case there was no headache, and I discovered no changes in the optic nerves. The patient was very healthy-looking, and except for the fits I found nothing the matter with him. I gave the dose of oil of male fern by routine.

### Remarks on Tongue Biting

In connection with this case I may mention tongue biting. It is no sign of " epilepsy " in particular. It is found in convulsions from uræmia and from cerebral hæmorrhage ; indeed in all cases of convulsion, *when the convulsion is severe*. It is, therefore, of no real diagnostic value. It simply signifies that the patient has had a severe fit. It is not often found in the convulsion of cerebral hæmorrhage—one reason being that it is not often looked for—as the convulsions are not usually so severe as are many convulsions otherwise caused. It is not a diagnostic point to be relied on, even in the convulsions of young patients. A convulsion in a young man is usually epileptic, *i.e.* usually depends on minute changes which will not lead to a fatal result. But tongue biting does not help us to that diagnosis.

It is not easy, it is usually impossible, to get a look at the tongue in cases of coma, but we can often infer that it has been bitten from the presence of blood on the gums and from bloody foam. (Bloody foam, however, is seen in some cases of rapidly fatal cerebral hæmorrhage without tongue biting ; it may come from the lungs.) We should always look at the tongue at post-mortem examinations of those who have died from cerebral hæmorrhage. We may find that there is bruising without laceration. The other day I made an autopsy with my friend Mr. Herman, on a woman who had died from cerebral hæmorrhage which set in with a convulsion, and we found a dark plum-coloured patch the size of half a bean on the left side of the tongue. An incision showed extravasated blood.

*Case 4.—Seizures, partial and severe, beginning in the right thumb. Arrest by ligature. Dyspepsia.*

A single woman, 22 years of age, consulted me, August 23, 1869, for fits.

Each fit begins by movement in the thumb of the right hand, and by degrees the whole arm is involved. The same side of the face is drawn, and the head is drawn towards the arm, which is raised to meet it. The patient's remark is, " it seems as if it wanted to draw the arm into the head." " It " goes to the leg after the face has begun to work, and then she becomes insensible ; the insensibility she ascribes to the severe pain in the muscles (" sinews " is the word she uses). This observation is of value as showing that the pain from the cramped muscles is severe. She foams at the mouth and bites her tongue. When she comes to herself she speaks well. She cannot walk well after the attack, but this is attributed to giddiness and headache. She says the right arm and leg are affected, but only slightly. There is at least no decided hemiplegia after the seizures.

The above, however, refers to severe fits, and the description is necessarily incomplete, as she becomes insensible as soon as the right leg is attacked. The probability is that in the severe attacks she is convulsed on both sides after the first (right) side is fully seized. She has slighter seizures, or, as she said at the next visit, November 1, " I have had no fits, but the hand has been very fidgety, and I have had to tie it up twice." December 14, she said she had had no fit for six weeks, but the hand had been " very bad," and she had had to " tie it up." She added, " But it (tying) makes me feel giddy."

Then on January 4, 1870, she had a fit of intermediate severity. To use her own words, she had had " workings of a fit," but did not become insensible. The spasm affected the arm and the side of the face a little. It did not get to the leg, and there was no drawing of the head to the right. The arm was " tied up " ; first a ribbon was tied tightly round the middle of the forearm, and, as this " would not stop it," the ribbon was next tied around the middle of the upper arm—" this kept it from taking my senses away." The arm was " tied up " for two hours ; for when untied " it drew up " ; when tied it kept quiet.

The bromide keeps the attacks off. When I saw her last she said the arm had been " very peaceable."

The foregoing is little more than physiology—medical physiology it is true, but still physiology. The important clinical facts are to be added that she is dyspeptic, and suffers very much from flatulence. It seems clear to me, from her spontaneous remarks at several visits, that when she is flatulent the arm moves more. This point will be again referred to with regard to the question of " cause." There is no heart disease. Her sister is far advanced in phthisis, and the patient herself is phthisical looking, has a cough, and her respiration is harsh over the clavicles. She is quite regular.

### Dyspepsia in Chronic Convulsions

Dr. Paget, of Cambridge, in a lecture on " Gastric Epilepsy," *Lancet*, April 11 and 18, 1868, says, p. 491 : " In epilepsy once established, whatever may have been its exciting cause, gastric disorder may, in the course of the case, become the ordinary exciting cause of the fits." He relates cases in which remarkable benefit followed care in dieting and remedies for dyspepsia.

I have been led to advise epileptics to limit their quantity of *flesh* food since reading Professor Haughton's researches on *The Relations of Food to Work*. The following quotation will serve to show how I suppose his work bears on the dietetic treatment of epileptics. " The hunted deer will outrun the leopard in a fair and open chase, because the work supplied to its muscles by the vegetable food is capable of being given out continuously for a long period of time ; but in a sudden rush at a near distance, the leopard will infallibly overtake the deer, because its flesh food stores up in the blood a reserve of force capable of being given out instantaneously in the form of exceedingly rapid muscular action."

### Arrest of Fits by the Ligature

Case 4 is specially interesting, because the patient gave a clear account of the use of the ligature. There can be no question that the ligature is a most valuable means of arresting such fits. I have known very great success from this procedure in Brown-Séquard's practice, and also from another plan he adopted, founded on the same principle, *viz.* circular blisters—a garter of blister round the limb.[1] Probably the ligature, etc., merely put off the explosions; and patients the subjects of this, as of other varieties of fits, very often say that they feel better *after* a seizure—after a full discharge of that part of the nervous system which is unstable. It indeed occasionally happens that an epileptic complains more to his doctor when his fits are diminished in number. It may be that when his serious troubles are lessened, he thinks of the smaller ones. But I suppose that before the abrupt explosion which constitutes the severe fit there are frequent minute discharges—too trivial to produce any visible effects, but enough to cause discomfort to the patient. Nevertheless it is a gain to put off the fit—to save the patient from the *effects* of the discharge, especially to save him from the sudden violent stoppage of respiration and its secondary effects on the circulation in the head. It is reasonable to suppose that, whilst the fits are kept off by treatment, we may, by much exercise, by purgatives, by care in diet and especially by giving a very simple diet (milk, vegetables and little meat), prevent the diseased part of the nervous system from arriving at that high state of tension which permits severe convulsions.[2] (See p. 15.)

I presume that the first outward spasm is the result of the beginning of the internal discharge. It is an interesting question how the sensation which so often precedes the spasm is related to the seizure, and how the ligature averts the seizure. It is quite certain that the ligature will avert fits when they depend on *organic* disease of the brain—" coarse " disease—(see Case 8); and in any case it is unreasonable to suppose that a local irritation starting from the hand is the *sole* cause of the seizure—that it can provoke discharge in a *healthy* nervous system. It is to Brown-Séquard that we are indebted for our precise knowledge of the relation of external irritations to the production of convulsive paroxysms. He finds that experimental injuries of the spinal cord of guinea-pigs—section of one lateral half is the most certain—produces after a few weeks a condition of the nervous system which results in a convulsion when an external irritation is applied to a certain part of the face. In the case of his epileptic guinea-pigs there are obviously *two* factors in the production of the paroxysm—first, a permanent lesion of nerve tissue; secondly, an external irritation. It may be supposed, then, that in such cases of convulsion

[1] Pulling against the spasm, *e.g.* opening the clenching hand, will sometimes put off the fits. In other kinds of seizures, when the fit begins by a general warning of confusion in the head, the patients can shake them off by walking about, stamping, etc. I have several times heard patients remark to this effect, " I nearly had a fit, but I managed to shake it off." " It nearly got the better of me." See an interesting article by Dr. Buzzard, " On the interception of the epileptic aura by blistering," *Practitioner*, October 1868.

[2] I find, however, that a great authority, Niemeyer, says: " On the whole, compression of a limb from which the aura seems to proceed is not advisable, even although we may avert a fit by so doing, since, in the first place, the patient feels worse after thus repressing an attack than if he had had one; and in the second, because his next seizure is apt to be one of unusual violence." I quote from the translation by Dr. Humphreys and Dr. Hackley, of New York. The observation of the patient (Case 4), that tying up the convulsed arm made her feel giddy, is interesting in this connection.

as I have described, there are also two factors, (1) an irritation starting from the fingers which travels to (2) the part of the nervous system unstable, and then determines the discharge.[1] I have now under my care a patient whose case seems to support such a view. He cut the palmar surface of his left index finger with a gouge. (There remains a hard scar to the present time.) *Nine months later* he had a severe convulsion, beginning in this and in the next finger. (I do not give the other particulars of his case, as they would be for all practical purposes a mere repetition of those given of Case 4. His fits always begin in the same way, and he has both full and partial seizures.) But cases are numerous in which external local irritations exist without the occurrence of convulsions of any kind. It seems most reasonable to suppose that the man whose case is just noted has permanent disease of the opposite side of his brain, and that, at the most, irritation from the injured finger acts on it only as the explosion of a gun cap does on the charge in the barrel.

It seems certain that external injuries bring about tetanic spasm, but then they very rarely do, and I think the inference is at least plausible that those in whom a local irritation develops tetanus have already some abnormal condition of the nerve centres for the local irritation to act upon.

The subject calls to mind cases I many years ago heard related by Mr. Paget, in a clinical lecture, of neuralgia, set up by injury, persisting when the nerve to the injured part was divided. It seemed as if the injury to the nerve had led to permanent changes in some connected part of the nervous centres, for the patient continued to " feel " pain in the injured part when it was quite anæsthetic from surgical division of the nerve trunks leading to it. Similarly it may be that the injury by the gouge, in the case of convulsion just mentioned, produced slowly the very changes in the patient's brain on which the convulsions depended.

I think, at all events, that other conditions determine the discharge in some cases, when the spasm is quite local. The unstable equilibrium of the patch of unstable nerve tissue may, I imagine, be upset in many ways (see p. 35), and possibly one way may be by an irritation starting from the region which is afterwards convulsed.

*Case 5.—Partial convulsion beginning in the right hand.*

This case has to me very great interest, because I witnessed the paroxysm. The march of the spasm was very deliberate : the time occupied was about ten minutes. Seven of these minutes were measured by the watch, the rest were guessed. The fit was incomplete, but from the observation of other cases I may safely state what the order of events would have been if the convulsion had gone on to a severe fit. The patient's head and both his eyes would have been turned to the right, the right leg would have been convulsed, the chest would next have been fixed, and then the convulsion would have " repeated itself " on the left side. The convulsion on the left side would, however, have been less severe, and the parts would have been affected, I believe, more contemporaneously. It is to be observed that the bilateral

[1] And as a corollary we may suppose that in health there is not only a relation by motor fibres from the corpus striatum to the muscles, but a relation by sensory fibres from the skin covering these muscles, and from the muscles themselves, to the (vessels of the ?) corpus striatum. This supposition seems to me to be but an amplification of Hilton's well-known hypothesis of the supply of skin and muscles from nerve trunks.

muscles of the face were involved in spasm as well as the unilateral. (See pp. 27 and 28.)

A man, 48 years of age, was admitted for convulsive attacks, which he described very minutely. They were, by his description, like that on which the following observation was made. One day when waiting his turn to be seen by the physician, his right hand began to twitch, the thumb and index finger taking the lead. The fingers were soon partially flexed in a curve, except the index, which was straight, but flexed at its metacarpal joint; the thumb was straight too, but flexed also at its metacarpal joint, and lay with the palmar surface of its terminal segment against the side of the index finger. Next the whole arm twitched, but it did not rise; the exact sequence of involvement of its several parts was not ascertained, as the man was dressed. In about two minutes from the first, the right side of the face began to twitch, but before movement of it was discernible the patient said he felt "it" in his face. The right eye was closed, the right cheek was drawn up, and both jaws came together. The mouth was drawn to the right (but whether before or after the meeting of the jaws was not noted), and its opening was ovoid, the wider end of the ovoid being to the right. The right ocular aperture was a little closer than the other, but both were narrowed. Both sides of the forehead were wrinkled upwards. There was no deviation of the head nor of the eyes; the leg was not affected, and the patient could talk in any part of the fit. He begged me to let the porter take hold of his hand—to unclench it—as the porter could manage it better. The fit ceased very suddenly. After the attack the arm, which was weak before the fit, was completely paralysed, quite limp, and fell forward when he stooped, and it had not recovered completely when he left the hospital fourteen days later. The patient's speech was not distinct before the fit, but it was worse after. It is not possible to say anything more definite about his speech than this, as the patient was a foreigner; what he said could be made out.

## Absence of Insensibility in Convulsions

In the above case there are many points of interest. I shall now speak only of the absence of insensibility in the seizure. These are the very cases of convulsions in which so often there is no loss of consciousness. As before said, these seizures occur in all degrees, and when they are partial the patient may be conscious, although sometimes speechless, throughout. So far as I can ascertain, the rule is, that (when the fit begins in the hand) consciousness is lost as soon as, or just before, the leg is seized, but sometimes the whole side may be affected, and even, I believe, the thoracic muscles slightly, without any loss of consciousness. It has been said by the late Dr. Addison, of Guy's, that absence of insensibility in convulsions is some evidence that the internal lesion is organic, such for instance as tumour. I have had no autopsy in any case of the class of fits which I describe in this paper in which I have not found organic disease. For all that, I cannot hold the opinion which this great physician has expressed. *Such convulsions point only to minute changes involving instability in the opposite hemisphere.* If the reader will not admit this, it suffices for the present argument to say that they point only to *local* changes of instability. They tell us nothing of the pathological processes by which that local instability results, or, in narrower terms, they give no information as to whether the changes are primarily minute, or secondarily minute, *i.e.* changes due to the irritation of a foreign body.[1] To tell whether the changes are diffused from a foreign body, such as a syphilitic lump, a tumour, etc., we have to consider a very different kind of evidence (see p. 31). If the patient have severe pain in the head—not the mere sequel of a convulsion,—if he have vomiting, above all if he have double optic neuritis, I should then think it probable that the convulsion depended on changes diffused from a foreign body in the brain. If he have no such symptoms, I should suppose the local change was not diffused from a foreign body.

Patients with minute local lesions of the brain are not likely to die under our care. A patient with a foreign body in his brain very often dies under our care. Partial fits—fits without insensibility—very often occur without symptoms implying a foreign body, and I can therefore place no value on absence of insensibility in such seizures towards the diagnosis of organic disease. If we work in the wards of a hospital only, where we find patients who are admitted for *severe* intracranial disease, we shall be misled. We must work also in the out-patient room, where we see patients year after year with fits of the kind above mentioned, and without any symptoms to lead us to suppose that there is " coarse " disease of the brain.

So far I have spoken of cases in which the fit begins in the hand, and it will have been observed that in some the fits began in the thumb and index finger. This is (as remarked at p. 10) the rule. I could, however, give several instances in which the fit has commenced in the little finger, but their recital would make the paper too long. These fits are, however, rarer. I next pass to cases in which the fit begins in the side of the face, or tongue, or both.

## Temporary Defects of Speech with Convulsive Seizures[2]

In all cases of convulsions beginning unilaterally, it is important to consider carefully the side of the body in which the fit begins. We find that when persistent *loss* of speech occurs with *hemiplegia*, the hemiplegia is nearly always of the right side. I have long observed of convulsions that when spasm begins on the right side there is defect of speech more marked than when it begins on the left. However, my facts on this matter depend very much on the observations of the patient or his friends. The friends of patients very naturally do not always distinguish betwixt mere inability to talk or defective speech, and insensibility or confusion of mind. The patient is sometimes said to be speechless for a time, and sometimes is said to talk badly. The patient very often remarks that as soon as the fit begins, he cannot speak. I must say that there is sometimes no complaint of defect of speech when the seizure begins on the right side. But I think it will be found that, when the spasm starts in the *face and tongue* of the right side, there usually is great defect of speech, and

[1] I use the term " foreign body," as I use also the term " coarse disease," to include glioma, syphilitic nodules, hydatid cyst, blood-clot, abscess, etc. It is used as the opposite of minute changes. When a patient comes to us for any symptom implying that there is disease of some kind inside his head, the first attempt is to find where it is; next to determine whether it be constituted by primarily minute changes, or by changes (softening) diffused from a "foreign body"; and after this is done, we try to find out the particular pathological nature of the foreign body, whether it be glioma, syphilis, etc.

[2] " There is a peculiar class of cases of epileptic hemiplegia, in which the exciting cause of the epileptic fit at the same time damages or greatly injures voluntary power and speech."—Todd, *Nervous Diseases*, Lect. XV.

that there usually is not when it starts in the *right hand or right foot*. It may be supposed that the loss or defect of speech is owing to locking of the articulatory muscles by spasm in the fit, or to palsy of those parts after it. We shall be able to settle this by observing if equally great defect results when the spasm begins in the *left* side of the face and tongue. It is unlikely that the speech defect after the seizure is owing to partial palsy of the articulatory muscles, since total palsy of the face and tongue on one side from disease of the portio dura and ninth nerves does not cause either the same kind or the same amount of difficulty of talking which we now and then find following a fit. My impression is that in the right-sided convulsion there is often considerable defect of speech, and in the left-sided convulsion at least rarely. I am obliged to use the word " impression " as I have not often had the chance of observing patients soon after these seizures. The subject is one on which it is particularly dangerous to draw hasty conclusions. I by no means urge its consideration with the hope of confirming the view held by many, that disease in the *left* hemisphere only, causes loss or defect of speech. (The fact of real significance is, that extensive disease in but *one* hemisphere can lead to total speechlessness.)

I beg those who have the rare good fortune to see patients in such seizures, or quickly afterwards, to note the nature and degree of the defect of speech. It is important also to set the patient, during the continuance of his defect of speech, to write, and we must not be satisfied with his writing his name or copying. Persons who have permanently lost speech from destroying lesions of the left hemisphere may do both when they cannot write to dictation, or anything " out of their own heads."[1] We should also ask the patient to read.

Another thing to be noted is, that in cases (see Case 2) where there is great defect of speech after a seizure we are sometimes told that the patient talked badly long before he was subject to fits, although he talks worse after a seizure. This does not do away with the significance of the defect of speech after the seizure. I suppose that the previous defect of speech implies a weak spot in the nervous system, and very likely the fits are the result of ingravescence of old-standing disease in the same region. This, however, is only a speculation.

[1] It is a great mistake to suppose that a speechless patient can write, that is, write in the sense of expressing himself, because he can sign his name, or because he can copy what is put before him. It is *a priori* incredible that a person who cannot speak should be able to write. For when we write we merely translate nascently revived words into written symbols. We have to speak " inside ourselves " first. (Cases of loss of talking from immobility of the articulatory organs are of course not here in question.) When a patient does not utter a word, and yet writes well, *and swallows well*—this fact showing there is no considerable palsy of the articulatory muscles—we may be almost certain (quite certain, I believe), that he—it is usually *she*—is pretending, or that the defect is " hysterical," whatever that word may mean.

The fact that an aphasic person cannot write must not be brought forward as *additional* evidence on his mental condition. It is the *same* defect as loss of speech in another manifestation. The speechless man cannot read, not even to himself. It is not that his eyes, or rather the parts of the brain which contain processes for the recognition of images of things, are affected, for he does recognise objects, and when he cannot read, can recognise headings (*e.g.* one of my patients could find in a magazine volume the continuation of a serial tale), and knows by the handwriting where a letter comes from. The difficulty is still one of loss of speech. Written and printed words, strictly, have no meaning. They are merely arbitrary signs of words. They require translation into words, and into an *order* of words. This translation the speechless man cannot effect, as he cannot revive words. He understands what we say to him, as, although *he* cannot revive words, the sounds of our words revive the motor symbols of words in his brain—*i.e.* in the undamaged side. For the speechless man is not wordless ; his defect is that he cannot revive words *voluntarily*.

*Case* 6.—*Convulsions beginning in the face. Defect of speech.*

Elizabeth F., 9 years old. June 25, 1866. The child was brought to the out-patient room by her mother on account of fits. Before I spoke to her the mother made a statement to the following effect, which I give as nearly in her words as I could write it down. " This child has had fits. The first was two months ago. It begins in the right eye ; then her mouth opens ; the face draws up to this side " (pointing with her finger to the child's right cheek). " Her hand draws up to her head, and her leg works. She cannot talk when it begins, and it has altered her speech a good deal." In reply to a question the mother said the child was not at all insensible in the attacks. I asked her how she knew that, as the child could not talk. She replied, because the child could tell her what had happened during the fits, instancing without questioning that the child knew who was there and what was done. She also said that during one fit she (the mother) being distressed shed tears, and when the fit was over the child spoke to her of her crying. In reply to an inquiry, she said the fits would last ten minutes, and on my expressing my incredulity she very quietly added that she had " timed them by the clock." (See Case 5.) I now made inquiries as to the details of the fit. It would begin in the midst of talking or singing. Although the face was the first to twitch, the fit began by an aching in the hand, and the arm " dropped." After the face had begun to twitch the arm drew up. She never bit her tongue.

The defect of speech continued after the fit had passed off. It was, she said, a sort of stammer, and would affect her sometimes all day after severe fits. She had never been subject to stammering before. She would sometimes have seven fits in the day ; would have two in the night, and might miss a day. After the fits there was weakness in the right side, so that she could not walk nor use the hand, and she always found the hand weak for writing.

She was a well-formed, good-looking, light-haired, intelligent child. She looked delicate, but she was fairly nourished, and I could find no signs of general ill health. She had walked when about 14 months old, and it is said that she talked when 18 months old. She had never had scarlet fever, nor rheumatism, nor measles, and a careful examination of her chest did not disclose any signs of pulmonary or cardiac disease. The optic nerves were normal. She had, however, " earache," [1] and now and then discharge from the ear, and sometimes complained of headache.

She had headache in a morning, but this symptom was not one which the mother mentioned without questioning. There was not that severe and continued headache which would lead to the suspicion of " coarse " disease. (See footnote, p. 19.) There had been no vomiting. Her temper was reported to be very good, and she seemed intelligent.

July 2. Yesterday the twitching came on " for a moment," it affected the

[1] We not very unfrequently find disease of the ear with " epilepsy," but it is rare to find it with fits like those considered in this paper. The attacks are scarcely ever well described, and we mostly only learn that the patient has occasionally a severe convulsion. This fact is of importance as being some evidence that loss of consciousness is the first thing, and as leading to the inference that the discharge is of parts at a distance from the motor tract. We know that disease of the ear leads occasionally to *abscess* of the cerebrum, or of the cerebellum, and I imagine that it may lead to *slighter* changes—of instability—in these regions, which changes may allow convulsive attacks. It is possible that this patient's fits (Case 6) may have such a causation. On this subject I have made remarks, *British Medical Journal*, June 26, 1869.

face and hand. July 16. No fit except many slight twitchings of the face and arm.

It is needless to go on with the report. On December 31 she still had the seizures, severe ones as well as slight ones, and I fear she has them still.

As the difficulty in talking was described as a " stammer," it may be said that it was not of an aphasic character, but " merely " a difficulty in articulation, and that it did not depend on disease of the left cerebral hemisphere. That such a symptom depends on temporary changes in some part of the Sylvian region I have no more doubt than I have that hemiplegia after such seizures is so dependent. I say nothing of the particular part of the hemisphere in fault, since even from cases of destroying lesions—*e.g.* clot—producing permanent *loss* of speech, I have only been able to conclude that the disease on which that loss is dependent is in the region of the corpus striatum, mostly, I admit, involving Broca's convolution. I am satisfied that the absolute distinction made between cases of " genuine " aphasia and certain cases of difficulty of articulation [1] is at the least arbitrary, and I think misleading. With decided and permanent hemiplegia of the right side, we find *all kinds and degrees of defect of speech.* We find all degrees of defect of speech, from difficulty of articulation to complete speechlessness, without any palsy of the articulatory muscles themselves. At least the articulatory muscles are not obviously paralysed, and they serve quite well in eating and drinking, swallowing, smiling, laughing, etc. We may reasonably expect, then, to find, after convulsions beginning unilaterally, all or many degrees of defect of speech, from difficulty of articulation to complete loss of speech, just as in these cases we find all degrees of loss of power in the arm from what the patient calls a " deadness," to utter immobility. I may fairly beg those who see patients who speak badly after such seizures to *describe* the kind of talk. To say it is " not of an aphasic character " is unsatisfying. To describe speech defects is, however, one of the greatest difficulties in clinical investigation. It is comparatively easy to set down on paper an account of the phenomena of a case of *complete* speechlessness, but it is very difficult to give a faithful picture of slighter defects. We usually observe in the difficulty of speech which follows a convulsion beginning unilaterally, that the patient hesitates, and slurs words ; his talk is mumbling. We hear ourselves that he talks badly, but when we attempt to put down on paper what the nature of the defect is it seems to melt into nothing. For of the above statement the reader may well say that hesitation, slurring, and mumbling are very common things. Even such a description is better than the use of such terms as, " he was manifestly suffering from great impairment of speech," or, " his speech was of an aphasic character." These expressions are only verbally definite. When, however, the patient

[1] I cannot believe that there is any adequate reason for the popular separation of symptoms into " mental " and " physical." Everyone admits that there are degrees of evolution of sensori-motor processes, from those which are comparatively simple to those which are exceedingly compound, and the terms " physical " and " mental " may be convenient, but only as names for large *degrees* of difference. I presume that defects of articulation and loss of speech occurring with hemiplegia, besides differing on account of the quantity of nerve tissue destroyed near the corpus striatum, differ also according as the part destroyed is, or rather was, one serving in simple or in highly compound processes.

Besides degrees of *loss* of speech from *destruction* of nerve tissue, there are to be considered degrees of *disorder* of speech from instability of nerve tissue. Loss of speech is analogous to hemiplegia. Disorder of speech is analogous to hemichorea. This is quite a different distinction from that into " ataxic defects " and " loss of memory for words."

does not talk badly when we see him, we must be content to put down what he or his friends tell us, and we shall be obliged to use loose expressions. But we must bear in mind that they are loose.

### Convulsions Beginning in the Foot

The next group is of cases in which the spasm begins in the leg, and it usually begins in the great toe. Sometimes, however, the patient will say it starts from the calf. I shall relate no cases of this kind.[1] They are rare, and I have never witnessed a paroxysm. The point of great interest is the march of the spasm. Fits which begin in the foot have a different march from those which begin in the hand, although in each the same muscles are ultimately convulsed. When a fit begins in the hand it goes *up* the arm and *down* the leg. (The sequence is not simple ; see p. 10.) Now patients who have fits beginning in the foot tell me that the spasm goes *up* the leg and *down* the arm. I have no doubt they speak accurately, as I ask no leading questions and different patients tell the same tale. In some, however, insensibility comes on just after the leg is fully affected—the last patient I saw with this kind of seizure used the expression, " when it gets to my heart." Here we have two seizures, in each of which the same muscles are engaged, but in each in different order. The two sorts of fits are " isomeric." Another matter to observe is the kind of hemiplegia which follows fits beginning in the leg. This is a rare sequel of such fits, and I have no notes of any such cases. The leg is often partially paralysed for a time after fits so beginning, but of the condition of the arm and face I can say nothing. On these points I ask for information.

Again, I have had no post-mortem examination of a patient who had had fits beginning in the foot, and I am very anxious to learn where lies the disease which causes such seizures. I suppose that in most cases we should *discover* no internal disease, but we are likely to discover changes when the fits have occurred in a patient who had suffered intense pain in the head, and who had had other symptoms implying " coarse " disease. In the fits which begin in the hand, I have found, when there has been intense pain in the head, etc., " coarse " disease of convolutions in the region of the middle cerebral artery. (See Case 7.) Is the disease on which fits beginning in the foot are dependent in the region of the thalamus opticus ?

Again, I think it of importance to consider the side of the body in which the spasm starting in the leg sets in. My reason is this, that mental defect (imbecility) sometimes occurs with hemiplegia in which the leg suffers more than the arm, and I believe that it occurs oftener when the left is the side paralysed. I fully admit that my facts on this matter are very few, and I therefore ask others to help me in this part of the investigation.

### The Cause of Convulsions Beginning Unilaterally

We now come to the question of cause. The word " cause " is used in various senses in medical language, and we shall therefore discuss the following points :

1st. The seat of the internal lesion.

[1] I have recorded a very striking case (*Lancet*, May 16, 1868), in which fits beginning in the great toe were stopped by rubbing the calf, etc. (See p. 6.)

2nd. The nature of the changes in nerve tissue on which the spasm *directly* depends.

3rd. The pathological process from which these local changes result.

4th. The circumstances which may determine a paroxysm.

1. *The Seat of the Internal Lesion.*

The fact that the symptoms are local implies, I hold, that there *is* of necessity a *local* lesion. I submit that one-sided spasm, or spasm beginning in one side, implies *local* change in the central nervous system as surely as one-sided palsy does. It may be plausibly asserted that there is no local lesion in those chronic cases of convulsion where the spasm is general and also contemporaneous, or nearly contemporaneous. But in a case like Case 4, where the fits always start on one side and always in the very same fingers, it is simply incredible that there is no persistent local lesion. The fact that the patient is seemingly quite well betwixt the paroxysms does not negative this view in the least. No fact is better recognised than that a large part of one cerebral hemisphere may be *destroyed* when there are no obvious symptoms of any kind.[1] Why, then, should the apparent good health of a patient betwixt his fits (see Case 3) lead us to conclude that his brain is healthy in the intervals of the paroxysms? He had a fit, let us say, a week ago, was hemiplegic after it, and is now seemingly quite well again. But it is next to absolute certainty that he will have another fit soon, perhaps next week, which will begin exactly as the last, will follow the same march as that did, and may again leave him temporarily hemiplegic.

I have no doubt that many readers will grant what I affirm, and will think it quite needless to try to prove that local symptoms imply local lesions. But I know well that others will say that the fits in many cases of unilateral convulsions are "caused by" disorder of the digestive organs, by fright, by overwork, by mental anxiety, and by like *general* conditions, and will assert that there is no local lesion. Similarly fright, which is a general condition—the whole body suffers—is said to be a "cause" of chorea. It cannot surely be the cause of hemichorea. They will affirm of such a case as Case 4, that the nervous tissue which explodes in the fits is healthy, and that its equilibrium is upset by general bodily disturbances which derangement of digestion, etc., produces. I assert, on the contrary, that there must of necessity be some *place* where the nervous system is diseased, or the spasm determined by causes acting generally would not be local.

The fact that palsy after convulsive seizures beginning unilaterally disappears quickly is certainly no proof that there is no permanent local lesion. In the first place it is notorious that in many cases in which we have observed transitory hemiplegia there is found post-mortem gross disease, say, syphilitic nodules, of the cerebral hemisphere. (See Case 7.) Disease in the hemisphere never causes palsy *limited to one side*, unless it also involves or squeezes the motor tract. It may, if very extensive, cause general weakness, and more weakness of one side of the body than of the other, but never distinct hemiplegia. It does not cause hemiplegia, that is, by *destroying* a large part of the

[1] This is, I believe, agreed on by physicians, but it may be well to refer to recent observations. See a most able paper in vol. i of the Pennsylvania Hospital Reports, by Dr. T. H. Andrews. Dr. Andrews relates a very important case which occurred in his own practice, and gives particulars of seventy-two cases. See also Callender, "The Anatomy of Brain Shocks," *St. Bartholomew's Hospital Reports*, vol. iii.

hemisphere. It very frequently *leads to hemiplegia by convulsion*, and in cases of coarse disease the passing off of the palsy shows that it did not depend on destruction of nervous tissue by the coarse disease, for the coarse disease remains. The palsy depends on secondary changes near the coarse disease, or rather on the " overwork " of nerve fibres by the excessive discharge on them which these secondary changes permit. The recurrence of the fit and of the hemiplegia shows that the secondary changes are there still.

It will be observed that the statement is not that hemiplegia does not *attend* lesions of the hemisphere ; it *frequently* does. (See Case 7.) The assertion is that hemiplegia does not result from *lack* of the part of the hemisphere *destroyed* by the disease. Niemeyer (*Medical Times and Gazette*, January 15, 1870) believes that hemiplegia does not result from lesions of the cerebral hemisphere and that hemiplegia *occurring with* lesions of the hemisphere is owing to the " secondary participation of the district of the corpus striatum and thalamus opticus."

Let us suppose that a square inch of convolution is diseased. If this part were destroyed, there need be no symptoms ; but if it be not destroyed, but unstable, there must be symptoms—for it will *discharge* on muscles when its tension reaches to unstable equilibrium. If the discharge be excessive, the nerve fibres will require some time to recover from this " overwork," and in the meanwhile the muscles which have been convulsed are paralysed.

Another objection will be advanced, *viz.* that in some cases of unilateral spasm we find no local change in the brain post-mortem. Many will think this argument conclusive. I have not yet seen an autopsy on any chronic case of convulsion beginning unilaterally without finding obvious disease in the brain, but I have had few post-mortem examinations in these cases, and I grant—not for the sake of argument only ; I will admit it—that in most cases, probably in nearly all those in which there is no severe pain in the head, no optic neuritis, etc., we should *discover* no changes post-mortem. I should still believe in their existence. I should not expect easily to discover the minute changes from which results only an *exaggeration of normal function.* It is the function of nerve tissue in health to " store up " force and to expend it in an orderly manner at the provocation of special excitations. The discharge of disease differs from the expenditure of nerve force in health, in quantity, and in that it is provoked by a more general excitation. And even in those cases where we *do* find a lump in the brain—in Case 7 for instance—we do not discover the *very* changes on which the discharge depends. The lump does not discharge, but some (" softened ") part of the brain near it—which part cannot be destroyed or it would not discharge at all, but which part must be diseased or it would not discharge so much, nor in so disorderly a manner, nor on slight provocation.

So far I have only attempted to prove that there is a local lesion, but incidentally proof has been advanced as to the exact locality of the lesion—that the disease is in the region of the corpus striatum. The fact that hemiplegia so often follows such fits is further proof. In some cases the palsy is exactly like that which follows plugging of the middle cerebral artery.

I have now to mention that when the fits begin in the hand (see Case 7), if we do discover a gross lesion, it is found in the region of the corpus striatum—in the region of the brain supplied by the Sylvian artery. It may seem to the reader that this fact is sufficiently conclusive to render unnecessary the former arguments. But I doubt not that many will not accept the fact. Some will reply that disease of *many* parts of the brain " will produce epilepsy." This is really irrelevant. I will not deny that disease in many parts of the encephalon " may produce epilepsy." I wish but to show that disease in the Sylvian region produces those convulsions which begin in one hand or in one side of the face, and which affect the side of the body they commence in, before the spasm spreads to the bilateral muscles, and to the unilateral muscles of the other side.

There is a more definite objection. It is held by some that the coarse disease, although it lies in the cerebral hemisphere, is quite as much an *eccentric* cause of a fit as is a worm in the duodenum ; and that in both the medulla oblongata and pons are the centres which discharge. (I do not deny that grey matter in these parts is *secondarily* discharged.) When we consider that the hemiplegia left by the fits I describe is like that following *destroying* lesions in the Sylvian region, and is not like that following destroying lesions in the pons or medulla oblongata, it becomes, I submit, infinitely more probable that the primary discharge is of grey matter in the region (Sylvian) in which the coarse disease is discovered.

Although to me the above arguments seem sufficient, I will consider certain objections.[1]

If a small number, or, let us say, a square inch, of convolutions were cut away by the knife, there would be no loss of power, no paralysis. This is admitted. How, then, can discharge of this square inch produce violent convulsions ? If lack of the part leads to no *loss* of function, how can discharge of that part lead to *excessive* function ?

As nervous processes ascend in complexity, the number of fibres of necessity increases, and at the same time the number of ganglion cells. Moreover, the ascent is not one of aggregation—different independent processes being tacked upon others. It is an evolution of the higher out of the lower, of course with additions. The facts supplied by cases of hemiplegia show that *each* part of the corpus striatum " contains " movements of the whole of the face, arm, and leg, although no doubt in each part the muscles of the face, arm, and leg are represented in different degrees, and are grouped in different order. In hemiplegia the loss is of a *certain* number of possible Simultaneous movements of the face, arm, and leg—the sum of a number of possible co-ordina-

[1] It is asserted by some that the cerebrum is the organ of mind, and that it is not a *motor* organ. Some think the cerebrum is to be likened to an instrumentalist, and the motor centres to the instrument ; one part is for ideas, and the other for movements. It may then be asked, How can discharge of part of a *mental* organ produce *motor* symptoms only ? I say motor symptoms only, because, to give sharpness to the argument, I will suppose a case in which there is unilateral spasm without loss of consciousness. But of what " substance " can the organ of mind be composed, unless of processes representing movements and impressions ; and how can the convolutions differ from the inferior centres, except as parts representing *more* intricate co-ordinations of impressions and movements in time and space than they do ? Are we to believe that the hemisphere is built on a plan *fundamentally* different from that of the motor tract ? What can an " idea," say of a ball, be, except a process representing certain impressions of surface and particular muscular adjustments ? What is recollection, but a revivification of such processes which, in the past, have become part of the organism itself ? What is delirium, except the *disorderly* revival of sensori-motor processes received in the past ? What is a mistake in a word, but a wrong movement, a chorea ? Giddiness can be but the temporary loss or disorder of certain relations in space, chiefly made up of muscular feelings. Surely the conclusion is irresistible, that " mental " symptoms from disease of the hemisphere are fundamentally like hemiplegia, chorea, and convulsions, however specially different. They must all be due to lack, or to disorderly development, of sensori-motor processes.

tions in Space. Similarly a convulsion on one side is the abrupt development of a certain number of possible Successions of movements of the face, arm, and leg—the sum of a number of possible co-ordinations in Time.

Now palsy results from destruction of *fibres*, and of course the *fewer* the fibres which go to a muscular region from a particular part of the nervous system,[1] the *more* that region is paralysed by a destroying lesion in that part. In the ascent from the comparatively simple processes of the corpus striatum to the highly complex ones of the convolutions there will necessarily be a great increase of fibres, and hence large destroying lesions in the hemisphere will result in no palsy, whereas palsy will follow lesions equally large in the corpus striatum. But the increase of complexity necessitates many ganglion cells, results in a large supply of explosive matter, and hence excessive discharge, producing severe convulsions, occurs, when this grey matter becomes unstable.

Then it may be said that one convolution will represent only the movements of the arm, another only those of speech, another only those of the leg, and so on. The facts above stated show that this is not the plan of structure of the nervous system. Thus, to take an illustration, the external parts, $x$, $y$, and $z$, are each represented by units of the corpus striatum. But the plan of representation is not that some units contain $x$ largely only, as $x_3$, others $y$ largely only, as $y_3$, but that *each* unit contains $x$, $y$, and $z$—some, let us say, as $x_3$, $y_2$, $z$, others as $x_2$, $y_3$, $z$, etc. When we come to the still higher evolution of the cerebrum, we can easily understand that, if the same plan be carried out, a square inch of convolution *may be wanting*, without palsy of the face, arm, and leg, as $x$, $y$, and $z$ are represented in other convolutions; and we can also easily understand that *discharge* of a square inch of convolution must put in excessive movement the *whole* region, for it contains processes representing $x$, $y$, and $z$, with grey matter in exact proportion to the degree of complexity.

Then it may be asked, Why, if the face, arm, and leg *are* represented *together* in the square inch, is the fit a sequence only? Why are not all these parts convulsed contemporaneously?

We are in the habit of considering degrees of range of paralysis—defects of co-ordination in Space—and too little degrees of disorderly succession of movements—disorders of co-ordination in Time. The two co-ordinations are obviously inseparable, but we may for analytical purposes consider each distinctly. Co-ordination in Space—the power of using several muscles together for one purpose—is brought about by groupings of fibres. Co-ordination in Time—the process by which one movement follows another—is brought about by relations betwixt ganglion cells. (See p. 36.) There must in health be fixed orders of simultaneous movements, and fixed orders of successions of movements. Not absolutely unalterable, but allowing variations within certain limits only, and in the hemisphere—mental processes being seemingly, but not really, without law—the possible variations will be greater than in parts representing automatic movements, *e.g.* those of respiration. In disease, the range of paralysis and the sequence of spasm will represent sums of fixed orders of co-ordinations. To take a case in which the convulsions

[1] It is not to be implied that all fibres run direct from the brain to the muscles. No doubt there are series of centres betwixt the convolutions and the muscles they move. Probably some fibres run direct.

are limited to one side : the spasm affects the forearm, then the upper arm, then the face, then the thigh, and lastly the foot. Such sequences will represent the sums of the fixed time-relations these regions have to one another in the part of the nervous system discharged. We see the same in the severest fits. The spasm is of the unilateral muscles of the first side, then of the bilateral of both sides, and then of the unilateral muscles of the second side. When records of cases in which the spasm extends to the second side are obtained, the presumption is that sequences will be disclosed, which will show the time-relations of physiological regions of the limbs of one side, to physiological regions of the limbs of the other side : for illustration's sake, such relations as we see in quadrupedal walking.

Then it will be said, How comes it that the bilateral muscles are affected on *both* sides in discharge of the convolutions, when a destroying lesion, even of the corpus striatum, produces no palsy of these muscles ? The usual explanation used to be that these muscles escape in hemiplegia because they are *un*connected with the corpus striatum. Broadbent has advanced an hypothesis which has thrown much light on this and on other points in the physiology of the nervous system. He supposes that the bilateral muscles of both sides, those muscles which must act together, are connected with each of the corpora striata, whilst the unilateral of each side are connected only with their corresponding (opposite) corpus striatum. (For details I must refer to his original paper, *Med. Chir. Rev.*, April 1866.) When but one of the corpora striata is *destroyed*, the bilateral muscles of neither side are quite paralysed, because they are governed by the opposite corpus striatum. When one of the corpora striata is *discharged*, or when convolutions discharge through it, the bilateral muscles should be put in action on both sides, if Broadbent's hypothesis be correct. They are put in action on both sides in some cases. The reason they escape in others is simply that the fit is partial. They are always involved at a certain stage of the fit. Parts serving for most varied uses—*e.g.* the limbs—will be those which are represented not only by most grey matter, but by most unstable grey matter, even in health. In the seizures they are convulsed first. The more automatic parts—*e.g.* the muscles of respiration—will obviously be represented in the cerebrum by more stable processes than those serving in the more " voluntary " actions. That Broadbent's view is correct I have no doubt, and I presume to have verified it by the observation of cases of hemispasm. (See *Medical Times and Gazette*, August 15, 1868 ; also Case 5, p. 17.)

But in severest cases (see p. 10), the spasm beginning, say, in the right hand, not only affects the unilateral muscles of this side (I call this the " first side ") and the bilateral of both sides, but next the unilateral of the left side (I call this the " second side "). But it is to be observed that the unilateral muscles of the second side (left) are affected less in degree (and I believe more contemporaneously), and, more important still, *after* those of the first side (right).

It may seem that the last-mentioned observations are contradictory to Broadbent's hypothesis. But I think they are at least in harmony with the *principle* of that hypothesis. Broadbent does not make an absolute distinction betwixt bilateral and unilateral movements. At all events I think there can be no doubt that the hypothesis is so far correct as this, that the more muscles of the two sides act together, the more equally are they represented in the two sides of the brain, and the less they are paralysed on one side from disease of the opposite side of the brain.[1]

I deduce from these facts that the unilateral muscles of the two sides are represented *fundamentally* on the same plan as the bilateral of the two sides. But whilst the bilateral of both sides are represented in each side of the brain nearly equally in quantity of fibres and cells, and nearly equally in degrees of instability of grey matter, the unilateral of both sides are represented in each side of the brain very unequally in quantity of fibres and cells.

2. *The Functional Nature of the Change in Nerve Tissue.*

I will now take it for granted that the fact of the muscles of the face, arm, and leg of one side being first and most affected, shows that there is disease of the opposite side of the brain in the Sylvian region. I say "affected," because so far as *localising* goes, it matters little *how* the muscles are affected—palsied, or in occasional spasm, or in frequent irregular movement. It is the muscular *region* affected which localises—or in other words, it is this which points to the organ damaged. In order to find out the *functional nature* of the damage of nerve tissue thus localised, we have to consider a totally different kind of evidence, *viz.* the *condition* of the muscles of the region affected.

From the *point of view of function*[2] there are two ways in which nerve tissue suffers. It may be destroyed, and then there is loss of function. It may be unstable, and then there is disorder of function—discharge.[3] In the case of nervous organs representing movements, we have palsy from destruction and we have irregular movements (chorea), occasional spasm, etc., from instability. The fit is occasional, because the unstable part requires time to "store up" force for its disorderly discharge, just as healthy nerve tissue requires time to store up force for its orderly discharge. Of course the two conditions may co-exist. Part of a nervous organ may be destroyed, and another part of it may be unstable. Thus we find that limbs partially paralysed are often attacked by spasm. (See Case 8.)

Functional changes must not be confounded with pathological changes, although of course the two necessarily co-exist. I will try to make clear what I mean by this seemingly contradictory statement. Many different pathological processes may lead to destruction, and many different pathological processes may lead to instability. To illustrate by *loss* of function from destruction of a motor organ. It is inaccurate to speak of hemiplegia (the common form of hemiplegia) as a symptom of any kind of pathological change —of cerebral hæmorrhage for instance. It is a symptom signifying *destruction* of the higher motor tract *however produced*, by clot, softening, tumour, lacera-

[1] In each of two cases of hemiplegia from disease of the pons Varollii now under my care, the chest on the side of the palsy of the limbs does not expand so much as on the other side, but the difference is slight.

[2] It is perhaps well to remark expressly that the word "functional" is not used in the text in the sense in which it is most frequently used. It is often used to imply a transient change in nerve tissue; and occasionally to imply that the lesion is very trivial, and one that admits of quick restoration. I use it to express what I presume is the real function of nerve tissue, *viz.* "to store up" and to expend force. It is true that this is the function of all organic matter, but it is *par excellence* the function of nervous matter.

[3] This distinction is, I believe, at the basis of classification of nervous symptoms, whether they be such as hemiplegia and hemispasm or dementia and mania, or loss of speech and disorder of speech (*e.g.* mistakes in words).

tion, etc. We find essentially the same kind of hemiplegia from these several destroying lesions—the face, arm, and leg are palsied on one side. Similarly, it is inexact to say that the hemispasm in Case 7 depends on syphilitic disease of the brain. It does so depend in one sense, but, methodically speaking, spasm depends on instability of nerve tissue, and this instability may attend any kind of lump, syphilitic or not, and may indeed occur from causes altogether different. I have seen unilateral convulsion in a case of meningeal apoplexy, and with syphilitic nodules in the cerebral hemisphere ; I have seen it following hemiplegia, the supposed result of embolism ; and I have seen it following blows on the head. And no doubt instability results from pathological processes which we cannot detect. So if I am told that hemispasm is " only a symptom," and may depend on " many causes," I admit it in the sense that various pathological processes may lead to that instability of nerve tissue which permits an occasional excessive discharge on muscles ; but *from the point of view of function* there is but one cause of convulsion, *viz.* instability of nerve tissue. Of course there will be varieties of range of convulsion, degrees of instability, degrees of quantity of nerve tissue unstable, and, more important than all, degrees of evolution of the nervous processes (nearer to and farther from the motor tract) which the pathological change renders unstable.

So far then I have concluded :

First, that convulsions beginning unilaterally point to disease of the opposite hemisphere.

Secondly, that the spasm depends on changes of instability there seated.

Now we come to consider the several kinds of pathological processes by which such local instability may be brought about.

### 3. *The Pathological Processes.*

I confess that in most cases we cannot conclude.

In Case 1, and in Case 2, I have not a particle of evidence to show what the pathological process may be. We need rarely be at a loss for the " cause " of a fit if we are satisfied with attributing the seizure to the nearest unusual circumstances in the patient's medical history, especially to the so-called causes to be mentioned under No. 4.

There are but two pathological processes which lead to the local instability above mentioned, of which I can speak with any confidence, *viz.* (*a*) changes produced by embolism, and (*b*) changes diffused from coarse disease.

(*a*) *Embolism.*—It is not very uncommon to find when a patient has recovered or is recovering from hemiplegia, the result of embolism of the middle cerebral artery, or of some branch of this vessel, that he is attacked by convulsion beginning in some part of the paralysed region, almost always, I believe, the face or the hand. I have not, however, yet made a post-mortem examination on a patient whom I knew to have had fits *of this kind* after supposed embolism. It will be safer, then, to say that such seizures occur in patients who have recovered partially, or seemingly entirely, from hemiplegia occurring with heart disease, or with the parturient state. And as I have made no post-mortem examination in any such case I will not relate any cases in illustration. I have recorded several cases of the kind in a paper on " Loss of Speech," in the first volume of the *London Hospital Reports*, 1864.[1]

[1] I think it very likely that in some cases of convulsion after embolism we should find post-mortem, aneurism of a branch of the middle cerebral artery. The autopsies I have had

Dr. John W. Ogle and Dr. Murchison have drawn attention to the fact that aneurisms of the larger cerebral vessels have been found in patients who have been subject to " epilepsy," that is, to chronic convulsive seizures before the fatal one due to rupture of the aneurism. Mr. Callender, *St. Bartholomew's Hospital Reports*, vol. iii, 1867, p. 426), has made the very important observation that " the epileptic attacks belong to aneurism of the middle cerebral artery." I have, in the volume above referred to, spoken of the significance of the fact of aneurism of the middle cerebral artery being attended by fits. But I know of no case on record in which the particular kind of fit has been described. I surmise that in these cases the convulsion begins on one side, but I have, I repeat, no facts on the matter.

I do not think as I then did (1864) that the *persistent* condition of nerve tissue on which the fits depend results from diminished supply of blood to healthy nerve tissue in this vascular region.[1] (See p. 4.) Plugging of small branches of the middle cerebral artery leads to congestion, and thus to over-nutrition, and consequent instability of the convolutions (and possibly of the grey matter of the corpus striatum). It is admitted that plugging of *small* arteries does lead to increased quantity of blood in the part to which the plugged arteries belong. Plugging of a large branch leads to softening and destruction, and consequently to palsy, but even in these cases we occasionally find also congestion[2] of parts of the convolutions and sometimes minute extravasations.

The occurrence of unilateral convulsions with conditions implying plugging of the middle cerebral artery is interesting as regards the *seat* of the changes producing or allowing this variety of convulsions.

(*b*) *Coarse Disease.*—I had prepared here remarks intended to show how we arrive at the conclusion that the convulsion is the result of changes of instability produced by a foreign body—by coarse disease. But I omit them, since they would be a digression. We may say generally that the symptoms are such as severe headache, in unusual places; urgent, purposeless, and perhaps bilious vomiting; and double optic neuritis. This remark requires careful qualification which space will not allow me to give. The symptoms mentioned merely point to the inference that there is a lump of something —a " foreign body," " coarse disease " (footnote, p. 19)—inside the head. They give no information as to its locality, whether, for instance, it be in the cerebrum or cerebellum, and no information as to its particular pathological nature, *e.g.* whether it be a glioma or a syphilitic nodule.

I will suppose that we have arrived, in a particular case (see Case 7), at the following inferences:

(1) Disease of the Sylvian region of one cerebral hemisphere, because the muscular region affected was the face, arm, and leg of the opposite side.

in cases of death by rupture of aneurisms of large cerebral vessels tend to confirm the view Dr. John W. Ogle has put forward as to the causation of aneurism by embolism. For facts in support of this view, see Dr. Church's admirable paper, " Contributions to Cerebral Pathology," *St. Bartholomew's Hospital Reports*, 1869.

[1] *Sudden diminution* of the supply of blood to a large tract of grey matter, as when the middle cerebral artery is plugged, will cause convulsion. Hemiplegia from plugging of the middle cerebral artery does not always come on suddenly, and then there is no convulsion, and probably convulsion does not occur when the vessel plugged is small.

[2] I have considered this subject (*Medical Times and Gazette*, March 6, 1869) in relation to the pathology of chorea, which symptom I suppose *most often* depends on changes produced by blocking *small* arteries in the region of the corpus striatum.

(2) That the disease is instability of the grey matter there situated, because the motor symptoms were *occasional spasm*.

(3) That the instability is the result of changes spreading from "foreign bodies" there placed, because the patient has had violent headache, etc.

Still, we have to find out what is the pathological nature of the foreign body. Is it glioma, syphilis, etc.? I can only glance at this part of the question. It is admitted that it may be of any kind, but it so happens that in nearly all the chronic cases on which I have had autopsies, the examination has revealed *syphilitic* disease of the hemisphere. The foreign body has been a syphilitic nodule. Indeed in most cases when this kind of convulsion is associated with *double* optic neuritis, there has been clear evidence of syphilis. These two symptoms are not decisive evidence of syphilitic disease within the cranium, but are at least warrant for the administration of iodide of potassium in large doses. (*Medical Times*, May 23, 1868.)

I have published three cases of this kind in the *London Hospital Reports*, vol. iv. In one of those cases, subsequent to the publication of the volume, I made an autopsy, and found syphilitic disease of each cerebral hemisphere. It may be said, then, that the optic neuritis and the unilateral spasm depended on disease of *both* hemispheres. But the following is a report of a case in which but one hemisphere was diseased.

I have a very lengthy account of the case, but the following brief note, which appeared in the *Lancet*, October 24, 1868, will suffice for my present purpose. I have recently made an autopsy on a man who had been under my care for several years with like symptoms. In his case there was syphilitic disease of the lower part of the ascending frontal and ascending parietal convolutions of the right hemisphere, but there was disease of the left hemisphere also.

*Case 7. Convulsions beginning in the left hand. Double optic neuritis. Syphilitic disease of the opposite hemisphere.*

A man aged 24 was admitted in January 1868, for convulsive seizures, each of which began in the left hand. After each severe fit he was weak on the left side. His sight was apparently good; but his field of vision was not tested. Nevertheless, he had double optic neuritis (descending).[1] His eyes were examined by several good ophthalmoscopists (Brudenell Carter, Soelberg Wells, and Clifford Allbutt, of Leeds). The patient had also severe pain in the head. Now the disorder of the unilateral muscular region and the "epileptic hemiplegia" showed plainly, Dr. Hughlings Jackson believed, that

[1] It will have struck clinical observers, and perhaps puzzled non-medical psychologists, that blindness often and deafness never attends disease of the cerebral hemisphere. We cannot suppose that the auditory nerves do not reach the cerebral hemisphere while the optic nerves do. No doubt the auditory and the optic nerves are represented in every part of it—not directly, but in *combination* for movements of speech, sight, etc. The fact is that no kind of disease of the cerebral hemisphere causes blindness. I mean that mere destruction of large parts of the hemisphere does not cause blindness nor even defect of sight. Indeed (see footnote, p. 24) it need not cause any symptoms at all. Coarse disease therein leads to changes in the optic nerves on which blindness may or *may not* follow. The patient (Case 7) had no defect of sight when his optic nerves were inflamed. My speculation is that optic neuritis occurs, not because a part of the hemisphere is *destroyed*, but because a "foreign body" therein—especially when, as in Case 7, grey matter is largely involved—leads to frequent contractions and relaxations of arterial branches supplying the optic nerves. (See *Medical Times and Gazette*, April 30, 1864.) It has long been observed that blindness attends tumours of the hemisphere. It very rarely—never in my experience—attends softening from embolism.

there were pathological changes in the corresponding cerebral hemisphere. The pain in the head and the optic neuritis showed that the local internal disease was " coarse," and the subsequent cropping up of a node on the right side of the head declared that the " coarse " disease was syphilitic. The fits continued at irregular intervals, and, besides, the muscles of the affected arm were the seat of a great variety of abnormal movements. It is important to observe that, after one severe fit, the right third nerve was palsied. The patient's sight failed a few weeks before his death (August 29), and on August 8 the eyes presented the appearances of the " swollen " disk. As was easily inferable during the patient's life, there was found at the autopsy a syphilitic mass, or rather a cluster of syphilitic nodules, growing from the dura mater, and seemingly pressing the pia mater before it into the right cerebral hemisphere. Iodide of potassium was given in large doses—ten and twenty grains—but did little good. The bromide was also given.

Although as a matter of fact the gross disease is most often syphilitic, it may be of any gross kind. In the following case the disease was possibly an abscess. This case was published in the *Royal London Ophthalmic Hospital Reports* (vol. v, part i).

*Case* 8. *Injury to the right side of the head. Convulsions and hemiplegia of the left side of the body.*

I first saw this patient when he was in St. Bartholomew's Hospital, under the care of Mr. Paget. By Mr. Paget's permission, the man was afterwards under my care at the Hospital for the Epileptic and Paralysed.

A man, now (1865) 23 years of age, was struck on the head, December 3, 1863, by a shovel ; the immediate result was a scalp wound, for which he was kept in a hospital in New York fourteen days, and was then discharged apparently well. A week later he began to be giddy, rambled about and talked nonsense, and was supposed to be going out of his mind. His head swelled, and he was told at the hospital that he had a " puffy tumour " on the right side of his head. He became comatose ; and on January 3 was trephined. He was afterwards told that this was done on the supposition that there was an abscess " pressing on the brain," and that at the operation " four or five ounces of matter were let out." He did not recover his senses, he says, until March 4.

[Here, out of order, I may state, to have done with the description of the organic disease, that there is now wanting a large tract of bone on the right side of the skull (4 in. by 4 in.), part of the frontal, part of the occipital, and nearly all the parietal bone.]

The first fit, or at least the first of which he knows anything, occurred on March 14, one hundred and one days after the injury, eighty days after

It thus contrasts very strikingly with loss of speech which is caused by destruction of brain structure by any kind of pathological changes. When the lesion is clot this may, some time *after* causing loss of speech in its character as a destroying agent, lead to optic neuritis in its character as a " foreign body." The optic nerves have direct nutritive relations, but very indirect functional relations, with the hemispheres. The auditory nerves have not, so far as we can judge by the distribution of arteries, direct nutritive relations with the cerebral hemisphere. It is also a significant fact that disease of (a foreign body in) *one* hemisphere can affect *both* optic nerves. It has not, however, a significance of the same kind as the fact that disease of but *one* hemisphere causes loss of speech.

These remarks are not really a digression, as the inference is strong that optic neuritis, and the changes on which convulsion, irregular pulse, etc., occurring with coarse disease of the brain, depend, are all really changes of the same kind. (See *Medical Times and Gazette*, August 15, 1868.)

the trephining, and ten days after recovering consciousness. The fit began in the fingers of the left hand, and it gradually ran up the arm, missed the neck, and affected the face. The face was drawn. After this he became insensible, and found on recovery that he had bitten his tongue on the left side. He was told that the fit lasted only two minutes ; he did not sleep after it, and in half an hour felt well, except that the arm and leg were weak, and they have been so ever since. He had in fourteen days a series of 5 fits, and for some time 4 or 5 at a time, about every fourteen days. At the end of about five such periods he had no more, until an operation on August 20. The bone came away on August 3, and on the 20th an unsuccessful attempt was made to bring the skin over the gap. He then had three fits. Since they have been much less frequent.

They all begin in the same way, *viz.* in the hand, and sometimes can be stopped by the ligature. The arm is now decidedly paralysed. He can *move* it, but he cannot *use* it for any purpose. The left leg is weaker than the other, but only slightly so. (*Vide infra.*)

This patient has atrophy of each optic disk; they are now pretty well margined, but there is slight irregularity at their edge, which makes me conclude that the condition of atrophy has followed neuritis. It is the condition into which neuritis ultimately passes. The vessels are not very much diminished in size. There is no loss of smell, and the patient is very intelligent. So long as he takes the bromide, so long is he free from fits.

To the time of the above report from the *Ophthalmic Journal* the patient was only partially paralysed. On March 3, 1866, he was struck on the head, and the same night or next day he became absolutely paralysed of the left side, and to this time—January 1870—the arm is quite motionless and rigid. He can walk, but for all that the leg is absolutely paralysed. He walks by swinging the leg from the hip—the muscles from the trunk to the leg only having much power. This happens more frequently than would be supposed. A patient may walk when he cannot move his toes, nor his foot, nor his leg at the knee. A patient may say he has got the use of his leg, when we find on examination that he has only regained power in the muscles from the trunk to the leg. The leg gets stiff, and the limb is not so much a muscular apparatus as a stiff crutch. But the point of interest with regard to my present subject is that the patient has had no severe fits since he was completely paralysed, although he has since taken no bromide. The only thing is, that when he is startled he has what he calls " drawings to the left." He shows me that his head and shoulder give a little twist to that side. These attacks are only momentary. He is now, although more paralysed, in a much better condition than before. I suppose the unstable part of his hemisphere which used to discharge has become somehow destroyed since the accident, and can discharge no longer.[1]

Dr. Pagenstecher, who was at the hospital the day this patient attended,

[1] Since the whole of this paper was in type I have learned from Mr. Bloxam, of St. Bartholomew's, that the patient was admitted into that hospital, March 8, 1870, and that he died there, March 17. He had been injured by a fall while intoxicated ten days before admission. Subsequently hernia cerebri occurred. Mr. Bloxam intends to publish details of a careful examination of the brain, but it will suffice for my present purpose to say that—as indeed was evident ante-mortem—there was found post-mortem disease of the surface of the right cerebral hemisphere in the region of the Sylvian artery. There was universal meningitis as well—most marked at the base and in the Sylvian fissure.

made an ophthalmoscopic examination, and agreed with me that there was atrophy of *both* optic nerves.

Cases 7 and 8 give still further proof that the seat of the disease in these seizures is the region of the corpus striatum. Although embolism, which I suppose to lead to this kind of convulsion, is a different pathological process from that which occurs in Cases 7 and 8, the result is the same, *viz.* instability of nervous tissue in the region of the corpus striatum. We now come to the

4. *Circumstances which determine the Paroxysm.*

Many things may discharge nerve tissue, *viz.* tearing up by blood clot, bleeding to death, and, as is supposed, poisonous conditions of the blood, *e.g.* uræmia. But I speak here only of chronic cases in which there is a persistent local lesion and an occasional discharge.

I think, as I have before remarked, that there are two factors in the production of a paroxysm—first, permanent local instability ; secondly, something which determines the discharge of the part unstable.

The part unstable " stores up " force, and when it reaches a certain degree of instability discharge of it is easily provoked. It may be that when by continuous nutrition it has risen to a certain degree of instability—it explodes, either " spontaneously," or in some normal periodical change in the body, or in some abnormal disturbance, the result, for instance, of fright or of flatulence. (See Case 4. For an account of the researches of M. Spring, on healthy periodicity, see *Lancet*, May 22, 1869.) It falls then to a state of stable equilibrium, and once more by continuous nutrition rises to its former undue instability, when another explosion can occur. It is, in short, an exaltation of ordinary nutrition and function. I suppose that the provoking agents may be various—that many things will upset the equilibrium of the highly unstable nerve tissue.

We may say of all nerve tissue, healthy and diseased, that it acquires by nutrition a condition of unstable equilibrium,[1] but discharge in health is a consequence of excitations which are *special*. The discharge of a *highly unstable* patch in disease may, I believe, be brought about by very *general* excitations. This is, I presume, the belief of those who attribute fits to excitement, flatulence, etc. (See Case 4.) All these general causes, I presume, act by altering the circulation in the head, during which alteration the equilibrium of the unstable patch is upset. I suppose this must be the explanation of the effect which dyspepsia, fright, etc., have in " causing " convulsion limited to one side. They can only alter the bodily condition generally. They cannot, at least, pick out one side of the brain. They must affect both its sides equally, and yet the equilibrium of the side diseased only will be upset, because on that side only is there nerve tissue which is in a condition to explode on slight and general provocation. I believe such general conditions are only exciting causes of the paroxysm—that they only determine the beginning of the discharge, which when begun leads to further and further discharges in the vascular region in which the unstable nerve tissue lies. I can, however, only

[1] Here I would refer the reader to Mr. Paget's paper " On the Chronometry of Life," read at the Royal Institution, April 8, 1859. The statements in the text appear to me to be an application of his doctrines on the time-regulated processes of health to the explanation of disorder of time-regulated processes in disease.

state the speculation on this matter in merest outline, as I have many times written on this subject elsewhere.

The usually accepted theory of the production of the paroxysm is that it is determined by contraction of arteries (Brown-Séquard). I have advanced the speculation that certain symptoms—*e.g.* optic neuritis, "cerebral fever"—follow the order of arterial regions, and that the *liability* to the convulsions which I have described in this paper—those at least beginning in the hand—is due to persistent changes in the region of the middle cerebral artery, and that the *paroxysm* itself is owing to a *local* vascular contraction.

It seems to me that the development of simultaneous movements and of movements in succession must depend on different processes both in health and in disease. As before said (p. 27), the separation here made is to a large extent artificial. It is, I think, of great importance to distinguish the two kinds of co-ordination. It will not, at all events, suffice to speak of co-ordination as a separate "faculty." Co-ordination is the function of the whole and of every part of the nervous system. And although each part co-ordinates different impressions in different time-relations, no doubt the process in every part is fundamentally the same—in breathing, walking and thinking. We are, I think, studying co-ordination in its simplest aspects when we work at regional palsy and sequence of spasm. The following is speculative, but may be of some value in suggesting lines of investigation.

Simultaneous movements are brought about by combinations of fibres and cells. Successions of different movements are developed by contraction of arteries. *Repetitions* of movements may be owing to repeated discharges of the *same* nervous process. But when one movement follows a different movement automatically, the discharge of the nervous process for the first movement develops the second movement by fibres to the vessels supplying the nervous process for that second movement.

I take it for granted that the arteries are arranged on some plan, or orderly nutrition would be impossible. I suppose the irritation of "coarse" disease in an arterial region produces abnormal and persistent changes of nutrition in the region of that artery, by frequent contractions and consequent relaxations of its branches; changes in convolutions, from which convulsions may result; and optic neuritis, from which blindness may result. A convulsive paroxysm is developed by a stronger and more continued contraction of the same branches, and one which probably spreads to branches supplying healthy nerve tissue. It is, I speculate, through the arteries that sequence of movements is developed, whether those movements be spasm passing up the arm and down the leg, or whether they be the orderly sequences of movements in health.

In concluding this paper I wish particularly to refer to important observations on "Hemiplegic Epilepsy," by Dr. Russell, of Birmingham, *British Medical Journal*, June 12, 1867.

# ON THE ANATOMICAL AND PHYSIOLOGICAL LOCALISATION OF MOVEMENTS IN THE BRAIN [1]

## PREFACE,[2] 1875

" FOUR years have elapsed since I published my opinion, supported by such facts as I could then state, that the *brain*, although the organ of consciousness, *is subject to the laws of reflex action ; and that in this respect it does not differ from the other ganglia of the nervous system.* I was led to this conclusion by the general principle that the ganglia within the cranium, being a continuation of the spinal cord, *must necessarily be regulated as to their reaction on external agencies by laws identical with those governing the spinal ganglia and their analogues in the lower animals.* And I was confirmed in this opinion by finding, after the investigation and collocation of known facts, that observations and arguments like those satisfactorily adduced in proof of the existence of the reflex function of the spinal ganglia may be brought forward in proof that the cerebral ganglia have similar endowments " (Laycock, *British and Foreign Medical Review*, vol. xix, January 1845, p. 298).

This paper deals with paralysis and convulsion as the results of experiments made by disease on the brain of man. As the title implies, its object is to show that we may, by the study of these motor symptoms, localise movements in this part of the nervous system.

In former papers I have considered convulsion as *a symptom of disease* of the brain ; and also, for the purposes of anatomy and physiology, *as an experiment made on the brain by disease.* This plan is complex. In the paper now republished, therefore, I considered convulsive seizures and certain cases of paralysis with regard only to the Localisation of Movements in the Brain. In this Preface I shall show that I have for more than ten years, and before the experiments of Hitzig and Ferrier were made, held that convolutions contain nervous arrangements representing movements. It is in accordance with this belief that I have long considered chorea,[3] and more lately convulsion, to be movements resulting from " discharges " of the cerebral cortex. The careful investigation of such motor symptoms, with a view to the localisation of movements, is a subject in which I have for some years felt deeply interested. So far back as seven years ago I suggested that the facts

[1] This was published by J. and A. Churchill as a pamphlet which had as an appendix a paper by W. Gowers on " Convulsions from Organic Brain Disease," reprinted from *British Medical Journal*, September 26, 1874. The substance of the paper originally appeared in the *Lancet*, 1873.

[2] This Preface has gradually outgrown legitimate limits, and is now larger than the paper it precedes. Moreover, it is itself in substance a reprint ; much of it has appeared in some papers on Epilepsy, published in the *Medical Press and Circular*.

[3] Thus *London Hospital Reports*, vol. i, 1864, p. 459, after suggesting that choreal movements result from changes induced in *convolutions* by embolism, I write : " There is no more difficulty in supposing that there are certain convolutions superintending those delicate movements of the hands which are under the immediate control of the mind than that there is one, as Broca suggests, for movements of the tongue [articulatory organs] in purely mental operations." I still think to the same effect, but should not now use such vague phraseology.

of convulsive seizures should be used for purposes of localisation. In the *Medical Times and Gazette*, August 15, 1868, I published a note on "localisation," various kinds of convulsive seizures being the facts brought forward. At that time, however, I believed the corpus striatum to be the part discharged in *convulsions* beginning unilaterally, although then and several years before I believed the convolutions also to contain processes representing movements. What at this time interested me most was, not so much the localisation of movements in the cerebral hemisphere, in the sense that, for example, the movements of the foot are localised here and those of the arm in another place, but the facts of the cases as they bore on a broad principle of localisation. I considered them as part of the evidence that the most special or most voluntary movements have the leading representation (see Section 10, p. 68). For in disease the most voluntary or most special movements, faculties, etc., suffer first and most, that is in an order the exact opposite of evolution. Therefore I call this the principle of Dissolution—dissolution as the opposite of evolution.[1] It is, indeed, as illustrating this principle, that the study of convulsion still interests me most. For in dissolution we have, I think, a principle of classification for all kinds of diseases of the brain (classification as distinguished from mere arrangement), and therefore a means of methodical investigation. It is referred to in several sections in the reprint. Ferrier's experiments confirm the broad principle mentioned, so far as the onset of the simplest kind of convulsive seizures illustrates it (see Section 9). Ferrier says (I refer especially to the parts I have put in italics)—" The proximate causes of the different epilepsies are, as Dr. Hughlings Jackson supposes, 'discharging lesions' of the different centres in the cerebral hemispheres. The affection may be limited artificially to one muscle, or group of muscles, or may be made to involve all the muscles represented in the cerebral hemispheres, with foaming at the mouth, biting of the tongue, and loss of consciousness. When induced artificially in animals, the affection, as a rule, *first invades the muscles most in voluntary use*, in striking harmony with the clinical observations of Dr. Hughlings Jackson."

The principle applies, indeed, to things so different as convulsions, cerebral palsies (hemiplegia for example), affections of speech, and to all kinds of mental disorders. It appears to me to put in a natural order the whole of the phenomena of cases of Aphasia (see Section 3), that is when they are regarded from an anatomico-physiological point of view.

The application of the principle of dissolution to aphasic cases (see Section 4) harmonises with one of the most important of Ferrier's conclusions from his experiments. It is a matter of extreme satisfaction to me to find that Dr. Ferrier has (at least with regard to the share the two sides of the brain have in what I call verbalising) come to a conclusion from the results of his experiments similar to that I have arrived at from clinical investigation of cases of aphasia. This is important, as the phenomena of cases of aphasia most clearly illustrate the nature of the duality of mental operations. If the view

[1] I have used as synonymous with dissolution, the expression " Reduction to a more Automatic Condition." The phenomena of dissolution, as seen in cases of " Diseases of the Mind," seem to me to illustrate in a very striking way Laycock's doctrines on the Reflex Function of the Brain and Herbert Spencer's doctrines on Evolution of the Nervous System. Insanity is dissolution, beginning in the very highest of all nervous centres, that is in the anatomical substrata of consciousness. In insanity there is always defect of consciousness. There is defective object-consciousness often along with increase of subject-consciousness.

I take as to the nature of the duality of verbalising be correct, it disposes of the statement that "cases of aphasia give proof that we can think without words." I may here quote one of my earlier statements of the hypothesis; the following is from an abstract of a paper "On the Physiology of Language," read at the British Association Meeting (Norwich, 1868). I quote the *Athenæum* report.[1]

"... The author showed next that, although patients cannot *speak* when they try, they may *utter words* when excited. Now it is to be carefully remembered that these patients are speechless, because but one side of the brain, generally the left, is damaged. They do not speak with the other; at all events they do not when they try. This alone shows that the brain is not a double organ, in the usually accepted sense of the expression. But the fact that the patients ejaculate, and that they can understand what is said and what is read to them, demonstrates that there are *motor* processes for words somewhere; for there must be subjective repetition [2] of words when we understand what is read to us. This 'somewhere' cannot, in a person who has lost language, be the left side, as damage of that side has made the person speechless. ... *They* cannot initiate the higher psychical *movements* [3]; yet, although they cannot rouse up *motor* processes, others can. The conclusion Dr. Hughlings Jackson has arrived at is briefly this: that in most people the left side of the brain is the leading [motor] side—the side of the so-called 'will,' and that the right is the automatic [motor] side."

Dr. Ferrier, however, uses the term "driving side," which is possibly a better expression than "leading side." I fear, however, that remarks on speech will not be considered to come fairly under my subject—the localisation of movements; but I shall show later on that I have, as indeed the above quotation shows, long held, that the anatomical substrata of words are nervous processes representing articulatory movements, and that this hypothesis agrees with the prior deductions of Bain and with certain of Ferrier's inductions from his experiments. Hence from my point of view the symptoms of aphasia are on their anatomico-physiological side disorders of motion; thus they are comparable with cases of chorea and convulsion.

The results of the now well-known experiments of Hitzig and Ferrier on the brains of lower animals are, for the purposes of localisation of particular movements, infinitely more precise than any "experiments of disease" are likely to be. The artificial movements I have seen Ferrier produce by locally applied faradaic currents to limited spots on the surface of the cerebral hemisphere of a monkey simulate the movements of health, whereas a convulsion is but a "clotted mass" of innumerable movements, produced by an excessive, sudden, and abrupt cerebral discharge. My opinion is that the experiments of Hitzig and Ferrier show, as they themselves believe, that parts of the cerebral hemispheres are centres for movements. In whatever way their experiments

[1] It will be observed that in the extract given the substrata of words are assumed to be *motor* processes; it will be seen that this also is in accord with one of Ferrier's conclusions (see p. 51).

[2] "Internal revival" I should now say, as the word "subjective" is used in several senses by medical men. (See last paragraph of Section 4.)

[3] I do not now defend the use of such expressions as "psychical movements." I should, however, be in very good company if I did, as I find that several distinguished physicians use an essentially similar expression, and one therefore equally open to criticism, *viz.* "Psycho-motor centres."

may be interpreted, they are of inestimable value for the furtherance of Clinical Medicine, Comparative Anatomy, and Physiology. Nevertheless, the experiments of disease are the only ones we can observe in the case of man. Of these the most important are convulsive seizures. So far as I know no attention has been paid to convulsive seizures in this regard. A word, as Lewes says, is not only a symbol of a thing, but is also a centre of association; the word "convulsion" has in most minds no anatomical or physiological associations. The statement that an epileptic discharge of a convolution caused "convulsion of the arm" rarely rouses what is really only another way of putting the same thing, the thought that that convolution contains processes representing "movements of the arm"; I mean not even in the minds of those who admit that movements are represented in convolutions. The convulsion shows a contention of innumerable movements; or, as I have already said in loose metaphor, it is a "clotted mass of movements." In still other words, we may say that it is a sudden development in a coarse, brutal way of the functions of some part of the brain.

No one feels more than I do the difficulty of observing convulsive seizures with suffiicent precision for anatomical and physiological uses, and the difficulty there is in defining at autopsies the exact parts of the brain damaged. The damage by disease is often coarse, ill-defined, and widespread. The facts I have up to this time obtained towards the "Localisation of Movements in the Brain" of man by observing cases of convulsion are, I admit, very few, and of a most general character; they scarcely deserve mention along with those obtained in the masterly investigations of Hitzig and Ferrier on the lower animals. Nevertheless, I repeat the experiments of disease *must* be considered in the case of man. We cannot have clear notions of convulsion as a symptom in epilepsy until we have studied it anatomically and physiologically.

I would therefore entreat physicians to contribute to the more and more exact "Localisation of Movements in the Brain" of man by the precise study of the symptoms of cases of convulsion [1] and paralysis, and by carefully defining the position of the diseased parts found in the brain after death. The interpretation of such observations will be very much aided by the results of the work Hitzig and Ferrier have done.

In order to render some parts of this paper intelligible, the reader must keep in mind that it is assumed throughout that the cerebral hemisphere is made up of nothing else than nervous arrangements for the co-ordination of impressions and movements; that, in other words, the unit of composition of this as of every other nervous centre (the "organ of mind," as well as the ciliary ganglion, spinal cord, etc.), is sensori-*motor*. To requote what Laycock wrote thirty years ago: "*The ganglia within the cranium, being a continuation of the spinal cord, must necessarily be regulated as to their reaction on external agencies by laws identical with those governing the spinal ganglia and their analogues in the lower animals.*"

Let one at once consider a possible misunderstanding. To say that the cerebral hemisphere is for mentation, that is, as a counter-statement to what

[1] The cases I have published have appeared in the Hospital Reports of the *Medical Times and Gazette*, during the years 1872 *et seq.*—Reports of cases of convulsion from organic brain disease, in which the Localisation of Movements is one of the objects of the reporter, are published by my colleague, Dr. Gowers, *British Medical Journal*, September 26, 1874.

has just been said, is simply irrelevant ; no one, nowadays, denies that the cerebral hemisphere is for mental operations. All I have asserted is that the *substrata* of mentation are sensori-*motor* processes. It is with these, the physical side of mentation,[1] that we are directly concerned.

The reader must never forget that an absolute distinction is made in this paper between mental states and their corresponding physical states, and that no attempt is made to explain the former by the latter. Whether there is such a distinction or not does not matter so much for anatomical and physiological purposes as may appear. As subsequent quotations will show, such a distinction is made by most. A parallelism being assumed, all that is attempted is to discover the nature and conditions of activity of those nervous arrangements which are assumed to be the substrata of states of mind. In other words, whilst admitting, as of course, that prior psychological analysis is necessary, we are directly concerned not with psychology, but with certain questions in the anatomy and physiology of the nervous system.

The following quotation will show what is meant by the distinction betwixt psychology and the anatomy and physiology of the nervous system : " Physiology is an objective science ; and is limited to such data as can be reached by observations made on sensible objects. It cannot, therefore, properly appropriate subjective data ; or data wholly inaccessible to external observations. Without questioning the truth of the assumed correlation between the changes which, physically considered, are disturbances of nerves, and those which, psychically considered, are feelings, it may be safely affirmed that physiology, which is an interpretation of the physical processes that go on in organisms, in terms known to physical science, ceases to be physiology when it imparts into its interpretations a psychical factor—a factor which no physical research whatever can disclose, or identify, or get the remotest glimpse of.

" The relations between nerve actions and mental states form a distinct subject, to be dealt with presently. Here we are treating of nerve-actions on their physiological side, and must ignore their psychological side. Doing this, we have no alternative but to formulate them in terms of motion " (Spencer, *Psychology*, vol. i, p. 48).

Tyndall writes : " . . . The passage from the physics of the brain to the corresponding facts of consciousness is unthinkable. Granted that a definite thought and a definite molecular action in the brain occur simultaneously, we do not possess the intellectual organ, nor apparently any rudiment of the organ, which would enable us to pass by a process of reasoning from the one phenomenon to the other. They appear together, we know not why." This quotation is given by Lewes, in his *Problems of Life and Mind*, vol. ii, p. 458. Lewes adds : " To the same effect, Mill, *Logic*, vol. ii, p. 436. Du Bois Reymond, *Über die Grenzen des Naturerkennens*, 1872, p. 17. Griesinger, *Maladies Mentales*, 1865, p. 7. Donders, in the *Archiv für Anat. u. Physiol.*, 1868, p. 658. Lotze, *Mikrokosmus*, 1856, 1, 161."

Mr. Lewes differs, as the following quotation serves to show : " That the *passage* of a motion into a sensation is unthinkable, and that by no intelligible process can we follow the transformation, I admit ; but I do not admit that there is any such transformation. When I am told that a nervous excitation is *transformed* into a sensation on reaching the brain, I ask, who knows this ? On what evidence is this fact asserted ? On examination it will appear that

[1] The word " mentation " was, I believe, introduced by Metcalfe Johnson.

there is no evidence at all of such a transformation ; all the evidence points to the very different fact *that the neural process and the feeling are one and the same process viewed under different aspects.* [Not italics in original.] Viewed from the physical or objective side, it is a neural process ; viewed from the psychological or subjective side, it is a sentient process " (*Problems of Life and Mind*, vol. ii, p. 459).

Mr. Lewes's view does not conflict with mine *in this inquiry*.[1] For all I have to urge in this paper is, that we should try to determine the anatomical nature of the neural arrangement, and this can be done regardless of any hypothesis as to the relation betwixt the neural process and the feeling. It is, I think, indeed convenient to make the distinction, even if it be purely artificial.

The reader will observe that I did not in the paper here reprinted try to *prove* that the convolutions contain processes representing movement. *I had for years assumed that convolutions contain processes representing movements and impressions.* In fact, I cannot conceive of what other materials the cerebral hemisphere can be composed than of nervous arrangements representing impressions and movements. I have long taken this for granted when considering what is commonly called the Physiology of Mind, especially with regard to speech, as well as when speaking of convulsions and chorea.

In a paper (*Royal London Ophthalmic Hospital Reports*, vol. v, part 4), published as far back as 1866, it is assumed throughout.[2] As I am anxious to show, for several reasons, that this notion had long ago become in my mind almost automatic, I will requote a footnote from a paper written five years ago. It had become so automatic, that although it is implied throughout that paper that the convolutions contain processes representing movements, my belief to that effect is only explicitly stated in the part here reproduced. I mention this to account for the statement appearing in a footnote. In fact, in every paper written during and since 1866, whether on chorea, convulsions, or on the physiology of language, I have *always* written on the assumption that the cerebral hemisphere is made up of processes representing impressions and movements. It seems to me to be a necessary implication of the doctrine of nervous evolution as this is stated by Spencer.

When speaking of convulsions (a mass of movements) as being owing to discharges of *convolutious* (" Study of Convulsions," *St. Andrews Medical Graduates' Transactions*, vol. iii, 1870, see p. 26), I say—" It is asserted by some that the cerebrum is the organ of mind, and that it is not a *motor* organ. Some think the cerebrum is to be likened to an instrumentalist, and the motor centres to the instrument—one part is for ideas, and the other for movements. It may, then, be asked, How can discharge of part of a *mental* organ produce *motor* symptoms only ? I say motor symptoms only, because, to give sharpness to the

[1] Mr. Lewes, under the head *Psychological Spectrum*, writes : " Every psychical fact is a product of sense work, brain work, and muscle work " (*Problems, etc.*, vol. i, p. 147).

[2] One quotation from that paper will show this : " So far as we can know anything definite of mind [the actions of the anatomical substrata of mind, I should have said], it is made up of sensory and *motor* phenomena—the functions of a series of anatomical possibilities in the cerebrum in correspondence with its wide environment," etc. Again, p. 290 : " On the evolution of movements I have spoken several times, especially as regards the arm-nervous-system—*i.e.* from nerve trunks supplying muscles directly to the corpus striatum." As the observation of Hilton on the method of nerve supply to skin, muscles, and joints shows, there is in the ultimates of the body rudimentary or incipient co-ordination. The following is a further quotation referring to the sentence last quoted : " If such an expression be permitted, there is a gradual increase in *intelligence* in movements from the lowest nerve trunks to the *highest centres*."

argument, I will suppose a case in which there is unilateral spasm without loss of consciousness. *But of what ' substance ' can the organ of mind be composed, unless of processes representing movements and impressions ; and how can the convolutions differ from the inferior centres, except as parts representing more intricate co-ordinations of impressions and movements in time and space than they do ?* Are we to believe that the hemisphere is built on a plan *fundamentally* different from that of the motor tract ? What can [the anatomical substratum of] an ' idea '—say of a ball—be, except a process representing certain impressions of surface and particular *muscular adjustments* ? What is recollection but a revivification of such processes, which, in the past, have become part of the organism itself ? What is delirium, except the *disorderly* revival of sensori-*motor* processes received in the past ? What is a mistake in a word, but a wrong *movement*—a chorea ? Giddiness can be but the temporary loss or disorder of certain relations in space, chiefly made up of muscular feelings. Surely the conclusion is irresistible, that ' mental ' symptoms from disease of the hemisphere are fundamentally like hemiplegia, chorea, and convulsions, however specially different. They must all be due to lack, or to disorderly development, of sensori-*motor* processes."

In innumerable places I have witten to the same effect explicitly or implicitly. To have long believed this is no proof of its truth ; but I think that, to say the least, it adds something of plausibility to the evidence in favour of the interpretation Hitzig and Ferrier give of the results of their experiments. I had been driven to the conclusion that the convolutions *must* represent movements and impressions long before their experiments were made. So far as I can imagine, there is nothing else they can represent. I cannot conceive what even the very highest nervous centres can possibly be, except developments out of lower nervous centres, which no one doubts to represent impressions and movements. These are audacious expressions, and therefore I am very anxious to show that my opinions are not mere after-thoughts. Let me give another quotation. In the *Medical Times and Gazette*, November 17, 1868, p. 526, I write (italics in original), " *The psychical, like the physical processes of the nervous system, can only be functions of complex combinations of motor and sensory nerves.*" I should not now use such vague phraseology, but this quotation, like the former one, shows that I have long had no doubt whatever that the cerebral hemispheres (the " organ of mind ") represent an element of movement. I shall give many quotations to the same general effect in this paper.

I found this conclusion, as I thought and as I still think, in entire harmony with the facts supplied by cases of choreal movements, convulsion, and aphasia. It is, then, something better than mere blind prejudice which leads me to accept the interpretation Hitzig and Ferrier have given of the phenomena observed in their experiments.

I am not forgetting the counter experiments of Dupuy and Burdon-Sanderson. There are, on the other hand, the valuable observations of Putnam in reply, to say nothing of the rejoinders of Hitzig and Ferrier themselves. It is at any rate permissible to assume as an hypothesis that the cerebral hemispheres contain processes for movements in order to investigate more methodically cases of chorea, convulsion, and other diseases of the mind—i.e. diseases of nervous processes serving in mentation. As the use of the word " hypothesis " implies, the assumption may be taken as provisional ; the facts of cases of disease may lead to disproof of it, although, I think, they are entirely in support of it, and will verify it.

To myself, who have for more than ten years been teaching that convulsions represent movements, it naturally comes easy to believe that the experiments of Hitzig and Ferrier are a demonstration that this is the anatomical constitution of certain of them. Those who have read the quotations above given will not accuse me of affectation when I say that I was surprised that anyone hesitated to accept the conclusions of the recent experiments.

There is one objection to the conclusion which must be mentioned. It has been recently asserted that the convolutions—let us say the convolutions near to the corpus striatum—cannot represent movements, because destruction of much of them produces no loss of movement. The theory of evolution accounts for the two superficially discordant facts. I wish to point out that I have faced this difficulty long ago, and, if I may use such an expression, I considered the objection before it was made. I raised the objection myself.[1] For example, in the " Study of Convulsions " (1870), (see p. 26) after adducing arguments to show that in convulsions beginning unilaterally the central discharge is of convolutions in the region of the middle cerebral artery, I write: " Although to me the above arguments seem sufficient, I will consider certain objections.

" If a small number, or let us say a square inch, of convolutions were cut away by the knife, there would be no loss of power, no paralysis. This is admitted. How, then, can discharge of this square inch produce violent convulsions? If lack of that part leads to no *loss* of function, how can discharge of that part lead to *excessive* function." I then considered the objection in detail. Whether I have succeeded in solving the problem is one thing. I wish to show by the quotation I have given that at any rate I did not shirk the difficulty.

Some time before I wrote the " Study of Convulsions " I had the objection to reply to. For as I held that choreal *movements* result from discharge of *convolutions* near to the corpus striatum, I was compelled to face the very obvious objection that parts of the cerebral hemisphere might, as I could not deny, be destroyed altogether without the production of any obvious symptoms of any sort. I stated what I now call the Principle or Hypothesis of Compensation as regards chorea in the *Edinburgh Medical Journal*, October 1868. In all the statements I have made of the principle, it is assumed that the cerebral hemisphere is made up of nervous arrangements representing impressions and movements.

The following is one of the earliest statements I have made of the " Principle of Compensation." I had been speaking of representation of movements in the corpus striatum, but had for mere simplicity of illustration spoken only

[1] In their masterly article on the Functions of the Cerebral Hemisphere in the *Archives of Physiology*, Nos. 3 and 4, 1875, MM. Carville and Duret say that all the authors, whom they enumerate, and of whom I am one, have not taken note of the law of " suppléance " of one part of the cortex for another. The quotations in the text show that I am not in fault here. I have stated the Principle of Compensation years ago. It was not possible that I could have overlooked it; for how otherwise could I have held that movements are represented in convolutions near to the corpus striatum when it is notorious that these convolutions may be extensively damaged in cases where there are no symptoms whatever? I have had to consider the Principle of Compensations, as regards the question of recovery from hemiplegia when the damage causing that hemiplegia is not restored, with regard to the therapeutics of one form of syphilitic hemiplegia, with regard to chorea, epilepsies, etc.

of movements of the arm.[1] From this quotation, also, the reader will observe that I long ago held that the " organ of mind " consists of nervous arrangements representing movements. The arrangement of nervous elements representing increasing complexity of movement is supposed to begin with the nerve trunks. (See on this point also the footnote p. 42.)

" Just as in the arm-nervous system there is a gradually increasing complexity, from the delivery of nerves to muscles through interweaving of nerves in the nerve trunks, to an interrelation so great in the corpus striatum, that damage to a small part of this organ weakens the whole of the limb, and yet destroys no single movement—so we may fairly infer that, continued from the corpus striatum, deeper in brain—further in mind—are still more complex arrangements of *motor* processes, reaching a minute degree of interrelation and a vast width of association with the complex *motives*—the sensation aspect of mind—of the hemisphere, and becoming at length so complete that a quantity of brain may be destroyed without any special [striking] mental defect resulting " (*Medical Times and Gazette*, December 21, 1867).

I reproduce another statement of the hypothesis, somewhat differently put. It is from the " Study of Convulsions." (See p. 27). This quotation also shows that I then (1870) believed the convolutions to contain processes representing movements, and that discharge of them produced convulsions.

" Then it may be said that one convolution will represent only the *movements* of the arm, another only those of speech, another only those of the leg, and so on. The facts above stated show that this is not the plan of structure of the nervous system. Thus, to take an illustration, the external parts $x$, $y$, and $z$ are each represented by units of the corpus striatum. But the plan of representation is not that some units contain $x$ largely only, as $x^3$, others $y$ largely only, as $y^3$, but that *each* unit contains $x$, $y$, and $z$—some, let us say, as $x^3$, $y^2$, $z$, others as $x^2$, $y^3$, $z$, etc. When we come to the still higher evolution of the cerebrum, we can easily understand that, if the same plan be carried out, a square inch of convolution *may be wanting*, without palsy of the face, arm, and leg, as $x$, $y$, and $z$ are represented in other convolutions ; and we can also easily understand that *discharge* of a square inch of convolution must put in excessive movement the *whole* region [face, arm, and leg], for it contains processes representing $x$, $y$, and $z$, with grey matter in exact proportion to the degree of complexity."

The two following quotations are from the *Medical Mirror*, October 1869. As in the former ones it is assumed that the cerebral hemispheres represent movements, and here the conclusion is stated that the whole of the gross movements of the body are represented in each cerebral hemisphere.

" The cerebral region, of which the corpus striatum is part, consists of units, each one of which represents movements of the whole of the so-called voluntary muscles of the two sides of the body ; although, no doubt, each unit will represent a different grouping of them. Thus we have arrived at a minute degree of interrelation of movements, and it is presumable that this is carried to a still greater extreme in the anterior and posterior lobes with processes of incoming sensations."

The following further quotation from the same article shows the application of the principle : " When in the cerebrum we have arrived at an interrelation

[1] As will be seen by later quotations, I suppose the whole of the body to be represented in the highest nervous processes.

so great that *each* part of that organ contains processes for movements of the *whole* of the body, we can, as aforesaid, understand that destruction of much of that organ may lead to no symptoms ; but if part of the *grey matter* of the organ be not destroyed but unstable, it is plain that there must be symptoms by its discharge."

The word " compensation " itself shows what is meant. A region of the body is not permanently paralysed when a part of the brain representing it is destroyed, because the neighbouring parts also represent the very same region. The principle applies, I believe, to partial lesions of all nervous centres, but more evidently the higher the centre. This is what we should expect on the principle of evolution ; for the higher the centre, the greater the number of *different* movements and impressions represented in it. This implies a greater number both of nerve fibres and cells. Now, of course, the more fibres in the centre, the less loss of movement will result from destruction of part of it ; and, of course, the more ganglion cells, the more over-movement from discharge of an unstable part of it. When we come to the highest centre, the cerebral hemisphere, it is notorious that destruction of much of it may occur without the production of any obvious symptoms. This is a fact which is forced on the attention of every surgeon or physician. And then, on the other hand, the discharge of a very limited part of it produces considerable external movement. I suppose I have stated the principle or Hypothesis of Compensation a score of times, and many times before the experiments of Hitzig and Ferrier were begun. I will not, therefore, state it again here, but will refer to an essentially similar hypothesis by M. Taine.

The Hypothesis of Compensation is the result of observation of cases of disease ; but the facts of experiments on animals have a similar bearing. M. Taine has, chiefly from these facts, but also from cases of disease, come to a conclusion which is very like the one I have come to. He says : " The brain is a kind of polypus, whose elements have the same functions." I think the same general truth is contained in the statement I have made of a subordinate centre, " that the corpus striatum is a mass of small corpora striata " (*Medical Mirror*, October 1869).

Referring to certain experiments by Vulpian, M. Taine says : " We see that, in the case of the frog, the *eighth part* of its brain supplied the place of the rest ; a larger portion would be required in the case of a superior animal ; and, when we come to the summit of the animal kingdom, the mutual dependence of the different parts of the brain is much greater. But the conclusion is the same ; the brain is a kind of polypus whose elements have the same functions."

I do not think the compensation is ever absolute (I speak of destruction of parts of the brain producing no *obvious* symptom). I think it probable that what is called loss of muscular sense in a limb is in some cases loss of the most special or, metaphorically speaking, " most delicate " *movements* in that limb. I say " movements," as I hold it to be as misleading an expression to say that the convolutions represent muscles directly, as it is to say that language is made up of letters.

In the same paper I go a step farther as to representation. I have long believed that not only the movements ordinarily so-called, but the movements of arteries and the viscera are represented in the cerebrum. I believe, indeed, that the very highest processes (the substrata of consciousness) are only the most multifold and complex of all sensori-motor processes, that they represent or re-represent *all* lower nervous centres, and thus the whole organism (the organism as a whole). They are the processes by which, physiologically speaking, the organism is adjusted to its environment, and, psychologically speaking, the subject to the object.[1]

In the *Medical Mirror*, October 1869, I write, except for a few verbal alterations, as follows: "We have now, then, to add to the constitution of the units of the cerebrum nerve fibres to the heart, vessels, and viscera, or rather probably to regions of the sympathetic system, from which these parts are supplied. The inference we have now arrived at is that the units of the cerebral hemisphere (in the region of the corpus striatum, at least) represent potentially the whole processes of the body. If this be so we can understand how it happens that in cases of epilepsy [beginning by loss of consciousness, *i.e.* the discharge beginning in the highest nervous processes], besides obvious convulsion, we have premonitory shivering, pallor of face, and increased flow of saliva, and in some cases vomiting. Thus, too, we see how it is that emotional manifestations accompany intellectual phenomena. Emotional manifestations are wide and yet temporary bodily states, and we have seen that the heart, arteries, and viscera, as well as the large muscles of the body, are represented in the units of the cerebrum."

The statement that muscle, viscera, etc., are represented in the "organ of mind," and in the very highest parts of that organ, at first glance appears extravagant. It is to be noted that it is in general agreement with independent statements of Laycock, Bain, and Lewes. Laycock says (*Mind and Brain*, vol. ii, p. 144) "The functions of the hemispherical ganglia, as the organs of thought and mental action proper, are in unity *with all the processes of life whatever, whether they be termed vegetative or animal*" (no italics in original). Bain writes that the organ of mind "is not the brain by itself; it is the brain, nerves, muscles, organs of sense and viscera." It accords with Lewes's statement that "every mental phenomenon has its corresponding neural phenomenon . . . *every neural phenomenon involves the whole organism.*" *The highest nervous processes are potentially the whole organism.* Moreover, the seemingly extravagant statement accords closely with what disease shows. I wish to say that I have not arrived at the above conclusion by reasoning that since emotional phenomena are (on their physical side) widespread agitations of the limbs, viscera and circulatory organs, there *must* be a representation of these parts in the highest centres, but from observing that gross disease, tumours for instance, of "the organ of mind," produce muscular, circulatory and visceral symptoms. Let us consider a striking case.

As it seems to me, slight cases of epilepsy, beginning by loss of consciousness (cases of *petit mal*), give almost a demonstration of the truth of the hypothesis that the highest centres represent all lower nervous arrangements, and thus the whole body. To say that an epileptic fit "begins by loss of consciousness" is a symptomatic statement, to which, anatomically and physiologically, corresponds the statement that the discharge begins in the very highest nervous arrangements. Now in such cases there is deep pallor of the face, increased flow of saliva, and a universal wave of movement. There is, in the excessive and sudden discharge of the highest nervous arrangements, affection of the

[1] The reader will observe that there is not the slightest implication from the remarks in the text that any explanation of consciousness is given by giving an account of the anatomical substrata of consciousness.

whole organism ; moreover, its parts are affected nearly contemporaneously.[1]

We must bear in mind that there is a case in which it is plain that a very small part of the body (the germ cell) represents the whole of the man it is detached from ; so much so that it " potentially contains " even the tone of his voice and tricks of manner.

I repeat that I cannot conceive of what other " materials " the " organ of mind " can be composed, than of processes representing both movements and impressions. Before giving the reasons for this belief, let us consider contrary views widely accepted. Let us see what are the views " in possession " as to the constitution of the cerebral hemisphere. We can do this most conveniently by considering how mental diseases are very often studied. There is a frequent confusion of mental states and physical states—betwixt Psychology and the Physics of the Nervous Systems (Neural Physiology). I freely acknowledge that I have in my earlier papers on nervous diseases used expressions which appear to illustrate this remark ; this is an additional reason why I should point out the evil results of the confusion.

Among those who believe that their method of studying those nervous diseases in which there are mental symptoms is anatomical or physiological, there are some whose method is neither, but practically psychological only. For they speak as if at some place in the higher parts of the nervous system we abruptly cease to have to do with impressions and movements, and begin all at once to have to do with mental states. There are motor centres, and above these are centres for ideas, for memory, volition, etc., which " play on " the motor centres. For example, there is supposed to be a centre for " memory " of words, and below that a subordinate centre for the co-ordination of the " movements " of words. Even admitting the truth of each of these statements, taken separately, the mildest criticism on the coupling of them is, that in one case psychological language is used, and in the other anatomico-physiological language. There are in use such expressions as that an " *idea* produces a movement." It would be a marvellous thing if there were any such sudden and total change in function. Supposing that we do [2] *begin* in the cerebrum to have to do with mental states, does it follow that we cease to have to do with impressions and movements ? For have we not to do with the nature of the *material basis* of the mental states ? Let us consider this point—the nature of the material basis—in some detail.

To say that mental states have parallel and, so to speak, subjacent physical states, is nowadays to utter a mere truism, which needs no comment. To say that the brain (in which physical states, having a mental side, occur) is made up of nerve cells and nerve fibres, is a morphological statement, and one accepted by all educated men, medical and non-medical—practically a truism too. Such a statement is not an anatomical, or, as it is usually called, a physiological statement. It is morphology only. So then, to speak of nervous " centres for ideas," of " centres for memory of words," etc., is to use not anatomical, but a

[1] Of all facts supplied by clinical medicine bearing on our subject, there is not one more significant than that slight epileptic vertigo, which is on its subjective side a defect of consciousness, is on its objective side a disorder of motion. Such vertigo is owing to a slight discharge beginning in the highest nervous arrangements, that is, in the substrata of consciousness.

[2] On the other hand, it would be a marvellous thing if we began all at once to have to do with mental states. Mr. Lewes thinks there is, attending the activity of the lowest nervous centres, a " sensibility " homologous with that consciousness attending the activity of the highest nervous centres. I think this hypothesis more probable than the current hypothesis.

mixture of morphological and psychological terms. Such statements are perfectly true, no one denies that the higher centres are for mental states; the statements are, nowadays, mere truisms. They are, however, used as if they were anatomical and physiological statements, which they really are not. To give a materialistic explanation of mind is not to give an anatomical one. Suppose that mind *is* a force, as some say, that is only the beginning of an investigation as to lines on which this force manifests its effects. We, in our character as medical men, have to ask the further question, What is the anatomy[1] of the centres for ideas? The anatomical expression as to the composition of the brain is, I consider, that it, although the "organ of mind," is, like the lower nervous centres, made up of processes representing impressions and movements. The co-ordinations of impressions and movements which the very highest centres, the substrata of consciousness, in the hemispheres effect, are only in very great degree different from those of the lowest nervous centres. This does not, as I have already remarked, exclude the other so-called "function" of the cerebral hemisphere, "ideation," "consciousness," etc. Sensori-*motor* processes are the physical side of, or, as I prefer to say, form the anatomical substrata of, mental states. It is with these substrata only that we, in our character as physicians and physiologists, are directly concerned.

Going into detail we have to find out where lie the anatomical substrata of visual, tactual, etc., ideas; and this is, as I think, finding where lie the *most special* and most widely associated nervous processes representing retinal impressions and ocular movements, hand impressions and movements, etc. We have not to investigate *why* we obtain ideas of objects, or of words, during active states of substrata so constituted.

Let us now illustrate these principles by two cases: (1) let us consider the nature of the Substrata of Words; (2) the nature of the Substrata of Visual Ideas. Repeating what I have said in other words, we are not trying to explain verbal and visual ideation; we are only trying to find out the anatomy and physiology of their material bases.

*Substrata of Words.*—We will assume, but only for the sake of illustration, the correctness of the usual statements that there is a higher centre for "memory[2] of words," and that, subordinate to it, is another centre for co-ordinating the movements of words. But the psychological expression must be rendered into an anatomical one. When we "remember" a word there is an excitation or discharge of cells and fibres in our supposed higher centre for verbal memory.[3] That there is a discharge of nerve cells and fibres in this active mental state is a mere truism, and applies to all active states of all parts of the nervous system. So far morphology and physiology only. Now for anatomy. The anatomical expression is, I think, that the cells and fibres excited or discharged, when we

[1] Otherwise put, What peripheral parts of the organism do their nervous arrangements of cells and fibres represent or re-represent? Or in still other words, What particular adjustments of the organism to the environment, or of parts of the organism to one another, do they represent? The answer to these questions will give the anatomy, which is the statics of the nervous system. Physiology is concerned with the dynamics of the nervous system, with the conditions and degrees of excitations or discharges of nervous arrangements.

[2] "To remember," "to be conscious of," "to think of," "to have an idea of," are used synonymously.

[3] I do not really believe in abrupt and arbitrary distinctions into motor and ideational centres. All nervous centres are centres of co-ordination of impressions and movements, differing only in the kind of impressions and movements they co-ordinate, and in the degree of complexity to which the co-ordination is carried.

remember words are components of nervous arrangements, which represent movements of the articulatory muscles, still more special, and still more widely associated, than those movements which the lower co-ordinating centre represents. The higher centre for " memory for words " is, I think, evolved out of the lower centre—out of the so-called co-ordinating centre for the movements of words; thus, it represents the same muscles, but in much more elaborate and special combinations, and in more definite associations. Briefly, the anatomical substratum of our memory of a word is, on this view, a highly special nervous arrangement representing certain definite articulatory movements; it is an arrangement so special as to have a particular organised connection with an equally special nervous arrangement of some other series.[1]

I wish to show that this view as to the nature of the substrata of words is, with me, an old one. I wish also to show that the same conclusion has been reached by three different and independent observers.

I have urged for years (*vide* p. 39), that the anatomical substrata of words are *motor* processes. Thus, in a paper read at Norwich (British Association Meeting, 1868), speaking on the physiology of language of the fundamental nature of the defect in cases of aphasia, I say (Abstract, *Medical Times and Gazette*): " It is the power of intellectual expression by movements of any kind, which is impaired—those most special, as of speech, suffering most; those of simple sign-making, least, or not at all." When we have an idea of a word, either in speaking aloud or in speaking to oneself, a nervous arrangement, representing articulatory movements, energises. In fact I adopt the principle of that part of Professor Bain's teaching which is embodied in a quotation which I shall give from one of his works.[2] It was quoted in a paper which I published on the " Physiology and Pathology of Language " (*Medical Times and Gazette*, June 23, 1866). The following is an extract from that paper: " It is not difficult[3] to show that ataxy of articulation, and so-called loss of memory for words, are really defects of the same kind and that the loss of the sign the speechless patient had for the thing is the loss of power to reproduce in his organs (in health, from his brain, through series of centres, to the end of his tongue) the *movements* he has learned for that sign, or, at least the ' motor impulse.' . . . The fact that people do not put their tongues in motion when they think may seem to be a great difficulty; but I hope to show that it is not so great a one as is imagined. This will be but a particular expansion of the views which Bain has long taught, and which, indeed, he has applied to speech. ' When we recall,' he says, ' the impression of a word or a sentence, if we do not speak it out, we feel the twitter of the organs just about to come to that point. The

[1] With, for example, the nervous arrangements forming the substratum of a visual idea. We may imagine that, during the discharge of the nervous arrangement for the word " ball," there arises an idea of that word. Next, as this word arrangement has an organic connection with the sensori-motor arrangement for the object " ball," the latter is secondarily discharged, and we have then an idea of the object " ball,"—of the thing of which the word " ball " is only the symbol.

[2] The following is a quotation from M. Fournie's work, *Physiologie de la Voix et de la Parole*, 1866. " Idea, considered as an element of thought, is a *movement* willed, defined by the intelligence, for the purpose of submitting to the intelligence belonging to it in a sensible form, its state of being (sa manière d'être) at the moment when it receives an impression through the senses." " Idea is something more than sensation; it is sensation transformed by the intelligence into a willed, decided *movement*. This *movement* constitutes the element of language." " To think is to reproduce subjectively these different movements and to establish relations between them."

[3] I should not now say, " It is not *difficult* to show, etc."

articulatory parts—the larynx, the tongue, the lips—are all sensibly excited; a *suppressed articulation* is, in fact, the material of our recollection, the intellectual manifestation, the *idea* of speech.' "[1] (The italics are in the original.)

In an important article, *Medical and Chirurgical Review*, January and April 1869, Dr. Bastian, referring to Professor Bain's opinion, and to my explanation of the phenomena of aphasia founded on it, combats the view that words are motor processes. Dr. Bastian thinks that words are revived in the cerebral hemisphere as remembered sounds.

Ferrier has come to a conclusion essentially like mine. He writes as follows: "Hence I should incline to the opinion that the organic centres of word memory are situated in the same convolutions as the centres which preside over the muscles concerned in articulation. If this be so, then we ought to have a hand memory, a face and eye memory, an ear memory; and thus we may ultimately be enabled to translate into their psychological significance, and localise phrenologically, the organic centres of various mental endowments. This I put forward only as a speculation, but numerous other facts which might be mentioned in connection with the concomitants of epilepsy give to the idea a certain degree of colour."[2]

Indeed, my conclusion and Ferrier's are very close. Thus, in a paper read at Norwich, 1874 (See *British Medical Journal*, December 19, 1874), he says: "The mouth-centre is the centre, not only for the movements of articulation, but also for the memory of articulation. What are words? Words are merely certain articulations effected under the guidance of the ear. The memory of words is the memory of certain articulations so effected." This is in complete harmony with the independent statement quoted from the paper in *Medical Times and Gazette*, June 23, 1866, and also with the following statement I have made, *Medical Times and Gazette*, October 23, 1869: "In the reproduction of a word in thought there will be, I presume, an excitation of the parts which were concerned in acquiring the word—the ear as well as of the muscles of articulation. This is the view Fournie has put forward. It is true that there is no obvious movement of the articulatory muscles, but there may be nascent movements of them, or nascent excitation of the highest of those nervous arrangements which in actual speech do move them."

Surely there is something of support to the belief that convolutions contain nervous arrangements representing movements in the fact that three persons—Bain, myself, and Ferrier—each from a totally different kind of evidence, and quite independently, come to an essentially similar conclusion on a point so special as that the anatomical substrata of words represent articulatory movements.

When we remember a word there is faint excitation in the highest centres for articulatory movements; when we remember and also say that word aloud the excitation is stronger and currents spread down to lower centres of movement, and thence reach the articulatory muscles.

Those who speak of "centres for memory of words," or of "centres for ideas" of any kind, as arbitrarily acting on and governing motor centres, are,

[1] *The Senses and the Intellect*, ed. 2, p. 345. The quotation does not give a full account of Professor Bain's views on the subject. He thinks that words as spoken are remembered partly as auditory impressions, and that in written language there is the addition of visible signs.

[2] "Experimental Researches in Cerebral Physiology and Pathology," by David Ferrier, M.D., *West Riding Medical Reports*, vol. iii, p. 76.

as regards their method, essentially like those who speak of the soul producing movements, etc. The difference is that the former practically talk as if the soul were a solid one, made up of fibres and cells. This psychologico-materialistic method practically ignores anatomy and physiology. It leads to verbal explanations, such as that an aphasic does not speak " *because* he has lost the memory for words " ; that " chorea is a disorder of volition " ; that " ideas are formed in the cortical grey matter of the brain, and produce movements by acting on lower centres " ; " that we combine two retinal impressions by a mental act " ; it leads to the free use of such phrases as " volitional impulses," " by an act of memory," etc.

It is sometimes objected that we cannot " understand " " how energising of nervous processes, representing *movements*, can give or share in giving us *ideas*." This is a very naïve objection. We cannot understand how any conconceivable arrangement of any sort of matter can give us mental states of any kind. Is it more difficult to understand why we remember a word during energising of cells and fibres because we believe those cells and fibres represent articulatory *movements* ? I do not concern myself with mental states at all, except indirectly in seeking their anatomical substrata. I do not trouble myself about the mode of connection between mind and matter. It is enough to assume a parallelism. That along with excitations or discharges of nervous arrangements in the cerebrum, mental states occur, I, of course, admit ; but how this is I do not inquire ; indeed, so far as clinical medicine is concerned, I do not care. If anyone feels warranted in assuming that physical states in the highest nervous centres and mental states are one and the same thing, he is just as much bound as anyone else to seek the anatomical nature of the nervous arrangements in which the psychico-physical states occur. *To give a materialistic explanation of mental states is not to give an anatomical one.* For clinical purposes it matters nothing whether we believe (1) that conscious states are parallel with active states of nerve fibres and cells, the nature of the association being unknown, or (2) that mental states and nervous states are the very same thing, or (3) whether we believe that there is a soul acting through a mere mechanism. I wish to insist that to hold any one of these beliefs does not one whit justify us in omitting anatomy. Betwixt our morphology of the nervous system and our psychology there must be an anatomy and a physiology. Morphology has to do with cells and fibres or with masses of them. Anatomy has to do with sensori-motor processes.

I have no doubt too much " taken it for granted " that the " organ of mind " is made up of processes representing impressions and movements. Let me give a prominent example. I fear that such expressions as that (which is only another way of making the statement that the organ of mind is made up of nervous processes representing impressions and movements) " we do not make enough use of cases of *convulsions* in our physiological studies of [the substrata of] *mind*" (*Medical Times and Gazette*, November 30, 1872) seem simply grotesque. But I submit that this may be owing to the prevalent confusion of psychology with the physiology of the nervous system to which I have adverted.[1] The confusion, I submit, is not necessarily on my part. The

[1] The expression " Physiology of Mind " is, strictly speaking, a very erroneous one, and is itself an example of the confusion spoken of. I have, therefore, intercalated the words " substrata of " in the quotation in the text. Neural physiology is concerned only with the varying conditions of anatomical arrangements of nerve cells and fibres—with the physics of the nervous system. Yet the expression is now almost universally used by medical men, and it is hopeless

objector may be thinking of mind only, and thus necessarily any statement of connection between mind and convulsion is grotesque to him. But I am thinking of the anatomical substrata of mind, and if, as I suppose, these substrata contain an element of movement, the statement is not absurd. We will suppose that there is a strong discharge of the so-called centre for "memory of words." To say that this produces convulsion of the face, tongue, and other parts serving in articulation, necessarily sounds strange to those who have given no thought to the nature of the *anatomical* substrata of words. But on my hypothesis, even if that hypothesis be an entirely erroneous one, the statement is, at any rate, intelligible. The two statements (1) that the anatomical substrata of words are motor processes, and (2) that excessive discharge of the so-called centre for memory of words results in convulsion of the face, tongue, etc., are in complete harmony, even if they be both fictions. We shall better consider the relation of convulsions to the study of the nature of the substrata of ideas after speaking of visual ideas.

We will now consider "visual" ideas, the most important of all ideas (that consciousness formed of visual feelings, the most developed part of perceptive mind—Spencer). We shall, I think, in doing this, discover how it is that the representation of movements in the convolutions has been ignored or denied by medical men; many appear to hold that the material substratum of mind is made up entirely of afferent nerves and their centres.

What is the anatomy and physiology, not of visual ideas, but of the substrata of these ideas? First, what is the anatomy? I wish principally to show that, as is asserted, Section 16, p. 75, these substrata must contain an element representing movement. "In all that regards visible movement and visible form, the muscular consciousness, it is now contended, is the indispensable element, the optical sensations merely guiding the movements" (Bain, *Fortnightly Review*, April 1869).

The common notion is that the anatomico-physiological process which goes on whilst we have, or let us say whilst we acquire, visual ideas of objects, is a purely sensory one. By a sensory process, however, we could only acquire a knowledge of the secondary, or, as Spencer calls them, the dynamical[1] properties of bodies. To obtain ideas of the primary or statical properties (size and shape) movement is absolutely necessary. Yet to some of those who have not thought on the matter it seems simply nonsensical to say that the anatomico-physiological process, which goes on whilst we obtain our visual idea of the *shape* of an object, is a motor one. It seems so perfectly clear that the shape and size of an object are known through the anatomico-physiological process of the object, as it were, printing itself on the retina, a sensory expansion continuous with higher centres in the brain. Now, I am not bound to prove that

to try to displace it. I am not answerable for it. Again, the term "psychology" and its derivatives are constantly used when speaking of the functions of the highest parts of the nervous system; they are used when dealing with those diseases of the *brain* which are attended by mental symptoms. There are such expressions as "Psychological Medicine," "Mental Pathology," etc. I use the term "Physiology of the Mind" because, as far as I know, *all* medical men use it.

[1] I believe that the secundo-primary or statico-dynamical properties of bodies are estimated by impressions and movements represented in the cerebellum. The "impressions" here, I think, are pressures, and the movements are tonic. We have actual and symbolical estimation. For example, the superficial extension of any object is estimated symbolically, by sweeping concomitant ocular movements, actually by tactual movements. Resistance is arrested locomotion. Resistance and depth, as also distance, are symbolically estimated by convergence, etc., of the two eyes (*vide infra*).

motion is really the essential thing, for that is the theory already in possession. So far as I know, it is most widely, if not universally admitted. I will simply quote Spencer's conclusion in his chapter (*Psychology*, vol. ii, p. 177) on the "Statical Attributes of Body." He says: "That whether visual or tactual, the perception of every statical attribute of body [shape, size] is resolvable into perceptions of relative position which are gained through *motion*." Again (vol. ii, *op. cit.*, p. 171): "Those motions of the eye required to bring the sentient elements of the retina successively in contact with different parts of the image, being themselves known to consciousness, *become components of the perception*."

Again (p. 172), that "the primitive element out of which our ideas of visible extension are evolved, is a cognition of the relative positions of two states of consciousness in some series of such states, consequent upon a subjective motion . . ."

If we *acquire* ideas of the primary or statical qualities of bodies by movements—if, when we "really" see an object, movement is essential—must there not be an element of movement represented in those anatomical substrata during excitation or discharge of which we see the object "ideally"?[1] For when we "think" of the object which is absent ("recollect" it, "are conscious" of it, etc.) we necessarily see it ideally of some shape, as well as of some colour. The inference is irresistible that there must be a motor, as well as a sensory, element in the nervous arrangement in the "organ of mind" which is faintly discharged when we "think of" an object. This notion is to many unfamiliar. It seems unlikely to be true, but apparently only because it is novel. "What can *movement* have to do with *ideas*? One is a physical process, the other a mental process." But, I repeat, that it is only said that movement enters as an element, not into ideas, but into the anatomical substrata of ideas. I merely wish to discuss the nature of nervous arrangements which all people admit to be in a state of activity when we have ideas. I do not know, nor as a physician do I care, how it is that the physiological process of nascent or strong molecular changes in a nervous arrangement representing movement, or representing anything, is attended by any kind of psychical state. Clearly, however, it does not seem to those who deny, or perhaps I should say ignore, the motor element (efferent nerves and centres) a strange supposition that we obtain ideas of objects from energising of our sensory (afferent) nerves and centres. We may infer that those who say nothing of the motor element believe that the anatomico-physiological process, which goes on whilst we have ideas of shape and size, is a sensory process merely. But we will speak of colour only. What I wish to point out is, that it is just as impossible to tell why we have the mental state, colour, during

[1] I beg the reader to observe that this is not an after-thought. I do not write this because Hitzig and Ferrier find that they develop movements of the eyes by electrical excitation of certain parts of the cerebral cortex. I believed that movements of the eyes must be represented in the cerebral hemispheres before their experiments were begun. Before it was surmised that movements could be produced by artificial excitation of the brains of healthy animals, I wrote as follows (*Medical Times and Gazette*, October 23, 1869) of the anatomical substrata of visual ideas: "In the organised forms which serve as the mental representatives of objects when the objects are absent, there will therefore be comprised not only impressions of surface, *but risidua of movements*. . . . The speculation supposes that we have particular visual impressions in fixed association *with particular ocular movements*." A convulsion in which the eyes are strongly deviated is owing to an excessive discharge of a part where the motor elements of the substrata of visual ideas are largely represented.

energising of certain sensory nerves and centres, as it is to tell why we have ideas of shape during energising of motor nerves and centres. It does not, at first glance, *seem so* difficult, because the word " sensation " is often used in two senses. It is applied both to a physical state and to the mental state that occurs along with that physical state (see Mill's *Logic*, vol. ii, p. 43). For example, it is used for colour (mental state), and for the molecular disturbances which occur in the optic nervous system whilst that mental state exists. This double use of the word leads to confusion.[1] It makes it fallaciously easy to " understand " how it is that we have mental states "*from*" the energising of afferent nerves and their centres, whilst no thought is given to the much simpler assumption that mental states may arise " during " the energising of efferent nerves and their centres. It makes it seem easy to understand that energising of nervous arrangements, representing only a sensory element, as a retinal impression, should give us visual ideas of objects, whilst it leads to difficulty in accepting the opinion that energising of nervous arrangements, representing articulatory *movements*, should give us ideas of words. The difficulty is just the same in the two cases. The real fact is that in neither case can we tell why, during energising of cells and fibres, we have ideas. This is so whatever they represent. For mental states arise during *molecular movements* in nerve cells and fibres, and there is no more difficulty in believing that they arise during molecular movements in the nerve cells and fibres representing muscular movements, than during molecular movements in those representing peripheral impressions. The comparison is not betwixt molecular movements in a sensory (afferent) nerve and molar movement *of a muscle*.

" Sensations," in the sense of " mental states," arise, I submit, during energising of motor as well as of " sensory " nerve processes—with the " out-going "[2] as well as with the " in-going " current. I say " arise during "; I have used no expressions which imply, even remotely, that in the penetralia of the highest centres, physical vibrations, however fine they may become, fine away into mental states—such as for example that molecular changes in optic nerves and centres turn into sensations of colour.

I believe this double use of the word " sensation " leads to errors of grave

[1] Starting only with molecular changes in nerves, we can easily build up an orderly scheme of mental operations out of " sensory units " if we use the word " sensation " now in one way, and now in the other. Physical states in this way evidently get so very fine that they " fine away into mental states " in the penetralia of the highest divisions of the nervous system. There is, I submit, a double error in such systems. Physical states do not *become* mental states, and the substrata of mind are *not* merely sensory (afferent) but sensori-motor centres.

[2] As will be inferred from these statements, I adopt, in great part at least, Bain's views on the " out-going " current. The facts of cases of vertigo, many ocular symptoms, but most strikingly the production of " ideal " movements by faradising stumps, have led me to agree with him. I have in a former paper (in the third volume of Crichton Browne's *West Riding Asylum Reports*, pp. 82, 191) tried to show two things—(1) that excitation of nervous processes representing movements is a factor in the physical side of ideation (as, for example, in the development of ideas of size and figure), and (2) that *nascent* excitation (excitation *limited* to the centre, or, otherwise expressed, a " motor impulse ") suffices in internal speech. In the cases spoken of there are feelings of movement from excitation of motor centres when the current developed in that excitation is physically debarred from reaching the muscles, there sometimes being no muscles. (*On Faradising Stumps*. See the masterly work of Weir Mitchell on *Injuries of Nerves*.) The evidence from faradising stumps is very striking. A man loses his arm by amputation just below the elbow; he knows nothing of anatomy, and yet when the end of his ulnar nerve is faradised (the stump being healed), he describes the *movements which we should see* if we faradised the ulnar nerve in a healthy man. Obviously these " *movements* " of the lost limb are the results of excitation of *motor* centres roused into activity by incoming currents from the sensory nerves contained in the ulnar nerve stump.

importance in medical science. A " sensation " attends giddiness, and thus giddiness is said to be a " sensory " symptom. Really giddiness is objectively a motor symptom, and the " sensation " it is attended by is a state of consciousness accompanying the " out-going " current. Numbness of the hand before an epileptic fit for example, coloured vision, nausea, pains of all kinds, are states of consciousness, very crude states, but as much states of consciousness as are thoughts about landscapes, or as the notion of justice is. Every one of them has physical substrata, and of these there is an anatomy and a physiology.

Now, we will take it as proved that the anatomical substrata of our visual ideas are not sensory, but sensori-motor arrangements. We may call them retino-ocular processes. So far anatomy. Now for physiology. The study of the degrees and conditions of excitation or discharge of nervous centres is a physiological study. Physiology deals with the *functions* of nervous arrangements. We have to consider what occurs in health when we have visual ideas —that is either when we see or when we remember objects.

Most of our ideas are latent. The equivalent physiological statement is that their anatomical substrata (sensori-motor arrangements) are unexcited. But we speak now of ideas actual, and correspondingly of their anatomical substrata as being excited, or in other words as being discharged. First, let us observe that we have in health vivid ideas and faint ideas. That is to say, we have ideas in two degrees. For example, we see objects, and we can afterwards think of them when they are absent. There is presentation and re-presentation. We can see them really, and can see them again ideally. First, for the vivid ideas.

When we actually see and *recognise* external objects we have *vivid* visual ideas. There is then strong excitation of the retina, thence to the highest centres in the cerebrum, and back to the ocular muscles. There is complete and strong sensori-motor (or, as we have said, retino-ocular) action. This is what is fundamental, even if only diagrammatic, however many intermediate centres we may like to suppose betwixt the afferent nerves, optic nerves and retina, and efferent nerves to the ocular muscles. Next for faint ideas.

When we have faint visual ideas (think of objects when they are absent— " recollect " them, etc.) there occurs essentially the very same physiological process as in vivid ideation. There is a discharge in each case. Moreover, the discharge occurs in the same anatomical series in each case. In faint ideation there is slight or nascent excitation (discharge) of those highest centres to which, when we actually saw the objects, the molecular impulses roused by the retinal impressions came, and from which the impulses to the ocular muscles departed.

There are two differences of degree. In thinking of objects (faint ideation) the central discharge is (1) slight, and (2) limited to the centre. In actually seeing them (vivid ideation) it is (1) strong, and (2) spreads from the periphery to the centre, and from the centre to the periphery.

Let me state these differences in another way by considering a popular view. Some speak and write as if, when we actually see an object, there is a physical process only, a lower centre, and the periphery being engaged, and that when we think of the object (remember it when it is removed) there is a mental process only, a higher centre being engaged—a centre for ideas. There is, however, I submit, a physico-psychical process in each case, and in each case a *central* change. When we see an object there is a strong and wide physical process, and an accompanying vivid mental state ; when we think of it there is a weak and central physical process, and an accompanying faint mental state.

Now we can state what is supposed to occur when the substrata of our visual ideas are strongly discharged in an epileptic seizure. In the illustrations to be given I do not speak of epileptic discharge of some *one* centre for visual ideas, because, as I shall mention later, I suppose the motor and sensory elements of the substrata to be represented, for the most part, widely apart in the brain.

I trust I shall now show more clearly than in the previous attempt (p. 52), that the statement about convulsions and the physiology of mind (p. 53) is not altogether absurd. But I must first remark that it must never be forgotten that the discharge in a convulsion is an *excessive* discharge. We shall call it an epileptic discharge. Not only is it very much more excessive than the discharge which occurs when we have faint mental states, but it is very much more excessive than that occurring in vivid mental states. Besides being excessive, it is of a limited part of the brain. It is rapid, and it is soon over. It is plain, then, that in such excessive discharges, as the epileptic discharge of the substrata of vast numbers of visual ideas, there could not be a development of ideas of objects ; neither of such ideas as occur in health, nor even of such as occur in delirium and insanity. Such discharges of the organ of mind have only the crudest mental sides, such as " balls of fire " before the eyes, numbness of the hands, and pain from the muscular contraction. We have, however, to do with what occurs physically. We have now to do with the physical results of epileptic discharges of those sensori-motor processes which are the anatomical side of ideation. The evidence as to discharge of the sensory element is necessarily indirect. There is, in some cases of epilepsy, evidence of excessive excitation of parts of the brain representing retinal impressions, as the patient tells us that he has clouds of vivid colour before his eyes. The results of discharge of the motor elements are visible. There occurs from an epileptic discharge that clotted mass of movements of the ocular muscles which we call spasm or convulsion (for example, strong lateral deviation of the eyes). In the first case there is, I believe, a sudden and excessive discharge of a limited part of the cerebral hemisphere, which part contains crowds of the sensory element ; and in the second of a part containing crowds of the motor element. The discharge begins centrally, as it does when we have faint ideas ; but the epileptic discharge, being very strong and rapid, spreads down to lower centres, and by these to the muscles ; because it is excessive, and because numerous nervous elements are discharged at once, it produces not successions of movements, but a struggle of many ocular movements ; in the tonic stage it jams innumerable ocular movements into one sharp struggle. The most special movements determine the position of the eyeballs ; there is lateral deviation of the eyes.

The same reasoning applies, *mutatis mutandis*, to the discharge of the anatomical substrata of tactual ideas, the chief of which are impressions of surface of the fingers and adjusted movements of the hand. An epileptic discharge of the anatomical substrata of these ideas would produce numbness and spasm of the hand and arm.

Similarly, an epileptic discharge of the so-called centre for " memory " of words on the left side of the brain results, I consider, in convulsion of the articulatory muscles. So, of course, would discharge of the corresponding part on the right side, for, as I have urged (see Section 4), there are motor processes for words on both sides of the brain.

The remark that lateral spasmodic deviation of the eyes, that spasm of the hand and arm, drawing of the face and torsion of the tongue, represent in a brutal way a development in vast numbers of the motor elements of the anatomical substrata of visual, tactual, and verbal ideas, will seem, I fear, mere extravagance to some of my readers. For it amounts to saying that convulsion is as much a symptom of disease of the " organ of mind " as delirium is. I have long thought so. I repeat what I said five years ago—" Surely the conclusion is irresistible that ' mental ' symptoms from disease of the hemisphere are fundamentally like hemiplegia, chorea and convulsions, however specially different. They must all be due to lack of, or to disorderly development of, sensori-*motor* processes." (See pp. 42 and 43.)

In Section 16, p. 75, I have spoken of the " translation " of visual into tactual ideas. Few things are so interesting physiologically and, indirectly, psychologically, as the illustration which certain cases of hemiplegia, and certain cases of convulsion, give of the organised anatomical relations in the higher parts of the nervous system betwixt movements of our eyes and movements of our hands. Again, the relation of the sensory element of the substrata of visual ideas to the sensory element of the substrata of touch may be best studied in the corresponding cases of hemianæsthesia with hemiopia (see second paragraph of Section 16).

I wish now to remark briefly on what is *most general* in localisation of the motor and sensory elements of the substrata of mind, that is, of the two elements anatomically corresponding to what are psychologically the primary and secondary qualities of bodies. I wish to show first that there is here also a harmony with Ferrier's conclusions.

I long ago reached the conclusion that the anterior is the chiefly motor, and the posterior the chiefly sensory region of the cerebrum. The sentences italicised in the following quotation state this belief. The first part of the quotation refers to the mode of representation of the optic, and inferentially of all the sensory nerves. I give it not only as an introduction to the sentences spoken of, but because it shows that I have looked full in the face a difficulty—a very superficial one, I think—in the way of the speculation that the posterior part of the cerebrum is the " chiefly sensory " region. I have long insisted on two things apparently contradictory: (1) that no kind of disease of any part of the cerebral hemisphere directly[1] produces either loss of sight or loss of hearing. Nevertheless, I have stated (2) my belief that these two nerves

[1] Observe that I say *directly*. It is well known that tumours and other adventitious products in the cerebrum produce blindness. But such kind of disease produces blindness in a very *indirect* way; it leads to acute changes in the optic *nerves*, on which blindness may or may not follow. There is not from clinical medicine a particle of evidence, so far as I can judge, to prove that *destruction* of any part of the cerebral hemisphere produces defect of sight. I do not speak of the optic nervous system (corpora quadragemina, optic thalami, etc.) It seems to me to be, *a priori*, as unlikely that destruction of any part of the cerebral hemisphere should produce loss of sight, as that destruction of any part of it should produce inability to talk from mere lack of power to move the tongue, lips, and palate. Dr. Ferrier, however, finds that destruction of certain parts on the two sides of the brain in animals produces *loss of sight*. This is, I admit, strong evidence against the view I take. But I repeat, so far as I know, there is *no clinical* evidence against it. It is irrelevant to reply that tumours of the brain nearly always produce defects of sight. I know it well, and have been insisting on it for many years. Were it that Ferrier's experiment produced *loss of Perception*, or loss of Recognition, the result would be quite in agreement with the results I have come to from clinical observations. I may fairly give the conclusions I have deduced from observations of cases of disease. I make four

are represented in the hemispheres. For besides other reasons, we have evidence of activity of sensory processes in the coloured vision, etc., attending what all would admit to be epileptic discharges. Why there should be no loss of sight from *destruction* of any part of the brain is explainable on the principle of Compensation (see p. 46). It is as to the *mode* of representation of the optic and auditory nerves that I now wish to advert. I wish to point out that I have suggested that disease of the posterior lobes, chiefly of the right one, although it does not produce loss of sight, does produce loss or defect of visual perception (imperception); or, as I now prefer to say, defect of recognition.[1] Unless this be borne in mind it might be supposed that certain of Ferrier's conclusions do not agree with mine. So far as I can judge, some of them harmonise closely.

The quotation is from an abstract of my second Gulstonian Lecture (*British Medical Journal*, March 6, 1869): " He does not think it, *a priori*, likely that the optic nerve, any more than the radial nerve, would be represented in any *one* part of either or of both the cerebral hemispheres, but in every part of each of them; and, excepting to an inconsiderable extent, only indirectly. Taking illustrations from disease, the kind of ' sensation disorder ' we should expect from disease of the cerebral hemisphere would be spectral illusions—a disorderly reproduction of *very complex impressions*, which differ from defects of sight as a mistake in a word does from a cramp in the tongue. On this higher level, however, there will, doubtless, be some kind of localisation, and its most general character may be inferred. Since—as Lockhart Clarke has pointed out—the structure of the anterior convolutions does differ from that of the posterior, they must serve differently in mind.

" *Facts seem to show that the fore part of the brain serves in the motor aspect of mind, and we may fairly speculate that the posterior serves in the sensory*."

This speculation seems to me to accord with one of Ferrier's conclusions from his experiments. The following is a quotation from a summary of his most recent researches (*Medical Record*, March 18, 1874): " The whole brain is considered as divided into a sensory and motor region, corresponding to their anatomical relation to the optic thalami and corpora striata and the motor and sensory tracts."

It will, I think, be seen that there is no discrepancy so far betwixt my speculations and Ferrier's conclusions from his experiments.

The following is an earlier statement of my hypothesis. The quotation refers also to differences in the two sides of the brain:

" If," as suggested (*Medical Times and Gazette*, August 15, 1868, p. 179), " both sides of the brain are educated in expression, although the left is the leading side, I would still advocate the view I brought forward in the *Lancet* [Nov. 26, 1864], that the right cerebral hemisphere is the seat of perception, with the important qualification that the right may be the *leading* side for perception—educated sensations.

. . . . .

" It would seem by certain observations of Gratiolet—which are embodied

statements: (1) destruction of no part of the cerebral hemisphere produces loss of sight; (2) *discharge* of parts of it (I think posterior part chiefly) produces coloured vision; (3) tumour in it leads to changes in the optic nerve (optic neuritis), in consequence of which defect or loss of sight may or may not follow; (4) disease of the posterior lobe (right) produces defect of perception.

[1] Because it implies duality in that process, of which the end or second half only is perception.

in the following extract from M. Baillarger's address before the Academy of Medicine—that there is 'crossed development of the brain,' if we may take the corpus striatum and thalamus as fixing the (chiefly) motor and sensory regions. The first part of the quotation refers to M. Trousseau's views on the possible explanation of the rightsidedness of the paralysis of speechless patients. [I omit this part of the quotation.]

"'Le second fait a été signalé par Gratiolet, ce professeur si éminent, dont la science déplore la perte récente.

"'Il m'a semblé, dit-il, par suite d'une série d'observations *consciencieusement étudiées*, que les deux hémisphères ne se développent pas d'une manière absolument symétrique. Ainsi le développement des plis frontaux paraît se faire *plus vite à gauche qu'à droite*, tandis que *l'inverse* a lieu pour les plis des lobes *occipitaux et sphénoïdaux*'" (Leuret et Gratiolet, *Anatomie du Système Nerveux*, p. 241). (*Medical Times and Gazette*, August 22, 1868.)

The following quotation from some remarks of mine in the Hospital Reports of the *Medical Times and Gazette*, May 4, 1872, state the opinions I hold as to the motor and sensory regions of the brain, by detailing the general condition of the aphasic patient, in contrast with that of the patient who has imperception (loss of recognition). One is damaged in the motor series, and the other in the sensory series. The object is to show that the two conditions are complementary. It will be observed that in this quotation the substrata of words and of images of objects are assumed to be sensori-*motor*.

"We have many facts as to the kind of mental affection (aphasia) which so often attends lesions in the region of the *left* corpus striatum, and it is legitimate to inquire if there be not symptoms as *special* from lesions in the neighbourhood of the *right* optic thalamus. The former, when speech is *lost*, consists in an inability to reproduce words and to reproduce them in propositional order; but in cases of loss of speech—in chronic cases at least—there is no difficulty in the reproduction of images of objects. The patient can recognise handwriting, although he cannot read; he can copy print into writing, but cannot express himself in writing; he may be able to play at dominoes or cards. In these operations speech is not concerned; the operation of *another* series of sensori-*motor* processes is required. Dr. Hughlings-Jackson believes his patient has, or has had, defect in this other series—in the sensori-motor processes concerned in the *recognition* of objects (not in *seeing* objects), and in putting images of things in 'propositional order,' so to speak. Such a defect, when extreme, would pass as one of imbecility, and in a minor degree as one of 'loss of memory.' Obviously the investigation of such cases will be very difficult indeed."

I wish now to consider what this geographical separation means physiologically, and then what is implied by it psychologically. In all centres the connection of sensation and motion is, I think, necessary.

In the lower centres there is a direct adjustment of few and simple movements to few and simple peripheral impressions. In the very highest centres also there is a similar adjustment, but then it is of exceedingly special movements (representing movements of the whole organism) to the most special of impressions from the environment. So far for resemblances; there is reflex action in each case. Now for certain differences. The difference is not that reflex action is the characteristic of the lower centres, but that exact and perfect reflex action is characteristic of them. In the highest centres, as Laycock long ago insisted, reflex action occurs, but it is imperfect. In the simple reflex actions of lower centres the movements follow the afferent incitations with no or with little delay. In the highest centres, if my speculation as to the motor and sensory regions be correct, the movements will not be immediate. For the speculation is, that there is in the cerebral hemispheres wide geographical separation, and thus probably delay in action. Again, in the lowest reflex action some particular movement is fatally necessary, and occurs rapidly after some particular impression. But in the highest centres it may be that there is not this absolute connection. This remark brings me to consider what is implied psychologically by the geographical separation. I believe it implies that the sensory and motor elements which enter into the physical side of what is, psychologically speaking, our perception of the statical and dynamical qualities of objects, can be, so to speak, transposed, can enter into new combinations. After seeing a red circle and a blue square, we can think of a red square and a blue circle. The separation is never absolute. It is impossible, for example, to think of redness. In accordance I speak of the *chiefly* motor and sensory regions. Yet we can think of red things of innumerable forms.

The principle is, I think, capable of extension in various degrees to all the higher mental operations—to all complex states betwixt the organism as acted on (chiefly sensation side), and the organism as reacting (chiefly motion side),[1] and accounts for what takes place, anatomically and physiologically, during the mental process, which beginning as metaphor ends in abstraction.

The separation betwixt processes representing sensation and those representing motion and consequent delay of action, or, generally speaking, imperfect action, in the very highest centres, seems to me to accord with certain speculations by Herbert Spencer. I intercalate some words in square brackets.

" For since all modes of consciousness can be nothing else than incidents of the correspondence between the organism and its environment, they must be all different sides of, or different phases of, the co-ordinated groups of changes, whereby internal relations are adjusted to external relations.

" Between the reception of certain impressions and the performance of certain appropriate motions there is some inner connection. If the inner connection is organised [lower centres] the action is of the reflex order, either simple or compound ; and none of the phenomena of consciousness proper exist. If the inner connection is not organised [higher centres], then the psychical changes which come between the impressions and motions are conscious ones ; *the entire action must have all the essential elements of a conscious action—must simultaneously exhibit Memory, Reason, Feeling, and Will ; for there can be no conscious adjustment of an inner to an outer relation without all these being involved* " (*Psychology*, vol. i, p. 495).

The following paper was occupied almost solely with a consideration of the representation of movements in the cerebrum. I believe, however, that all the muscles of the body are represented in the cerebellum, as all are in the cerebrum but in different order. I spoke chiefly of the representation in the cerebellum of movements of the eyes, and at the same time for the sake of contrast of the representation of ocular movements in the cerebrum. I quoted Adamük and Donders to show that the parallel[2] movements of the

[1] All modes of consciousness can be nothing else than incidents of the correspondence betwixt the organism and its environment (Spencer).

[2] Unfortunately I said " side to side " movements instead of " parallel."

eyes which Hering and Donders think are for direction, are represented in parts of the corpora quadrigemina different from those parts of these nervous centres, where movements of adduction and abduction of the eyes, which they suppose to be for estimating distance, are represented. I suggested that the former, which I consider to be the movements for estimation of extension, are *re*-represented in the cerebrum. It has, indeed, long been well known that lateral movements of the eyes are represented in the cerebrum (Vulpian, Prévost, etc.). I suggested also that the movement for distance,[1] and I would now add for depth and resistance, are re-represented in the cerebellum (see Section 17).[2] These two orders of movements occur together in health, but disease separates them. Thus there is loss of the lateral movements of the eyeballs in some cases of disease of the cerebrum ; from extensive disease of one side of the cerebrum we have loss of *one half of* the lateral movements of the two eyes. In order to understand loss of one half of the ocular movements for estimation of distance by disease of one side of the cerebellum, we must note that there is something more than mere convergence. The movement of the eyeballs in estimating distances is a complex one. Besides alteration in the size of the pupil, and difference in tension of the ciliary muscle, there is convergence and divergence of the visual lines.[3] It must be particularly noted that in convergence the eyes are directed slightly downwards, and in divergence upwards. Now it is an old-established fact that, as is stated in Section 17, in lesions of the (right) middle peduncle of the cerebellum there is a skew deviation of the eyes. The right eye is turned upwards and outwards, the left downwards and inwards. This seems to me to be loss of *one half* of the movement for the estimation of distance. Only one half, for there is a one-sided lesion only. It will, I think, be seen that the speculation as to the representations of these ocular movements (see Section 17, p. 76) is verified by some of the results of Ferrier's experiments on the cerebellum. And the further speculation (Section 17, p. 76) that these movements are by nervous arrangements in the cerebellum associated with movements of locomotion goes also with Mr. Spencer's hypothesis that the cerebellum is the organ for doubly compound co-ordination in space.

## On the Anatomical and Physiological Localisation of Movements in the Brain[4]

### (1) *Paralysis and Convulsion are not only "Symptoms of Disease," but supply Evidence bearing on the Localisation of Movements and Impressions in the Brain.*

For some years I have studied cases of disease of the brain, not only for

[1] Ferrier's experiments seem to me to show that this speculation is correct.

[2] These ocular movements are supposed to be *symbolic* of distance, depth, and resistance (statico-dynamical property), estimated by locomotor movements. I use the word "locomotor" in an unusually wide sense. When I put out my hand to feel the surface of a book, my putting forth the hand is, I consider, an act of locomotion, and it is, I think, a cerebellar movement. The movements of my finger ends over the book (tactual) are cerebral movements, and serve in the physiological process of giving me notions of superficial size and shape. The former go with an act of convergence of the eyeballs, the latter go with the concomitant sweeping movements of them.

[3] It seems to me that Loring's experiments demonstrate that the external recti are *in action* in looking into the distance. Indeed, it would be a very exceptional thing if there were not action of both external and internal recti, both in divergence and in convergence. There is, as Duchenne points out, a co-ordination of antagonism as well as a co-ordination of co-operation.

[4] This is the original paper to which the previous 25 pages are the Preface.

directly clinical, but for anatomical and physiological purposes. Cases of paralysis and convulsion may be looked upon as the results of experiments made by disease on particular parts of the nervous system of man. The study of palsies and convulsions from this point of view is the study of the effects of "destroying lesions" and of the effects of "discharging lesions." And for an exact knowledge of the particular movements most represented in particular centres, we must observe and compare the effects of each kind of lesion. It is just what the physiologist does in experimenting on animals; to ascertain the exact distribution of a nerve, he destroys it, and also stimulates it. Indeed, this double kind of study is essential in the investigation of cases of nervous disease for physiological purposes. For limited *destroying lesions* of *some* parts of the cerebral hemisphere produce no obvious symptoms; whilst *discharging lesions* of those parts produce very striking symptoms. By this double method we shall, I think, not only discover the particular parts of the nervous system where certain groups of movements are most represented (anatomical localisation), but, what is of equal importance, we shall also learn the order of action (physiological localisation) in which those movements are therein represented.

### Movements Lost from "Destroying Lesions"

(2) *The Order of Loss of Movements, Faculties, etc., is from the Special or Voluntary to the General or Automatic; Illustrated by Hemiplegia*

I begin by speaking of destroying lesions, and take the simplest case—hemiplegia of the common form from lesion of the corpus striatum. A blood clot which has destroyed part of the corpus striatum has made an experiment, which reveals to us that movements of the face, tongue, arm, and leg are represented in that centre. This is the localisation of the movements anatomically stated. Physiologically we say that the patient whose face, tongue, arm, and leg are paralysed has lost the most voluntary movements of one side of his body, and it is equally important to keep in mind that he has not lost the more automatic movements. The study of cases of hemiplegia shows that from disease of the corpus striatum those external parts suffer most which, psychologically speaking, are most under the command of the will, and which, physiologically speaking, have the greater number of different movements at the greater number of different [1] intervals. That parts suffer more as they serve in voluntary, and less as they serve in automatic operations, is, I believe, the law of destroying lesions of the cerebral nervous centres. It may be illustrated in the hemiplegic region itself: that limb which has the more voluntary uses—the arm—suffers more.

I have illustrated by a case of hemiplegia of limited range from a lesion of moderate gravity. But from lesions of different degrees of gravity we have hemiplegia of very different ranges, varying gradually from palsy of the face, tongue, arm, and leg of one side, to universal powerlessness.[2] Or, physiologically speaking, there are all degrees, from paralysis limited to the most voluntary

[1] I shall use (and, after the physiological definition, without any psychological implication) the words "voluntary" and "automatic." It is not to be implied that there are abrupt demarcations betwixt the two classes of movements; on the contrary, there are gradations from the most voluntary to the most automatic.

[2] Of course, the term "hemiplegia" becomes a misnomer when there is universal powerlessness. I shall have more to say of the universal powerlessness which occurs from disease of but one side of the brain when I consider convulsive seizures.

parts of one side of the body to paralysis of the most automatic parts of the whole body. The movements of the heart and respiration are less frequent, and the temperature is abased (soon after the seizure, of course, is meant). The patient, to put it in the shortest way, *is reduced to a more or less automatic condition*, according to the gravity of the lesion.

It must be added, that degrees of hemiplegia are not simple degrees; that is to say, they are not either degrees of more or less loss of power only, nor degrees of more or less range only, but of both. They are Compound Degrees. For example, if there be paralysis not only of the *most* voluntary parts of the body—face, tongue, arm, and leg—but also of those next [1] most voluntary, *viz.* loss of certain movements of the eyes and head and side of the chest, we find that the most voluntary parts (face, arm, and leg) *are very much paralysed*. In other words, the graver the lesion not only the more are the most voluntary parts paralysed, but the further spread to automatic parts is the paralysis.

From these facts, supplied by cases of destroying lesions of the centre producing *loss* of movements, we may conclude that the physiological order of representation of movements in the corpus striatum is such that action in health spreads from the automatic to the voluntary; or rather (the unit of action of the nervous system being a double unit—a molecule of two atoms) that there is *first* action spreading from the automatic to the voluntary, and then action spreading in the reverse order.[2] The spreading of healthy movements is best illustrated by degrees of "effort," as in lifting weights. There is first fixation of the more automatic parts of the arm, side of chest (and still further in automaticity according to the preconceived degree of heaviness of the object), before the most voluntary part, the hand, grasps the weight and then lifts it. The heavier the weight, not only the more strongly are the most voluntary parts used, but the further does the movement spread to the more automatic parts. This compound spreading of healthy movement corresponds to the compound degrees of hemiplegia.

### (3) *The Order applied to the Movements and Motor Impulses of Speech* (*applied to Cases of Aphasia*)

I will try now to show that the physiological order of gross movements applies to the movements of speech. I say *movements* of speech advisedly,

[1] Or, in equivalent terms, of those next least automatic.

[2] That the unit of action of the nervous system is double the unit of composition is inferable from the fact that the whole nervous system is double. This conclusion runs physiologically parallel with the psychological law that all mental operations consist, fundamentally regarded, in the double process of tracing relations of likeness and unlikeness. The lower parts of the nervous system are plainly double in function, and it would be marvellous if the higher parts were not so too. The most automatic of the visible movements of the body "practically" constitute a single series, although we see that they are in duplicate. The two sides of the chest act so nearly together in time and so nearly equally in range that there is "practically" but one movement. But the very highest movements—those for words—are *apparently* in single order too, but for the very opposite reason. It is because we only consider the *end* of word processes (speech), and neglect altogether the prior automatic reproduction of words. In the double action, of which the second part is speech, there is first, I suggest, the automatic and unconscious reproduction of words. Later in this paper will be given facts which tend to show—(1) that the unit of action of the nervous system is double the unit of composition; (2) that the higher the nervous processes are the more unlike become the two components of the unit of action; (3) that the unlikeness is first in time, one acting before the other; and second in range, one being in stronger action than the other.

as I think the abrupt distinction made in the expressions " loss of memory for words " and " ataxic affection of speech " is arbitrary and misleading.

The physiological order applies to the classification of the whole of the phenomena of cases of so-called aphasia : to the positive—the inability to speak ; and to the passive—the ability to understand speech. Taking an ordinary case of entire *loss* of speech, we find that the patient has lost the most voluntary form of expression (speech), and has not lost the most automatic (emotional manifestations). We find that pantomime, which, bordering on gesticulation, stands half-way, suffers little. We find that the exception to the statement that the patient is speechless (for he can usually *utter* some one or two words) is frequently the exception proving the rule. He has lost speech altogether, *except the most automatic of all propositions—" yes " and " no."* Even these real words are often only of interjectional value ; they can often be used only along with emotional manifestations—can be used, that is to say, automatically only. And, curiously, we find occasionally that the patient who can *reply* " No " correctly may be quite unable to *say* " No " when told. Another occasional exception proves the same thing : he may *utter* oaths or other ejaculations when excited which he cannot *say*—cannot repeat—when he tries to do so. Occasionally he gets out ejaculations of a less automatic character (less general in the sense of being suitable to fewer occasions). Thus he may say " Thanks," " Good-bye," on fit occasions, but not when he tries. In a narrow corner we see the same thing ; he may be unable to put out his tongue when he tries, and yet move it well in all automatic operations.

### (4) *The Order accords with the Hypothesis that the Left Side of the Brain is the Leading Side for Words, and the Right the Automatic Side*

But there is a far wider and far more important illustration to be given.

Coining the word " verbalising " to include all the modes in which words serve, we see that there are two great divisions or rather extremes of verbalising : one is the voluntary use of words (speech) ; the other is the automatic use of words, as in receiving speech of others. Now in the ordinary " specimen " of loss of speech the former is lost, and the latter is intact. The patient cannot speak at all, but understands all we say—on simple matters, at any rate.

That he cannot write is simply loss of speech in another form. For the physiological reality of speech it matters nothing whether the proposition be uttered aloud or to ourselves ; it is enough that certain nervous processes *be excited, and excited in definite order :* if they be strongly excited, there is external speech ; if slightly, there is internal speech. So that internal speech and internal reproduction of words are not synonymous : there is a voluntary internal reproduction of words in new and propositional forms (as occurs when we write) ; and there is an automatic internal reproduction of words in old and acquired forms, or in forms given us, as when we receive and understand words in propositions spoken to us.

### (5) *The Order applied to Mental Symptoms*

This physiological order will, I think, be of great use in the investigation of Mental Diseases proper. It seems to me to apply, at any rate, to some comparatively simple mental symptoms which occur in a general physician's practice. After some epileptic or epileptiform seizures, the patient becomes strange or outrageous, and acts queerly or violently. My speculation is, that in these cases he is reduced by the fit to a more automatic mental condition. Thus I have recorded the case of a man (the *Lancet*, March 18, 1871) who walked eight miles in a state like that of somnambulism. He was subject to fits, beginning by a subjective sensation of a disagreeable smell, and depending on (as, I suppose, *petit mal* always does) changes in the region of the anterior cerebral artery. Now, just as after a fit of unilateral convulsion a patient is often reduced to a more automatic condition, so far as his *physical* state goes—he is paralysed of one side,—so I suppose this patient was reduced to a more automatic condition, so far as his mental state was concerned.[1]

Possibly it will be objected by some readers that I speak in one article of several things which are very different. The reply is, that the same principle is displayed in each of them. That a hemiplegic patient's arm suffers more than his leg; that an aphasic patient cannot put out his tongue when he tries, although he moves it well in swallowing; that he cannot speak, and yet is able to understand all that we say; that a patient in *petit mal* loses consciousness and behaves strangely and outrageously—these are evidently facts of different kinds, but they are all facts of the same order. In each instance there is reduction to a more automatic condition.

## II. Movements Developed by "Discharging Lesions" of Convolutions

I pass now to speak of symptoms resulting from "discharging lesions" of the brain. The movements in chorea, as well as those in convulsion, are the result of abnormal discharges; but I shall speak in this paper only of convulsions ordinarily so called. Here, again, it may be objected that I consider still another topic; but I think it will be seen that the facts to be pointed out illustrate the same principle as do the symptoms already spoken of as resulting from "destroying lesions."

### (6) *The Nature of the Morbid Discharge in Convulsion*

The nervous discharge in a convulsion differs from the discharge which occurs in a healthy movement in that it is sudden, excessive, and of short duration. The discharge being of the grey matter of processes for *movements*, there is caused by it a development of movements in the related and connected external regions. But the development of the movements is so abrupt, and the number of movements developed at once is so great, that the visible result is apparently a mere heedless struggle of muscles, in which at first glance it seems unlikely that we shall trace any kind of order. If we take for first investigation cases of *general* convulsions (such as are sometimes called "idiopathic epilepsy"), we shall, I believe, make little out. The paroxysms are too sudden, too quickly universal, and of too short duration for precise investigation. But if we take simple cases we shall, I think, accomplish a great deal. Most unquestionably the simplest cases of convulsion are

[1] In cases of slow deterioration of brain, the disposition "alters"; I fear it is that the natural disposition has its way, and that our more animal, our more instinctive habits and desires are no longer subordinated. There is reduction to a more automatic condition; there is dissolution, using this word as the corresponding opposite of evolution. The weaker the mind the more do the more automatic desires have their own way. In a few cases of intracranial hæmorrhage the patient becomes violent and swears; resembles the "drunken man," whose "natural disposition comes out"; the condition expressed by the proverb *in vino veritas* is equivalent to a Reduction to a More Automatic Condition in which the natural impulses have freer play.

those in which the spasm begins deliberately on one side of the body and affects that side only, or affects it more than the other. Such fits are often very limited in range, and then the patient is not unconscious, and can describe the seizure. As they begin deliberately, and as they may last many minutes, we are able, if we are present at a paroxysm, to note the place of onset and the order of spreading of the spasm. But even these simple convulsions represent the healthy movements contained in the region discharged only in outline and, so to speak, in caricature. For besides the facts already mentioned (that the discharge is sudden, excessive, and soon over) the discharge is of a *limited part of the brain*—of a part picked out, as it were, somewhat at random, by disease. The presumption is that there are no more isolated discharges of parts of the brain—an *excessive* discharge of a small part—*in health* than there are movements of single muscles in health. (Movements of single muscles, except perhaps in the face, are, Duchenne insists, only producible artificially—that is, by galvanism.)

### (7) *Convulsion beginning Unilaterally, the Mobile Counterpart of Hemiplegia*

These seizures I used to call unilateral convulsions, but since the spasm (although it affects one side first and most) may *become* universal, it is more correct to call them " convulsions beginning unilaterally." Indeed, as is well known to careful clinical observers, they occur in all degrees, from twitching of a finger to universal convulsion. It is important to bear this in mind, especially as the same patient may have fits of several degrees ; unless we do, we may erroneously suppose that he has several *varieties* of convulsions. Convulsions beginning unilaterally depend on disease of the same *cerebral* region as does hemiplegia of the common form, but hemiplegia depends on " destroying lesion " of the corpus striatum, the convulsion on a " discharging lesion " of the convolutions near to this body—convolutions in the region of the middle cerebral artery. We have, indeed, not only " a corpus striatum paralysis," but a " corpus striatum convulsion." To prove that the convulsion is one of the mobile counterparts of hemiplegia, we find both in the same case. After a severe fit which has begun in the hand, we occasionally find hemiplegia like that which is so often produced by a clot in the corpus striatum, like it in degree and in range, but unlike it in being transitory. When the convulsion is partial, the palsy left by it is partial too. Thus I have recorded the case of a patient who had paralysis limited to the arm after a convulsion of that limb dependent on tumour in the hinder part of the first (superior) frontal convolution.[1] (There was a tumour in each lobe of the cerebellum as well.) There can, in short, be no doubt that these convulsions are the mobile counterparts of hemiplegia.

### (8) *The Convolutions near the Corpus Striatum re-represent the Movements represented in that Centre*

When in such cases we do discover disease of the brain, we do find it in the region of the corpus striatum, but occasionally no local morbid change is found in any part of the brain. Nevertheless, the very fact that the convulsion has been one-sided, or has begun on one side, warrants the inference that there *is* in such cases also a local lesion, although we are unable to detect it. The lesion

[1] See *Medical Mirror*, September 1869.

—when a lesion is discovered—involves more or less of convolutions which are near to, and, I suppose, *discharge through* the corpus striatum. I suppose that these convolutions represent over again, but in new and more complex combinations, the very same movements which are represented in the corpus striatum. They are, I believe, the corpus striatum " raised to a higher power." *Discharge*[1] of the grey matter of these convolutions *develops* the same groups of movements which are *lost* when the corpus striatum is *destroyed.*

### (9) *The most Voluntary or most Special Movements first and most affected by the Discharge of Convolutions*

But there are several varieties of convulsions beginning unilaterally. They may be classified according to the places of onset of the spasm. There is nothing more important than to note where a convulsion begins, for the inference is, that the first motor symptom is the sign of the beginning of the central discharge.

There are three parts where fits of this group mostly begin : (1) in the hand ; (2) in the face, or tongue, or both ; (3) in the foot. In other words, they usually begin in those parts of one side of the body which have the most voluntary uses. The order of frequency in which parts suffer illustrates the same law. I mean, that fits beginning in the hand are commonest ; next in frequency are those which begin in the face or tongue, and rarest are those which begin in the foot. The law is seen in details. When the fit begins in the hand, the index-finger[2] and thumb are usually the digits first seized ; when in the face, the side of the cheek is first in spasm ; when in the foot, almost invariably the great toe.

### (10) *Leading Movements ; Compound Order of spreading of Spasm*

In each of these varieties there must be some difference in the situation of the grey matter exploded. In one part the movements of the hand have the leading representation, in another part those of the cheek and tongue, and in a third those of the foot. I say *leading* representation because spasm of the hand, etc., is only the *beginning* of the seizure. I had under my care a patient whose fits always *began* in his left thumb. [Case recorded *Medical Times and Gazette*, November 30, 1872.] We found, after death, a tubercle the size of a hazel-nut in the hinder part of his third right frontal convolution. Now

[1] It is supposed that in the part which is occasionally discharged the grey matter is highly unstable. This, indeed, seems to me to be a truism ; the difficulty is to discover the *pathological process* by which that instability results. In the cases I shall mention later on it has been *associated with* tumour ; the tumour does not discharge, but in some way it leads to changes involving instability of grey matter. My speculation is that, speaking in chemical language, the highly unstable grey matter of disease remains of the same Constitution as the comparatively stable grey matter of health, but that it is of a different Composition ; and a further speculation is that the phosphorus ingredient is replaced by its congener nitrogen—that the nervous matter is more nitrogenised, and therefore more explosive. If this be so, we see that although the nutrition of grey matter is carried on abnormally, in cases of convulsion, chorea, etc., we cannot say without much qualification that its nutrition is *defective*. The supposed therapeutical value in nervous affections of the other member of the group of triads (arsenic) is significant.

[2] Perhaps it may be well here to mention again that the word " voluntary " is used for a part like the hand, which has the greater number of different movements and the greater number of different intervals of movements, and that the word " automatic " is used for a part like the chest, which has the greater number of nearly similar movements and the greater number of nearly equal intervals. The hand is a more " voluntary " part than either the cheek (or articulatory organs altogether) or the leg. Indeed, the hand is the most important part of the body from any point of view. Hence the significance of the fact that in disease of the highest centres it usually suffers first and most.

in this case the most that one could say was, that in the convolution or region first discharged there lay processes for movements in which the thumb had *the leading part*. For although the spasm *began* in that digit, it went up the arm, and at length probably all over the body.

Besides, since the movements of the thumb and fingers could scarcely be developed for any useful purpose without fixation of the wrist (and of parts further and further in automaticity according to the force required), we should *a priori* be sure that the centre discharged, although it might represent movements in which the thumb had the leading part, must represent also certain other movements of the forearm, upper arm, etc., which serve subordinately. These remarks have partly anticipated the next topic—the march of the spasm.

### (11) *The Order in which Movements are developed by Discharge of Convolutions. The March of Spasm*

After noting the part in which the fit begins, we have to observe how the spasm spreads (the " march of the fit "), and this for two purposes. We have not only to learn *how much* of the body is ultimately involved by the spasm, but also to note the *order* in which the several parts involved are affected. For example, we have not only to report of a case that the spasm " affected the whole of one side of the body," but also that " the spasm began in the hand, spread *up* the arm, next took the face, and then passed *down* the leg." We have to note not only the range of a fit, but the *order* of development of movements one after another in that range. Or, speaking now of the nerve centres, we have to study convulsion not only to learn what particular movements are represented in a nervous centre (anatomical localisation), but also to learn the particular order in which those movements are therein represented (physiological localisation).

As already remarked, the movements first developed in a fit probably represent those which take the lead ; those next developed are, we may suppose, the subordinately associated movements. Let me illustrate by a healthy movement. When we grasp strongly, although the flexors take the lead the extensors must be in subordinate, and yet in associated action, or the grasp would not be vigorous ; and the more strongly the hand is used, the farther up the arm does the movement spread. The observation therefore of the order of development of spasm will enable us, it is reasonable to hope, to determine the association of leading with subordinate movements. For example, if a fit begins in the thumb and index-finger, there will probably [1] be developed as the spasm spreads that series of movements which in health serves subordinately when the thumb and index-finger are used. Of course we can only make very rough observations, as in a convulsion a great number of movements are developed all at once.

It is to be observed that, just as degrees of hemiplegia are compound degrees, so the order of development of spasm is a compound order. For example, when the fit begins in the hand, the spasm does not leave the hand when it involves the rest of the arm. Two things occur : the spasm of the hand becomes more powerful, and the spasm spreads up the arm. This compound order—as are degrees of hemiplegia (*ante*, No. 2)—is roughly in accordance with the order of development of movements in increasing strains, as in lifting

[1] In the case mentioned we had no opportunity of noting the march of the spasm.

things of different weight (in what is technically called " effort "). It is important to note this compound order, especially when we consider that it implies that increasing discharge of a centre has not only the effect of intensifying movement, but also the effect of increasing the range of movement. It has an important bearing on the method of mental operations. For brevity and clearness, we shall, however, in what follows, speak of the spreading of spasm as if it were simple.

### (12) *The Same Muscles represented in Different Order in Several Places*

To show, further, the importance of noting sequence as well as range, I would mention that there are two varieties of fits, in each of which, so far as I can learn, the same muscles are involved, but in each they are involved in a different order. The range is the same ; the sequence is different. Thus one man's fits begin in his hand, go up his arm and down his leg ; another man's begin in his foot, go up his leg and down his arm. But, though the same muscles are in action in each of the two fits, the fact that parts of both limbs are involved in different order, and probably in very different degrees, renders the inference irresistible that the two fits depend on discharge of two different centres. For the nervous centres do not represent muscles, but very complex movements in each of which many muscles serve. In each of the two centres discharged the *very same muscles* are represented in two different orders of movements. In one there are represented movements in which the arm leads and the leg is subordinate ; in the other, movements in which the leg leads and the arm is subordinate. The very same notes are made up into two different tunes ; in chemical metaphor, the fits are isomeric.[1]

My impression is, that the face is differently affected according as the spasm *begins* there and then goes to the arm, or comes there after the arm has been first seized. In the former case the spasm, I believe, begins in the mouth (both sides of the lips, or in the cheek near the angle of the mouth), and spreads all over the face. When the spasm begins in the hand, I believe the orbicularis palpebrarum is the part of the face first in spasm. If the order be as I suppose, the muscles of the face will be represented in movements of different orders, and therefore in several parts of the nervous system.

Thus, then, the three fits may be looked upon as experimental stimulations, each of some different part in the region of the corpus striatum, and as showing us (1) what movements have the leading representation in each part ; (2) the movements which are sequent and subordinate to those having the leading representation. It is freely granted that no definite results have as yet been obtained on the second point. Very few cases have been carefully observed, very few autopsies indeed have been obtained on cases which *have been* observed carefully ; and, lastly, as I shall point out very prominently later on, there are complications which impede our attempt to draw exact conclusions. It is for the very reason that so little has been done that I urge the careful investigation of these seizures.

[1] I have recently had two patients under my care whose fits begin in the foot. When the spasm does get to the arm in these cases, it begins in the fingers and goes up the limb ; but even in these cases the centre discharged must be a different one from that discharged when the fit begins first of all in the hand.

### (13) *Movements of the two Sides of the Body represented in Each Side of the Brain*

We have now to consider the method of representation of movements on the largest scale. Just as there are from *destroying lesions* of different gravities in the region of the corpus striatum ranges of paralysis from weakness of the face, arm, and leg of *one* side to universal powerlessness, so from *discharging lesions* in this region there are all ranges of spreading of spasm from the most local to universal convulsion. Let us consider a severe convulsive paroxysm. The spasm begins, we will suppose, in the right hand, affects the *right* side (the face, arm, and leg), then *both* sides of the trunk, and next the face and limbs of the *left* side. What I wish to draw attention to prominently is, that from destroying or discharging lesions of but *one* side of the brain there results paralysis or convulsion of *both* sides of the body. This seems to me to warrant the inference that movements of the *two* sides of the body are represented in each side of the brain. Some years ago Dr. Broadbent put forth the hypothesis that the bilaterally-*acting* muscles of the two sides are equally represented in each side of the brain. That this is so I have proved by observations on cases of convulsion; and, as above stated, I believe that the muscles of the *limbs* of both sides—the muscles of those parts, that is to say, which can act independently of their fellows—are represented in each side of the brain.[1]

I must consider both the *universal powerlessness* from a *destroying* lesion of one side of the brain, and the *universal spasm* from a *discharging* lesion of one side of the brain. (We shall, for verbal convenience, suppose, throughout these remarks, that the left is the side of the brain damaged.) I begin with *universal powerlessness*. I believe this to be really two-sided paralysis. (That the right side should be paralysed presents no difficulty, of course.) Universal powerlessness is the result of a grave[2] lesion. Now this grave lesion is usually a

[1] My colleague, Dr. Gowers, has kindly drawn my attention to the following remarks by Sir Charles Bell: "It is a fact familiar to pathologists that, where debility arises from affection of the brain, the influence is greatest on those muscles which are, in their natural condition, most under the command of the will. We may perceive this in the progressive stages of debility of the drunkard, when successively the muscles of the tongue, the eyes, the face, the limbs, become unmanageable; and, under the same circumstances, the muscles which have a double office—as those of the chest—lose their voluntary motions and retain their involuntary motions; the force of the arms is gone long before the action of breathing is affected" (*Nervous System*, 3rd ed., p. 165). With regard to one point in the above, it is interesting to observe that in some cases of hemiplegia the two sides of the patient's chest move equally in quiet breathing, whilst in voluntary breathing there is less expansion of the paralysed side. As to another point, we have to account for the *increase* of power (the excitement) in the drunkard who has lost *voluntary* power. I believe it to be a fact of the same order as the increased excitability of a nerve after its division, and of the same order as the increased reflex excitability of the lower segment of the cord when cut off from the brain. (The last-mentioned fact has been used by Dr. Thompson Dickson to illustrate his views on epilepsy, the paroxysm of which, he believes, results from a loss of control.) I believe that the outrageous and violent conduct which occasionally occurs in an epileptic patient who *has lost consciousness* is a fact of the same order—that after *sudden* loss of voluntary power there is an increase of *automatic* action. In hysteria there is loss of voluntary power, and yet there is often excitement. The contradiction disappears if we can establish that the excitement is of lower and more automatic processes from lack of inhibition by the higher and more voluntary.

[2] The word "gravity" is used as inclusive of two factors, *quantity* of nerve tissue destroyed and *suddenness* of destruction. Suddenness is a most important factor; hence a difference betwixt cerebral embolism and cerebral thrombosis; betwixt the symptoms of cerebral hæmorrhage and cerebral tumour; betwixt bleeding an animal to death slowly and suddenly (in the latter there are convulsions). It *seems* to make a difference even in the *kind* of symptoms, for as Prévost says of the lateral deviation I have so often mentioned in this paper, "C'est surtout dans les attaques *brusques* que s'observe cette déviation." Of a large clot we have to observe that it destroys, that it destroys suddenly, and that it squeezes widely and suddenly.

bulky clot, and thus it may be said that the palsy of the left side of the body results because the clot on the left side of the brain squeezes the opposite side of the brain ; or again, that, as the patient is deeply insensible, the left side of the body only *appears* to be paralysed. I confess that I have no satisfactory proof that the left side of the body has been palsied from a hæmorrhage limited to the left side of the brain in a patient who was conscious at the time I examined him. I have, however, only to show that the left side is *weak*, not that it is as much palsied as the right. For whilst wishing to prove that movements of the left side of the body *are* represented in the left side of the brain, I wish also to prove that they are *less* represented therein than are the movements of the right side. It is only to be expected that the left side will suffer for a short time. There is an order of recovery in cases of hemiplegia, and I suppose in all other palsies ; it is that the more automatic movements are regained first. Thus, in hemiplegia (right side, we suppose), the leg recovers before the arm, and if there be at the outset a further degree of paralysis—*viz.* lateral deviation of the eyes and head—these deviations are usually transitory. It is then only reasonable to suppose, when there is yet a further degree of paralysis—namely, of limbs of the left [1] side—that this will pass off first of all.

But there is proof that fibres pass from the left corpus striatum down into the left side of the cord, as well as into the right side ; there are " direct " as well as " decussating " fibres. That there is a " decussating paralysis " from lesion of the left corpus striatum, no one doubts ; but the existence of direct fibres, I think, supports the inference that there is also a transient " direct paralysis " from extensive lesion of that centre. After old lesions of the left corpus striatum there is Wallerian wasting of nerve fibres, traceable from the seat of disease not only down into the *right* side of the cord, but also into the left. This splitting of the bundle of wasted fibres on entering the cord is, I think, demonstrative evidence that *both* sides of the body are represented in the left corpus striatum. Does it not show that movements of the *left* face, arm, and leg are represented in the *left* corpus striatum by the *non-crossing* fibres, as well as that movements of the *right* face, arm, and leg are therein represented by the *crossing* fibres ? It may, however, be urged that these non-crossing fibres are solely for the bilaterally acting muscles (" muscles of the trunk "). But if now we consider the phenomena of a severe convulsion, and find that from a discharging lesion of the left side of the brain the muscles of the face, arm, and leg of the left side are convulsed (after those of the right side), it is, I think, most reasonable to conclude that the non-crossing fibres are for the movements of the muscles of the left face, arm, and leg, although perhaps chiefly for those of the left side of the trunk.

[1] Here it may be well to advert to a difficulty, a very superficial one, in the use of the words " voluntary " and " automatic " ; one which would equally attend the use of the words " special " and " general," " independent " and " dependent." Perhaps the best words would be, " varied " and " similar." Those movements of the left side of the body which are supposed to be represented in the same (the left) side of the brain (and from *sudden* lack of which there results transitory left-sided palsy) are called automatic. It seems contradictory to call movements of the *limbs* automatic. The speculation is that those movements of the left side which are represented in the left side of the brain are automatic, or subordinate to those of the right side of the body, which also are represented in that left side of the brain. Put otherwise, the muscles of the limbs of the left side are, in the right side of the brain, represented in movements from the voluntary to the automatic, and in movements from the automatic to the voluntary in the left side of the brain.

## (14) *Nature of Duality of Brain—the Two Halves not mere Duplicates (see Section 4, p. 65, on Leading and automatic Sides of Brain)*

From these facts we may conclude that the movements of both sides of the body—those of the limbs as well as those of the trunk—are represented in each side of the brain. The inference is that the units of the nervous system are double units, as the whole nervous system itself is double. In chemical metaphor, the unit of action is a molecule of two atoms. But it is not meant that the double unit is a mere duplicate. For, again referring to the *whole nervous system*, we see that *its* highest halves are not *mere* duplicates. Saying nothing of right-handedness, of the fact that disease of but *one* [1] hemisphere can make a man speechless, and of the statement of Gratiolet that the left frontal and right sphenoidal and occipital convolutions are developed earlier than their fellows, there is the striking fact that the convolutions of the two hemispheres are not symmetrical. These differences in form imply differences in function.[2] This is the more significant when we find that the asymmetry becomes greater the higher we go in the animal kingdom, not only from lower to higher animals, but from the lower to the higher races of men. According to Dr. Todd, there is greater asymmetry in the convolutions of intellectual men. We see, then, that the higher in the scale of intellectual life the less of a duplicate are the two halves of the highest and most important divisions of the nervous system. It is reasonable to suppose, then, that the two elements of the units which enter into the composition of the highest centres are not mere duplicates.

## (15) *Movements of the Two Sides of Body represented in Different Order in Each Side of Brain (?)*

Whilst insisting that movements of the two sides of the body are represented in the left side of the brain, it has been pointed out that they are not equally represented ; the movements of the left side are *less* represented in the left side of the brain, for they suffer less from a destroying lesion (and, as I have said, it may be urged that they do not suffer at all), and they suffer less in convulsion. The fit which begins in the right side, and passes at length to the left, affects that second side less, and for a shorter time, and, I believe, the parts of this side are affected more contemporaneously. But besides this difference in *quantity* of representation, there are other differences. The left side suffers *later* than the other. This difference is quite as important as any. It is as necessary to know

[1] The fact of most significance is, not that disease of the *left* hemisphere mostly makes a man speechless, but that disease of but *one* hemisphere can make him speechless. I have suggested that one hemisphere is for the automatic, and the other for the voluntary and automatic, use of words. It is well known that speechless patients may sing ; on this point, and on the singing of imbecile children, I have remarked in the *Mirror* of this journal (*Lancet*), February 17, 1866, and again in a subsequent *Mirror*, where I quote Dr. Langdon Down. There is in this month's number of the *Edinburgh Medical Journal* a valuable paper by Dr. Ireland, in which he says that in mere taste for music idiots are not much behind other children. Music is probably one of the most *automatic* of higher mental operations ; hence the significance of the existence of musical faculty in those who have little higher mental faculty. It is a fact of the same order as many stated in the text. Spencer (*Psychology*, vol. ii, p. 471) says (when speaking of inherited experiences) that faculties, *as of music*, which scarcely exist in some inferior human races, become *congenital* in superior ones.

[2] It is possible that the asymmetry may be such that whilst the third left frontal convolution is, so to say, the " yellow spot " of speech, some other convolution on the right is the chief seat of word-processes. I think this is probable because in one seizure dependent on disease of the third *right* frontal convolution, the discharge was *first* on the muscles of the thumb, and not on the parts for the exteriorisation of speech.

that in certain centres movements of different parts are represented in different order as it is to note that they are represented in different degrees.

We have, then, two things to bear in mind—(1) that movements of the right and left limbs are represented in the left side of the brain ; and (2) that the right are represented more than the left, and so represented that they are developed at a different time. Are there other differences ? Other facts supplied by the Wallerian wasting, already spoken of, warrant us in seeking further differences. For descending wasting occupies different tracts of the cord. The fibres wasted in the right side of the cord (crossing fibres) are those of the posterior part of the lateral column, those in the left side (direct fibres) are in the anterior column near the middle line (as before stated, the lesion is supposed to be of the left corpus striatum). These facts justify the inference that the two sides of the body are not represented in each half of the brain in the same way. To suppose otherwise would be to hold that the two different parts of the cord had the same function. We have already spoken of difference of quantity of representation (the left side being less represented). Will not the difference we are now in search of be one of *order* of representation ? We find that, speaking generally, the order of representation in the right side is from the voluntary to the automatic movements.[1] Is the order on the left side from the automatic to the voluntary ? It will be observed that it is not supposed that the two different strands of fibres in the cord represent different *muscles* on the two sides of the body ; but that each strand represents the corresponding muscles of the two sides of the body, but made up into movements of different degrees and orders. Thus, to put it roughly, the speculation is, that on the right side the order is from the limbs to the trunk, on the left from the trunk to the limbs.

I have, I regret to say, no useful observations of the order of spreading of spasm on the *left* side. As I think it very important to make observations thereon, I will write down certain questions. 1. Does the spasm of the left side begin in the leg ? 2. Does it go *down* or *up* these limbs ? 3. Does it affect the extensors more than the flexors, or vice versa ? 4. Is the spasm more tonic than on the other side ? (The fit is supposed to begin in the right hand.)

Of course, since our object is to learn the plan of representation of movements, we must also study healthy movements, taking the simplest of these. I have several times spoken of " effort," using the word in its technical sense. In lifting objects of increasing heaviness with the right hand we bring into play movements spreading from the most voluntary to the most automatic. At a certain stage the left limbs are engaged ; the left arm is lifted away from the side, the forearm is more or less extended, and the hand is open ; the leg is held off the ground somewhat stiffly from the hip. I think it probable that the spreading of spasm to the left side will conform roughly to the spreading of movement in effort to the left side. We shall be assisted in investigating the order of representation of movements by considering the play of the limbs in walking. Thus, when the right leg comes forward, the right arm goes backwards and left forwards. Probably, however, these movements have their representation in the cerebellum ; but somewhere the order, as well as the degree, of these movements will be represented.

[1] Strictly this is the order of the *loss* of movements from breaking up of nervous processes. The representation of movements in the healthy organ will be in the reverse order.

### (16) *Certain Correlations of Movement—Lateral Movements of Eyes and Movements of Tactual Organs represented in the Cerebrum*

Both in hemiplegia and in convulsions beginning unilaterally we note certain associations—*e.g.* affection of the orbicularis palpebrarum along with affection of the limbs. Donders' researches give an explanation of this association. The most important, however, is the association of affection of *certain* movements of the eyes with affection of those of our limbs. Significantly (and in accordance with the principle spoken of throughout this paper) the movements of the eyeball which are first affected are the *lateral*. We can overcome a prism of from 20–30° with its base placed outwards, and one of 6–8° with its base placed inwards ; but few persons can overcome more than a prism of 1° or 2° with its base turned upwards or downwards. There is then greater variety or independence in the lateral movements of the eye. (The internal rectus is the strongest of the ocular muscles.) In association with this greater independence of the lateral movements we may note that the sensibility of the retina diminishes less rapidly outwards than upwards and downwards. That the movements of our chief tactual organs should have close and direct associations in the *highest* nervous centres with certain movements of the eyes is what one would expect if, as Spencer says (*Psychology*, Part 24, p. 358), " tactual impressions are those into which all other impressions have to be translated before their meanings can be known." I suppose visual impressions and ocular movements may be said to " stand for " tactual impressions and movements in the sense that the strong excitation of the nervous processes of the former leads to *faint* excitation of those of the latter (movements of the hands, etc.). The study of cases of hemiplegia and convulsion shows us, not only that there is an association, but the *order* in which eye movements and limb movements are associated. Of course a coarse lesion of a nervous centre, or a sudden discharge of one, is not a very neat experiment. In hemiplegia the parts suffer in degree, I believe, in the following order : arm, leg, side of face and tongue, orbicularis palpebrarum, lateral movements of eyes, lateral movements of head. The difficulty obviously is that several systems are damaged all at a blow—the movements of lifting, by which we have ideas of weight, the eye to hand movements of writing, the movements of speech, etc.

I have observed cases of hemiplegia complicated with hemiopia. I have as yet had no autopsy on a case of this kind ; but I think it important to draw attention to the association because I think it is a very significant one, especially as there has been a very persistent and a very unusual amount of loss of sensation in the hemiplegic region ; and in one case under my care the power of estimating weights is very much affected. I believe the lesion to be in the thalamus opticus. It is very significant that a *lateral* loss of vision occurs with hemiplegia. In these cases the patient cannot *see* to the paralysed side ; this condition is the sensory analogue of that of the hemiplegic patient who, having lateral deviation of the eyes, cannot *look* to the paralysed side. Since the sensori-motor processes which form the anatomical substrata of our ideas of objects are [highly special arrangements representing] retinal impressions and ocular movements, the study of deviations of the eyes and corresponding limitations of the fields of vision has an important bearing on mental physiology.

(17) *Certain Movements of the Eyes for Estimation of Distance represented in the Cerebellum along with Locomotor Movements*

There are other conjugate deviations of the eyes besides lateral. Thus in lesions of the right middle peduncle of the cerebellum the right eye is turned upwards and outwards, the left downwards and inwards. Just as there is an association of lateral movements of the eyes with movements of our tactual organs for ideas of objects, so we may suppose that there will be associations of ocular movements of convergence and divergence (the former especially downwards, the latter especially upwards) with those movements of the spine, legs, and arms in locomotion, represented in the cerebellum, for ideas of distance; hence the importance of studying particular ocular deviations in association with accompanying disorder of movement. That the two sets of ocular movements are to a large extent separately represented seems clear from the researches of Adamük. He finds that the anterior tubercles of the corpora quadrigemina rule the side-to-side movements of the two eyes, whilst irritation of the posterior part of either the right or left eminence produces strong convergence, lowering of the visual lines, and contraction of the pupil. The cerebrum contains processes of eye movements and tactual movements for seeing objects; the cerebellum, we may suppose, contains processes of the eye movements and locomotor movements for estimation of distance. I shall shortly try to show that facts of disease and experiment support this inference. The association of ocular deviations with circus movement, rotation, and rolling, is well known, and is obviously very significant with regard to what has just been said.

# OBSERVATIONS ON THE LOCALISATION OF MOVEMENTS IN THE CEREBRAL HEMISPHERES, AS REVEALED BY CASES OF CONVULSION, CHOREA, AND "APHASIA"[1]

THE results of the recent researches of Ferrier briefly stated by him, *British Medical Journal*, April 26, 1873, and those of Fritsch and Hitzig, to which he refers, are highly important from several points of view. To me they are interesting, especially because they demonstrate, in a novel and very striking way, the truth of what I have long urged, *viz.* that discharges of *convolutions* develop *movements*, notwithstanding that destruction of limited parts of the brain produces no obvious loss of movements. The discharges I have studied have been those causing epileptiform seizures *in man*, and in particular those simple cases where the spasm developed begins unilaterally, in the hand or face or foot. The value of Ferrier's researches, and those of Fritsch and Hitzig, as showing by an *artificially* induced discharge of convolutions the "homologous convulsions" in lower animals, is very great. The extreme importance of their facts for physiology proper, and for comparative anatomy, is too obvious for comment.

I have, however, written so many times on convulsions, and so much recently, that I cannot here, without undue recapitulation, consider the direct bearing of Ferrier's experiments on the anatomical and physiological part of our Clinical Study of Convulsions. I may refer, however, to recent papers in the *Lancet* (January 18, 1873, *et seq.*, see p. 62), in which some of the points are illustrated. Epileptiform seizures are there looked upon as experiments on the brain made by disease, and as revealing to us, although necessarily *in the rough*, the localisation of special classes of movements in the cerebral hemisphere. I may refer also to a paper (*British Medical Journal*, May 10), written since Ferrier published brief abstracts of his main conclusions, which is in great part devoted to a consideration of the direct bearing of his experiments on medical anatomy and physiology.

In this paper—partly preliminary to two others—I try: (1) to show that convulsions, choreal movements, affections of speech, and other motor symptoms, are not *only* to be thought of as "symptoms of disease," but can be considered also as results of experiments made by disease revealing in the rough the functions of cerebral convolutions; (2) to urge that the study of such *motor* symptoms is of direct importance for *mental* physiology; (3) to show that if we do our work anatomically and physiologically, and reduce the very *different* symptoms to their lowest terms, to movements, for example, we shall find that there are certain *fundamental* principles common to them all—common to symptoms so specially different as "aphasia" and a convulsion of one side of the body.[2]

[1] *West Riding Lunatic Asylum Medical Reports*, vol. iii, 1873, p. 175.

[2] Since writing the chief part of this paper I find that there is more recapitulation from former papers than I expected. I have acknowledged this in part by giving quotations from former papers and by footnotes.

The most important matter I have to urge is the study of the localisation of movements on the *double* plan—by comparing the effects of destroying and discharging lesions on the brain of *man*. The following quotation, especially the parts I have italicised, will show my meaning on this point more plainly. It is the opening paragraph of a paper in the *Lancet*, January 18, 1873 (see p. 62).

" For some years I have studied cases of disease of the brain, not only for directly clinical, but for anatomical and physiological purposes. Cases of paralysis and convulsion may be looked upon as the results of *experiments made by disease* on particular parts of the nervous system of man. The study of palsies and convulsions from this point of view is the study of the effects of ' destroying lesions ' and of the effects of ' discharging lesions.' And for an exact knowledge of the particular movements most represented in particular centres, we must observe and *compare the effects of each kind of lesion*. It is just what the physiologist does in experimenting on animals ; to ascertain the exact distribution of a nerve, he destroys it, and also stimulates it. Indeed, *this double kind of study is essential* in the investigation of cases of nervous disease *for physiological purposes*. For limited *destroying lesions of some parts of the cerebral hemisphere produce no obvious symptoms ; while discharging lesions of those parts produce very striking symptoms*. By this *double* method we shall, I think, not only discover the particular parts of the nervous system where certain groups of movements are most represented (anatomical localisation), but, what is of equal importance, we shall also learn the order of action (physiological localisation) in which those movements are therein represented."[1]

In the *St. Andrews Graduates' Transactions*, vol. iii, 1870, " A Study of Convulsions " (see p. 8), I have considered convulsive seizures first from a clinical, and secondly from an anatomical and physiological point of view. I have indeed written on " Convulsions beginning Unilaterally," innumerable times during the last ten years, but I will only refer the reader to the two papers just mentioned. The earlier papers, and perhaps those above referred to as well, are full of crudities. It may be remembered in extenuation that my investigations of epilepsies have not been from orthodox points of view. I have not simply repeated accepted doctrines with slight variations and new illustrations. Working on a novel method, I run continual risk of making novel blunders. But in thinking for one's self there are certain kinds of blunders which almost must be made. And it is always easy to avoid appearing to go far wrong if one does not go far from the beaten track. Let me speak more particularly.

As will be seen stated at some length in what is to follow, I do not in any case of convulsion, or occasional loss of consciousness, endeavour to see if there be an approach to a certain clinical standard—to " genuine epilepsy." I try in each case to find the seat of the " discharging lesion," and also the pathological process which has led to it. The first question in my mind is *not*, " Is it a case of epilepsy ? " but " Where is the lesion permitting occasional excessive discharge ? " Hence the presentation of the facts to those who do not look at cases of epilepsy from so novel a standpoint seems strange and unreal. My method is *just the opposite* of the common method. It is a small matter to me whether a case of convulsions or other paroxysmal nervous seizure is to be called epileptic or not. What I labour to find out is the *part*

[1] " On the Anatomical and Physiological Localisation of Movements in the Brain," *Lancet*, January 18, 1873, *et seq*. (See p. 62.)

of the brain of the functions of which the convulsion is the brutal and sudden development. For example, to quote from a former paper,[1] " We *do not care* to say that a tumour of the brain (or minute changes near it) had ' caused epilepsy,' but that changes in a particular region of the nervous system—say in the region of the left middle cerebral artery—led to convulsions, in which the spasm began in the right hand, spread to the arm, attacked next the face, then the leg, etc."

The new method has, I think, the advantage of showing the relations of different " diseases " or symptoms. This is a matter of importance when symptoms are to be looked on as the results of the experiments of disease. To give examples of the relations of different symptoms : there are several *mobile* counterparts of hemiplegia. There is hemichorea, there are certain cases of hemispasm, and there is what I may call hemi-contracture, a mixture of palsy and spasm. I call these one-sided mobile symptoms " Hemikineses." I believe that each of them depends on disease of the same *internal* region as does hemiplegia—the region of the corpus striatum. For the same *external* region is affected in each. To obtain a knowledge of the movements represented in the cerebral district mentioned, we have to study each one of these symptoms carefully. As some evidence that this method of study is practically useful, I may adduce Dr. Radcliffe's testimony. In his article on chorea,[2] after stating the reasons I have advanced for the localisation of the changes producing chorea in convolutions near to the corpus striatum, he writes, " for most assuredly the difficulties which beset any attempt to localise the choreic lesion in the nerve centres, are not a little simplified by thus insisting upon the clinical relations between hemichorea and hemiplegia, as a ground for believing that the region of the corpus striatum is the part affected in both disorders."

The old method, however, deals with circumscribed entities. It *looks* simpler. Thus many students, I find, are interested in being told that a case is one of *true* epilepsy, or of *real* chorea, or of *genuine* aphasia, who show no interest in the description of a paroxysm of convulsion, not even the simplest ; who have never tried to form a clear conception of the *sort* of movements they can see in a choreal child, and who, whilst they are interested in such discussions, as whether a particular case is one of *genuine* aphasia or not, take no pains to obtain a realistic account of what that patient's condition was—what he really could say or could not say. They have been taught to study cases as the symptoms show *approaches* to certain clinical standards, and not as they show departures from healthy states. The latter plan (to illustrate by a simple case of convulsion) requires a more minute study of the paroxysms, and further, it demands more *extensive* knowledge of *other* nervous diseases or symptoms. Those who only wish to know whether a given convulsion is epileptic or epileptiform have an easy task. Those who wish to know whether the discharging lesion is of convolutions in the region of the middle cerebral artery or not have a much more difficult task. They have to note carefully the muscles convulsed, in order to see if they are the same as those paralysed in cases of the common form of hemiplegia, which symptom is well known to be due to lesion in this

[1] *St. Andrews Reports*, vol. iii, 1870. After speaking of a case supposed to be carefully investigated, on its own merits I remark as above.

[2] Reynolds' *System*, 2nd ed., vol. ii, p. 199. (Passage not in first edition.) I give comparison of hemiplegia and hemispasm on p. 334 of *West Riding Lunatic Asylum Medical Reports*, vol. iii (see p. 103).

region. And in order to be able to note this, they must know thoroughly beforehand the symptoms of the several degrees of hemiplegia, as, for example, that with a lesion of a certain degree of gravity there is deviation of the head and eyes.

One reason for the complexity of part of the work I have done in cases of epilepsy, chorea, etc., is that I have written of cases from several points of view. For example, not only have I urged that convulsions beginning unilaterally point to *disease* in the region of the middle cerebral artery— a clinical statement—but I have urged the study of them for purposes of Localisation of Movements—a physiological statement.[1] To make cases of convulsion of use for the latter purpose, much minute work and great patience are required. And after all the fear is that to many whose opinions are to be esteemed it will seem a sheer waste of time to note the movements developed in a fit so minutely as is done, for example, in the following remarks[2] on a case of very partial convulsion. The extract, however, only gives a summary of what was observed in several seizures: "The order of involvement was that the mouth all round was first in action, then the mouth was drawn to the left, then both eyes to the left (the head to the left), then the eyelids of both sides (the left the more) closed. The thorax was affected early, and the arm late."[3]

But it is possible to observe many partial seizures precisely, for some of them last a long time. I have witnessed one limited to the arm and face which lasted ten minutes.

Why should not a carefully observed convulsion of the right arm, associated with central disease so local as a tumour in the hinder part of the uppermost frontal convolution on the left side, be considered as an anatomical and physiological experiment, although a rough one, on part of the brain? But the idea of using cases of convulsions or of hemiplegia for anatomical and physiological experiments is entirely unfamiliar—and to many unfamiliarity is the same thing as unreality. I would here repeat what I have said in the *Lancet*, January 18, 1873 (see p. 63), to the effect that *there is no other way* of ascertaining the localisation of movements in the cerebral hemisphere of *man*, than by the study of his convulsive seizures. But let us take a simpler illustration. Let us take the very simplest of all cases of paralysis—hemiplegia from a *destroying lesion* of the "motor tract." Why should not the effects of an experiment which a clot makes on the corpus striatum of *man* be recorded in works on physiology, as well as the effects of intentional experimental injury to the

[1] See note "Localisation," *Medical Times and Gazette*, August 15, 1868. See also *St. Andrews Reports*, vol. iii, 1870, from which I quote the following: "In hemiplegia the loss is of a certain number of possible *simultaneous movements* of the face, arm, and leg—the sum of a number of possible co-ordinations in space. Similarly a convulsion on one side is the abrupt development of a certain number of possible *successions of movements* of the face, arm, and leg—the sum of a number of possible co-ordinations in time" (see p. 26).

[2] See *Medical Times and Gazette*, January 6 and 27, 1872.

[3] It may be well to give the concluding paragraph of the remarks on this case, as they embody the main facts of the autopsy: "In this case the lesion was not sufficiently local to enable one to conclude that fits beginning in the face show damage to any particular convolutional region. For instance, the fits may have been owing either to discharge of the grey matter of the convolutions of the temporo-sphenoidal lobe, or of the island of Reil. In most cases of convulsion beginning unilaterally the cerebral lesion is very extensive. I shall shortly, however, report a case of convulsion beginning in the left thumb, in which there was a tubercular tumour, the size of a hazel-nut, in the hinder part of *one* convolution—the third right frontal convolution. [See report of that case, *Medical Times and Gazette*, November 30, 1872, p. 597.] By numerous observations of this kind we may confidently expect to arrive at clearer notions on localisation of movements."

corpus striatum of *a rabbit*? It is our fault. The physiological part of our clinical work is not sufficiently methodical; we have medical knowledge, and we have separately physiological knowledge, but our medical knowledge is not sufficiently physiological. On this matter I may quote from a lecture on hemiplegia published some years ago, and I do so none the less willingly because part of my own medical physiology in that lecture deserves criticism.

". . . Our School Physiology and our Medical Physiology do not very well harmonise; and this is particularly so of the corpus striatum and thalamus opticus. An eminent physician and physiologist, in his valuable textbook of physiology, says that the corpora striata are not peculiarly concerned in movement, and he adds that 'the recent experiments of Schiff, confirming and in many respects correcting those of Magendie and others, show that when they are removed in rabbits, sensation is unimpaired, *and the power of movement complete*.' But I suppose no physician denies that disease of the corpus striatum in man produces paralysis of a great part of the muscles on the opposite side of the body."[1]

To urge that the study of *convulsion* from discharge of *convolutions* is most important for *mental* physiology, as has been already done by implication, will seem more than strange to those who hold that the convolutions are parts of the "organ of mind," and are for "ideas," and that the subjacent "motor tract" is the only part of the brain for movements.

This—the notion that the cerebral hemisphere being for ideas, consciousness, etc., is not for movements—accords with the prevailing theory of epilepsy. The motor symptom, the convulsion, is ascribed to discharge of the medulla oblongata, and the loss of consciousness—the mental symptom—to sudden and almost contemporaneous anæmia of another part, the "organ of mind." There are supposed to be necessarily *opposite* states of two separate parts—"une inertie totale (*cerveau*) et une suractivité fonctionnelle (*bulbe*)."[2] I shall give reasons for believing that all the symptoms in cases of "epilepsy," even as that term is used by the most rigid authorities, are owing to *one* state, one discharge, and that probably of a single cerebral hemisphere. (See *West Riding Lunatic Asylum Medical Reports*, vol. iii, pp. 328–9, and Appendix II, on Loss of Consciousness, p. 107.)

In the case of partial convulsions instanced (p. 80), it is surely significant for mental physiology that disease in the uppermost frontal convolution did by some process, by any process, produce frequent occasional spasm of the arm; when it is remarked that the disease was seated deep in the "organ of mind" (far from the motor tract), and that the part convulsed is the most specialised part of the whole body.

There seems to be an insuperable objection to the notion that the cerebral hemispheres are for movements. The opinion I have brought forward, that chorea may be due to disease of the corpus striatum, has received some favour (chiefly that of being disputed), but the suggestion that choreal movements may more probably depend on disease of *convolutions* near to that centre has scarcely been mentioned. The reason, I suppose, is that the convolutions are considered to be *not* for *movements*, but for *ideas*. In another paper I hope to show clearly that there is no contradiction in supposing that the convolutions are for

[1] *London Hospital Reports*, vol. ii, 1865, p. 301. See *West Riding Lunatic Asylum Medical Reports*, vol. iii, p. 342, Appendix II, p. 109.

[2] Jaccoud, *Pathologie Interne*, p. 386.

ideas and for movements too. I shall try, indeed, to show that *sudden discharges* give *proof* that sensori-*motor* processes are the *anatomical substrata of ideas*. And in the case of chorea, if the very great speciality both of the parts most moved and of the movements themselves be considered, there is nothing unreasonable in supposing that the sensori-*motor* processes which are affected are of *convolutions* in the region of the corpus striatum and are those for " ideas " of touch, weight, etc., in *acquiring which ideas*, movements of the hand and arm were necessarily concerned. It is, indeed, most important to note the great speciality of the movements in cases of chorea ; they should not be dismissed as " disorders of co-ordination " ; as if there were a " faculty " of co-ordination. Wherever nerve fibres meet in ganglion cells, there is a centre of co-ordination ; what is anatomically a sensori-motor process is physiologically " a co-ordination."

The great speciality and the separateness of the movements in cases of hemichorea is quite as strong evidence of their dependence on discharging lesions of very highly " evolved " centres (convolutions of the brain), as is that supplied by the fact that the parts affected (face, arm, and leg) are the parts affected in hemiplegia, which symptom is undoubtedly owing to a destroying lesion of a very highly evolved centre. The following quotation[1] shows that these opinions are not hastily formed :

" It is not denied that ' disorderly movements ' occur with disease in many parts, probably in most parts, of the nervous system. What I wish to show is, that *certain* irregular movements—often affecting the face, arm, and leg of one side only—occur from disease of the higher centres of movement, viz. *of the convolutions* near to *the corpus striatum*. It is especially to be observed that they differ from the jerky movements of the arm occasionally seen in severe cases of locomotor ataxy. They are not mere spasms and cramps. They are an aimless profusion of movements of considerable complexity, much nearer the purposive movements of health."

. . . . . . .

" Now it is clear that close upon the corpus striatum lie the rudimentary arrangements of fibres and cells for the highly complex and widely associated movements of speech, and it is, I think—independently of other arguments—at least plausible, that corresponding movements of the arm—*which may be called, according to our standpoint of thought, either rudimentary psychical, or highly developed physical movements—should have their centres here too*."

" Although I have instanced series of comparatively simple movements of single parts analogous to ataxy of articulation, there are, in some cases of chorea, *movements* of much wider range, implying, I imagine, changes deeper and wider [?] in the hemisphere, just as there are probably movements (*i.e.* misuse of words or incoherence) dependent on changes deeper in the left hemisphere than the parts close to the corpus striatum."

. . . . . . .

" But we must begin our studies of *mind* by a consideration of the more rudimentary phenomena, *although we should not make arbitrary distinctions betwixt those which are grossly motor and those sensori-motor impulses which we speak of as being mental*."

[1] *Edinburgh Medical Journal*, October 1868.

It will probably seem to some a very abrupt change to speak of "aphasia" after speaking of convulsion and chorea. I think myself it is the very relation in which the fundamental nature of loss of speech can be most methodically considered. In some cases of convulsion beginning unilaterally there is affection of speech. But this is not the best reason for considering them together. The reason is that in affection of speech there is an affection of a *highly special class of movements*, exactly as there is of other special classes in cases of convulsion and chorea. Observations of cases show that with *right* hemiplegia there *are* all kinds of defects, from ataxy of articulation to mistakes in words. Both are really motor defects. There is no *abrupt* distinction made by disease betwixt articulatory movements and words, and it is not well to make a clinical entity of aphasia by paring away a difficulty of articulation at one end of a series of defects and incoherence at the other end.

The following extract [1] will show that changes of opinion on this matter were forced on me by observations of cases of disease. I give the quotation as I wish to point out that the opinions I here put forward have not been formed hastily:

"When my attention was first drawn to the class of cases (Class II) I am discussing, I thought there was a fundamental distinction betwixt the mistakes of words and 'ataxy' of articulation—the mistakes of muscular movements. I used to suppose there was a part for words, and, besides, a distinct co-ordinating apparatus for the movements of words, and that Broca's convolution was a sort of cerebellum for articulation. It is quite true that the defects I have recently mentioned ('ataxy' of articulation and mistakes in words) are very different, but then they are not altogether different. It was forced on me that the separation was one which observation of cases did not justify, and I soon concluded that, to use a crude expression towards the end of my first paper,[2] 'the ataxy of articulation was a quasi-mental defect—an inability to combine muscular movements in a particular mental *act*.' Again, in a subsequent paper,[3] speaking of defects accompanying right hemiplegia, I remarked that 'it was hard to say where obviously motor symptoms ended and mental ones began.' I have long believed it to be not only hard, but impossible, even using the words 'motor' and 'mental' in the popular sense. I now think that the only differences in ataxy of articulation, mistakes of words, and disorder of ideas are differences of 'compound degree.'"

It would be marvellous if there were *not* all degrees of defects. For is it not accepted doctrine that nervous processes *gradually* increase in complexity, in independence, and in speciality? If so, is there anything at all wonderful in the fact that damage low down in the series of sensori-motor processes (close to and of the corpus striatum) should produce a defect of a comparatively simple nature—ataxy of articulation—and that damage high up in the very same series should produce one of a highly elaborate nature—"loss of memory" for words?

In friendly controversies my opponents imply (because I say that from a physiological point of view a certain defect of *articulation* is a *rudimentary* defect of *speech*, or that "loss of memory for words" is loss of sensori-*motor* processes for words) that I am not aware of the differences betwixt the two

[1] *Medical Times and Gazette*, September 26, 1868.
[2] *London Hospital Reports*, 1864, p. 471.
[3] *Medical Times and Gazette*, January 28, 1865.

defects.[1] Attempts are made to assist my imagination by such remarks as, "*That* contains an *idea*; the other is the agent, executive, etc." I do not really think I particularly need *these* helps. I used to make that distinction myself, as the quotation given (p. 83) shows. A little consideration would make it plain that it is impossible for anyone to overlook the difference betwixt a sort of stammering talk and saying "orange" for "onion." But is it not just possible to trace *fundamental* resemblances without ignoring exceedingly striking and very superficial resemblances. Do I not know as well as an ignorant man that a whale is *very* unlike a bat, although I steadily insist that in fundamental characters they are far more alike than a whale and a fish? And is it not possible without contradiction to hold that an ataxic articulation and a mistake in a word are *fundamentally* defects of the same kind and yet *very* different in speciality? Is it not likely *a priori* that the two symptoms are owing to damages of *one* series of sensori-motor processes—the damage being of sensori-motor processes respectively low and high in evolution.

Psychology is older than mental physiology, and thus when we come to that arbitrarily limited part of medical physiology which deals with defects of mental operations, we use psychological terms, not only to describe but also to explain abnormal physiological phenomena. But in order to make our work at cases of aphasia a *methodical part* of our work at other cases of disease of the brain, we must reduce the symptoms to their lowest terms—to the same terms to which many of the coarser symptoms are reducible, that is to say, to movements (sensori-motor). We must study affections of speech, so far as is practicable, in the same manner as we do cases of chorea, convulsion, and hemiplegia. The distinction into "loss of memory for words" and "loss of movement for words" (speaking of cases of damage to the brain), looks clear and orderly, but it will not work. On the other hand, to say that there are all degrees, from difficulty of articulation to mistakes in words (and there are), looks indefinite. But there need be no trace of indefiniteness in the work to be done except what is the outcome of the workings of our own minds. The defects of speech occur in *cases* which can be investigated with any degree of minuteness.

As some evidence of the merging of the several defects into one another, one listens with interest to discussions on cases of defects of speech. One speaker will take the view—the patient being present—that the defect is *only* one of articulation, another urges that there is at least *some* aphasia. Is not this good evidence that at the lower extreme the defects merge? Again, it is occasionally discussed whether a man's abnormal way of talking is of an aphasic character or is owing to a mental defect. Does not this show that at the other extreme there is no abrupt demarcation? Does it not show that a person has not mind *and* speech, any more than he has speech *and* movements of articulation? There are no absolute separations betwixt either. All phenomena of the organism—whether they be such as walking or such as thinking, have for their anatomical substrata sensori-*motor* processes, and for the condition of their development excitation of nerve cells and fibres.

[1] It is very important to bear in mind that, besides paralytic difficulty of articulation from disease of the nerve trunks to the articulatory muscles, or of their immediate centres in the medulla oblongata, there is a difficulty of articulation (I call it ataxic) in which paralysis of the lips, tongue, and palate is not discoverable. In the latter the patient has usually some difficulty in expressing himself in writing—showing that the ataxy is a rudimentary defect of *speech*. It occurs with right hemiplegia. I have seen it in one case of disease of the pons Varolii.

Disease *appears* occasionally to respect the two divisions; there are cases of little more than ataxy of articulation, and cases of mistake of words only. They appear to be very distinct things. The explanation, however, is, I believe, simply that different pathological processes tend to damage different parts of the region of the corpus striatum. Thus either clot or softening (from embolism or thrombosis) may produce entire loss of speech. But what is to the point is that each of them can, when the damage is limited, produce *defect* of speech. Now if there be *defect* of speech with softening, it, as I have long noticed,[1] more often consists of mistakes in words. But in cases of cerebral hæmorrhage, the defect of speech (if it is only defective) is more likely to be one of articulation (it is an ataxy of articulation). In the former case the pathological process is one which can affect convolutions directly, and that without at the same time extensively damaging the motor tract; the pathological process in the latter affects chiefly the motor tract (as we are considering *defects* of speech we are concerned with *limited* damage). But to speak of convolutions and motor tract here is not to speak in terms sufficiently safe. It encourages the notion I am trying to disprove throughout this article, that there is an abruptly separate part for *ideas* and another separate part for *movements*. (The anatomical substrata of ideas can be nothing other than processes for impressions and movements.) We now say, then, that whilst in each kind of defect the very same series of sensori-motor processes is damaged, there is in the former (mistakes in words) damage where the series is comparatively high in evolution, and in the latter (ataxy of articulation), where it is low in evolution. To the above differences correspond important clinical differences. In the former, if there be hemiplegia, it is usually slight and transitory; in the latter the hemiplegia is usually decided and persistent. The bearing of these two facts is obviously in accord with what has been said. Another fact, I think, is, that the more the leg and the less the arm suffer in cases of right hemiplegia, the less defect of speech there is.[2]

The objection that when we speak internally, as, for instance, when we express ourselves in writing (and we must speak before we express ourselves in writing), there *is no movement* of the articulatory organs, is not of weight. To remember a word is to have a faint excitation of the sensori-motor process of that word.[3] The objection tacitly assumes that the convolutions, being for *ideas*, cannot be for *movements*. It is only supposed that in internal speech there is *faint* excitation of those *central* sensori-motor processes which for external speech require to be strongly excited. There is as much speech when I say " Gold is yellow " to myself as there is when I say it aloud. We cannot surely suppose that different sets of sensori-motor processes are concerned when we " think " " gold is yellow " and when we " talk it." Of course

[1] *Medical Times and Gazette*, June 23, 1866, p. 662.

[2] I have put forward the opinion that mistakes in words are analogous to choreal movements in so far as this. I mean here that they are the results of *over* action of nervous processes, and thus that they (degrees of *disorders* of speech) differ fundamentally from degrees of *loss* of speech, the analogues of degrees of paralysis. This opinion I do not discard. But I now think, as was several years ago suggested to me by Mr. Herbert Spencer, that there is in some of the cases of mistakes in words, the mistake of making a more general for a more special symbol. Thus, a patient seeming afraid of a kitten put on her lap, said, " Take little fur child away." When so, the cases evidently come in the category of palsies; they conform to the law of destroying lesions—the patient is, in his speech, " reduced to a more automatic condition." The analogues of choreal movements will be the utterances of more special for more general symbols.

[3] See *Principles of Psychology*, 1st ed., p. 359; Spencer on Memory, etc.

there is a vast difference in the degree, and, what is equally important, in the extent of the excitation. In one there is a "motor impulse"; in the other actual movement. Perhaps the most striking way of putting it will be to assert that the patient who has lost power over his articulatory organs from disease in the medulla oblongata, and who cannot, therefore, get a word *out*, has no affection of speech. The proof is that he continues able to express himself in writing, *and he could not write unless he spoke internally.* There is, indeed, no more reason why a patient who has become unable to *talk* because his tongue, lips, and palate will not move should not *speak* internally than there is that a person who has *become* blind should not see *internally* ("ideally," "subjectively," etc.). And that the man who has become blind does see *internally* by central excitation is plain, since he dreams of objects. Doubtless (although I have put no questions on the matter to such persons) those who have lost articulation, but not speech, dream of talking (aloud).

The following quotations concerning Laura Bridgeman bear on several foregoing matters. The first of them I have used before[1] to show that there is good authority for the belief that in deaf-mutes a set of educated *movements* (those of their hands) serve as our articulatory movements do in internal as well as in external speech. It was used also to show that, in deaf-mutes, there are very special ("mental") movements of the hands, which serve immediately in mental operations. I do not, however, suppose it to be likely that deaf-mutes think in images of "raised letters," if that be what the archbishop means. This and the quotation from Whately also show that *central* excitation of nervous processes for hand movements suffices for the internal speech of deaf-mutes—motor impulses instead of actual movements.

Laura Bridgeman, when she dreamed, "talked" to herself in finger-language, and doubtless she thought by aid of the nervous processes for signs she made with her fingers. As we generally think by help of symbolic movements of our articulatory organs, or rather of the nervous impulses to move them, so she thought by help of symbolic finger-language.

Dr. William Thomson, the present Archbishop of York, writes[2]: "Those among the deaf and dumb who have been taught by the pains of an enlightened humanity to converse and to think, must use, instead of the remembered words which we employ, the remembered images of hands in the various combinations of finger-speech [here the italics are mine] *as the symbols of their thoughts.* The deaf and blind, taught the names of objects from raised letters, must think, not by associations of sound, but by touch."

Whately, speaking of Laura Bridgeman, says:

"The remarkable circumstance in reference to the present subject is, that, when she is alone, her *fingers are generally observed to be moving*, though the signs are so slight and imperfect that others cannot make out what she is thinking of. But if they inquire of her, she will tell them.

"It seems, that, having once learnt the use of *signs*, she finds the necessity of them as an *instrument of thought*, when thinking of anything beyond mere individual objects of sense.

"And, doubtless, everyone else does the same; though in *our* case no one can (as in the case of Laura Bridgeman) *see* the operation; nor, in general, can

[1] *Medical Times and Gazette*, June 23, 1866, p. 662.
[2] *An Outline of the Necessary Laws of Thought.*

it be *heard* ; though some few persons have a habit of occasionally audibly talking to themselves, or, as it is called, 'thinking aloud.'"

There is, from another department of clinical medicine, proof, although indirect, of the opinion that faint and central excitation of sensori-*motor* processes suffices in thought. It is necessary to give this at some length, as we shall thus obtain facts bearing on the way in which *movements* serve in higher mental operations, facts which will make clearer what has been said on the relation of "mental" to "physical" operations.

In a case of sudden paralysis of the right external rectus, when the patient tries to turn the eye outwards, that is, to the right, "l'organe n'obéit plus à la volonté, il s'arrête à moitié chemin et les objets *paraissent se déplacer à droite, bien que l'œil et les images rétiniennes qui s'y produisent ne changent pas de position.*"[1]

In a case of *paresis* of the external rectus there is evidence of disorientation ; in striking at an object held on the paralysed side, the patient's hand goes beyond the object. To bring the eye upon the object, the patient has to "send down" as much "force" as would in health be enough to carry the eye beyond it. In the case supposed, the defect is in the conducting nerve trunk, not in the energising centre. It is in the transmission of force, not in there being a less amount for transmission ; an unusual amount *is* transmitted part of the way, but it cannot all get to the muscle. The patient judges by the strength of the central excitation, not by what that actually accomplishes.[2]

Of the case of *paralysis* Helmholtz says : "L'acte volontaire *ne se traduit par rien en dehors du système nerveux*, et cependant nous jugeons la direction de la ligne visuelle *comme si la volonté avait exercé ses effets normaux*" (op. cit., p. 764 (no italics in original). These facts seem to me to give striking corroboration of the view that central[3] excitation suffices for internal speech, and indirectly that there are in internal speech, or "memory of words," motor impulses—rudimentary or incipient movements.

We must now remark very briefly on certain other ocular motor symptoms, with the same intentions. (I assume that the reader is well acquainted with all the symptoms I speak of. They are nearly all common ones.)

In some cases of hemiplegia there occurs a symptom which shows that there are in the brain, at any rate in the corpus striatum and adjoining convolutions, sensori-motor processes for highly special movements of the two eyes. These very special ocular symptoms are conveniently considered after speaking of the strange "mental" effects occurring in cases of palsy of a nerve *trunk*. The symptoms are, turning of the two eyes *from* the side paralysed in hemi*plegia*, and, correspondingly, turning of the two eyes *to* the side convulsed in cases of hemi-*spasm*. This lateral deviation of the eyes (first described by Vulpian and Prévost[4]) seems to me to be the motor analogue of hemi-opia. The ocular

[1] "Helmholtz." French translation, by Javal and Klein, of the *Physiological Optics*, p. 764. (No italics in original.)

[2] These facts explain the patient's giddiness, in the production of which, contrary to what is commonly supposed, double vision has little share. Vertigo, I would define to be taking as accomplished a movement which is only strongly attempted—in which there is only a strong or wide *central* excitation. This is the physiological definition ; the pathology of vertigo is another matter.

[3] If we impress the retina with a scarlet object, and thus obtain a negative image, that negative image will appear to us to enlarge as we look into the distance. Under atropine, objects appear to be smaller. One of my epileptic patients told me to-day that when his fit sets in, the wall seems "to come nearer," and, again, that distant objects seem "clearer."

[4] In this country by Humphry, Lockhart, Clark, Hutchinson, Broadbent, Russell Reynolds, and myself.

movements lost are *as special* as the articulatory movements lost in certain cases of affection of speech. Put otherwise, we say that lateral deviation of the eyes differs as much from paralysis of the third or sixth nerve, as ataxy of articulation does from defective articulation owing to paralysis of the tongue, palate, and lips.

The occurrence of this symptom from disease of the brain is of very great importance for mental physiology [1]; *movements* [2] *of the eyes enter into the anatomical substrata of our visual "ideas."* The significance of the occurrence of this symptom (in severe lesions and strong discharges) along with affection of our chief tactual organs, is very great. Donders supposes, with Hering, that there are movements of the eyes together for *direction* (upwards, downwards, inwards, and outwards), and also of adduction and abduction for *distance.* He shows from Adamük's [3] experiments that " au moins chez le chien et chez le chat, les deux yeux ont une innervation commune, qui part des tubercules antérieurs des corps quadrijumeaux. L'éminence droite régit les mouvements des deux yeux vers le côté gauche, et vice versâ. En irritant des points différents de chaque éminence, on peut provoquer le mouvement dans une direction quelconque, mais toujours les deux yeux se meuvent simultanément et en conservant entre eux une relation déterminée." But such movements are also represented in the corpus striatum and adjacent convolutions (perhaps I should say, re-represented), *and in direct relation with movements of our chief tactual organs.* The movement is lost in hemiplegia, and is developed at a certain stage in convulsion beginning unilaterally. I was long puzzled by the fact that in the lateral deviation of the eyes in hemiplegia and convulsions beginning unilaterally the eyes were parallel. As the act of accommodation (in which the eyeballs are converged) is a very important one, I expected to find the movement of convergence the *first* of the ocular movements to suffer. For, as I shall mention more particularly in my next article, the most special movements suffer first in cases of cerebral lesions. (See *West Riding Lunatic Asylum Medical Reports*, vol. iii, pp. 315–16; see p. 90.) But I now see that convergence, as it has to do with distances, belongs to the locomotor series (cerebellum) and not to the tactual series (cerebrum). The movements for carrying the retinæ over objects are just as special in the cerebral series as those for convergence are in the cerebellar series. I say " cerebellar series," because my inference has been that the movements of convergence are chiefly represented along with movements of our spine, arms, and legs for locomotion. At any rate, according to Donders and Adamük, the two kinds of movements are *differently* represented in different parts of the corpora quadrigemina. I continue the quotation: " Par l'irritation de la partie postérieure, soit de l'éminence droite, soit de l'éminence gauche, on obtient une forte convergence, avec abaissement simultané des lignes visuelles et rétrécissement de la pupille." In the corpora

[1] I am surprised that Vulpian's important statements on this ocular symptom have received so little attention in this country. Lateral deviation of the two eyes is valuable clinically as evidence of a gross lesion in cases of apoplexy ; enabling us sometimes to tell cerebral hæmorrhage from drunkenness (Prévost). I have found it a most important help towards completing the parallel betwixt hemiplegia and hemi-spasm (see *Lancet*, February 16, 1867). Thirdly, as suggested in the text, the symptom is one of extreme importance for mental physiology.

[2] See Spencer's *Psychology*, 2nd ed., vol. i, chap. xiii.

[3] I take these extracts from a translation of a paper by Donders in *Robin's Journal*, September and October 1872. In a very brief statement in the *Lancet* (February 15), of what is given at more length above, I represented Donders as speaking only of the *lateral* movements of the eyes.

quadrigemina we should not expect any very great differentiation of the two classes of movements, any more than of movements for articulation and deglutition in the medulla oblongata. But betwixt the mode of representation of movements in the cerebrum and in the cerebellum, we should expect the differentiation to be carried to its extreme.[1]

In healthy looking at near objects, of course, both classes of ocular movements will be developed. The eyes must be adjusted ; when " fixed together " so as to " reach " the object, they can be carried over the object ; the retinæ can then " feel " it.

I have urged the doctrines stated in this paper many times ; I have urged them in places where at first glance they seem out of place, as in the *Ophthalmic Hospital Reports*.[2] But the object I have had has been one. I have wished to show that there are for those who study muscular disorders of the eye, for those who study hemiplegia and chorea, and for those who study diseases of the mind certain simple and yet fundamental principles, which give a harmony to their very different facts. If we work anatomically and physiologically (not at clinical entities) we shall, I think, make more progress than we do ; we shall work together without confusion. Above all, to make our studies of mental diseases part of our scheme of studying nervous diseases in general, our method must be anatomical and physiological—not psychological. I conclude this paper by a quotation from an article I wrote some years ago. " Special work at diseases of the mind should, I feel convinced, be begun only after a large real experience of all the special phenomena of motion and sensation that damage to any parts of the nervous system may give rise to. I say a real experience, as I suppose a collection of numberless facts, however accurately gathered, is not held to be of itself a real experience. Unless a man can put the particular phenomena he himself sees under more general laws, or unless he tries to do this, he can scarcely be said to know or to be studying a thing in any very valuable sense. The knowledge the ophthalmologist has of muscular disorders of the eye, the knowledge the physician has of defects of articulation, of chorea, and of epilepsy, and that the psychologist [alienist physician I should have said] has of incoherence and delusions, should aim to be Physiological Units,[3] each different, but each related to a wide common knowledge of such laws—present or in progress—as those of the Evolution of Sensation and Movement in organisms."[4]

[1] As will be pointed out later from larger illustrations, it does not follow that movements represented in a lower centre are not also represented in the higher centre. Are we to believe that the movements by which a headless frog rubs vinegar off its back are not also represented, and that more specially in the detached head ? Here the fact I have insisted on, that discharging lesions produce motor symptoms when destroying lesions of the same parts do not, obviously bears closely.

[2] *Vide infra.*

[3] " Physiological unit " is a term introduced by Mr. Herbert Spencer. (See his *Principles of Biology*.)

[4] *Royal London Ophth. Hospital Reports*, vol. v, Part iv, 1866.

# ON THE ANATOMICAL, PHYSIOLOGICAL, AND PATHOLOGICAL INVESTIGATION OF EPILEPSIES[1]

In the investigation of Epilepsies, or of any kind of case of nervous disease, we have three lines of investigation. We have :

1. To find the Organ damaged (Localisation).
2. To find the Functional affection of nerve tissue.
3. To find the alteration in Nutrition.

There is, in brief (1) Anatomy, (2) Physiology, and (3) Pathology[2] in *each* case. The third part of the inquiry will be only incidentally considered. (See p. 96.) It is a very distinct part. As to the first, I shall speak of the localisation of lesions in epilepsies scarcely more than is necessary to illustrate the second, that is, the physiological, part of the investigation. The reason is, that on the simplest "epilepsies,"[3] which have to be first studied for principles of localisation, I have already written very many times.

There is one matter, however, which must be alluded to here. In these simple cases of convulsion there is well exemplified an important principle, which, I presume, applies to all symptoms of the *cerebral* series. This principle is of essential importance in unravelling the complexities of cases where mental symptoms occur after epileptic discharges. It will also, I trust, help us to a more realistic view of that important symptom, loss of consciousness. The principle is that those parts are wont to suffer first and most which serve in the more voluntary (special) operations, and those last and least which serve in the more automatic (general) operations. Briefly to illustrate this, I quote from a paper I published in the *Lancet* (February 1, 1873) (see p. 68). The quotation refers only to the mode of onset of the fits. *The mode of onset is the most important matter in the anatomical investigation of any case of epilepsy.*

" There are three parts where fits of this group mostly begin : (1) in the hand ; (2) in the face, or tongue, or both ; (3) in the foot. In other words, they usually begin in those parts of one side of the body which have the most voluntary uses. The order of frequency in which parts suffer illustrates the same law. I mean, that fits beginning in the hand are commonest ; next in

[1] *West Riding Lunatic Asylum Medical Reports*, vol. iii, 1873, p. 315.

[2] This division will be clearer if I anticipate the definition to be given (p. 100) of an epilepsy—an occasional, sudden, excessive and rapid discharge of grey matter of some *part* of the brain. The functional alteration (No. 2) is plain, for the very existence of repeated paroxysms tells us that there is a " discharging lesion." Under anatomy (No. 1) we try, from a study of the paroxysm, to find where the discharging lesion is—to localise. And under pathology (No. 3) we try to trace the steps of the abnormal process of nutrition by which the discharging lesion resulted. We have also a fourth heading for " causes " (fright, etc.) determining the discharge.

[3] I had written out for this paper some account of the paroxysms of these simplest cases (convulsions beginning unilaterally), but I withhold it, as its publication would be merely recapitulating what I have already said many times before. I refer the reader to a paper, " Study of Convulsions," in the *St. Andrews Reports*, vol. iii, 1870, p. 8 ; and for a summary to the report of a " Case of Epileptiform Seizures, beginning in the Right Hand " (*Medical Times and Gazette*, December 23, 1871). See also the *second* edition of the *second* volume of Reynolds' *System of Medicine*, art. " Convulsions " (*Class 1. The Convulsion begins Unilaterally*, p. 277.)

frequency are those which begin in the face or tongue, and rarest are those which begin in the foot. The law is seen in details. When the fit begins in the hand, the index-finger and thumb are usually the digits first seized ; when in the face, the side of the cheek is first in spasm ; when in the foot, almost invariably the great toe."

The fits begin, it will be observed, in those parts which suffer most in the common form of hemiplegia.

It is very interesting to me to find that Ferrier's independent researches confirm the general principle above stated, so far as experiments on lower animals can be supposed to be comparable with the experiments disease makes on man.

The following remarks will show the bearing of the above statements of the mode of onset of convulsive seizures : on the principle mentioned. In this group of fits the spasm " prefers," so to speak, to begin in those parts which have the more voluntary uses ; in other words, in those parts which have the more leading, independent, separate and varied movements ; in other words still, in those parts the movements of which are last acquired (" educated "). In strict physiological definition, a voluntary part—the hand, for example—is one which has the greater number of *different* movements at the greater number of *different* intervals ; shortly, the more " varied " uses. An automatic part—the chest, for example—is one which has the greater number of similar movements at the greater number of equal intervals ; shortly, the more " similar " uses. Hence, convulsions which begin in the hand usually begin in the thumb and index-finger—in the most " voluntary " parts of the whole body.

It is not supposed that there are abrupt demarcations betwixt the two classes of movements. Movements of the shoulder (intermediate betwixt the arm and the thorax) may be considered as " voluntary " when compared with those of the chest, and automatic when compared with those of the arm. To illustrate : it is just as a metal is positive or negative, according as it is considered in relation to the one before it or to the one after it, in the electro-chemical series.

Each of the three varieties of fits is supposed to depend on discharge of more or less of the sensori-motor processes of some particular series. The mode of onset gives us a clue to the series. Thus, those fits which begin in the hand are supposed to depend on discharge of a part of the cerebrum where the hand is largely represented in movements to which other movements (those of the face and leg) are sequent and subordinate. Again, in fits beginning in the foot, the internal part discharged contains processes for certain movements of the foot and lower limb, to which certain other movements (those of the upper limb) are sequent and subordinate. In *this* series the foot is the voluntary (special, etc.) part. Hence the remark that the mode of onset is the most important matter in the paroxysm for our consideration. It points to the part of the brain which discharges, or where the discharge begins.

As a more definite illustration, I will mention that in fits beginning in the right cheek, there is often temporary defect of speech. The fit (for it usually, the patient tells us, affects the tongue also) begins in the parts for the exteriorisation of speech. There is, *after* some of these seizures, epileptic aphasia,[1] analogous to epileptic hemiplegia.

[1] After some fits, beginning in the hand (right), there is occasionally temporary defect of speech.

The main object of this article, however, is the topic to which I now come, *viz.* the Physiology of Epilepsies—the second line of investigation.

As I would define it in its application to the investigation of Epilepsies, Physiology is concerned with the *function* of nerve tissue. What I call a " discharging lesion " is *one* of the two morbid modifications of the function of this tissue. It will, however, be impossible to limit the remarks rigidly to this line of investigation. It will be necessary to consider not only the discharging lesions themselves, but, for illustration, we must speak of the different phenomena (different kinds of seizures) which differently placed " discharging lesions " produce—of the localisation of the discharges, a topic which strictly belongs to the Anatomical division of our inquiry. Our particular task, however, is the consideration of a certain functional change in nerve tissue.

Before I speak of abnormal functional *changes*, I must expressly point out that I do not use the word " functional " in senses in which it is frequently used. It is sometimes used as a name for minute changes, or for those the existence of which we are obliged to infer because nervous symptoms are present, but which we do not expect to discover post-mortem. For instance, it is said that epilepsy and chorea are functional diseases, it being meant that the changes on which the symptoms depend are so slight that they do not involve alteration of structure, but only of function. This is, I think, an inconvenient way of using the word. The real meaning is little more than that the changes spoken of are as yet undiscovered. In the second class of what I shall call functional changes, the changes are slight, but their slightness is no essential part of the definition to be given.

The term is used more loosely still. Thus, when a patient has a transient and imperfect paralysis—for instance, slight hemiplegia—lasting a day or two only, the internal changes may be declared to be functional *simply because the external symptom presented was a slight and transitory one.* In reality, the slightness and transientness of a paralytic symptom depend on the *extent* of the lesion of the nervous organ, not on the *nature* of the affection of nerve tissue of that organ. If there be a limited lesion the patient will recover quickly ; and his recovery does not always follow, if indeed it ever does, because the damage to the motor tract is repaired, but simply because he has lost only a small *quantity* of that tract. For it is manifest to those who make post-mortem examinations that recovery from paralysis will occur when a part of the motor tract is permanently wanting. Nor will this be strange to those clinical observers who *do not* make post-mortem examinations, if they consider the facts bearing on the plan of structure of nervous organs (Appendix II, p. 106), and that when recovery follows in a case of paralysis it observes a particular order—it is from that of the more automatic parts to that of the most voluntary. Recoverability from paralysis is chiefly a question of the *size* of the lesion—quantity of nerve tissue destroyed. As lesions differ in size in all degrees—for example, lesions produced by clots from the size of a pea to that of a hen's egg—there are all degrees of paralysis and all degrees of recoverability. There is no need to explain a transient paralysis by a state of nerve tissue. Transientness of paralysis cannot be taken as evidence that nervous *structure* has not been *destroyed.* That parts of the cerebral hemisphere may be destroyed when there are no obvious or striking symptoms is well known. But it is so of the motor tract also. I shall have again to insist on this class of facts (Appendix I, p. 105).

Another objection to a not uncommon use of the word is, that under it two very distinct things are confounded, viz. functional changes and the pathological processes which lead to them. This is, I think, particularly unfortunate ; physiology and pathology are mixed. I will here remark on the difference of the two things by quoting from an article on " Hemichorea " I published in the *Edinburgh Medical Journal*, October 1868.[1]

" Just as loss of function—for instance, palsy—follows destruction of nerve tissue, *however produced*—by clot, by tumour, by injury, etc.—so *disorder* of function—(discharge) for instance, chorea or spasm—results from instability of nerve tissue, *however produced*—by mechanically produced anæmia (?), and, as I think, by embolism." [2] There is a still further objection to the common use of the word.

I have for some years used the term " functional " to describe the morbid alterations of *the normal function of nerve tissue.* Therefore, before I speak of these alterations, we must notice what the normal function of nerve tissue is. Its function is to store up and to expend force. It is true that this is the function of *all* organic matter, but it is *par excellence* the function of nerve tissue. There are *but two* kinds of alteration of function from disease. Saying nothing of degrees of each, there is on the one hand loss of function, and on the other over-function (not better function). In the former, nerve tissue ceases to store up, and therefore to expend force. In the latter, more nerve force is stored up than in health, and more is therefore expended ; the nerve tissue is highly unstable. Under the first head come palsies (akineses), anæsthesiæ ; under the second, chorea, epilepsies, tetanus (hyperkineses), neuralgia, etc. In a not uncommon way of using the word " functional " no distinction is made ; this is the further objection just mentioned. The changes which produce paralysis (provided the symptoms be slight in degree or transitory), as well as the changes which produce tetanus, chorea, etc., are spoken of as being functional. The term is, in short, used for two opposite states of nerve tissue.

I used to consider these two states of nerve tissue to be degrees of but one

[1] One reason for quoting *that* article is, that I may correct a misapprehension under which most of those labour who have criticised my opinions on the pathology of chorea. The remarks quoted in the text, taken with the statement of the second division of my hypothesis on an earlier page of the article quoted from—" That this local instability is *frequently* brought about," etc.—show that I have not undertaken to defend the doctrine that embolism is the *sole* cause of chorea (cause of the instability of nerve tissue in chorea). The fault, however, is my own ; I freely admit this. By a clerical error which I ought to have corrected, I am made in the *Mirror* of the *Lancet*, November 26, 1864, p. 606, to say " limited *to* softening " of the brain instead of " limited softening " of the brain. I have, however, corrected it by implication. In a report of the Obstetrical Society (*Medical Times and Gazette*, August 1, 1868), I say : " This instability, although *frequently* the result of anæmia [hyperæmia I now think] from blocking, *might doubtless be induced in other ways*, as in the choreiform movements which sometimes occur during recovery from epileptic hemiplegia, the secondary results of coarse disease of a cerebral hemisphere." In the *London Hospital Reports*, 1864, vol. i, p. 459, I write : " I think, from many circumstances, that embolism is a *frequent* cause of chorea." I believe, however, that embolism (or blocking of arteries by some process) is *almost* the sole cause of chorea. Nay, speaking in the very strictest sense, I do not believe that two *different* pathological processes would damage an organ in absolutely the same way ; from two pathological processes leading to instability of convolutions near to the corpus striatum, I should expect slight, even if insignificant, differences in the movements resulting.

[2] The functional change of nerve tissue in epilepsies, in chorea, and in tetanus also, is supposed to be the same.

condition. I will stay to remark on this point, although its consideration belongs strictly to pathology. The remarks will, however, scarcely be digressive, as two important facts will be incidentally disclosed which are required for a later development of the physiological part of our subject.

One reason I had for thinking these two states to be degrees of one condition was suggested by the very striking clinical fact that paralysis is frequently associated with convulsion. For example, hemiplegia not unfrequently follows convulsions beginning on one side; it is the epileptic hemiplegia of Dr. Todd. I now explain this remarkable sequence by the supposition that the paralysis is caused by the strong discharge in the fit. But here it must be mentioned that there is occasionally hemiplegia (partial hemiplegia) *before* the first fit, and when the attack is on we see that those parts which have been *paralysed* are first and most *convulsed*. This puzzles students. They think it contradictory that *paralysed* parts should be the very ones which are "picked out" for spasm. And in trying to "remember" on which side a patient was convulsed, a student will occasionally really *infer* the side convulsed, as is shown by his saying, "It *must* have been his left side, *because his right side was paralysed*." I used, as above mentioned, to explain the association by the notion that the condition of nerve tissue which caused the paralysis was a more extreme degree of the same condition as that which caused the spasm. But I think a more satisfactory explanation can be given (see Appendix II, p. 106).

To return now to the two kinds of functional changes. In the first class of cases nerve tissue is frequently actually destroyed, as when it is broken up by a clot; but, at any rate, its function is lost. In the second class nerve tissue is unstable, it energises too much—it discharges on slight provocation, and discharges strongly. It matters nothing for the definition how the destruction or instability be effected—by what pathological process. Destruction (loss of function) of nerve tissue may be the result of tearing up by blood clot, of slow wasting (as in spinal amaurosis), or it may probably be the result of a strong discharge, as in cases of epileptic hemiplegia (*vide supra*).[1] Then as to instability; it may, I believe, be produced by hyperæmia consequent on blocking of vessels (see p. 97), by "irritation" of a tumour, and probably in many other ways.

The mode of *production* of the discharging lesion (of unstable nerve tissue—grey matter) belongs to pathology. Something will be said under this head (pp. 96, 97).

Using somewhat curiously compounded but convenient terms, the two kinds of functional changes may occasionally be called "destroying lesions" and "discharging lesions."

Epilepsies are the results of the second class of functional changes; they are, speaking briefly, "discharging lesions." But there are many varieties of discharges. Defined from the paroxysm, an epilepsy is a *sudden*, *excessive*, and *rapid* discharge of grey matter of some *part* of the brain; it is a *local* discharge. To define it from the functional alteration, we say there is in a case of epilepsy grey matter which is so abnormally nourished that it *occasionally* reaches very high tension and very unstable equilibrium, and therefore occasionally "explodes." The two definitions are of different faces of the same thing.

[1] As here implied, one does not mean necessarily physical destruction, nor *permanent* loss of function.

It will be observed that the " discharging lesion " of epilepsy is supposed to be a *permanent* lesion ; there is grey matter which, since it is permanently under conditions of abnormal nutrition, is permanently abnormal in function. That this permanent abnormality is a varying state has been said ; it has been remarked that the grey matter *occasionally* reaches high tension, and therefore *occasionally* discharges (or is discharged). There are waves of stability and instability. It follows from this that the first fit is supposed to be a discharge of a part which has *for some time* before been in a state of malnutrition ; and a still further inference is, that such " causes " of epilepsies as fright are only determining causes of the *first* explosion. Many of the " premonitory symptoms " of a first attack are probably results of slight discharges [1] ; they are miniature fits.

There is not, I think, nowadays much difficulty in understanding that from a *permanent* abnormality of nutrition there can result *occasional* disorderly exhibition of function. The process in epilepsies roughly corresponds to what is supposed to occur normally in the ganglia of the heart ; there is, it seems to me, only a particular application of certain physiological doctrines long since put forward. Thus, I quote from Baker's edition (seventh) of Dr. Kirkes' *Physiology* (p. 141) : " Why these nervous centres " [nervous ganglia of the heart] " should issue impulses for rhythmic rather than for continuous action, is still a debatable point. The most philosophical interpretation yet given of it, and of rhythmic processes in general, is that by Mr. Paget, who regards them as dependent on rhythmic nutrition—*i.e.* on a method of nutrition in which the acting parts are *gradually raised*, with time-regulated progress, to a certain state of *instability of composition*, which then issues in the discharge of their functions, *e.g.* of nerve force in the case of the cardiac ganglia, by which force the muscular walls are excited to contraction. . . . *All organic processes* seem to be regulated with exact observance of time ; and *rhythmic nutrition and action*, as exhibited in the action of the heart, are but well-marked examples of such chronometric arrangement." (No italics in original.) Schrœder van der Kolk writes, as his fourth conclusion on epilepsy, that " The special seat and starting-point of these convulsive movements is situated in the ganglionic cells of the medulla oblongata, which, as reflex ganglia, possess the peculiar property that, when once brought into an excited condition, they may more or less suddenly discharge themselves and communicate their influence to different nervous filaments. After their discharge a certain time is again required to bring them to their former degree of excitability, and to render them capable of fresh discharges, just as we see to be the case with electric batteries, or in the phenomena of an electrical fish.[2]

So long as a patient has one-sided *palsy*, we do not doubt him to have a " destroying lesion " of his " motor tract." Similarly, so long as a patient has recurrences of one-sided convulsion, so long has he, I believe, a " discharging lesion " of convolutions near to the motor tract.

Of course it is not denied that *healthy* nerve tissue can be made by certain very abnormal provocations to discharge so strongly as to produce convulsions. Thus, convulsions occur during rapid tearing up of nervous substance in large

[1] The other day I congratulated a mother on the fact that her son had not had a severe fit. She, however, regretted it, saying that the severe fit " cleared his system," whilst the slight fits rendered him, from their frequency, unable to go to business.

[2] *Sydenham Society's Transactions*, p. 283.

hæmorrhages, either when the bleeding is in the cerebral hemisphere or in the pons Varolii. They are producible in healthy animals by *rapid* bleeding to death, as Kusmaul and Tenner's experiments show. Besides, there are the very striking results of direct action on the brain in the experiments of Fritsch, Hitzig, and Ferrier. I speak of cases in which fits are either one-sided, begin by a very local aura, or of cases where the fits recur.[1] In these cases there must be a local and persistent lesion.

Symptoms of instability in disease are, I suppose, an exaggeration with caricature of the effects of healthy discharges. Of some this is easily seen. In chorea the movements are often only awkwardnesses—only slight departures from health; the poor child is occasionally beaten by his parents for clumsiness. The following remarks, referring to healthy discharges, would, with a few slight modifications, apply to some of the trifling degrees of instability of disease. "The longer repair goes on unopposed by appreciable waste, the greater must become the instability of the nerve centres, and the greater their readiness to act; so that there must at length come a time when the *slightest impressions* will produce motions."[2] In fact, there is, at the time Spencer is speaking of, a healthy and yet random discharge. "On awakening from refreshing sleep, there commonly occurs an involuntary stretching of the muscles of the whole body, showing an immense undirected motor discharge."[3] Then a sneeze is a sort of healthy epilepsy.

Before I close the remarks on the functional nature of the lesion in epilepsies, I will consider briefly the pathology of discharging lesions in general, taking as a starting-point the remark made on p. 93, that I used to believe the two functional states of nerve tissue were degrees of one condition. At that time, following Radcliffe, Handfield Jones, and Anstie, I considered that the nutrition of nerve tissue was *imperfect* in unstable nerve tissue. In a certain sense I think so still. Recently, indeed, I have been led to think that the view I now hold is in some respects simply a modification of the one they have long taught. I say this, however, to acknowledge an obligation. The reader will, of course, judge of the views of these physicians from what they have written themselves, and hold me responsible for what I now write.

There are, I submit, two ways in which nutrition may be imperfect—in quantity and in quality. I believe that nerve tissue in discharging lesions is over-nourished in the former sense and worse-nourished in the latter. In order to make my meaning clearer, I will take chemical illustrations and use chemical nomenclature. Two bodies may be of the same Constitution, but yet of very different Composition. For example, the constitution of acetic acid and of the chloracetic acids is the same; but they differ in composition, as in the latter hydrogen has been replaced by chlorine. The "structure," however, is unaltered.[4]

[1] If we are called to a patient in his first convulsion, and if that convulsion be "general," we often cannot tell to what it is owing; whether, for instance, it be owing to some local cause, acting on a previously healthy brain—as rupture of an intracranial aneurism—or be owing to explosion of some part of the brain which has long been getting into a highly unstable condition. I do not deny that it is easy to guess; we should mostly guess rightly. All I mean is that we do not make a diagnosis worth calling one if, when we are called to a person who has had a severe convulsion, and of whose case we have no history, we turn out to be right in having said, "It is a case of epilepsy."

[2] Spencer, *Psychology*, vol. i, p. 90.

[3] Spencer, op. cit., vol. i, p. 90.

[4] Perhaps a better illustration may be the formation of that highly unstable substance, gun-cotton, from stable cotton by the process of substituting 3 atoms of hydrogen by $NO^2$.

I believe, then, that the highly unstable nervous matter of disease (in a "discharging lesion") differs in composition, but not in constitution, from the comparatively stable grey matter of health. The alteration in composition is of course such that the nervous substance formed is more explosive. We must suppose that there is some order in this Substitution-Nutrition, and we must infer that it is in the direction of explosiveness, or instability. The following is a speculation as to the kind of alteration of composition. One striking constituent of nervous matter is phosphorus. It belongs to the chemical class of triads of which other members are nitrogen and arsenic. My speculation is that in the abnormal nutritive process producing unstable nervous matter the phosphorus ingredient is replaced by its chemical congener, nitrogen. There is a substitution compound; the replacement probably occurs in different degrees, as it does in the three differing chloracetic acids. If nitrogen be substituted as supposed, we can easily understand that the substance produced would be more explosive. The supposed value of arsenic in certain nervous affections is significant; it is another member of the group of triads. The nutrition is, therefore, assumed to be defective not in quantity but in quality, in those functional alterations I call "discharging lesions."

I think these speculations have a practical bearing on the dietetic treatment of epileptics. I advise epileptics not to eat much meat (not much nitrogenised food), nor, indeed, much of anything. I was, however, led to give this advice in another way, not by the speculation just mentioned, but by the following remarks of Dr. Haughton:

"The hunted deer will outrun the leopard in a fair and open chase, because the force supplied to its muscles by the vegetable food is capable of being given out *continuously for a long period of time*; but in a sudden rush at a near distance the leopard will infallibly overtake the deer, because its flesh food stores up in the blood a reserve of force capable of being given out *instantaneously* in the form of exceedingly *rapid* muscular actions."[1]

I think a great part of the "weakness" and languor of some of those persons who suffer what is popularly called "nervous debility," and who are often hypochondriacal, is explainable on the supposition that their nervous tissue is over-nourished in quantity, and yet so imperfectly nourished in quality that it is explosive; or, let us use in this simple and not uncommon condition of ill health, the expression, more irritable nervous matter. They often keep up this irritability by frequent eating and drinking. My colleague, Dr. Andrew Clark, insists that the most successful treatment of such persons is putting them on a very simple unstimulating diet, alcohol in particular being forbidden. My speculation is, that the good results are owing to the formation of less explosive or less irritable nervous substance—one of a *more normally stable composition*. The excitability of these patients reminds one of the fact that the nerves of a weak animal are found, experimentally, to conduct with greater velocity than those of a healthy one.

The above speculations seem to me to harmonise with certain doctrines on the *pathology* of discharging lesions in some cases. Thus, I believe that chorea frequently, and epilepsies sometimes, are produced by embolism or thrombosis. The cases spoken of (p. 94), of convulsions *following* hemiplegia, and affecting first and most the parts already partially paralysed, are, I believe,

[1] *Address on the Relation of Food to Work*, p. 28. No italics in original.

cases in which there is usually plugging of branches of the middle cerebral artery. That plugging of vessels can lead to local *destruction* of nerve tissue is plain enough. But I think there is a strong presumption that it can lead to *instability* of grey matter. When (as stated p. 94) I held the doctrine that the two functional states of nerve tissue were degrees of but *one* condition, I was under the mistaken impression that plugging of vessels led always to local anæmia. But it can lead to local hyperæmia: this bears most significantly on the production of unstable nervous matter. It is to be observed that, though there is in hyperæmia thus caused *more* blood, there is less change of blood; hence the nutrition will be of a more general kind. That there is less change of blood is a very important departure from the normal circulation of the brain, as one peculiarity of this organ is that a large quantity of blood passes *through it*; it has a great *change* of blood.

I may most conveniently state the further points on this matter by the following quotation from a paper I contributed to the *Medical Times and Gazette*, March 6, 1869. Although it was written *a propos* of chorea, it applies to the discharging lesions of other symptoms (epilepsies, etc.):

" It has been often urged as an argument against embolism being the cause of chorea, that *anæmia* from plugging of vessels can scarcely lead to *increased* expenditure of force. If arteries be plugged, it seems certain that the nutrition of parts they supply will be *defective*; still, it does not follow that it will be *decreased.* For, according to certain physiological experiments, it seems that plugging of a small artery does *not* always cause *anæmia* of the capillary region to which the vessel should deliver arterial blood. On the contrary, it may cause *congestion*, and may even lead to extravasation. I must, for the facts and arguments of this question, refer the reader to MM. Prévost and Cotard's work, *Études physiologiques et pathologiques sur le Ramollissement cérébral* (Paris, 1866), and especially to a section (p. 38), ' De la congestion qui accompagne infarctus.' I will only quote the last of the three conclusions from their experiments (italicising some words): ' Consécutivement aux *oblitérations artériales* il se produit habituellement de *l'hyperémie* et de la tuméfaction,' etc. Dr. Ivan Poumeau has also published very interesting statements on the effects of plugging of vessels—*Du Rôle de l'Inflammation dans le Ramollissement cérébral*, 1866. To explain how increase of blood results from *blocking* of an artery is a very difficult thing. The first step towards an explanation lies in determining whether the increase of blood is of the venous or arterial kind. Rokitansky thinks the local congestion is produced by increased pressure on the collateral arteries; Virchow thinks it is owing to return of blood from the veins. It is impossible to decide without further evidence when such men differ, except, perhaps, by the clumsy expedient of fitting the two views together —*viz.* that in the periphery of the congested spot there is arterial congestion, and in the centre venous congestion. As it seems to me, the local increase in quantity of blood, at all events, has an important bearing on the production of chorea *and other symptoms implying increased expenditure of force.* If it be venous, we may suppose that, although nutrition may be carried on faster, it will lead to *more imperfect and more easily decomposable nervous matter*; or, if we suppose the nerve force is supplied from the blood to the nervous structure in the same way as recent investigators believe force is supplied to the muscles, the increase in the quantity of blood is still significant when associated with increased expenditure of force, I suppose we may fairly say that the general character of blood, which is stagnant or slowly changed, will be venous rather than arterial."

I believe then, as Dr. Russell Reynolds says, that " the proximate cause of convulsions is an abnormal increase in the nutritive changes of the nervous centres " ; but I also think that the nutrition is carried on on an inferior level. I suppose that if the nervous matter cannot get enough phosphorus, it takes nitrogen, provided it is under conditions favourable to some kind of nutrition—just as a plant will take soda when it cannot get potash.

Let us now consider " discharging lesions," with a view to a more formal definition of epilepsy in the sense in which I use the term in this paper. It will, however, be convenient to state first what things are not essential to the novel definition.

*First.*—Epilepsy is not one particular grouping of symptoms occurring occasionally ; it is a name for any sort of nervous symptom or group of symptoms occurring occasionally from local discharge. Whether the discharge puts muscles in movement or not—that is, whether there be a *convulsion* or not—matters nothing for the definition. A paroxysm of " subjective " sensation of smell is an epilepsy as much as is a paroxysm of convulsion ; each is the result of sudden local discharge of grey matter.

*Secondly.*—It does not matter for the definition whether there be Loss of Consciousness or not ; loss of consciousness is a fundamental thing in most of the accepted definitions. If there be no loss of consciousness, there is, according to most physicians, not epilepsy, and then the term " epileptiform " is used. But even when using the term " epilepsy " in the ordinary sense of the word the separation into cases where there is and where there is not loss of consciousness has no *physiological* warrant. It is an arbitrary distinction of psychological parentage. Loss of consciousness is not an utterly different thing from other symptoms. It is not to be spoken of as an epiphenomenon, nor as a complication. Consciousness has, of course, anatomical substrata as much as speaking has. The sensori-motor processes concerned in consciousness are only in degree different from others. They are the *most* special of all special nervous processes, the series evolved out of all other (lower) series.

To lose consciousness is to lose *the use of the most special of all nervous processes* whatsoever.[1] If those parts of the brain be first affected by strong discharge where the most special of all nervous processes lie, there will be loss of consciousness *at the outset.* If processes of a subordinate series be discharged, loss of consciousness of course occurs later. For example, in cases of convulsions beginning in the hand, consciousness is in most cases lost as soon as or just before the leg is reached by the spasm. In these cases the internal process will be that consciousness is lost as soon as the most special of all processes *are reached* by the internal discharge, or (since the sensori-motor processes underlying consciousness are evolved *out of* lower series : see Appendix II, p. 106) when a large quantity of a subordinate and yet important series is put *hors de combat.*[2] But, of course, one does not locate consciousness so geographically as the mere words we must use seem to imply. If a patient

[1] I say to " lose the use," because the use of sensori-motor processes will be temporarily lost *during discharge,* causing their excessive excitation, as much as it is permanently lost when they are implicated by gross lesion.

[2] Much depends on the rapidity of the discharge ; the more rapid the spasm of the arm the sooner is consciousness lost. It is not to be inferred from the foregoing that other factors, as asphyxia, are not concerned.

suddenly loses by any process the use of *any large part* of either of the two *highest* divisions of the nervous system, he will lose consciousness.

*Epilepsy is the name for occasional, sudden, excessive, rapid and local discharges of grey matter.*

That the epileptic attacks are *sudden*, needs no showing ; that the discharge is excessive is plain enough in those cases where convulsion occurs ; and in all cases the inference is irresistible that the morbid discharge is far greater than the corresponding healthy discharge. In those fits which begin in the hand the discharge is so strong that the pain from the cramped muscles is very great.

It is convenient to speak next of the *occasional*, or paroxysmal occurrence of epileptic discharge. There are discharges which are *not* occasional ; and thus the word " occasional," in my definition of epilepsy, excludes the " interrupted continuous " discharges of chorea [1] and the almost uniform stream of discharges in tetanus.

The next point is as to the discharge being *local.* I will quote [2] Voisin, to show that (using just now the term Epilepsy in its commonly accepted sense) epileptic attacks in the same patient are stated by one good authority to be like one another. If so, the discharge in each fit must be in the very same internal part ; yet attacks differ in different patients, and thus the internal discharges causing them must differ in locality.

At page 595, op. cit., Voisin writes :

" Axenfield a fait remarquer que les attaques se reproduisent le plus souvent avec une uniformité absolue, avec leurs auras, leurs caractères propres et leurs complications. Il s'établit une sorte d'habitude d'après laquelle tel individu sentira toujours la même aura, poussera toujours un cri et le même cri, tombera sur le même point du corps, le front l'occiput se blessera de la même façon, présentera les mêmes mouvements convulsifs, se mordra la langue au même point, se luxera toujours une même épaule, sera toujours pris de délire après l'attaque."

This being so, those who hold that the medulla oblongata is the part which discharges in epilepsy have, as well as others, to note *paroxysms* with great care, in order to find out how it is that in one patient there are fits of a certain kind, and in another of another kind, however much the seizures in the two patients may agree in the most fundamental characteristics required by the ordinary definition of epilepsy.

But, as stated, numerous and very different nervous symptoms may be epileptic in my definition of the term. And as any part of the grey matter of the cerebrum may become unstable, there will be all varieties of epilepsy,

[1] I would strongly urge that it is as important to note differences in the *time rates* of discharges, as in the speciality of the movements those discharges develop. For example, the dog's chorea differs from that of the child, not only in that the former is almost a repetition of *one* movement, whilst in the latter there are mostly successions of *different* movements, but also in that the choreal movements in the dog are nearly rhythmical, whilst in the child the intervals of the movements are varied as the movements are.

[2] *Nouveau Dictionnaire de Médecine et de Chirurgie Pratiques*, art. " Epilepsie." This is an article of great value.

I give Voisin's definition of epilepsy : " L'épilepsie est bien une maladie et non pas un symptôme, malgré ce que peuvent dire certains auteurs, qui ne me paraissent pas avoir suffisamment vécu au milieu d'une population d'épileptiques " (Voisin, op. cit., p. 581). He thus defines epilepsy : " Profitant des travaux de ces maîtres (Trousseau, Th. Herpin, B. A. Morel), nous pensons donc que l'on doit définir l'épilepsie une *maladie chronique, apyrétique, caractérisée par des attaques convulsives, des vertiges, des absences, qui frappent l'individu d'une façon irrégulière, au milieu de la santé, souvent, en apparence, la plus parfaite* " (Voisin, op. cit., p. 581).

according to the exact position—according to the extent of the grey matter altered—and there will be all degrees according to the degree of instability. But, for illustration, we shall give a list (*vide infra*). I wish first to speak of cases of limited seizures, or, if the expression be preferred, of partial seizures. I wish to point out that we must not take *degrees* of epilepsies for *varieties* of epilepsies.

It is obvious that there are all degrees of epilepsies. A fit which is limited to the hand is not a fit of a different *kind* from one which begins in the hand, and then *spreads* all over the body, and is, after a certain stage, " attended by " loss of consciousness. The latter seizure is but the result of a much stronger discharge. A fit which begins in a part like the hand, and *becomes* universal, *is* different from one in which the convulsion is nearly universal at the very first ; a different area of grey matter must be discharged in each. Another illustration as to degrees of seizures is that a patient may one day have transient loss of consciousness only, who, on another day, has this instantly " followed by " convulsion. There are here again differences of degree only depending on the strength of the initial discharge. For, as already remarked, the processes put *hors de combat* during the discharge which causes loss of consciousness are not *fundamentally* different from sensori-*motor* processes, discharge of which produces convulsion. The former are highly special sensori-*motor* processes, evolved out of—as it were, continuous with—lower sensori-*motor* processes.

There will, however, be a compound result from increasing strength of discharge. We see, externally, that the stronger the spasm is the *wider* spread it is—the stronger the internal discharge the further it will spread. There are *two* ways of spreading. The discharge will not only explode healthy *lower* centres, but will probably spread, as it were, laterally, to healthy associated centres in the brain. My speculation is, that the lateral spreading is by arteries [1] and their vaso-motor nerves ; the spreading is in arterial regions.

The following are epilepsies :

(1) A sudden and temporary stench in the nose, with transient unconsciousness. (2) A sudden and temporary development of blue vision. (3) Spasm of the right side of the face and stoppage of speech. (4) Tingling of the index-finger and thumb, followed by spasm of the hand and forearm. (5) A convulsion almost instantly universal with immediate loss of consciousness. (6) Certain vertiginous attacks.

All these six seizures are alike in that each results from an occasional and excessive discharge of unstable grey matter. This is the one functional alteration of nerve tissue underlying the different phenomena.

The investigation does not end here ; rather it begins here. The very general nature of the physiological statement *necessitates* most careful method in the anatomical part of the investigation. For, obviously, all the six epilepsies,

[1] On arterial regions in the brain I have often written, with regard to the interpretation of epilepsies ; *one* factor in the internal change causing the paroxysm being, I think, arterial contraction. See *London Hospital Reports*, vol. i, 1864, p. 466. The scheme of arterial supply is, no doubt, as definite and as purposive as are the arrangements of nerve fibres and cells. Very little consideration shows that the more special nerve centres become the more independent must be their nutrition, and this necessitates an increasing limitation of arterial areas. I believe the arteries have to do with developing *sequences* of movements. It is a matter of significance that the arteries of the cortical grey matter have no anastomosis ; they are " terminal arteries."

notwithstanding their *physiological* likeness, are very unlike *anatomically*—that is, in their Localisation. The area of grey matter altered in each must be in a different place, or the phenomena could not differ. In a word, although the functional alteration is the same in all epilepsies, the seats of those functional alterations are various.

No one can admit more fully than I do the difficulties in the localisation of "discharging lesions." The very method I work on keeps the difficulties well before me. I know well that in most of the six cases I cannot localise the discharging lesion. But this failure is no objection to the method. I still urge that we should go on trying to localise; and we should, so far as is practicable, work in the same realistic manner as we do in cases of paralysis. Surely it is as important to localise "discharging lesions" as it is to localise "destroying lesions." Every physician attempts the latter. If a man be hemiplegic, we observe the region affected by palsy to find where the central destroying lesion is. But, in cases of convulsion, the region affected by spasm is scarcely ever methodically studied in order to find where lies the central destroying lesion. Some most practical-minded men show great interest in discussions as to the particular muscles of the face most implicated in cases of hemi*plegia*, but no zeal in investigating the particular muscles of the face first and most implicated in cases of hemi*spasm* (convulsion beginning unilaterally). The question often put is, Is it a case of epilepsy? or is it only an epileptiform seizure? The question should be, Where is the discharging lesion in this case? The plan of studying cases of disease, so far as they show *approaches to certain clinical entities*, is, I feel convinced, an unfruitful one. To show that I have long held this view, I will quote from a paper I quoted from in my former article. The case referred to in the subjoined extract was one of amaurosis associated with convulsion beginning unilaterally:

"And I ought here to remark more particularly that I do not say simply that amaurosis in Case XX occurs with epilepsy. Not that this, according to a common use of terms, would be a wrong phrase, but because the term 'epilepsy' has not a sufficiently precise meaning. Besides, this expression has not vitality in itself. It is extremely important *to describe* the sort of fit an amaurotic patient may have; to call it 'epilepsy' gives the symptom too elastic a meaning, and careless people might think they had disposed of this part of the case by saying 'the amaurosis is complicated with epilepsy.' This classification would, I think, be an approach, under the cover of a conventional and yet an unreal preciseness, to the analogous looseness of saying 'the amaurosis is complicated with paralysis,' leaving it doubtful what sort of palsy there was. We want positive information as to how a convulsion is a *departure* from health of muscles and muscular groups and health of nervous organs and tissues, and not as to how far it *approaches* our idea of the almost metaphysical conception 'genuine' epilepsy. . . . there are to be found on record scarcely any positive statements of what has really happened in particular convulsive paroxysms—a process which sometimes occurs under our very eyes. I am fully aware that there are admirable accounts of the worst fits as types, but some of these accounts are descriptions more of dramas of great human interest, than calm and cold scientific observations in an orderly sequence of the outward phenomena of an inwardly suffering nervous system." [1]

One fruitful method of study is by seeking symptoms resulting from

[1] *Royal London Ophthalmic Hospital Reports*, 1866.

"destroying lesions"[1] which correspond to those the results of "discharging lesions." I will illustrate this method, but only in outline.

If we consider the effects of a destroying lesion of the corpus striatum, we find paralysis of the face, arm, and leg. There are paroxysms of convulsion which correspond, and which depend on discharges of convolutions near to this body[2]; we will illustrate by lesions of the *left* side of the brain.

FIRST DEGREE

| *Corpus Striatum Palsy.* | *Corpus Striatum Epilepsy.* |
|---|---|
| Mouth turns to left. | Mouth drawn to right. |
| Right arm paralysed. | Right arm convulsed. |
| Right leg paralysed. | Right leg convulsed. |

This is, however, only a comparison with the first degree of paralysis. A graver lesion of the corpus striatum produces the symptoms named in the next list, and there is a further degree of convulsion which corresponds.

SECOND DEGREE

| *Corpus Striatum Palsy.* | *Corpus Striatum Epilepsy.* |
|---|---|
| Head turns to left. | Head drawn to right. |
| Two eyes turn to left. | Two eyes drawn to right. |
| Face turns to left. | Face drawn to right. |
| Trunk muscles weaker on right. | Trunk muscles in spasm on right (?). |
| Arm and leg paralysed on right. | Arm and leg in spasm on right. |

THIRD DEGREE

But there is a still further degree of hemiplegia: a very grave lesion in the region of the corpus striatum of *one* side will produce palsy of *both* sides of the body; then, of course, the term "hemiplegia" is, strictly speaking, a misnomer. Similarly, the convulsion which begins on one side—in the hand, for example—will spread at length to the other side; it *becomes* universal. I believe, however, that a fit which thus *becomes universal* depends on discharge in but *one* hemisphere; for facts seem to me to show that each half of the brain represents movements of both sides of the body,[3] but that it represents the movements of the two sides in different degrees and orders. I have, however, had few opportunities of watching convulsions which, beginning in one side, have reached the other. One of my patients, whose fits began in his *right* ulnar fingers, said that once, after the right side of the body had been involved, "it" went across his chest to the *left* arm; it went *down that* arm, but did not reach the fingers.[4] One dare not trust much to a patient's observation on such a matter; but, as a hint, it is of very great value.

The points I wish to observe about the *second* side are:

1. Is the arm or the leg first affected?
2. What part of either of the two limbs does the spasm first reach? Does

[1] See "Remarks on Hemikineses," *West Riding Lunatic Asylum Medical Reports*, vol. iii, p. 178. (See p. 79.)

[2] I say nothing of the tongue, as I have not been able (except in one case) to make any observations on it in convulsions.

[3] See remarks on this point, *Lancet*, February 15, 1873. (See p. 71.)

[4] See report of his case, *Medical Times and Gazette*, December 23, 1871.

it first reach their upper parts (shoulder and thigh), or their lower parts (hand and foot) ?

3. Does it especially affect any group of muscles—*e.g.* the extensors or flexors ?

There are all degrees of palsy, from destroying lesions in one half of the brain, and there are corresponding degrees of convulsion ; the above examples are taken simply for illustration. Another thing we have neglected is the *order of spreading* of the spasm. Still another is that the bilateral muscles of both sides are involved when the unilateral of but one side are well engaged. The following extracts from the report of a case will show my meaning. There was injury to the head ; the *first* set of motor symptoms was, palsy of the right arm and turning of both eyes and of the head to *the left* ; a second set came on later.

The case is of interest for several purposes of this paper. It was published [1] under the title, *Case of Corpus Striatum Epilepsy* (*Hemispasm*), and chiefly, as will be seen, to illustrate Broadbent's Hypothesis.[2]

" There was blood in the arachnoid ' cavity ' on the left side. The bulk of it, however, lay in one spot over the frontal convolutions, and was so placed as, I imagined, to squeeze the corpus striatum, which body at the autopsy seemed to be otherwise undamaged.

. . . . .

" The right arm was in spasm, so was the right cheek ; so was the right orbicularis palpebrarum, and the head and eyes were turned to the right. So far, then, omitting consideration of the leg, which did not move, the unilateral muscles which the left corpus striatum governed were involved. Now for the bilateral muscles which *each* corpus striatum governs in health, which *one* will govern when its fellow is damaged, and which are put in action when *either*, being ' unstable,' is discharged.

" The bilateral muscles of the thorax were fixed, both masseters were tightened, both cheeks moved (the right being drawn up), and both orbiculares palpebrarum were involved and both sides of the occipito-frontalis acted. With regard to the last-named muscle, its action was, on the right side, partly counteracted by the orbicularis palpebrarum, the eye being closed ; but on the left there was a more even struggle between the two. According to Broadbent's hypothesis, the orbicularis palpebrarum should be most represented in its corresponding (opposite) corpus striatum, as it is a muscle which we can use on one side only ; but still it will be represented in each, as we generally close both eyes at the same time. Now I have noted that in some cases of hemiplegia the patient may be able to close the eye on the non-paralysed side alone, but not the eye on the paralysed side, on which side he can only close the eye by a ' bilateral effort '—*i.e.* when closing both. This small fact I had noticed [3] before I had heard Dr. Broadbent's hypothesis, which seems to account so well for the singularity. The differing degree of spasm in the case above given is still further confirmation."

[1] *Medical Times and Gazette*, August 15, 1868.

[2] See Broadbent's Paper, *Med. Chir. Rev.*, April 1866. The hypothesis is stated clearly in Watson's *Practice of Physic*. See Appendix I, p. 105.

[3] *London Hospital Reports*, vol. ii, 1865, p. 309.

## APPENDICES

### No. I

There are many things in the two foregoing papers which require more development than has been given to them. Most of them would come under an explanation of the superficial paradox, that whereas *destruction of part of a nervous organ may produce no loss of movements* (no obvious or striking loss is of course meant), *discharge of that part may bring about excessive movements.* I have already in many places urged that, without observing the effects of discharging, as well as of destroying, lesions, we cannot methodically investigate the functions of certain parts of the brain. It will be well here to give particular illustrations, and the illustrations of most point will be those I have already used.

Speaking in the Gulstonian Lectures (1869) of Broadbent's Hypothesis (already referred to at p. 104), I remark [1]:

"This complementary study of the effect of absence of function and 'over-function' of nervous organs is important for several reasons, and notably for this reason, that—in one instance at least—the muscles put in action when a nervous organ is 'discharged' are not only those palsied when that organ is destroyed."

I think the principle is of very great importance for direct *clinical* purposes. I give an illustration, and purposely choose one which shows how the application of the principle in question widens our schemes of investigation. There are cases of disease of the ear (attended by discharge) with which epileptic or epileptiform convulsions occur. I believe the accepted explanation would be that these seizures are reflex—the results of irritation starting from the ear. My speculation is that the local instability on which they depend is the result of infarction of veins; it is, I suppose, a result of a minor degree of the same process as that which leads to cerebral or cerebellar abscess. Now, cerebral abscess from ear disease occurs mostly in the middle lobe of the brain, and I infer that the changes of instability—the discharging lesion—producing convulsions in those who have epilepsies in association with organic disease of the ears are in that lobe also. But in the case of abscess (nerve tissue destroyed) there usually *are no motor symptoms*—no paralysis, or no local palsy at least. We have not, then, a basis for the kind of comparison which was illustrated on pp. 102–103. And it might even be assumed that the middle lobe does not contain processes for movements, because there is no loss of movements (no obvious loss is of course meant), from the destroying effects of abscess occurring therein; and as a necessary inference that minute changes in this part could not lead to *development* of movements (convulsion); investigation would be stopped.

But to quote from the report of some remarks [2] I made on the group of cases referred to:

"It does not follow that, because *destruction* of a part of the nervous system

[1] *Lancet*, Abstract, February 27, 1869. Broadbent's principle of the double representation of those movements which are bilateral in the sense that they must act together, or mostly do act together, is a very important contribution to physiology and scientific medicine. I believe, however (as stated p. 101, and for reasons given more at length, *Lancet*, February 15, 1873, p. 71), that all orders of *movements* of both sides of the body are represented in each side of the brain, the most voluntary very unequally, the more automatic very equally.

[2] *British Medical Journal*, June 26, 1869, p. 591.

leads to no symptoms, the part destroyed had no functions. The middle lobe of the cerebrum and the cerebellum of course have functions, and there must be symptoms when these parts *discharge*—where the nervous tissue is not destroyed, but is unstable. A man can *do without* a certain quantity of his cerebrum, cerebellum, or corpus striatum, just as he can do without a certain quantity of his lung or his liver. It is altogether a different thing when, instead of being destroyed, a quantity of his nervous system is unstable and discharges occasionally. Hence it comes to be a matter of importance to study as a first step, with all the precision the subject admits of, the seizures which occur with discharge from the ear, especially when the offensiveness of the discharge implies diseased bone. When we have put the symptoms in groups—in some kind of order—we may cautiously speculate further, and see if there be plausibility in fixing the blame for their occurrence on instability of those regions of the brain in which disease of the ear sometimes leads to abscess."

## No. II

### On Evolution of Nervous Centres

After the above preliminary remarks, which, I trust, show satisfactorily the importance, both for anatomy and physiology as well as for clinical medicine, of the *complementary* study of the effects of the *two* kinds of functional lesions, we can consider certain other points alluded to in the foregoing papers. In the first paper (*West Riding Lunatic Asylum Medical Reports*, 1873, p. 181. See p. 81) there is a quotation to the effect that removal of the corpora striata does not, in the rabbit, cause loss of movements of the limbs. Let us, however, take instead the following much wider illustration, given by Vulpian in his *Physiology of the Nervous System*.[1] The case is that of a rat from which the cerebral hemispheres, corpora striata, and a great part of the optic thalami had been removed :

" Vous voyez qu'il est dans l'immobilité la plus complète. Je vais répéter l'expérience que j'ai déjà faite devant vous. Je fais un bruit d'appel avec les lèvres : vous avez vu le rat tressaillir et sursauter brusquement. Les sensations auditives se produisent donc bien encore chez cet animal. Je pince l'extrémité d'une de ses pattes ; il crie aussitôt. Ces cries paraissent bien être des indices de douleur."

The following is even more important :

" Voici un jeune lapin auquel on a enlevé aussi les hémisphères cérébraux et les corps striés. Vous le voyez se tenant très-bien dans l'attitude normale, criant d'une façon plaintive lorsqu'on pince un de ses membres ou sa queue, faisant alors quelques pas, puis redevenant immobile. Ce lapin, ainsi que vous pouvez le constater, fait parfois quelques pas d'une façon tout-à-fait spontanée en apparence, et évidemment, très-régulière ; le voilà même qui court ; il va se jeter sur le rebord saillant de cette table, et, après un effort pour avancer, il reste de nouveau tout-à-fait immobile." [2]

I have a double purpose in considering this kind of experiment. (1) To put forward once more a speculation to account for the fact that a destroying lesion of a part may produce no obvious symptoms when a discharging lesion of that part may produce very striking symptoms. (2) To consider an objection to the view that the cerebral hemispheres are the seats of epileptic discharges,

[1] P. 666. [2] Op. cit., p. 680.

which is often inferred from the statement (the correctness of which I will admit) that epileptic fits are producible in animals whose cerebral hemispheres have been removed.

Since a rat or a rabbit, mutilated as described by Vulpian, does make adapted movements when noises are made, or cries when pinched, and since a pigeon, similarly mutilated, turns its head after a moving candle, it is plain enough that in the *lower* centres of these animals there are sensori-motor processes for the adjustment of *very general* movements to *very general* impressions. But the inference is not that these very same kinds of impressions and movements are not also represented in the *higher* parts removed. Rather the very same processes are in the higher centres *re-represented* in greater complexity and speciality. Let us take a still more striking case. A headless frog will rub vinegar off its back with a hind-leg. But can we suppose that these very movements are not also represented in a more special manner in the frog's encephalon? Co-ordination in the higher centres is the co-ordination in the lower "carried a stage farther."[1]

The conclusion I have arrived at from the study of cases of disease is, that the higher centres are evolved *out of* the lower—receiving intercalations as they ascend from the spinal cord to the cerebrum. The higher centre re-represents more specially the impressions and movements already represented generally in the one below it. The co-ordinations are continually being re-co-ordinated; for example, those of the pons and medulla are reco-ordinated in the cerebrum.[2] There are in the lower centres sensori-motor processes for very *general* purposes, but in *their* higher representatives for the more special. A rude symbolisation would be to suppose the pons Varolii to represent the simpler sensori-motor processes of the cord raised to the "fifth power," and the cerebral hemispheres these processes suddenly raised again, let us say, to the "fiftieth power."

If such be the plan of structure of nervous organs, we can understand how it is that part of a highly evolved organ—part of the brain, for instance—may be wanting, with only a very special and not an obvious loss of movements or faculty. Or returning to our very rough illustration, many terms may be

[1] The two following quotations bear on this matter very directly, each from a very different point, however:

"It does not follow, as it at first seems to do, that feelings are never located in the inferior nervous centres. On the contrary, it may well be that in *lower* types the *homologues of these inferior centres are the seats of consciousness*. The true implication is, that in *any case* the seat of consciousness is that nervous centre to which the *most heterogeneous impressions* are brought; and it is not improbable that, in the course of nerve evolution, centres that were once the highest are *supplanted* by others in which *co-ordination is carried a stage further*, and which thereupon become the places of feeling while the centres before predominant become automatic" (Spencer, *Psychology*, vol. i, chap. vi, p. 105). (No italics in original.)

"Je viens de vous dire que l'influence du cerveau proprement dit sur les mouvements volontaires était d'autant plus grande en apparence que les animaux opérés *appartenaient à une classe plus élevée*. Vous pouvez en juger par vous-mêmes. Voici un chien sur lequel on a détruit en partie un hémisphère cérébral; il y à une paralysie très-incomplète des membres du côté opposé, et l'animal est très-affaibli. Voici, au contraire, un pigeon sur lequel un hémisphère est entièrement enlevé; il semble être presque dans son état normal. L'influence de l'opération serait de moins en moins appréciable, au fur et à mesure qu'on passerait des oiseaux aux reptiles, des reptiles aux batraciens, et de ceux-ci aux poissons" (Vulpian, op. cit., p. 677). (The parts I have italicised are very important for the whole of this subject.)

[2] "This progress (see *Principles of Psychology*, vol. i, p. 67) from co-ordinations that are small and simple to those that are larger and compound, and to those that are still larger and doubly compound, is one of the best instances of that progressive integration of motions, simultaneously becoming more heterogeneous and more definite, which characterises evolution under all its forms" (Herbert Spencer).

lacking in the highest ranges of evolution without producing loss of any one power, as of $x$, or of $y$, or of $z$, as each of these will be represented in innumerable other remaining terms. There will be loss only of certain highly special or, metaphorically speaking, *delicate*, processes in which $x$, or $y$, or $z$ is leading. And such a loss could not be very obvious. In this way we can understand how it is that recovery occurs from hemiplegia, notwithstanding that part of the corpus striatum (see pp. 92 and 94) is permanently lacking ; the rest of the corpus striatum also represents the very same muscles, although made up into somewhat different movements. We can also understand how it is that a part of the brain near the corpus striatum may be wanting, without obvious loss of movement.

The above-stated conclusions seem to me to be essentially the same as those deductively arrived at by Spencer. I give quotations from his work, italicising some parts of them to make prominent their bearing on my subject.

In his *Psychology*,[1] speaking of the cerebrum and cerebellum, he says : " We may regard them as organs of *doubly compound co-ordination*—organs which have for their common function the *re-combining* into *larger* groups, and into countless *different* orders, the *already* complex impressions received by the *medulla oblongata* ; and which have the further function of so arranging the *already* complex motor impulses issuing from the *medulla oblongata* as to form those *far more* involved aggregate actions," etc.

He then suggests that the cerebrum is for " doubly compound " co-ordination in Time, whilst the cerebellum is for " doubly compound " co-ordination in Space. After stating the evidence, he says : " There is complete harmony between the hypothesis and the seemingly-strange facts that these centres may be *partially destroyed* without causing *obvious* incapacity, and that they may be *wholly removed* without destroying the ability to co-ordinate the *less complex impressions and acts*."

But if it be granted that the hypothesis of Evolution accounts for absence of loss of movements (of local palsy), in cases of limited destroying lesion of a nervous centre, there comes the question, " How does the hypothesis account for the *development* of a large mass of movement (spasm) in corresponding limited discharging lesions ? " A little consideration will show that the plan of structure, which permits *destruction* of part of a highly " evolved " nervous organ without any but the most special loss of the movements or " faculties " that organ represents or shares in representing, is the very one which necessitates the presentation of a great volume of movement when that part *discharges*. For the more elaborate the structure of a nervous organ, that is to say, the greater the number of *different* co-ordinations it effects—the more grey matter there must be, that is to say, the greater quantity of explosive material. To quote Spencer again :

" Each vesicle, or each portion of grey matter that establishes a continuity between the central termini of fibres, is not *merely* a *connecting* link ; it is *also* a *reservoir* of molecular motion, which it gives out when disturbed. Hence, if the composition of nerve is determined as above indicated, it follows that in *proportion to the number, extensiveness, and complexity of the relations*, simultaneous and successive, that are formed among different parts of the organism, will be the *quantity* of molecular motion which the nerve centres are capable of disengaging.[2]

[1] Vol. i, p. 60. [2] *Psychology*, vol. i, p. 35. (No italics in original.)

" . . . The *quantity* of molecular motion evolved in the nervous centres will become great in proportion as the nervous relations increase in *integration and heterogeneity*."[1]

Hence, in the convolutions there is not only elaborate structure, but, *as a consequence of this*, there is a large quantity[2] of explosive material.

Now we can consider the objection that in epilepsy " les effets convulsifs de l'excitation bulbaire sont indépendants de l'influence cérébrale, *ils peuvent être produits avec des caractères identiques quand les hémisphères du cerveau sont enlevés*."[3] Kusmaul and Tenner[4] write of their well-known experiments: " Convulsions in epileptic attacks sequential to the abstraction of red blood, do not proceed from the cerebrum properly so-called, but from the motor centres situated behind the thalami optici, the excitation being induced by a sudden arrest of nutrition." Their experiments show that removal of all parts in rabbits up to the thalami optici does not exercise any influence upon the production of general convulsions. But I think the speculation I have advanced shows that in less differentiated animals than man discharge of the lower centres would be enough to produce severe universal convulsion. For the condition of the mutilated rat and rabbit (see quotations, p. 106) shows that they have much grey matter left in the lower centres, the centres not removed. For, as stated, very general actions are performed by these mutilated animals. I grant, however, that it is an argument against my view that the convulsions in the mutilated rabbits are *as violent* as they are in the non-mutilated. But the lower in the scale of animals the less differentiation there is—the *less* the cerebrum has to do with the movements, and the more the pons, medulla and spinal cord have to do with them. The quotation from Vulpian given on p. 107 (footnote) shows this clearly.

We have now to consider how it can be asserted that discharge of but *one* hemisphere can produce convulsion of *both* sides of the body, as I suppose it does in most of those cases commonly called idiopathic epilepsy. I can only speak of this in mere outline. In the *Lancet* (February 15, 1873. See p. 71) I have advanced reasons for the belief that movements of the *two* sides of the body are represented in *each* side of the brain. Hence there is convulsion of both sides of the body from discharge of but one hemisphere. We saw this at p. 103, when speaking of convulsions beginning in one hand and becoming universal (*of Corpus Striatum Palsy, and Spasm*, 3rd Degree). But there are cases in which the convulsion is nearly universal to *begin with*, and nearly equal on the two sides. Yet it is significant that the spasm of the two sides is rarely, if ever, absolutely contemporaneous, and rarely, if ever, absolutely equal. The first conspicuous movement in the cases where the fit begins most nearly universally (least *one-sidedly*) is usually turning of the head and eyes to one side; I suppose the discharge to be of some part of the opposite cerebral hemisphere. I believe these cases differ from those simpler ones just mentioned: first, in that the discharge is more sudden and rapid (the fit does occur more suddenly and is more quickly over); second, in that the sensori-motor processes discharged

[1] Spencer, op. cit., vol. i, p. 55. (No italics in original.)

[2] The statement, it is to be observed, is not that the material (in health) is more explosive, but that there is a great quantity of explosive material. I have, I now think, erred in saying that the more automatic processes are in health more stable than the voluntary or special (*St. Andrews Reports*, vol. iii, 1870).

[3] Jaccoud, op. cit., p. 385.

[4] *Sydney Society Transactions*, op. cit., p. 69.

are more highly evolved ; the evidence for the last statement is that loss of consciousness is the *first* thing, or it is lost *very soon* after a most *general and vague warning*.

So far we have spoken of ordinary gross movements. Now, in epilepsies, especially in those in which loss of consciousness is the first thing, or in which it occurs very early, there are " vital " symptoms as well as spasm of the limbs and trunk. But it is plain that the cerebrum (which I suppose to be discharged in such seizures) represents the " vital " processes of the body. Alterations of pulse, respiration and temperature, constipation, vomiting, " *tache cérébrale*," occur in some cases of cerebral tumour, and in cases of large cerebral hæmorrhage. These symptoms are owing to affection of the most general or most automatic processes of the body. They show that the units of the brain do represent (potentially contain) *all the lower processes* of the nervous system, as well as the higher or more special. In cases of epilepsy we have during or at the beginning of the paroxysm pallor of the face as well as convulsions.

The sensori-motor processes which underlie consciousness will be the most complex and special of all nervous processes ; they will be evolved out of and re-represent all lower series. " *The seat of consciousness is that nervous centre to which, mediately or immediately, the most heterogeneous impressions are brought*." [1] The statement is not of the most *numerous* impressions, but most heterogeneous (see definition of voluntary or special movements, p. 91). To the seat or seats of consciousness impressions of *all orders* are brought, and from it issue motor impulses of all orders. It will perhaps be safer to limit this remark by saying that " all gradations will exist between wholly unconscious nervous actions and wholly conscious ones " (Spencer). It is to be observed, however, in disease we feel pain in the most automatic parts—for example, in cases of colic and angina pectoris.

The facts that those very epilepsies in which consciousness is *first* lost, or is lost very early, are the cases in which the convulsion is nearly universal, in which the two sides are more nearly equally convulsed ; and that it is in these cases that there is at the very first much pallor of the face, tend to confirm the conclusion that the sensori-motor processes concerned in consciousness are evolved out of and potentially contain all other (lower) series. It is, indeed, most significant, whatever the explanation may be, that there are slight cases (*petit mal*) in which, with transient loss of consciousness, there is deep pallor of the face (and body ?) and a slight wave of universal movement.

The following quotation from Spencer has important bearings on several things discussed in this appendix. It is given here particularly to oppose the notion that the sensori-motor processes concerned in consciousness are fundamentally different from, and as it were tacked upon, lower series. Why during the excitation of any set sensori-motor processes, will, memory, etc., arise is unknown. The nature of the connection betwixt physiology and psychology is, so far as we can now see, an insoluble problem.

" Memory, Reason, and Feeling, *simultaneously* arise as the *automatic* actions become complex, infrequent, and hesitating ; and Will, arising *at the same time*, is necessitated by the same conditions. As the advance from the simple and indissolubly-coherent psychical changes, to the psychical changes that are involved and dissolubly coherent, is in itself the commencement of Memory, Reason, and Feeling ; so, too, is it in itself the commencement of

[1] Spencer, *Psychology*, vol. i, p. 105.

Will. On passing *from compound reflex actions* to those actions so highly compounded as to be imperfectly reflex—on passing from the organically determined psychical changes which take place with extreme *rapidity*, to the psychical changes which, not being organically determined, take place with *some deliberation, and therefore consciously ; we pass to a kind of mental action which is one of Memory, Reason, Feeling, or Will, according to the side of it we look at.*

" Of this we may be certain, even in anticipation of any special synthesis. For since all modes of consciousness can be nothing else than incidents of the correspondence between the organism and its environment, they must be all different sides of, or different phases of, the co-ordinated groups of changes whereby internal relations are adjusted to external relations. Between the reception of certain impressions and the performance of certain appropriate motions, there is some inner connection. If the inner connection is organised, the action is of the reflex order, either simple or compound ; and none of the phenomena of consciousness proper exist. If the inner connection is not organised, then the psychical changes which come between the impressions and motions are conscious ones ; *the entire action must have all the essential elements of a conscious action—must simultaneously exhibit Memory, Reason, Feeling, and Will ; for there can be no conscious adjustment of an inner to an outer relation without all these being involved.*" [1]

[1] Spencer's *Psychology*, vol. i, p. 496. (No italics in original).

# ON THE ANATOMICAL INVESTIGATION OF EPILEPSY AND EPILEPTIFORM CONVULSIONS[1]

In his valuable paper in the *Journal* of April 26, 1873, p. 457, Dr. Ferrier has drawn attention to some investigations[2] I have made concerning the bearing of cases of convulsion on the localisation of movements in the cerebral hemispheres. It is very satisfactory to me to find that the results he has obtained from the new method of investigation—the artificial rousing up of the functions of particular parts of the encephalon in lower animals by direct faradisation—agree with the general conclusions I have come to from observing cases of paralysis, convulsion, chorea, etc., in man. The importance of his novel facts, and those of Fritsch and Hitzig to which he refers, for anatomy and physiology, is obviously exceedingly great. But for what is called the *pathology* of convulsions in man they haye a remarkable value.

What is above called pathology would, however, be more conveniently named anatomy or physiology. Such convulsions, as I shall mention later in this article, are really experiments on parts of the human brain analogous to those Ferrier has made on the brains of dogs, cats, and rabbits—they are experiments made by disease. Indeed, very much of our clinical work is a study of quasi-anatomical and physiological *experiments*. For example, a large part of our investigations into cases of hemiplegia, convulsions, chorea, etc., is so. I think it is important to bear in mind that much of our clinical study of disease is *not* pathology ; from not doing so, our notions on the " causes " of epilepsy, chorea, etc., are confused. Thus the word " cause " is used by medical men in different senses. It is used for the seat of a lesion, as when it is said that " hemiplegia is caused by disease of the corpus striatum " ; for the functional nature of the lesion, as when it is said that " epilepsy is caused by increased excitability of the medulla oblongata " ; and for the pathological process when it is asserted that " loss of speech is caused by local softening." But, strictly, the *three* lines of inquiry should be pursued ; the causation is to be studied triply in *each* case of nervous disease. It is an anatomical inquiry to seek the organ or part damaged (the seat of disease, the localisation as it is more technically called). It is a physiological inquiry to search into the defective working of the nervous tissue of the organ damaged—the functional affection. It is a pathological inquiry to trace the processes by which the nutrition of nervous tissue is altered. (Strictly, I suppose, we should speak of pathological anatomy, pathological physiology, and pathological nutrition ? ) Reversing the order, and putting these three things in the most abstract form, there are abnormalities in the absorption, in the expenditure, and in the distribution of force.

In the study of epilepsy and of epileptiform seizures, it is of very great

[1] *British Medical Journal*, vol. i, 1873, p. 531.

[2] " On the Anatomical and Physiological Localisation of Movements in the Brain," *Lancet*, January 18, February 1 and 15, 1873 (see p. 37) ; also " Study of Convulsions," *St. Andrews Reports*, vol. iii, 1870. (See pp. 8–36).

importance to keep these several lines of investigation distinct; often it is not possible. The importance of doing so is that we shall more easily trace the fundamental resemblance of different symptoms in spite of their superficial differences. For example, a convulsion affecting one side, hemiplegia and hemichorea are alike in that the same muscles are affected, and, therefore, inferentially alike in that the same internal region is damaged; again, a convulsion and a sudden stench in the nose are alike, in that both depend on the same functional alteration in nerve tissue, they are alike in disorders of function; thirdly, epistaxis, hæmorrhage in the retina and cerebral hæmorrhage are alike in that they are accidental results of the same pathological process in arteries—results of the same abnormality of nutrition. A further advantage of further differentiating our investigation is that we shall learn more exactly *where* our knowledge is deficient.

In this paper I shall speak of the first line of inquiry—anatomical, and almost solely with the intention of showing the bearings of Ferrier's researches on the methodical study of the *seat of the lesion* in epilepsies. In future articles I shall consider the physiology of epilepsies and their pathology. As in this article the illustrations I give are from cases of *convulsions*, I can defer the definition I have to give of the term "epilepsy" as I use it.

It is to be hoped that Dr. Ferrier will make careful comparisons of the effects of the local discharges he artificially induces in animals and those artificial or, at any rate, abnormal discharges induced by local disease in human beings. Of course, the inference is not to be drawn that the phenomena in the two cases are alike. The differences in external conformation of animals imply differences in the normal functions of their nervous centres.[1] These differences will assert themselves, even under excessive and unnatural excitation, whether it be by faradisation or by disease, as surely as they assert themselves during healthy activity. But, although this is what one would expect *a priori*, Dr. Ferrier's experiments have the great value of *demonstrating* special differences in different animals. He concludes that "striking differences corresponding with the habits of the animal are to be found in the differentiation of the centres." "Thus," he continues, "the centres for the tail in dogs, the paw in cats, and the lips and mouth in rabbits, are highly differentiated and pronounced." In fact, we have in Dr. Ferrier's researches a starting-point for a "comparative physiology" of the convolutions. For, so far as comparative anatomists have ascertained homological cerebral structures, so far, it is to be hoped, will he be able to develop the homological functions.

Before we pass to speak of convulsion in man, it is necessary to speak of certain principles as to the constitution of nervous centres.

The nervous centres represent movements, not muscles; chords, not notes. This is evident from the effects of destroying lesions of the corpus striatum. From a *small lesion* of this body there does not result paralysis of *a small part* of the arm, nor of any such group of muscles as flexors, or extensors; there results *partial paralysis of the whole arm*, the most special parts of it suffering most. There is loss of a certain *number of movements of the limb*. Let us take a more striking example: in cases of *very grave* lesion of the corpus striatum (that is, of a centre far above the supposed deep origins of the ocular motor-

[1] I would here refer the reader to an article I contributed to this *Journal* in October 1869, p. 371, in which I have considered certain symptoms the result of disease or experimental injury of the brain in dogs, etc., in relation to corresponding symptoms in man.

nerves), there is, besides palsy of the face, arm and leg, an ocular palsy. Now this palsy is not of the sixth nerve nor of the third nerve, nor of the fourth, nor of any one muscle, nor of any random grouping of muscles. It is a *loss* of a highly special and widely associated movement ; the patient has lost power *to look* to that side on which his body is paralysed ; there is what is commonly called lateral deviation of the eyes. Similarly in convulsion there is a *development* of *movements*. In a convulsion beginning in the hand, the spasm creeps up the whole limb, developing first the movements of the most special parts of it, but not picking out such groups of muscles as flexors or extensors. Among other movements, there is at a certain stage a *development* of that of the eyes for "looking" to one side. In this case the two eyes are *turned to* the side of the body convulsed. We must, however, draw attention to a very important qualification with which the expression "development of *movements*" is to be used.

Both in Dr. Ferrier's experiments and in cases of convulsion from disease in man, the results of the discharges (since they are sudden, excessive, and very local) are only exhibitions of the movements represented in the parts discharged in the rough. A great number of different movements are developed at once.[1] And it must not be forgotten that not only are the discharges unnatural in being excessive, sudden, and temporary, but also in that they are very local. We are reminded of the effects of putting one muscle into strong action by faradising it ; the result is a mere caricature of a normal movement. Duchenne insists that a muscle is never singly in action in health, except perhaps in the case of the facial muscles.

But in spite of these drawbacks, the study of discharging lesions, whether induced by faradisation or by disease, is of great value. My own opinion is that *there is no other way* of finding out what movements parts of the convolutions near to the corpus striatum represent. The reason for thinking so is that the other process of experimentation—that by *destruction* of small parts of the cerebral hemisphere—produces no obvious symptoms—no obvious loss of movements, or no special loss at any rate. But it would be a great error to infer that the part *destroyed* did not represent special movements. The bearing of Ferrier's researches is very direct on this matter. For if we discharge that part, destruction of which produces no *loss* of movement, there will be a presentation of a mass of movements. See, then, the clearing of the paradox. Disease of the convolutions sometimes does, and sometimes does not, produce symptoms. The word "disease" is used vaguely ; so far as it involves destruction there are no symptoms, but there are symptoms from discharge. The speculation I have put forward (*St. Andrews Reports*, vol. iii) to explain these paradoxical results is as follows. (See p. 26.)

To begin with a "motor" centre. The study of cases of hemiplegia shows the constitution of the corpus striatum to be such, that *each* part of it represents movements of the *whole* of the parts which that organ governs. So to speak, the corpus striatum is a mass of corpora striata, each one of which represents faintly, and each in some slightly different manner, the whole of the parts which the corpus striatum in full represents in greater degree. Now, to pass to the hemisphere. The convolutions in the region of the corpus striatum *are* the corpus striatum "raised to a higher power." Each part of the

[1] In chorea, which I believe to depend on repeated small discharges of convolutions near to the corpus striatum, there is a succession of independent and quasi-purposive movements of great speciality.

brain in this region re-represents the whole of the movements which have been represented in the corpus striatum ; so then, if *any* one part of the brain in this region be *destroyed*, there is no obvious loss of movements, because the movements it represented are still represented in each neighbouring part, although in different degrees and orders. But for this very reason, if any *one* part be strongly *discharged*, vast numbers of movements are developed.[1]

I now mention illustrative cases. Although I can only take enough space to give a mere outline of the cases, I think they show plainly that some of the " experiments of disease " on man are, notwithstanding the *special* differences I have insisted on, *fundamentally* like the experiments of physiologists on animals ; that a large and definite part of the study of nervous diseases, of convulsion in particular, must be put on an anatomical and physiological basis ; and that Ferrier's researches will be a most valuable help in thus methodising our work—in making it less empirical and more scientific.

The first illustration is an outline of a case I have already published (*Medical Times and Gazette*, November 30, 1872). A man had convulsions, each of which *began* in his *left* thumb. He died : we found no other disease in his brain than a tubercle, the size of a hazel-nut, in the hinder part of the third *right* frontal convolution. It will be particularly interesting to me to know what effects Dr. Ferrier will obtain by faradising the homologous part of a monkey's brain, for he tells me that these animals will shortly be subjected to experiment. Theoretically, I should not expect an identical convulsion, but an homologous one. I will, before giving the second illustration, remark on this point, and, at the same time, state some facts which show that the study of cases of convulsion bears on what is conveniently, if not correctly, called the physiology of the mind. One constantly hears, however, that the convolutions are not for *movements*, but for " ideas," " memory," etc. Yet those who use psychological phraseology to describe symptoms of disease—" loss of memory for words," " chorea the result of disorder of volition," etc.—have as much as other people to seek the anatomical and physiological substrata of mental phenomena.[2]

[1] I have stated some of the facts on which this speculation is founded, and the speculation itself in a brief manner, in the *Medical Times and Gazette*, December 14 and 21, 1867. In a note, August 16, 1868, op. cit., the bearing on this principle of localisation of the facts supplied by cases of convulsions beginning unilaterally is more particularly considered. (At that time, I supposed that such convulsions depended on discharges of the corpus striatum itself.) The study of numerous different kinds of disease of the brain leads me to the conclusion that not only are the gross movements of the whole body represented or re-represented in the convolutions, but also the so-called " vital processes." A slow pulse and a lowered temperature are among the results of a large cerebral hæmorrhage. In epilepsies, we have pallor of the face and alterations of the secretions, as well as convulsions. In this article, I do not, however, speak of " vital " symptoms. They are best studied in some cases of cerebral tumour.

[2] Of what " substance " can the organ of the mind be composed, unless of nervous processes representing movements and impressions ; and how can the convolutions differ from the inferior centres, except as parts representing *more* intricate co-ordinations of impressions and movements than they do ? Are we to believe that the hemisphere is built on a plan *fundamentally* different from that of the motor tract ? What can the anatomical substratum of the " idea " of a ball possibly be, except a process representing certain impressions of surface and particular muscular adjustments ? Why, then, is there anything remarkable in the fact that discharge of a part of the " organ of mind " produces spasm of the arm and deviation of the two eyes ? What can occur physiologically in recollection, but a faint revivification of such processes which, in the past, have become part of the organism itself ? What is delirium, except the disorderly *revival* of sensori-motor processes organised in the past ? What is a mistake in a word, but a wrong movement, a chorea ? Surely the conclusion is irresistible, that " mental " symptoms from disease of the hemisphere are *fundamentally* like hemiplegia, chorea, and convulsions, however *specially* different. They must all be due to lack, or to disorderly development, of sensori-*motor* processes.

Among the fits which *begin unilaterally*, the commonest are those in which the spasm starts in the index-finger and thumb. This is significant. It is an illustration of what I believe to be the law of the effects of lesions in the brain. In evolution (development, education, etc.), the progress is from the general to the special. In the opposite process of dissolution the more special parts suffer first. I generally use the term " voluntary " instead of " special " ; it is a convenient counterpart to the term " automatic." In physiological language, a voluntary part—the hand, for example—is one which has the greater number of *different* movements at a greater number of different intervals—shortly, the most varied uses ; an automatic part—the chest, for example—is one which has the greater number of similar movements at the greater number of equal intervals—shortly, more similar uses. In brain diseases parts suffer the more as they are voluntary, and the less as they are automatic. Now, the thumb and index-finger are the most voluntary or specialised parts of the body ; hence the suggestiveness of the case I mention. The thumb in man has a distinct flexor longus pollicis. In the *Anthropomorphia*, Huxley (*The Anatomy of Vertebrate Animals*) says : " The *flexor pollicis* is more or less closely connected with the *flexor communis perforans*, or with that part of the muscle which goes to the index digit." On the intellectual importance of this muscle Duchenne insists strongly. " En somme, ces faits cliniques demontrent que le long fléchisseur du pouce est l'un des muscles qui sont essentiellement destinés, chez l'homme, aux usages manuels les plus delicats ; à tenir et à conduire la plume, le crayon, le pinceau, l'aiguille, etc. ; qu'il aide, en un mot, à l'exécution des travaux manuels qui sont à la hauteur de son intelligence supérieure " (*Physiology of Movements*, p. 251). And in his work on *Electrisation*, he says that when the small muscles of the thenar eminence are atrophied, the hand loses its distinctive human character and approaches that of the monkey. The thumb in the monkey is less specialised than in man. If, then, we discover in a monkey the homologue of the part discharged in my patient, we shall expect from *its* discharge a fit of less special kind ; for example, not a fit beginning in its pollex, but more likely one beginning in the whole of its five comparatively little differentiated digits at once, if not in the whole arm.

I have yet to publish the case of a woman who had fits beginning in her left great toe (where fits beginning in the foot nearly always start) ; there was a small tumour in her right hemisphere. My colleague Dr. Gowers made a careful examination of the brain for me ; he found that the tumour involved the lower part of the ascending frontal convolution. Although there were other lesions in this woman's brain—local indurations—there is a strong probability, amounting almost to certainty, that the fits depended on discharge of that part in which lay the tumour. Here, again, I await Dr. Ferrier's further researches in comparative physiology of the convolutions.

In the *Medical Mirror* of September 1869, I published the case of a man who had fits affecting the *right* arm. In this case there was a tumour in the hinder part of the first (uppermost) frontal convolution of the left hemisphere. (There was also a tumour in each lateral lobe of the cerebellum, to which I traced no symptoms). I did not see this man in a fit ; his arm was paralysed after the first seizure.

Lately I was allowed by Mr. Soutter to see a patient of his who had literally innumerable fits limited to the right arm. Mr. Soutter witnessed many ; I saw several. The spasm passed down the arm except in the later fits, then it passed up. Shortly before the patient's death she had, Mr. Soutter tells me, universal convulsion. Here I correctly predicted disease of the hinder part of the first (uppermost) frontal convolution—not from physiological knowledge, but because of what I found in the other case just mentioned. Once more I ask, What would be the homologous parts in a series of animals lower and lower in the scale ? [1]

[1] The significance of the fact that the hand is the part in which convulsions, beginning unilaterally, most often start ; that the arm suffers first, or most, or both, in the greater number of motor affections from brain disease (hemiplegia, chorea, paralysis agitans), will be better realised after reading Herbert Spencer's remarks on lacteal organs, in chap. viii, vol. i, p. 359, of his *Psychology* (second edition), from which I give these extracts.

He points out and shows the significance of the " striking instances which the animal kingdom presents of unusual sagacity co-existing with unusual development of organs, which, by the help of complex muscular arrangements, give complex tactual impressions." After remarking that it will perhaps be difficult to understand why *touch*, the simplest and earliest sense, should in its higher forms be more than any other sense associated with the advance of intelligence, he says : " The explanation lies in the fact that tactual impressions are those into which all other impressions have to be translated before their meanings can be known." Of the human hand : " All that we need here notice is, the extent to which, in the human race, a perfect tactual apparatus subserves the highest processes of the intellect. I do not mean merely that the tangible attributes of things have been rendered completely cognisable by the complex and versatile adjustments of the human hands, and that the accompanying manipulative powers have made possible those populous societies in which alone a wide intelligence can be evolved. I mean that the *most far-reaching cognitions, and inferences the most remote from perception*, have their roots in the definitely combined impressions which the *human hands* can receive." (No italics in original.)

The study of cases of disease of the nervous system appears to me to offer continual illustrations of the correctness of many of Spencer's deductions.

## REMARKS ON SYSTEMIC SENSATIONS IN EPILEPSIES[1]

THE order of frequency in which the higher senses suffer in epilepsies is, Dr. Hughlings Jackson believes, sight, smell, hearing. An aura of taste is very rare; a "sting," or other nongustatory aura from the tongue, is not so uncommon. It is not easy to say where touch comes.

In our investigation of epilepsies, we must not pass over those sensations which Lewes calls systemic sensations, and which Bain calls organic sensations. Speaking of the error of restricting sensations to the reactions of the five senses, Lewes says: "Physiology teaches us that there is another, and, indeed, far more important class of sensations, arising from what I have proposed to call the systemic senses, because, distributed through the system at large, instead of being localised in the eye, ear, tongue, etc. . . . they make up the greater part of that continuous stream of sentience, on which each external stimulus raises a ripple." It is probable that the "aura" from the neighbourhood of the epigastrium (sensation referred there, that is) is a crude and excessive development of visceral and other systemic sensations. However, if so, it seems strange that these sensations should, as is most common, occur in those cases of epilepsy in which loss of consciousness is, next to such warning, the first event in the paroxysm. For it implies that systemic sensations are first and most represented in the highest processes. Epilepsy, in which loss of consciousness is the first, or one of the first, events, is often preceded not only by development of systemic sensations, but is attended by pallor of the face. Indeed, the experiments of disease seem to show that the very highest processes (those underlying consciousness) sum up and re-represent all lower processes of the body. The epigastric sensation, so-called "aura," is variously described by patients. Some speak of it as a "fear"; a woman, 19 years of age, said it was "a frightened feeling, as if I had done something wrong." Another patient said it was "an indescribable feeling of horror." Women at the change of life and other persons will complain that they feel depressed, and as if they had done something wrong; and, when asked the seemingly ludicrous question, "Where do you feel it?" will put the hand over the epigastrium. The local physical sensation usually described as a "sinking." These are, probably in most cases, referred sensations; but, probably, organic changes in the abdominal viscera will provoke mental depression in the predisposed; it is, indeed, almost proverbial that dyspepsia goes with melancholy, and some times with uncertainty of temper.

For what is called the physiology of the mind, the development of all kinds of sensations in cases of epilepsy, from the most impersonal (as of sight) to the most personal, the systemic, deserves serious consideration. To show the importance of the systemic sensations, we will quote again from Lewes's *Problems of Life and Mind*, p. 134. After remarking that "their immense superiority as *motors* has been singularly overlooked," he writes: "They make up by far the larger portion of our sentient material, since from them issue the emotions, sentiments, etc.; combined, indeed, with the objective sensations, but subordinating these as means to their ends, inasmuch as we only see what interests us."

[1] *British Medical Journal*, February 7, 1874, p. 174.

# ON TEMPORARY MENTAL DISORDERS AFTER EPILEPTIC PAROXYSMS [1]

In the wards of a general hospital we meet with many cases of insanity—mostly temporary. For example, patients are brought in by their friends or by the police for sudden attacks of mental disorder occurring after epileptic fits. Then there are cases of severe wounds, self-inflicted by lunatics ; and, of course, temporary mental disorders occasionally occur in patients who have been some time in the hospital for non-mental diseases. Besides, there are cases of delirium tremens, and all degrees of delirium in patients with acute disease—rheumatic fever, pneumonia, erysipelas, etc. So far I have spoken of active or positive mental symptoms. In cases of intra-cranial tumour, cerebral hæmorrhage, softening, etc., all grades of the negative condition of imbecility are seen.

At this moment there is in the hospital a patient who is maniacal after severe injury to the head and erysipelas. There is a woman maniacal of whose antecedent history nothing certain is known, but from her high temperature, from the state of her tongue, and the nature of her stools, she is supposed to be suffering from typhoid fever. [So it turned out.] The woman came herself to the hospital saying that she had had a " fit " ; possibly it was simple fainting. There is another maniacal woman who may possibly be just recovering from typhoid fever, but of her history nothing is known. These patients are not simply delirious, but delirious with violent action—requiring restraint. A man is in the hospital who is just recovering from a self-inflicted wound in the throat ; he is subject to slight fits, and his account that he knows nothing of the infliction of the injury is credible.

I think, then, the study of mental diseases may be well *begun* in general hospitals. We have there the advantage of seeing transient and very slight mental disorders—simple cases which are comparatively easily studied. Especially do we see or hear of many degrees of slight and transient disorders of mind after epileptic paroxysms, in the wards and in the out-patient room.

There are few diseases of more practical interest than epilepsy. Reynolds says that 7 per cent. of nervous diseases are epileptic. Besides this and other good reasons for the assertion, there is the fact that epilepsy is often associated with insanity. Indeed, according to Bucknill and Tuke, 6 per cent. of persons in asylums owe their insanity to epilepsy. It is not asserted merely that 6 per cent. of insane patients have epileptic fits, but that epilepsy is the cause of insanity in 6 per cent. of insane persons.

We have even stronger grounds for the assertion. The insanity of epileptics is often of a kind which brings them in conflict with the law. We have not only to treat epileptic patients, but we have occasionally to declare whether an epileptic is or is not responsible for certain quasi-criminal actions. The epileptic is beset with troubles ; besides the calamity of fits, and besides such ill chances as severely burning his face by falling into the fire, there is the possible further calamity that he may be punished for " crimes " he has committed

[1] *West Riding Lunatic Asylum Medical Reports*, vol. v, 1875.

unconsciously directly after a seizure. We may help them here as well as by treatment of their malady.

Epileptic insanity is usually violent, and the violence may take the form of crime from purely accidental circumstances. Falret says that all authors have noted the excessive violence of the acts of epileptic maniacs. I suppose this remark is made of asylum cases, of patients so bad that they require continued restraint.

Not being an alienist physician, I mostly see cases in which the mental symptoms after epileptic attacks are comparatively slight; often they are merely grotesque actions. I purposely dwell most on the slightest cases of all. I shall, I hope, give good reasons for doing so. In all the cases I relate, even in those where the symptoms were severe, the patients, prior to the outbreak of their temporary post-epileptic insanity, were in supposed good mental health; of their real mental condition I can know nothing accurately; at any rate, they were well enough to be at their occupations. A goodly number are brought to the hospital from workshops or from the street. Again, the symptoms in the cases I see are often very transitory.

Let me at once relate a case in order to show the kind of case of epileptic insanity we often see at the London Hospital, and the difficult circumstances in which we sometimes see it. I do not mind confessing that I have more than once found it hard to tell whether a patient's violent conduct was owing to an epileptic attack, to drunkenness, or to meningeal hæmorrhage. In some cases of fatal meningeal hæmorrhage, the patient is not apoplectic but uproarious. It is so also in some cases of severe and fatal injury to the head. We occasionally see maniacal patients without any history whatever; we sometimes cannot tell whether the patient has had a fit of any kind or not.

A man was brought to the hospital about six o'clock p.m., said to have had a fit, and to have been extremely violent. When first seen he was struggling with the police who had brought him in, but as soon as freed he appeared sensible but irritable. He dressed himself and looked about sensibly. He then attempted to leave the room, and on being prevented became very violent, hit out blindly, and had to be held down. After this he could not, or did not, give his name, and when asked his address said Bethnal Green. He asked for his bag (he was a postman), and was much disquieted until he got it, when he appeared thoroughly satisfied. Subsequently he repeated his attempt to leave, and his blind violence when prevented. An hour and a half later he gave his name and address, said that he was accustomed to have fits, and that on several occasions he had lost his senses for half an hour, or for several hours; at this time he said he felt perfectly well again and fit for duty. His wife said that he was generally violent after the fits, that he had threatened her life, and that she was much afraid of him in the fits.

As I speak of epileptic insanity, I ought perhaps, before I go further, to say what I mean by epilepsy; for my opinions as to the nature of epilepsy are accepted by very few physicians. But for my present purpose I will adopt the accepted definition of epilepsy. I can properly do this, as the definition is symptomatic. The genuine epilepsy of authorities is but one epilepsy (according to my definition of the word "epilepsy").

According to authorities, epilepsy is a chronic disease of which the characteristic symptom is a sudden loss or trouble of consciousness occurring occasionally. The affection of consciousness is sometimes accompanied by evident spasm of muscles, and sometimes occurs without obvious spasm. The essential thing, according to this definition, is the paroxysmal affection of consciousness. It should, however, I think, be the occurrence of affection of consciousness very early in the paroxysm.[1]

There are three varieties of epilepsy as it is above defined. This division of course is arbitrary, although it is convenient. In fact, these are not so much varieties as degrees of the same thing. The three are called (*a*) vertigo, (*b*) *le petit-mal*, (*c*) *le grand-mal*. Not only is there affection of consciousness in each of these, but it is, I repeat, the first, or nearly the first, thing in the paroxysm; this must be borne in mind. There are three other things about epilepsy to be kept vividly in mind.

(1) That there occur all degrees of obscuration of consciousness, not loss only, in cases of epilepsy. From temporary confusion of thought (which is "defect of consciousness") to deepest coma there are all gradations. In fact, the patient who is subject to "genuine" epileptic attacks may have had (what he will probably call "sensations" or "turns") abortive seizures without any affection of consciousness before he ever had a full attack; for example, he may have had paroxysmal epigastric sensations only.

(2) That there are all degrees of severity of epileptic paroxysms, from giddiness attended by trivial confusion of thought, to a full violent seizure with universal convulsion and deep coma. This is indeed almost a repetition of the former statement, and it is repeating that the three so-called varieties or degrees are really arbitrary separations.

(3) And, most important, that cases of epilepsy in which there are the slightest attacks are the worst for mind. We must not forget this for two reasons: (*a*) the importance of these attacks is unfortunately often underrated because they are slight; (*b*) the attack being slight and transitory it is liable to be overlooked, and attention may be paid exclusively to its sequelæ, that is, to the patient's grotesque actions, raving, etc. These may in a woman be erroneously attributed to hysteria, and in a savage man to criminal intent. The gravity of these cases is not because the paroxysms are slight, but because the "discharging lesion," in cases in which such slight fits often occur, is of the highest and most intellectual nervous arrangements (substrata of consciousness).

I intend to speak only of temporary insanity *after* epileptic paroxysms. There are two other ways in which mental disorder is related to epilepsy. There is not only (1) the sudden and transient mental disorder after one or a few fits, but also (2) more lengthy infirmity after a rapid succession of numerous fits; and again (3) the persistent deterioration (imbecility),[2] the result of fits repeated for months or years.

[1] The distinction into cases of epilepsy with, and cases of epilepsy or epileptiform seizures without, loss or trouble of consciousness is useful for practical purposes. But, scientifically, it is arbitrary and has no rational basis. It is an empirical distinction of psychological, not of anatomical or physiological, parentage. The epilepsy of authorities is to me but *one* epilepsy; the paroxysms in it are, I consider, results of "discharging lesions" beginning in the *very highest* nervous centres of the cerebral hemisphere. Other epilepsies (such seizures, for example, as are commonly called epileptiform) differ in that in them the "discharging lesion" is of nervous arrangements of subordinate centres in the cerebral hemisphere. In them consciousness is lost late or not at all. But even empirically and for practical purposes (that is, from the symptomatic or from the clinical point of view), the distinction should not be into genuine epilepsy and epileptiform seizures; it should be into cases in which loss of consciousness is the first event and cases in which it occurs early, cases in which it occurs late, or not at all.

[2] Falret concludes that "delirium chiefly occurs as a consequence of epileptic attacks, recurring at short intervals after a prolonged suspension of the disease."

Cases of epileptic insanity have, of course, been long well known to alienists. For the first, and also I believe the best, scientific account we are indebted to Falret. Trousseau has given an account of the subject in one of his lectures. The third part of Trousseau's lecture is made up almost entirely of quotations from Falret's book. A most valuable case of " masked epilepsy " has been reported by Dr. Thorne Thorne, *St. Bartholomew's Hospital Reports*, 1870.

I intend to consider not only cases of violent doings, but cases in which the patient simply acts oddly, as, for example, such cases as that of a patient who after a paroxysm blew his nose on a piece of paper, cases in which there is no direct medico-legal interest. The latter have nevertheless an important *indirect* medico-legal interest. It is convenient to have one name for all kinds of doings after epileptic fits, from slight vagaries up to homicidal actions. They have one common character—*they are automatic* ; they are done unconsciously, and the agent is irresponsible. Hence I use the term *mental automatism.* I say mental, as the doings are probably external signs of crude mental states,—external signs of " epileptic dreams."

Every one of the cases I have to relate is an illustration of Laycock's doctrine of Reflex Cerebral Action ; in fact, I hope the cases will show that this hypothesis of Laycock, nearly forty years old, is one of inestimable value, both for scientific and practical purposes.

I have spoken of mental automatism as occurring *after* the paroxysm, but I must mention that according to some, I believe most, alienist physicians that degree of it which is called epileptic mania, although it usually occurs *after* a fit, does not always do so. It sometimes " replaces " a fit. A patient who is subject to ordinary epileptic attacks may, on this hypothesis, have, as it were, *instead* a paroxysm of mania. There is what is called the *masked* epilepsy, described by Falret. It has been said that the patient who is subject to attacks in which there is convulsion of muscles may at another time have an attack in which there is " convulsion of ideas," and corresponding excess of external action (mania). I used to adopt the hypothesis of masked epilepsy. But I do not now think it possible that a nervous discharge at all comparable in degree to that which causes convulsion would cause even such caricatures of normal action as occur either in epileptic mania or in slighter cases of mental automatism. I now think another hypothesis is preferable. I think it probable that there is a transitory epileptic paroxysm in every case of mental automatism occurring in epileptics before their mental automatism sets in. I am fully aware, and freely admit, that occasionally no signs of a prior fit are *discoverable*. The patient who at other times has ordinary convulsive seizures may become suddenly maniacal, although even when under observation he presented no physical change to indicate a paroxysm before the raving begins. To acknowledge this fully let me give an example. I wish to show that I look the difficulty full in the face. A very intelligent medical man came up to town with an epileptic patient of mine. He afterwards told me that the patient became suddenly, without any premonitory symptom to indicate an epileptic paroxysm, very much excited, struggling more or less violently with his attendants for twenty minutes. Nevertheless, I think it more probable (I think it a smaller hypothesis) that in this and in every case of sudden mental automatism in epileptics there has been a prior slight and transient paroxysm. I believe there is in such cases, during the paroxysm, an internal discharge too slight to cause obvious external effects, but strong enough to put out of use for a time more or less of the highest nervous centres. The mental automatism results, I consider, from over-action of lower nervous centres, because the highest or controlling centres have been thus put out of use. The automatism in these cases is not, I think, ever epileptic, but always post-epileptic. The condition after the paroxysm is duplex : (1) there is loss or defect of consciousness, and there is (2) mental automatism. In other words, there is (1) loss of control *permitting* (2) increased automatic action.[1]

I cannot discuss this matter here ; for medico-legal purposes it may, however, be assumed either that mental automatism always occurs after, or that in some cases it replaces, an epileptic seizure. In most cases there is clear proof that it does occur after the seizure.

Scientifically, the slighter degrees of post-epileptic mental automatism are the more important, for these cases are simpler experiments on the organ of mind. Moreover, the study of them is desirable, as they give us a clue to the nature of the severer degrees. I use the word " slight " as the opposite of violent or severe, for cases in which there is great raving, etc. It is not enough borne in mind that the more imperfect and the shorter the paroxysm, the more likely is it that *elaborate* delirium and correspondingly *elaborate* automatic actions will follow. This is, however, what on Laycock's hypothesis of Reflex Cerebral Action and Spencer's hypothesis of Nervous Evolution, we should expect *a priori*. Hence the transitory slight seizure may be overlooked or not inquired for at all, and an opinion as to the nature of the case may be formed from one part of it, from the more persistent, elaborate, grotesque post-epileptic action.

Our first task in such an inquiry as this is to show that, what I have called elaborate, but what are better called highly compound actions, can be done automatically—*i.e.* unconsciously. *It is not simply a question of the social importance or violence of the actions, but of their degree of complexity*. This must not be forgotten. Here again I would urge the importance of the slight fits. It seems to me to follow of necessity that the slighter the fit the more complex the mental automatism will be.[2] Again, it is not so much a question of the

[1] I believe that there is a double condition in insanity, whether acute and temporary, as in epileptic mania, or chronic, as in insanity ordinarily so-called ; there is a positive and a negative condition. I find that this opinion was stated long ago by Dr. Monro. The principle it illustrates was formulated by Laycock ten years earlier. The increased action (positive state, *i.e.* the raving, etc.) is owing to what, metaphorically speaking, is loss of control of lower centres by the highest centres, of which the function is lost or impaired (negative state, defect or loss of consciousness). This principle of over-action of lower centres as a consequence of loss of control from inaction of higher centres was stated by Anstie in his *Stimulants and Narcotics*. It was stated quite independently with regard to the epileptic paroxysm by Dr. Thompson Dickson. In this application of the principle I do not agree, but I think it applies to the very different condition of epileptic mania to which also Dr. Thompson Dickson applied it. See also Rutherford, *Lancet*, April 29, 1871. My own hypothesis is, that the epileptic discharge " removes control " by temporarily paralysing the highest centres. The highest centres are temporarily exhausted, paralysed, or put out of use by the strong discharge, just as a subordinate nervous centre (corpus striatum ?) is by a discharge of convolutions near it in cases of hemiplegia after convulsions beginning unilaterally. (Epileptic Hemiplegia of Dr. Todd.) It must never be forgotten that in post-epileptic insanity the " control " has been removed very suddenly. This fact bears, I think, on the interpretation of the violence which often characterises epileptic mania.

[2] At least it follows on the principle of Dissolution, and on the supposition that the discharge begins in the highest centres, as I believe it to do in the cases we have here to do with where there is loss or defect of consciousness at or very soon after the onset of the paroxysm. Of course I use the term Dissolution as the opposite of evolution. Nervous evolution is from the general to the special, from the simple to the complex. The highest nervous arrangements, the climax of the evolution, are the substrata of consciousness. The reverse process of dissolution, when it begins in these highest centres, will be from the most special to the general, from the

enormity of the actions as of their absurdity. On this view the recital of cases in which, after epileptic paroxysms, actions in themselves trumpery occurred, is relevant medico-legally as well as scientifically.

But even before speaking of slight automatic actions *developing* after epileptic seizures, one may remark that if a slight fit occurs while the patient is already employed in something which is largely automatic, as, for example, playing a well-practised tune, he may go on doing that automatic thing—may continue playing correctly whilst unconscious. The automatic action had, so to speak, possession of the mind, and consciousness was not concerned in it before the paroxysm occurred. Everyone has seen a person play a simple well-learned tune when talking of something else ; a transitory lack of consciousness might not interfere with his performance. In the following cases, however, *new* automatic actions were developed, or those actions going on were altered when the epileptic paroxysm had removed control. It is very interesting, however, to note that the alteration is sometimes not in the " form " of the action, but in the " contents " of that form. (See cases below.)

The first few of the following cases read almost like unscientific curiosities, but their indirect medico-legal interest is really very great indeed ; their scientific value is also very great.

A patient who had consulted me for epilepsy, whilst standing taking leave turned of a leaden white and looked very ghastly for a short time. He swayed a little, but did not totter. After a moment he came to himself, but he did not remember[1] that he had just before this attack given me my fee. This instance is not much to the point, but it leads up to another. On the next consultation, after replying properly to a series of questions, he gave no answer to one. I waited a little time, and then, looking at him, I saw that he was grinning as if amused at something. Next, whilst sitting quietly in his chair, he tore a piece off a packet of prescriptions, and put it in his mouth. I took it away, but he picked up another piece from the floor and began to chew it. In about a minute more he came to himself, and then spat out into the fire a pellet of chewed paper.

The following is a note of the case of a patient under my care in the London Hospital, who had several degrees of seizures. He had little attacks (*le petit-mal*) and grave attacks (*le grand-mal*) of epilepsy. " I was sitting on his bed taking his history, he sitting by my side holding the inkstand. After asking him a question, and getting no answer, I looked at him. He remained sitting, but his head was a little drooped, and his face slightly pale. He still kept hold of the inkstand, and after a moment moved as if to put it down. I tried to get hold of it as it was tilting, but he pushed me away with the other

most complex to the simple, or (using terms which are in this connection somewhat lax) from the most voluntary to the automatic. It is obvious, then, that the shallower the dissolution (the slighter the fit) the more highly compounded will be the consequent mental automatism. For, the shallower it is, the more are the nervous arrangements, next in speciality and complexity to the very highest, spared.

[1] On a minute scale this is an illustration of what is very often noticed, *viz.* that in failing memory recent events soonest fade away. Indeed, to some extent this occurs, I submit, daily. Our very highest processes are " swept clean " by sleep ; there is a daily oblivescence. Probably the unconscious cerebration (reflex action of Laycock) is active during sleep. There are two halves of thought, tracing resemblances and noticing differences. The former is the more automatic. This is the duplex form of all thought whatever. I think that the first half, tracing resemblances, is that which is active in sleep. It is, I think, to exaggeration of this half of thought, the resuscitation of ideas one after another by organised resemblances, that delirium and insanity, etc., are constituted.

hand. He was well again in about half a minute." The fact that this man's mental automatism was on this occasion of no importance to himself or to others, does not destroy its significance. Trivial as the affair was, his pushing me away shows most plainly an adjustment of actions done unconsciously, or, at any rate, with obscured consciousness, to external interference. We shall see the bearing of this later on.

Another epileptic patient of mine, when in an omnibus, blew his nose on a piece of paper, presumably after a slight fit. When he got out he gave the conductor £2 10*s.* instead of the usual coppers. This man was subject to both little and great seizures. It is important to note that the " form " of these actions was correct.

A patient of mine was seized with a fit whilst feeling a gentleman's pulse; when he came round, in another room, he began to feel his sister's pulse, she being near him.

I have another patient under my care, who, his friends say, as soon as the fit starts runs out as fast as he can. He is also subject to temporary mental confusion, in which he is supposed to be intoxicated. On one occasion he took a fellow-workman's coat, and was accused of robbery.

In an earlier part of this article, page 122, I mention the case of a patient who became maniacal in a railway carriage. The following is an account of one of his slight attacks as recorded by a medical man who witnessed it:

" Just after a walk, and whilst sitting down, K. had an attack in the garden. Head turned to the left; eyes the same. He was pale, and made three or four clucking noises; cheeks looked hollow and pale. He rubbed his nose, made odd grabs at his trousers, boots, etc.; moved his hands in a rubbing manner. Then, after sitting quiet, he looked round, examined a letter, and seemed to want to fix his whereabouts. I asked him the name of the town we were in. He did not know. Twenty minutes after he said he did not remember the attack, but remembered the incidents of the moment before."

For some years this patient *invariably* looked at his watch immediately after each attack. He has not done this recently; but one day lately, some time after returning from the water-closet, he found the candle extinguisher in his waistcoat pocket. I suppose this was because " he " had taken the extinguisher for his watch during the loss of consciousness. The grabbings at his trousers, the taking out the watch, are evidently automatic actions: of course unconscious, and of course therefore irresponsible. It is, in one sense, grotesque to talk about such trumpery actions being irresponsible. But see how the consideration of such slight symptoms bears in this very case. Since all the above facts were written out, the patient became suddenly unruly, striking lamps in a place of public amusement, and afterwards in the street; when going home, he struck his medical attendant; next a boy who was passing, and also an interfering bystander. Now if this patient were suddenly and without provocation to injure someone seriously, we might show that he was really irresponsible, because we could bring evidence of former elaborate and yet non-criminal actions done unconsciously, and therefore irresponsibly, as well as evidence of the comparatively trivial outrages on public rights last mentioned.

The following case is the most valuable one I possess of post-epileptic mental automatism. Several years ago an educated man, 31 years of age, was under my care at the Hospital for the Epileptic and Paralysed for epileptic seizures—using, as I do, throughout this lecture, the term " epileptic " according to the accepted definition. He became unconscious, and bit his tongue in his severe fits, and slept several hours after each of these. He had had about 60 severe attacks. But he had also very frequently what he called slight "seizures." It is of these I wish to speak. These slight seizures were of different degrees. He used the words "slight," "strongish," and "strong" to describe his fits in the lists he supplied me with. After the slight attacks he did not sleep; we may almost say that instead he dreamed only, or was somnambulistic. The following is a note written by him. The italics represent parts he underlined:

"20th. Unconscious? for perhaps three-quarters of an hour, remember *ordering* dinner, but not *eating*, or paying for it, but did *both*, and returned to the office, where I *found myself* at my desk feeling rather confused, but not otherwise ill; *was obliged to call at the dining-room to ask if I had been ill, and if I had had any dinner*. The answer was *no* to the former, and *yes* to the latter question."

At my request he again asked the landlady and waiters if he had been ill, but they had noticed no peculiarity. He ascertained, too, that "My fellow-clerk, who usually goes to dine when I return to the office, says he did not observe any peculiarity, nor was I gone longer than usual." The landlady told him "that three weeks ago I paid for my dinner with half a sovereign, that she gave me the change, which I put into my pocket, and very soon afterwards I went to her and tendered a shilling in payment for the dinner, when she told me I had already paid for it, but that I did not appear to remember having done so."

The following is the instance which makes the case most valuable. All the details are important:

"My wife and her sister being present, had been talking about supper, when it was agreed that my wife and I should have some cold fowl, and the sister some cocoa if there were any fire. She went into the kitchen to see, and reported that there was one. Soon after I began to feel chilly after being so warm with gardening, and I said I would go down to the fire. I did so; and after standing there a few minutes, I felt symptoms of an attack, and sat down, I believe, on a chair against the wall. And here my recollection failed, the next thing I was conscious of being the presence of my brother and mother (who had been sent for as they lived opposite), and I have since been informed by my sister-in-law that she came into the kitchen, and found me standing by the table mixing *cocoa* in a dirty gallipot, half filled with bread and milk intended for the cat, and stirring the mixture with a mustard-spoon, *which I must have gone to the cupboard to obtain*.

"This caused them to send for my friends, to whom I talked, showing no surprise that they were there, and entirely unconscious of what I had been doing until told this morning. After I had recovered, I partook of some bread and butter, and a glass of brandy and water. I went to bed, where I passed a good night, though I woke early and could not go to sleep again."

The bearing of this case is that if the automatism, instead of being a caricature of innocent normal actions, had been "criminal" and equally elaborate, the patient would have had a bad chance of escaping punishment. As the facts stated under date of 20th, page 126, show, he had fits which were too slight to attract attention; the case indeed illustrates what was said (p. 123, that the slighter the fit the more complex the automatism after it. What form a man's mental automatism will take depends, I think, very much on what his natural disposition is. A savage and suspicious man would, when a fit had temporarily removed his highest faculties, more likely have killed someone than have mixed cocoa. And just as this poor fellow went to the cupboard for a mustard-spoon, so, had he been a savage man, he might have gone to another room for a poker when his sister-in-law came in. The value of the case is that it shows very elaborate actions done unconsciously. We must not underrate the mental automatism because what was done, not being violent, was unimportant. I repeat, the significant thing is the *complexity* of the action. Had an equally elaborate action ended in murder, it would have looked intentional. True, it would have been equally *absurd* had he killed his sister-in-law; but when emotions are strongly excited, most of us are not logical. If a man or woman killed a beloved child, we, as scientific men, have to do with the question of absurdity or insanity of that action rather than with its enormity. It might easily have happened that the prior suggestion had not been about supper and cocoa, but about burglary. He might have been reading or hearing accounts of robbery which should be justifiably resisted. He might have automatically killed his sister-in-law instead of automatically mixed cocoa for her in a dirty gallipot.

Let me at this juncture mention a case in which also there was proof of external suggestion modifying post-epileptic automatism. One of my epileptic patients would, after an attack of epilepsy, get up unconscious and go about as if looking for something, or he would walk about unconsciously with his tools in his hands. Such things are, however, not much to the point; they are very common. But it was said that he would talk after a fit of what he had been reading. Thus, one day he had been reading in the newspapers of the Queen's way of bringing up her children; after his next fit he said that the "children were all put under the Queen's shawl, and were going up above"—a grotesque and childishly-poetical statement of maternal solicitude, and its recompense if "above" meant heaven.[1] We shall again have to speak of the influence of external suggestion before the paroxysm itself, or indeed occurring in the paroxysm,[2] and before the mental automatism sets in. I would now add to the statement that the slighter the fit the more highly compounded the actions permitted, the statement, "and the more are they developed by external circumstances occurring just before, during, or after the paroxysm."

I now state cases with a criminal aspect, but essentially similar scientifically, in order to illustrate how the trivial cases bear. I begin with trifling crimes. I had a boy under my care who was subject to fits, beginning by a "subjective" sensation of smell; he would turn pale.[3] To use his mother's expression, he would often after the seizures "go right out of his mind." He

[1] An aphasic patient under my observation made many mistakes in speaking; he made one which reminds me of the epileptic's observation mentioned in the text. He said, "Where is your little chapel?" instead of "Where is your prayer-book?"

[2] By external suggestion "occurring in the paroxysm" I allude to developments of sensations of colour, smell, at the outset of the seizures, etc., and to hurts received in falling; all are practically external.

[3] It was an interesting and important fact that he would hold his nose when the fit began. No doubt as his consciousness became obscured "he" believed the smell was of something actually outside. It is, perhaps, too strong an expression to say "*he* believed," for where is the "*ego*" when a man is unconscious or partly so? We may say that the smell developed an epileptic dream. I had a woman under my care who at the beginning of an attack had "subjective" sensation of smell, who said, "What a dreadful stink there is in the place!" She believed the smell was of something in the room.

was a shoe-black ; and once after a seizure threw his blacking-box at a policeman. This was the "crime." For this he was taken before a magistrate, and fined five shillings. One evening after a fit he got into a rage, and said that a gentleman in the street had offered him five shillings to clean his boots. Later, he was taken to a lunatic asylum.

The following is an account written by an epileptic patient's mother. She begins by speaking of her son's fits. "When I first observed them he became suddenly senseless, and remained in the same position as when he was first seized. Sometimes, if he had an attack when standing, I have known him fall on his knees ; also he has had fits in the night, when he foamed at the mouth and bit his tongue. [He had *le petit-mal* and *le grand-mal*]. On one occasion he had a fit at a place of worship during the sermon and took off his coat, sitting like that till he recovered his senses. At another time he was taking his tea alone when my servant heard the front door opened and shut. He had left the house without his hat, and was away about three-quarters of an hour. When he recovered himself, he found he was walking round the church near our house. This occurred at night. On many occasions he has gone out in a similar way, and *he invariably now rises and unbuttons his waistcoat and trousers*. Last Sunday he had a fit at another place of worship, and took off his boots. He has had many in the street. His memory is always very bad for some time after an attack."

Here is an account of another attack written by the patient himself :

"I was in a shop at Twickenham seeking an order for wines ; I suddenly fell on my back—the first time I have fallen in a fit for six or nine months. The shopman at once came from behind the counter, and with the assistance of a friend raised me. I instantly threw my arms about and shook both off, but they caught hold of me again and led me out of the shop, when the friend left and I again made my escape from the shopman, leaving my hat and order-book behind. The shopman then got a man to mind his shop, and he and two policemen went in search of me, all going different ways.

"He first discovered me a quarter of a mile away, *asking for my hat at all the shops, but not having recovered my senses, nor did I until I got to the railway ten minutes after*."

That he asked for his hat at the shops before he gained consciousness is important, as showing normal actions done unconsciously. Had he committed a "crime" when apparently so much himself, but when really so unconscious, one would have little hope of convincing a magistrate of the poor fellow's irresponsibility.

On one occasion he unbuttoned his trousers when there were four women present (see the part of his mother's letter italicised). It is quite clear that this poor fellow will run great risk of being indicted for an indecent offence. Fortunately the four women were members of his own family. It would be hard to convince a magistrate or a jury that he was not fully aware of what he was doing if he unbuttoned his trousers in the park under certain circumstances. It is possible that this action arises from the notion that he has to make water, and not from any sexual excitement. His condition after a fit to be next mentioned might, I imagine, have been easily altered into a quasi-criminal one had he been roughly interfered with, or had he been naturally of a savage disposition. I gathered the following from him at a visit to the hospital. I copy from my case-book :

" A few days ago, he went into the back parlour as he felt he was going to have a fit. His mother followed him, and found that he had taken a knife out of his pocket and was grasping it, not by the handle, but by the blade. His mother took it away, shut it up, and put it behind the bookcase. He went to the bookcase, got it again, and then kept waving it about, but it was now closed. His mother then got assistance, and the knife was again taken from him."

His taking the knife and his getting it again when it had been taken from him are medico-legally very interesting facts, showing elaborateness ; on the other hand, taking the knife by the blade was absurd.

As some evidence of this patient's general competency, I may say that his father threatens to turn him out-of-doors for not supporting himself. He is an intelligent man, seems very calm and sober-minded, and, in spite of what his mother says, appears to be in good general health. In the intervals of his fits his memory is impaired, but not to any great extent. Yet the fact that he is occasionally for a short time incompetent from an attack, renders him unable to keep his situations. He has been a traveller for orders, and when walking he " loses himself," but goes on walking. In one fit he lost himself at Blackfriars, and came round again when at the Elephant and Castle. He has been knocked down by an omnibus, and has once nearly walked into the Thames. He remarks, and this is worthy of consideration, that he is quite safe in these walking attacks if he is alone. This, I think, supports the speculation that if roughly interfered with in the fit in which he was waving the knife about, his doings might have altered to graver actions.

I now pass to speak of cases in which the patient's doings were violent, a separation which is arbitrary, although convenient. The violence and outrageousness of the seizure depend doubtless very much on the natural disposition of the patient who suffers from the attack. There was no criminal action in the case I relate, but the " material " for crime was abundant. This case is of a very common kind, and therefore I need the less regret that my notes of the non-mental part of it are meagre.

A man, 47 years of age, had been subject to severe fits for seven or eight years when I first saw him. At first he used to sleep after his fit ; but after the first few " he raved instead." This was his own expression, and is no doubt essentially correct. He dreamed instead of sleeping deeply, as is most common after fits, and his raving was the external sign of his dream. After a fit at the hospital he was asleep or comatose for awhile before he raved. The order of events in the paroxysms was this—(1) coloured vision ; (2) convulsion (sometimes, I was told, of one side, sometimes of the other) and insensibility ; and (3) after the paroxysm raving. He had a fit at the hospital one day. I was called to him. He was out of it when I saw him, was very dark, and breathing hard as if half suffocated. I left him after awhile, but was called again soon, and found him up shouting, looking *alarmed*, and yet apparently lost to what was about him ; he struggled with us, but did not look at us. His fears were evidently of something else, of something in " a dream," no doubt. This state of things lasted about a quarter of an hour. He then seemed simply stupefied and despondent, but could answer simple questions.

As he seemed an intelligent man, I asked him to write out an account of his coloured vision, for indeed this is the part of the case which then interested me most.[1] The words in square brackets are replies to questions I put to him after reading what he had written, or observations of my own :

" Before having a fit I have a throbbing light of various colours [green, yellow, and red], in the right eye, which lasts sometimes 15, 20, or 30 minutes, which takes my sight and senses away, and then I go off into a fit, making a loud noise as if I were frightened. I then lie very quiet. I am much convulsed, sometimes for 20, 30, 40 minutes [no doubt a succession of fits], and when I am coming to out of the fit, I rave like a maniac, and gradually come to my senses in about half an hour [of course this is what he was told]. I sometimes have those throbbing colours in my right eye, which last a few minutes and stop suddenly, and then I do not have a fit, only feel giddy for a short time. I mostly have a fit about every four or five weeks.

" Saw the doctor on Monday, February 16. The next day (Tuesday, 17th), had pains at back of ears ; had those colours in my eye, which lasted about five minutes and stopped suddenly ; felt as if a fit was coming on.

" February 26. About ten o'clock in the morning was taken very bad with the throbbing in the right eye ; could see various colours floating about, and lasted so until twelve. It then went off into a fit which lasted about an hour, was very much convulsed, came to a bit, and raved very much ; got gradually better and got my senses about three o'clock ; my eyes been very much bad with throbbing, and bad-sighted since."

This patient's case has only an indirect medico-legal interest ; I mean, it is for this purpose too simple, as the man was *known* to be subject to severe epileptic fits. But were the man to have killed someone in his first maniacal attack, the prior paroxysm not having been witnessed, he would possibly have been hanged.

We have sometimes in the same patient post-epileptic doings of different degrees, from a sort of quiet somnambulism to violent struggling. Seven years ago I had under my care a boy, 19 years of age, who had abnormal mental states after epileptic seizures, which illustrate this remark. The following is an account his father gave me. The exact onset of this condition was not noted in the symptoms to be first described, but in other seizures his father said that " the lad's eyes are open, he gets stiff, grinds his teeth ; the next [no doubt post-epileptic] is trying to get away, struggling," etc.

Last time he had a fit and went to bed, and when in bed said, " Wait a bit, Bill. I am coming." He went downstairs, he unbolted the doors, and went out in his night-shirt. He came to himself just as he was stepping on cold stones, and then his father touched him. He said that he had had a dream :

[1] The coloured vision was the subjective side of what was objectively the beginning of the cerebral discharge, which, increasing in strength, and therefore spreading, led to convulsion. Sometimes the discharge does not increase in strength, and does not spread. Sometimes it did not in this case ; the patient had occasionally attacks of coloured vision only. Similarly a man subject to fits beginning in his index-finger and thumb may have sometimes twitching of those digits only, and sometimes this twitching will lead on to a one-sided, or even further, to a universal convulsion.

I believe that this patient's seeming alarm in the post-epileptic raving was the result of some terrible dream developed in him by the coloured vision. I believe that the colour first developed in epileptics, when colour is the first symptom (warning or aura), is usually red ; it is not always so. I find that this is not a novel observation. Falret has pointed out that a premonitory symptom or beginning of an epileptic seizure is often red vision, but he adds " or purple." Again Falret, speaking of epileptic maniacs, says, " They constantly see luminous objects, flames, circles of fire ; and what is worthy of *remark, the colour red or the sight of blood* frequently predominates in their visions."

"It's all right, I have had a dream." He went to bed, and had not been in bed five minutes when he began again talking of Bill (an acquaintance in the volunteers), saying, "You are in a great hurry to get your coat on." His father went into his bedroom again, called his brother, and got the patient into bed. Then a fit, so his father says, began (I suppose it to have been post-epileptic automatism), and they were obliged to get a policeman. The policeman, I was told, got on the patient's chest, the others got hold of his arms and legs. The struggling only lasted about three or four minutes, but returned many times during four hours. This struggling was evidently mania.

The following case is the one of most direct medico-legal interest. I have to thank Mr. Rivington for permission to use it. It was a case of self-mutilation under his surgical care, in January 1874. I have to thank Mr. Mercier for taking notes of it for me. I beg attention to all the details Mr. Mercier gives; they are all important, either medically or legally. Any imperfection in the report is, I think, owing to difficulties in getting information. For any imperfections otherwise caused, I am at least fully responsible, as I frequently saw the patient with Mr. Mercier. I read his notes carefully from time to time. In January 1875, Mr. Mercier called on the patient, and obtained clearer accounts of some things in the case; but it will be well to give the report, showing how the case appeared when she was admitted, January 1874—a year before. It is most important to remark that many of our hospital patients or their friends, as do many of our private patients, give imperfect, erroneous, or confused accounts of their former conditions.

*Family history.*—A woman, aged about 35. Patient's maternal grandmother was in a lunatic asylum. Her maternal uncles and aunts died young. Her mother was melancholy, taciturn, and suspicious, and used frequently to say that she had "hosts of enemies." There is no history of cerebral disorder on the father's side. The patient's children are all healthy in mind and body; the second died of convulsions.

*Personal history.*—The patient herself has never exhibited any signs of madness before the present outbreak, but she has always been irritable and passionate. She never did odd things. (*Vide infra.*)

*Patient's own account.*—She was married thirteen years ago. Before her marriage she used now and then to faint away; she would fall down and lose consciousness, but never had convulsions. About a year after her marriage she began to have "fits," attended by loss of consciousness and convulsions. When the fit came on she would fall suddenly and remain unconscious for an hour, more or less. These fits recurred at intervals of about a month, and came on chiefly at the menstrual periods. She also had them during pregnancy.

*History of present illness.*—On the afternoon of January 19, 1874, the patient was cutting bread for her children's tea, when she suddenly sent them all out of the room, and was found a short time after lying in a pool of blood with a deep gash in the left arm, which divided all the structures in front of the elbow, and laid the joint open. It was then found that she was out of her senses; she was at once brought to the hospital, and was then in the following condition.

*Patient's state on admission.*—She had evidently lost a great deal of blood; her face was extremely pale, her lips livid, her radial pulse at first wholly inappreciable. Her face had a most peculiar, wild, horror-struck expression, due to her eyebrows being raised, and the upper eyelids lifted quite away from the upper edge of the cornea ; to her nostrils being much dilated, and her lips drawn in. She was excited, maniacal ; she tossed her arms about, tried to get off the stretcher, asked for her husband, who had been dead some months, confused the people around with her acquaintances. She seemed to feel no pain from her arm, although she occasionally looked at the wound and said it was cruel. *She accused different people of doing it.*

*Gradual subsidence of mania.*—Her wound was dressed, and she was put to bed, where she soon became much calmer, and the peculiar expression before noticed disappeared from her face. Several times, however, it suddenly returned, and she struggled to get out of bed. She asked for water once or twice, but except this uttered no rational sentence. During the night she slept for several hours.

*Return of sanity on the morning after—Relapse at night.*—January 20, second day. She appeared utterly different, her face was flushed, her lips natural red, her face was composed, and she was conscious and rational. She remained quiet and sane throughout the whole of the day, but at night was raving violently, trying to get out of bed and do herself an injury.

*Variations in mental state.*—For the next two days the patient remained quiet, conscious, and rational. On the morning of the fifth day she appeared uneasy ; she looked anxious, and said that she was surrounded by enemies. That night she was raving and furious ; it took two people to hold her down. All her violence, however, was directed against herself. The next morning she explained that she had seen things about her ; when asked what things, she said, " Wolves." During the sixth and seventh days she was quiet and rational, but had a remarkable expression of face ; she looked half frightened and half suspicious, as if she anticipated harm. In the evening of the seventh day I was told that she was wild again. I found her lying in bed, not struggling, but crying out, " The world is coming to an end, cut my throat, let me choke myself " ; and this she endeavoured to do. On speaking to her firmly and peremptorily, she immediately answered rationally, and replied to numerous simple questions quite correctly. (Such questions as the day of the week and month, the ages of her children, etc.) She had then been raving about a quarter of an hour. She remained quiet for about five minutes, and then began again in exactly the same style, saying that the world was at an end, and that we were all at the bottom of the sea, and desiring to have her throat cut. When she is very excited she will not answer a question, but when only moderately so she will break off from exclaiming that the world is at an end, to reply to a simple definite question, or to perform any action that she may be told to—*e.g.* to shut her eyes, put her tongue out, etc. She would even in reply to questions tell a definite connected story about her children. The next moment she was raving as before. Her tongue was at this time strongly deflected to the left. There was no convulsive action of any part before the attack. Ten minutes later she was quiet and rational.

*Subsequent history.*—Since that time she has had no outbreak of such violence ; but she often expresses the utmost anxiety about her children, fancying that they are secreted somewhere about the hospital ; or about herself, fearing that she will be sent away or not allowed to go, or some other equally reasonless fear. She sometimes has visual, but does not have auditory, spectra.

The wound healed well, and the patient got into apparent good health, mental and physical.

*A year later, January* 10, 1875.—Emily A—— has had very good health since she left the hospital. She has had numerous " fainting fits," in which she loses her senses for a few minutes, but none of the long spells of unconsciousness that she used to have. She had always contrived that no one should see her in the fits, so that no particulars were to be obtained from others, but she herself says that she never does odd or strange things after the fits now. She says, however, that before she entered the hospital she used frequently after the fits to do very strange things. She would " turn the house upside down," and " pull the beds to pieces," and then wonder afterwards who could have been doing it. She has never harmed herself or anyone else, except on the one occasion when she came to the hospital. With regard to that fit she states that she felt very bad all the morning, and that she went to a doctor's in consequence. In the afternoon she felt so bad that she had to lie down ; and shortly after, when her son came and asked her for some bread and butter, she went downstairs, took a knife out of the drawer, and then feeling very ill came and lay down again without cutting the bread.

After this, she remembers no more until she was brought to the hospital.

*Present state of her arm and hand.*—The muscles on the palmar aspect of the forearm are atrophied, as are the thenar muscles. The interossei do not look wasted. The thumb and two outer fingers are livid, cold, and the skin is smooth and shining, unlike the others, which look normal. The nails of those three digits also are distorted.

The position of the two inner fingers is normal. The proximal phalanx of the two outer is extended beyond a right line with the dorsum, and the two distal phalanges are flexed. The thumb lies along the index and she cannot extend it. The wrist is strongly flexed and cannot be extended, owing to contraction of flexor muscles.

Sensation on thumb and two inner fingers dulled but not lost, and localisation is imperfect.

She is stout, florid, and looks in good general health ; does hard work.

That this was a case of mental disorder following an epileptic seizure, was, I think, practically certain. She had had slight attacks, faints, etc., which were no doubt *petit-mal*, and also convulsive seizures. I should believe that she had had a slight attack of *petit-mal* before she sent her children out of the room, for it is to be repeated that elaborate mental symptoms more commonly attend those cases of epilepsy in which there are little attacks (*le petit-mal*). In Mr. Mercier's second account (1875), *vide* p. 133, there is a history of strange doings after attacks (" pulling beds to pieces," etc.) The suddenness and the grotesque absurdity of the action are complementary evidence. The action was more important than the cocoa-mixing (see p. 126), but scientifically it was about on a par with it—that is to say, it was about an equally highly compounded action. It also was developed by external circumstances ; the knife was in her hand, for she was about to cut bread when taken ill.

Self-mutilation is itself a crime. It is no great stretch of imagination to assume that it was a sort of accident that the woman did not cut the throats of her children instead of her own arm. A case thus presented would not be easy to the laity. It was not known that she had had fits. It was the woman's first outbreak of mental disorder, or rather the first striking attack ; this would have told against her. Her case well illustrates the importance of studying grotesque actions as well as violent actions. There was seeming method in what she did. She sent the children out of the room. This is analogous to the act of the cocoa-mixer, p. 126, who went to the cupboard for a mustard-spoon. It might have fared badly with her had she sent out an elder son and cut the throat of a little child. Moreover, her subsequent raving, although genuine, was of a common, wild, very incoherent sort, and might have looked like pretence to a suspiciously minded layman's " common sense."

I have already given evidence from the mental automatism of simple cases, that elaborate and highly compound actions may be gone through when a patient is unconscious—presumably after an epileptic seizure. I have also shown that the mental automatism may be developed by suggestion, or altered thereby. She was cutting bread when, as I suppose, the fit (or, as she would say, " faint ") took her.

In a legal inquiry, the facts as to heredity are exceedingly important, but their bearing is so obvious that I should be wasting time were I to dwell on their importance in such a case. The *nature* of the insanity in the mother must be mentioned ; she was suspicious, and had, she thought, " hosts of enemies." The patient herself was irritable and passionate. Her accusation of others when she came to the hospital is noteworthy. Her mental condition at that time might easily have led people to suppose that she had been injured by some-one else, except indeed for the nature of the injury. Then her subsequent mental condition was significant—she was " surrounded by enemies."

# ON EPILEPSIES AND ON THE AFTER-EFFECTS OF EPILEPTIC DISCHARGES (TODD AND ROBERTSON'S HYPOTHESIS)[1]

In the article in vol. iii of these *Reports* (" The Anatomical, Physiological, and Pathological Investigation of Epilepsies ") I spoke almost solely of the *direct* effects of epileptic discharges. It is very important, however, to study carefully the after-effects of these discharges—the condition of the patient when the discharge has ceased. I am not now speaking of what is commonly called the inter-paroxysmal condition, but of the temporary state of the patient immediately after the paroxysm—which will be called the post-paroxysmal condition. This has not, so far as I know, been studied methodically. We have descriptions of loss of consciousness or coma remaining after severe epileptic seizures, but the physical phenomena have not been carefully analysed even in these cases. We have, too, accounts of mania after epileptic seizures (" epileptic mania "), but I submit that the accepted interpretation of this important sequence is not in accordance with facts. The after-effects of epileptic discharges of subordinate cerebral centres causing limited convulsive seizures have commonly received least attention. Yet these cases are by far the most profitable for investigation of the after-effects of excessive nervous discharges (epileptic discharges) in general. If we arrive at an explanation of the causation of post-epileptic hemiplegia, we shall then more easily explain post-epileptic loss of consciousness with mania (epileptic mania). The clinical nomenclature is confusing : thus the mania in epileptic mania is not a thing analogous to hemiplegia in epileptic hemiplegia ; for besides other obvious differences, the former is a positive condition, the latter is a negative one. Some preliminary remarks on epilepsy are needed.

An epileptic discharge was defined (see p. 94) as an occasional, sudden, excessive, rapid, and local discharge of some *part* of the cerebral hemisphere—a discharge of some *part* of the cortex which has become highly unstable. There is what I call a " discharging lesion." These lesions are, as above said, supposed to be always local, notwithstanding that their discharge, when in the highest centres (as in so-called genuine epilepsy), may produce convulsion of all parts of the body nearly contemporaneously. As above defined, the term " epilepsy " is not the name for any one grouping of symptoms, but for any set of symptoms whatever presented paroxysmally from discharge of some *part*

[1] *West Riding Asylum Medical Reports*, vol. vi, 1876.

I find that the explanation which I thought I was the first to give of the effects of strong epileptic discharges in producing temporary paralysis has been given before, as the subjoined quotation shows. I fully acknowledge the priority of Todd and Alexander Robertson by giving the quotation and by placing their names in the title of this article. Thus I may proceed in the text in my own way. This article was written before I came across the following or before it attracted my attention : " But I am inclined to think that the late Dr. Todd was correct in supposing that severe and protracted convulsions may themselves in some instances be causative of palsy of a few hours' or days' duration, through simply the exhausting influence exerted on the cells of the central ganglia without much, if any, appreciable change of tissue. This explanation is especially applicable to some cases of hemiplegia following epilepsy in which the paralysis passes away in a few days " (Alexander Robertson, *Edinburgh Medical Journal*, December 1869).

of the cerebral cortex. Whether consciousness be lost or not matters nothing for this definition.

What is to come will be unintelligible unless the reader bears in mind:

(1) That it is assumed that all nervous centres, from the lowest spinal centres to the very highest centres (the substrata of consciousness), are made up of nothing else than nervous arrangements representing impressions and movements. The fact that movements are not produced by slight galvanic or faradaic currents applied to the cortex beyond Hitzig and Ferrier's region, does not disprove this. I do not see of what other "materials" the rest of the brain can be made. The term "impression" includes all cases where a peripheral effect (skin, tissue, or viscera) disturbs a nervous centre, and the term "movement" is used in an unusually extended sense, to cover not only effects produced by nerve centres on muscles (including arterial coats, muscular fibres of intestine, etc.), but on glands and effects by inhibitory nerves.

(2) That states of consciousness, although always parallel with, are utterly different from, nervous states, which in the higher (the cerebral) centres are, as in the lower, concerned with impressions and movements. It is not said that mind is made up of nervous arrangements for impressions and movements, but that the substrata of mind are thus constituted. Hence we do not say that any kinds of mental state *arise from* nervous discharges, but that they *occur* during nervous discharges.

Partly to enforce these remarks, I will repeat, but I hope with more precision, what I said (see p. 99) as to the kind of distinction I make betwixt cases of epilepsy where there is loss of consciousness and cases where there is not. Let me remark first that the presence or absence of consciousness in an epileptic paroxysm is not even the *empirical* distinction which I make betwixt different kinds of epilepsy. The empirical distinction is into cases where consciousness is lost first of all in the paroxysm, soon after the onset, late, or not at all. The distinction scientifically is that consciousness is lost at the onset of the paroxysm, or almost at the very first, when the discharge *begins in the very highest nervous centres*, these centres being the substrata of consciousness. Consciousness is lost late when the discharge begins in a subordinate centre—in some part of Hitzig and Ferrier's region for example. In epileptic discharge of these centres consciousness may not be lost at all; all depends on the momentum of the discharge, and therefore on how far it spreads. How it is that consciousness is lost during epileptic discharges of some *part* only of the highest cerebral centres will be explained later.

In very slight epileptic discharges, even of the highest centres, there may be only slight defect of consciousness, with only slight confusion of thought. Briefly, whether consciousness be lost or not depends on the *seat* of the discharging lesion and on the momentum of the discharge.

Another thing (a corollary from the foregoing) never to be forgotten is that the affection of consciousness is not a "symptom" comparable with any kind of abnormal physical state. One reason for this remark is that in my former article (see p. 99) I wrote: "Loss of consciousness is not an utterly different thing from other symptoms." This was a very blundering statement, but the context showed clearly, I hope, that what was meant was that cases of epilepsy, with loss of consciousness at the onset, depend on discharge of sensori-*motor* centres, just as do cases of epilepsy (or, as they are commonly called, epileptiform seizures) in which there is no affection of consciousness, the *difference* being not in the kind of constitution of the centres, but in their degrees of evolution. The following statements are, I hope, free from such blunders.

Suppose that from an epileptic discharge of a subordinate motor centre we have convulsion of the arm ; we do not compare this with loss of consciousness in a case of *le petit-mal*, where there is epileptic discharge of nervous arrangements in the highest centres. We compare the spasm of the arm from discharge of the subordinate cerebral centre with spasm of arteries (as signified by facial pallor), of the eyes, hands, arrest of respiration, etc., from discharge of the highest cerebral centres. That consciousness ceases during the latter discharge, and not during the former, is not the thing of moment in an anatomico-physiological inquiry.

According as the seat of the discharging lesion varies the symptoms of the paroxysm vary. And since the cerebral centres—even the highest of them—represent or re-represent all parts of the body, we have all kinds of symptoms in the paroxysms from differently seated discharging lesions. Let me give a rough list of some of the more important of them : increased flow of saliva ; pallor of face ; shivering, with *sensation* of cold ; arrest of respiration with *sensation of suffocation ; coloured vision ; noises in the ears ; nausea* (and other less definite *sensations* referred to the epigastrium) ; movements of the eyes with *vertigo* ; convulsion of the limbs, etc. The words in italics are names of mental states (sensations) ; the physical states corresponding to them are of course meant and are in some of the cases mentioned. Which of these symptoms occur, or which preponderate, or in what order any of them occur in co-existence or in sequence, depends on the seat of the discharging lesion and on the momentum of the discharge. In other words, every epilepsy is a development, but a brutal development, of the functions (1) of some *part* of the cerebral cortex, the cells of which part by some pathological process have become highly unstable ; and (2) especially when the momentum of the discharge is great, of collateral and lower healthy centres. From this it follows that there is, scientifically speaking, no entity to be called epilepsy ; but innumerable different epilepsies, as there are innumerable seats of discharging lesions. And as the first symptom in the paroxysm is the first effect of the discharge of the centre unstable, any two paroxysms *beginning* differently will differ throughout, however little. For practical purposes, it is convenient to have arbitrary types—definitions by type—but these are of no use in scientific investigations.

Recent experiments seem to show that what has been called " menial " work is part of the work of the cortex cerebri. " A relationship has been observed between the brain surface and the secretion of saliva, the beat of the heart, the action of vaso-motor nerves, and other organic functions ; but on these points the results of various observers are by no means constant " (Foster's *Physiology*, p. 441). It would be a very remarkable thing if the organic functions *were not* represented in the cortex cerebri. It would be very remarkable if the highest centres, the substrata of consciousness, did not represent the whole organism, the tissues, viscera, arterial system, and muscles. The physical phenomena occurring with transient loss of consciousness, in cases of *le petit-mal* would be unintelligible if the " organic functions " were not represented in the very highest centres. It would be most remarkable if the heart were not represented in every unit of the very highest centres.

For a fit to begin with loss of consciousness is for the epileptic discharge to begin in the highest centres (see p. 136). As regards two symptoms showing disturbance of "organic functions," increased flow of saliva, and deep facial pallor, it is to be observed that they will occur from the very slightest epileptic discharges of the highest centres; that is to say, in cases of *le petit-mal*. Herpin writes: "L'accumulation de la *salive* dans la bouche et dans la gorge est un des signes les plus constants des accès d'épilepsie. *On le retrouve même dans les simples vertiges*" (*Epilepsy*, p. 432).

Crichton-Browne (these *Reports*, vol. iii, p. 157) writes: ". . . Among the phenomena of the fit itself, pallor of the face is perhaps the earliest and most constant." Speaking of some cases of *le petit-mal* he says (op. cit.): ". . . This pallor is *the only* outward sign of the fit, and corresponds with the momentary unconsciousness or loss of perception and volition in which it consists."

It is to be noted, too, that emission of urine and fæces often occurs in slight cases of epilepsy due to epileptic discharges beginning in the very highest centres—*le petit-mal*. Herpin (op. cit., p. 433), writes: "Vomissements, selles, vents, ne sont montrés au milieu des accès que dans des crises fort légères." My own opinion is, however, that these symptoms do not occur *in*, but *after*, the paroxysm; they are too co-ordinated movements to result directly from epileptic discharges; there is, I think, a duplex condition: (1) negatively, loss of control; (2) positively, increased activity of healthy lower centres. Nevertheless, the association, or sequence, is very significant.

Equally unintelligible would be the occurrence of the bodily manifestations observed in normal emotion, or in the abnormal [1] emotion of hysteria.

These manifestations are exhibited in "all parts of the moving system, voluntary and involuntary; while an important series of effects is produced on the glands and viscera—the stomach, lungs, heart, kidneys, skin, together with the sexual and mammary organs" (Bain, *The Emotions and the Will*, p. 4).

I do not found these statements, however, on any recent experiments, properly so called, but on the experiments of disease. In the *Medical Mirror*, October 1869, I write, except for a few verbal alterations, as follows: "We have now, then, to add to the constitution of the units of the cerebrum nerve fibres to the heart, vessels, and viscera, or rather probably to regions of the sympathetic system, from which these parts are supplied. The inference we have now arrived at is that the units of the cerebral hemisphere (*in the region of the corpus striatum, at least*) represent potentially the whole processes of the body. If this be so, we can understand how it happens that in cases of epilepsy [beginning by loss of consciousness, *i.e.* the discharge beginning in the highest nervous arrangements], besides obvious convulsion, we have premonitory shivering, pallor of face, and increased flow of saliva, and in some cases vomiting. Thus, too, we see how it is that emotional manifestations accompany intellectual phenomena. Emotional manifestations are wide and yet temporary bodily states, and we have seen that the heart, arteries, and viscera,

[1] I believe, however, that there is a duplex condition in emotional states—negative (loss of control) and positive (over-activity of lower centres). I have seen somewhere, but where I cannot now remember, a remark on the strangeness that experimental irritation of the "centre" for an animal's tail should be the same centre as that for the secretion of saliva. Although I do not believe in such abrupt localisations, I see nothing remarkable in the association; the salivary glands will be in vigorous action when a lamb is sucking; its tail moves about in a ludicrous manner during that operation. Both parts are in action together during one emotional state.

as well as the large muscles of the body, are represented in the units of the cerebrum." I should now omit the words italicised, believing, as repeatedly stated, that the substrata of consciousness, the highest cerebral centres, as well as those in the region of the middle cerebral artery, represent the whole body. All the work of the cerebral cortex is "menial" if the secretion of saliva or the movement of a limb is menial work. During the highest kind of ideation there is menial work; for when we think of an object there is, on the physical side, an excitation of nerve cells and fibres representing retinal impressions and ocular movements.

These assertions would be strange indeed if they are taken to mean that nervous arrangements representing muscles, viscera, etc., constitute consciousness; but that inference has been repudiated. It is only said that they constitute the anatomical substrata of consciousness. No one knows why energising of any cells and fibres representing (1) muscles, tissues, viscera, etc.; or of cells and fibres representing (2) things in general; or of cells and fibres representing (3) nothing at all; or of cells and fibres representing (4) nothing in particular, is attended by any sort of psychical state. But although active nervous states are not psychical states, there is parallelism, and what we have to do in a medical inquiry is to discover the anatomy and physiology of the various nervous states *that go along with* various psychical states; and we have to note the *physical* manifestations when consciousness ceases during epileptic discharges. And those physicians who believe that nervous states and psychical states are one and the same thing are as much bound to take note of the physical manifestations which occur from discharges of "ideational centres" as those are who hold the commonly received doctrine that psychical states are utterly different from, although they always occur along with, nervous states.

From the above remarks it will be inferred that by highest centres we do not mean geographically highest, but anatomically highest. The highest centres are those which represent the most complex and most numerous different co-ordinations of impressions and movements of all parts of the body.

The symptoms of an epileptic paroxysm may be motor (convulsion), or there may be evidence of discharge of sensory centres. The hypothesis, I hold, is that the anterior part of the brain is *chiefly* motor, the posterior *chiefly* sensory. The evidence as to epileptic discharges of sensory centres obviously can only be indirect. We see nothing: the patient can only tell us of the mental states which occur along with them; he tells us, for example, that he has numbness or coloured vision. From this kind of evidence we *infer* discharges of sensory centres. The coloured vision, the numbness, etc., are crude psychical states; the corresponding physical states are the nervous discharges of sensory centres. Moreover, the patient can only tell us of crude psychical states occurring with the beginning of the epileptic discharges of sensory centres, although the discharge of sensory centres may doubtless continue long after his consciousness is lost. Hence the evidence as to discharges of sensory centres is not only indirect, it is also limited. However, in some cases of migraine, which in my nomenclature are epilepsies, the development of sensations during discharges of sensory centres is slow and deliberate, and consciousness is not lost. In these cases states of sensory centres corresponding to the sensations may be studied; we can, however, only infer them. But motor symptoms, *e.g.* convulsion, are far more easily studied. Here again we must insist on the distinction betwixt psychology and the anatomy and physiology of the nervous system. It is a most unfortunate thing that the word "sensation," the name of a state of consciousness, is of the same derivation as "sensory," the name given to afferent nerves and to centres to which afferent nerves go; it fosters the confusion that a physical state in a sensory centre *is* a sensation. "It is usual, indeed, to speak of sensations as states of body, not of mind. But this is the common confusion of giving one and the same name to a phenomenon and to the proximate cause or conditions of the phenomenon. The immediate antecedent of a sensation is a state of body, but the sensation itself is a state of mind" (Mill's *Logic*, 8th ed., vol. ii, p. 436). The fact is that "sensations" (which are not physical states of any kind) attend energising of motor as well as of sensory centres. Using here mixed psychological and anatomico-physiological language (and legitimately because we are at this moment speaking both of psychical and physical states), we may say that there are not only sensory sensations, but motor sensations. In healthy psychico-physical operations they are conjoined. Thus, whenever we see an object, we have the sensory sensation of colour, and the motor sensation of shape (relations of positions). "It may be said that *all* the senses are not physically sensori-motor. I think they are. Thus the auditory nerve has evidently (as the symptoms of Menière's disease show, and anatomy confirms) very extensive motor associations. I have tried to show this."[1]

In disease we may have more nearly pure sensory or motor manifestations than we can have in health, because the sensory and motor elements are for the most part geographically separate (p. 139) although physiologically connected. Taking for comparison a morbid sensory sensation and a morbid motor sensation from the same class—the visual—as in the illustration just given, we have in one case of epilepsy almost purely the motor sensation of vertigo (a sensation during extreme energising of ocular motor centres), and in another case almost purely the sensory sensation of colour (a sensation during energising of centres representing retinal impressions). But I do not think we ever have even in disease absolutely pure sensory sensations or absolutely pure motor sensations. Thus, in the ocular phenomena of migraine there is often a zigzag outline, and with epileptic spasm of the hand there is commonly abnormal sensation referred to the skin. The zigzag or fortification outline implies excitation of motor elements; of those, I suppose, which serve in giving us ideas (symbolically of tactual ideas) of roughness (minute shapes), and which are so immediately, inevitably, and deeply organised with their corresponding retinal impressions that roughness and colour seem to be one sensation. Then the "balls of fire" at the onset of some epileptic seizures must be of some shape. To say that by the constitution of the mind the patient is obliged to think of them as of some shape is true; but what is the physical side of this obligation?[2] It is excitation of centres for ocular movements.

Since the cerebrum is the "organ of mind," it might be supposed that *elaborate* mental symptoms would occur from, or rather *occur during* epileptic discharges, if these be, as I suppose, discharges of the cerebral cortex.

[1] *Medical Times and Gazette*, August 7, 1875.

[2] By the "constitution of his mind," "by an act of volition," a migrainous patient of mine can vary the size of his ocular spectre, but to do so he must, at the same time, alter his accommodation; the spectre is about four feet across when he looks at the window, a distance of eight or nine feet, and the size of a sixpence when he looks at the page of a book, ordinary reading distance.

As will be insisted on later, elaborate mental states do not occur during an epileptic discharge—as a *direct* result of that discharge, we mean. During epileptic discharges we have only crude mental states, such as " balls of fire before the eyes," noises in the ears, etc., and then only at the onset of the discharge when it is presumably *comparatively* slight and slow. Yet these incipient discharges will be far stronger than those of health if we may suppose the strong impressions of the patients (" balls of fire," etc.) imply vividness of sensation. It is possible to show by experiment that we can have more vivid sensations of colour " subjectively " than any that are caused by the presentation of outward objects. (See *Helmholtz's Popular Scientific Lectures*, p. 256.) But this admission does not involve the admission that we have such *elaborate* mental states as spectral illusions or " voices."

As was urged in the article on "Temporary Mental Disorders after Epileptic Paroxysms " (see p. 123), elaborate mental states occur only during activity of centres which, except for slight over-activity, slightly increased discharges " from loss of control," *are healthy*. There is a duplex condition ; negatively loss of function of the highest, and positively increased function of lower, centres. Elaborate mental states imply special, and complex, co-ordinations in co-existence and succession of vast numbers of sensations, which are to the elaborate states as raw material to elaborate structure. Mere increase in vividness of one or of many sensations is not an elaborate mental state.

Except at the onset of an epileptic seizure when there are crude mental states, such as coloured vision, there occur *no psychical* states of any kind *during*, but only *physical effects from*, the excessive local discharge, whatever the part of the " organ of mind " may be in which the " discharging lesion " is seated.

We have in all discharging lesions of any parts of the organ of mind a brutal development of the impressions and movements represented in the part discharged, and no elaborate mental states attend these developments. The elaborate mental states called intellectual auræ (spectral illusions, " voices," etc.) do not occur during epileptic discharges. They occur, I think, during over-activity (slightly increased discharges) of lower nervous arrangements not yet reached by the epileptic discharge. A spectral face is a mental state infinitely more elaborate than " balls of fire." In some cases of epilepsy we have the double warning of (1) coloured vision, so to speak, " turning into " (2) spectral visions of faces. Abandoning this misleading metaphor, I think the relation is that whilst the coloured vision is the result of, or rather occurs *during*, the onset of the epileptic discharge, the spectral face occurs *during* the springing into activity of the next lower nervous arrangements, which are healthy, except for excitement from loss of their higher " controlling " nervous arrangements put out of use by the epileptic discharge. But the epileptic discharge, mostly, but not always—for the fit may stop at the stage of the spectral faces—soon involves also the lower nervous arrangements, and, maybe, produces universal convulsion. Similarly for warnings of noise in the ear, followed by " voices." [1]

[1] The term " voices " is inaccurate when applied to cases in which the patient has the delusion, or illusion, or hallucination that someone is speaking to him. The so-called " voices " imply activity of the sensori-*motor* substrata of words, and of those substrata which are in health concerned in *receiving* speech ; these substrata lie chiefly, I think, on the right side of the brain. This explanation is not a verbal one, for the ordinary opinion seems to be that the auditory centres or sensory perceptive centres only are concerned. Again, the ordinary opinion is that

We shall consider in this paper, to begin with, cases of epileptic discharge of cerebral motor centres, that is, cases of convulsion. We shall select cases in which the discharging lesion is in subordinate motor centres ; we say *subordinate*, meaning thereby centres in Hitzig and Ferrier's region, because, as we have said, we believe all, even the very highest, nervous centres to be made up of nervous arrangements representing impressions and movements. There is in these cases excessive local movements, *i.e.* local spasm, for a short time. When the discharge has ceased and the convulsion is over, we very often find paralysis of the parts which were convulsed—or rather, which were first and most convulsed—of those parts first and most discharged upon. For example, after a convulsion beginning unilaterally, there is very often hemiplegia. Hemiplegia so occurring was called Epileptic Hemiplegia by Dr. Todd. There are other after-effects of epileptic discharges of other subordinate centres. There is an " epileptic aphasia." This and the local palsies are the after-effects of excessive discharges of subordinate motor centres (in Hitzig and Ferrier's region). Further, after severe epileptic discharges, beginning in the very highest centres, there is a very wide physical prostration ; this is *attended by* loss of consciousness, or rather *during this state* consciousness ceases. Or there is coma, according to degree of the discharge, and subsequent prostration. Although empirically we may compare the " loss of consciousness " with hemiplegia, it is obvious, from many prior statements, that the condition which we scientifically compare with epileptic hemiplegia is not loss of consciousness or coma, but the prostration of more or less of the organism, *during which consciousness ceases*. Similarly epileptic aphasia should be post-epileptic exhaustion of more or less of those highest articulatory nervous arrangements which are not words, but the substrata of words, and the substrata of those words which serve in speech. We shall, however, use the empirical expressions until we deal particularly with the states referred to.

It is better to speak of post-epileptic hemiplegia, post-epileptic aphasia, and post-epileptic loss of consciousness. For there are two opposite conditions of nerve centres, under which the use of parts is lost. We have already stated fully what, for another purpose, we now state briefly again, and with some new illustrations more directly to our purpose. The use of parts is lost *during* those excessive discharges which we call epileptic of their centres. *During* convulsion of the arm, as much as during paralysis of it, the patient has no use of that limb. This seems a pedantic refinement. But the principle is gravely important when applied to cases of aphasia and to cases of loss of consciousness. During the epileptic discharge of the centres which are the substrata of speech, there is loss of speech ; *during* the excessive discharge of the centres which are the substrata of consciousness, there is loss of consciousness. This sounds contradictory ; it seems like saying, that during " excessive function " there is " loss of function." It is so in effect. It is certainly true that what is erroneously called " mental *function* " ceases *during* excessive discharges ; and *from* excessive discharge of nervous centres the *proper use* of the parts excessively innervated is lost. It is evident enough in some cases ; the migrainous

speech is a single linear process—that an automatic reproduction of words does not precede speech. The view I take is that speech is the end of a process of " verbalising " of which the automatic reproduction of words is a necessary first part. Speaking generally, all nervous processes are dual, and there is a corresponding duality in all mental processes ; very evidently in perception, as cases of simple delirium (imperception) show.

patient can see nothing in the part of the field covered by his spectre ; his visual nervous centres are otherwise engaged.

All active bodily phenomena in health imply nervous discharges ; when we think of an absent object, as well as when we grasp it or see it, there is a nervous discharge. During the most refined emotional state, without obvious outward change, there are nervous discharges, as well as when we laugh or shed tears. But in epilepsy the discharges are excessive ; during the *rapid* discharges of *vast numbers* of the elements of the substrata of consciousness there could arise no conscious states. *Time*[1] *is required for consciousness.* What ensues on *excessive* discharge of a part of the brain is a development of the impressions and movements represented in that part ; there is not a development of mental states, but only a brutal development of the functions of the *substrata* of mental states ; during this consciousness ceases. Thus (speaking of the motor elements only), in epileptic discharges of centres for visual ideas we should have spasm of the muscles of the eyeballs ; in epileptic discharges of the centres for tactual ideas we should have spasm of the hand ; in epileptic discharges of the centre for speech we have spasm of the articulatory muscles. In epileptic discharges of the highest centres, which are the substrata of consciousness, we have implication of the whole organism. But no ideas of objects, of words, nor any kind of states of consciousness occur during these *excessive* discharges excepting crude sensations at the onset.

We now speak of post-epileptic loss of function, and we begin with the simplest cases—post-epileptic loss of function of subordinate cerebral, and probably often of still lower centres, for movements of the limbs.

In most cases there is, I think, temporary exhaustion, or, more technically speaking, temporary loss of *function* of the nervous centres in which the discharge began, and of centres through which the nerve currents developed passed. In an article in vol. iii of these *Reports* I urged that there were two great divisions of functional changes : (1) those of *loss* of function ; and (2) those of *over*-function. As there stated, the term "functional" is not used for slightness of pathological change, nor applied clinically to cases when symptoms are trifling and transitory. It is, when used medically, limited to the description of the morbid alterations *of the proper function of nerve tissue*, which is to "store up" and "expend" energy.[2] We must not confound functional states (abnormal physiological conditions) with the morbid nutritive processes leading to them (pathological conditions). In cases of convulsion followed by temporary hemiplegia there are both functional states. There is first over-function (excessive discharge signified by the convulsion), and next, loss of function (exhaustion after, of nerve tissue signified by the hemiplegia), the after-effect of the excessive discharge. There is in these cases a destruction of the function of nerve fibres, not a destruction of fibres. That is to say, there is no breaking up of structure, but the fibres cease to be nerve fibres in effect, so long as they are unable to "carry" nerve currents. The destruction of function after an epileptic discharge is only temporary. But however

[1] "In the internal perception of a series of mental operations, a certain time, a certain duration, is necessary for the smallest section of continuous energy to which consciousness is competent. Some minimum of time must be admitted as the condition of consciousness" (Sir W. Hamilton's *Lectures*, vol. i, p. 369, quoted in *Mill on Hamilton*, p. 277).

[2] I would here remark that I use such expressions as "store up energy" in the sense that the nerve cells are nourished by nutrient fluids containing potential energy ; such expressions as "currents passing," etc., are used conventionally, and not as implying any particular hypothesis.

slight and however recoverable, the physiological condition is, so long as it lasts, fundamentally the same as when nerve fibres are broken up. It is a most unfortunate error to confound losses of function with the pathological processes leading to these losses of function. Increased excitability of the medulla oblongata is said by most authorities to be the *pathology* of epilepsy; but increased excitability is an *abnormal physiological* condition. The pathological question is, by what disorder of the nutritive process do nerve cells become unstable or excitable?

I do not say, however, that there may not be coarse disease of the brain in these cases, and thus physical destruction of cells and fibres. In post-epileptic hemiplegia there very often is tumour. All I say is that the paralysis is not necessarily the result of that destruction. In some of these cases we discover post-mortem a tumour, involving convolutions near to the corpus striatum. The tumour *has* destroyed more or less of the cortex; this is admitted. But it would be most misleading to conclude in such a case that the tumour has necessarily "caused" paralysis when that paralysis followed convulsion. Certainly it does "cause" it, but not always directly. It does not cause it because it has *destroyed* so much of the brain. It causes it in a doubly indirect way. As a "foreign body" it is the initiator of abnormally increased nutritive changes (pathological process) from which results the abnormal physiological condition of over-function—instability of neighbouring grey matter (instability of cells constituting a "discharging lesion"). The unstable grey matter discharges excessively and suddenly, and the final step is supposed to be exhaustion of the part discharged, and more important still, of lower centres out of which the centre (which has become unstable) is evolved.

We have already (see p. 108) drawn attention to the fact that destruction of parts of the convolutions in the neighbourhood of the corpus striatum may produce no obvious paralysis, whilst the epileptic discharge of those parts would produce severe convulsion. These facts show that movements are largely represented in parts, destruction [1] of which parts causes no permanent loss of movement. The seeming discrepancy is explainable on the principle of Compensation. The higher a nervous centre the more tolerable is a given "quantity" of destruction, and the more intolerable an equal "quantity" of instability. Another thing, well brought out by Charcot, Lepine, and Landouzy, is that so far as the difference betwixt the corpus striatum and the convolutions in Hitzig and Ferrier's region are concerned, the more limited in range is the paralysis from destruction, the higher the centre. This is not, I think, because the centre destroyed does not represent, or rather re-represent, *all* the movements represented in the corpus striatum, but because it represents some very specially, and represents others generally, that is, in common with all neighbouring centres. Thus, to take an arbitrary and limited illustration, supposing one centre in Hitzig and Ferrier's region to represent specially

[1] Referring to previous remarks of mine to this effect (*British Medical Journal*, May 10, 1873) Dr. Day, of Stafford says (*St. Andrews Medical Graduates' Transactions*, vol. vi) that I endeavour "to prove, by *speculation*, that although the movements will take place even when the parts in which the function is believed to reside are destroyed, yet in spite of, or rather notwithstanding this, these parts *do* represent the special movements referred to. Thus making it appear that the movements can take place either with or without this portion of cerebral substance, or, in other words, that these particular anatomical conditions are, for the purpose in question, *supernumerary*." As stated in the paper Dr. Day is criticising, the explanation is that there is in other centres a representation, although a less special one, of the movements most specially represented in the centre destroyed.

the hand, another specially the face, another the foot, I should believe that each one of them represented all the movements of the chest.

I put forward the doctrine which I now call the principle of Compensation in an article in the *Medical Times and Gazette*, December 21, 1867. I mention this particularly, because it has been implied in some quarters that I am not aware of the " suppleance " of one part of the hemisphere for another. Since, in the article referred to, I write, " so the speculation is, that although each movement *is everywhere represented*, there are points where particular movements are specially represented," it would have been less erroneous to assert that I have applied the principle too audaciously.

The tumour does not produce the hemiplegia because it has destroyed so much. It destroys slowly. There is often no paralysis from *such* slow destruction of convolutions, or no notable paralysis. I say " no notable paralysis," because I do not think compensation is ever absolute. There is evidence of compensation from experiments on the brains of animals. It has been found that in cats and dogs extirpation of some part of the cortex, which Hitzig and Ferrier have shown to represent a given set of movements, is not followed by permanent loss of those movements. There is temporary paralysis only, after which, as I would express it, there is compensation by neighbouring centres. I have never believed in what I call abrupt localisations. I do not believe that there is any part, or example, where the movements of the hand are solely represented ; but that there are numerous parts where these movements have special or leading representations ; there being in each, as the term " leading " implies, a representation of other parts serving subordinately with the leading movement. I have never acceded to the opinion that speech is to be localised in any one spot, although I do believe most firmly that the region of Broca's convolutions is, so to speak, " the yellow spot " for speech, as the macula lutea is the centre of greatest acuteness of vision, although the whole retina sees. Even in the highest centres I hold that each of the component units represents the whole organism, although each unit represents it differently from all others, however slight the difference may be betwixt many of them. In the case of tumour the destruction is very slowly effected, hence often no discoverable palsy. The experimental destruction is rapid, hence decided palsy for a time. The difference of rapidity is an exceedingly important difference. The temporary palsy in the experiments results not from lack of *the part extirpated, but from sudden loss of it.*

Nevertheless, I will not deny, as I have formerly done, that permanent paralysis may result from *widespread* destruction of certain convolutions, and especially am I inclined to admit it after reading the physiological evidence adduced by Hitzig and Ferrier, and the clinical and pathological evidence of Charcot, Lepine, and Landouzy. But I do not think that *paralysis after epileptic convulsion* is thus explicable, as I shall try to show.

Let me now formulate the general principle. It is—" *Parts of the Central Nervous System are temporarily exhausted by Epileptic* (*that is, excessive*) *Nervous Discharges.*" Just as after great but healthy exercise there is fatigue of nerve centres and muscles, so, after the outrageously violent " exercise " in a convulsion, there is an excessive fatigue—a fatigue to that degree which we call paralysis. We begin by the simplest problem, that is, with limited convulsions, followed by paralysis of the parts first and most convulsed ; in other words, we begin by the consideration of excessive nervous discharges of *subordinate* motor centres, followed, according to the hypothesis, by exhaustion of the centre discharged, and of nerve fibres and cells of those lower centres which the current has reached or through which it has passed. We limit ourselves to the after-effects of epileptic discharges as these are seen in muscles ordinarily so called. In some cases there is, as there is after the nervous discharges of a rigor, a flaccidity of arteries ; a paralysis or paresis of their muscles (muscular coat) after their spasm. We speak of the effects seen in muscles of course in order to infer the condition of motor centres for those muscles. Unless we begin by these simple cases, I do not see how we are to find any principle to explain the more difficult cases of post-epileptic aphasia and post-epileptic loss of consciousness accompanying epileptic mania.

There is not always local paralysis, or at any rate *obvious* local paralysis, after limited convulsion. Paralysis is found when the discharge has been very severe, its severity being estimated by the severity of the convulsion. In such cases those parts which have been first and most convulsed are temporarily paralysed.

Logically there ought always to be *some* paralysis after every nervous discharge which is in excess of healthy nervous discharge, and no doubt there is. There will at any rate be the primary exhaustion from loss of energy of the unstable cells which constitute the " discharging lesion," even if no secondary exhaustion of collateral and subordinate healthy nerve cells and fibres. For even after discharges of health there follows exhaustion, evidently if the discharge be a little above the common ; hence fatigue, and in the case of vision the negative after-image following a positive after-image.[1]

In cases of epileptic discharge of centres representing retinal elements during which a vivid colour arises, we should expect, on the hypothesis stated in this paper, that the patient would be unable to recognise the colour of objects of that colour when the discharge had ceased ; that the central anatomical elements corresponding to it would be much exhausted. I have never tested this. Dr. Alexander Robertson has (*British Medical Journal*, April 18, 1874). " In this case the subjective reproduction of red as a distinct aura was followed by a temporary inability to recognise that colour for a time."

Practically speaking, there is no motor paralysis except after *severe* epileptic discharge.

[1] Many cases in which there really is exhaustion are misinterpreted. As several times mentioned in this article (see p. 138) a patient's symptomatic condition is often duplex ; negative and positive ; often the positive symptomatic condition attracts exclusive attention. In some cases it seems to me to be evident that contemporaneously with the loss of function of a centre, there is a rise in activity of the next lower centre. (Thompson Dickson's " Principle of Loss of Control.") I shall have very often, for various purposes, to show the wide bearings of this principle. I believe that it applies in the explanation of the occurrence of complementary colours—there is here also a duplex condition, negative and positive. To take a particular case : exhaustion of some of the nervous elements which are the substrata of the colour red is contemporaneous with, or is soon followed by, increased activity of those elements which are the substrata of blue-green ; such increased activity being a consequence of the exhaustion ; there is " loss of control " on a minute scale. The blue-green arises when, the eyes being closed, no light enters the eye, and thus that complementary colour is owing to " spontaneous " activity of the central substrata for that colour ; is not caused by fresh peripheral excitation. Further, I would suggest that the same occurs on a minute scale in ordinary vision ; that in seeing any colour, there follows not only a trifling exhaustion, or let us use here the less strong word, " fatigue," but also a trifling rise in activity of the substrata of all other colours probably in some order. The obvious objection is that we have no conscious states, no colours corresponding to this hypothetical rising in activity. But we cannot know any one colour except by comparison and contrast with other colours, and hence *a priori* we should assume that, although there is no vivid consciousness of the other colours, there is some consciousness—a " sensibility " of them, to use Lewes's term.

The reader will observe that it is not said that those parts which have been convulsed, but that those which have been first and most convulsed, are those left paralysed. The paralysis varies in two ways—in range and in degree. In these respects it is the correlative of the convulsion which it follows. Convulsions beginning locally in the hand, face, or leg attain all ranges, and are of all degrees of severity ; the post-epileptic palsy varies similarly. As to range there may be palsy of the hand only after a convulsion beginning there and affecting little more than that part, or there may be hemiplegia after a severe and universal convulsion beginning in the hand, and affecting the side it began in most. As to degrees ; after a slight and partial convulsion there may be either only such slight loss of power as prevents a patient picking up a pin, although he can strike a blow, or after a severe convulsion there may be absolute paralysis of an arm, or leg, or there may be as much hemiplegia as a large clot causes. When the fit has been very slight the patient may speak only of numbness, or use less definite expressions, as that " the hand feels queer." The numbness is, I think, owing to the loss of use of nervous arrangements for innumerable minute or limited movements, " delicate movements " which, associated with correspondingly minute skin impressions, give us ideas of infinitesimal shapes such as roughness of surface ; there is loss of use of some of the nervous arrangements for those innumerable minute movements which fill up, so to speak, the interstices of larger movements, such as those by which we tell whether cloth is rough or not. (An explanation in all respects similar to that given on p. 140 of the spectre in some cases of migraine is intended.)

In the third volume of these *Reports*, p. 103, I compared three degrees of convulsion beginning unilaterally with three degrees of the hemiplegia which is producible by destructive lesions (such as clot and softening) of different " gravities " of the corpus striatum. The part of the brain destroyed is only *chiefly* motor, as the posterior part of the brain is only chiefly sensory (see p. 139). The degrees are arbitrary ; the correct expression is that the graver the lesion (1) the more in degree are the most voluntary or special parts affected, and (2) the farther in range does the paralysis spread to the less special or less voluntary, *i.e.* more automatic. There is an increase of paralysis in Compound Degree. There are degrees of Dissolution,[1] using this term as the opposite of Evolution. It will be seen that the principle of Dissolution harmonises with the principle of Compensation.

The first degree of hemiplegia (paralysis of the face, arm, and leg) is often seen after a unilaterally beginning convulsion when that convulsion has been severe. There is hemiplegia *exactly like that which a clot in the corpus striatum so often produces or like that resulting from plugging of the middle cerebral artery* ; that is to say, like it in *range and degree*, unlike it in being transitory. This long since led me to the belief that unilaterally beginning convulsive seizures depend on disease in the region of the middle cerebral artery (*London Hospital Reports*, vol. i, 1864, and many places in *Medical Times and Gazette*). I noticed that

[1] Here, for the first time in this article I use the term Dissolution, I most gratefully acknowledge my vast debt to Herbert Spencer. What I have to say of the constitution of the nervous system appears to me to be little more than illustrating his doctrine on nervous evolution by what I may metaphorically speak of as the experiments of disease. I should make more definite acknowledgments were it not that I do not wish to mislead the reader, if, by any misunderstandings of his doctrines on my part, I impute to Mr. Spencer particular opinions he might not endorse. Anyone interested in diseases of the nervous system should carefully study Spencer's *Psychology*.

those parts which were first and most involved in the convulsion were the parts which were paralysed when the corpus striatum was injured by clot. I was much struck also by the confirmatory fact that, occasionally after a severe convulsion, beginning unilaterally, the same parts were temporarily paralysed.[1] Sometimes after a severe convulsion there is the second degree of hemiplegia (see p. 103), that is, there may be paralysis not only of the face, arm, and leg, but in addition all lateral deviation of the eyes and head.

Here, bearing in mind the principle of Compensation,[2] I would say that the eye and head movements escape in the first degree of hemiplegia—first degree of Dissolution—not because they are unrepresented in the destroyed units of the corpus striatum, but because they were still represented in every unit of the parts intact.

Each unit of the corpus striatum is a corpus striatum in miniature,[3] representing slightly the whole of the parts which the entire corpus striatum represents in greater degree. But it is not supposed that each unit represents the

[1] " I do not assert that ' epilepsy ' is due to disease of [the brain in the region of] the middle cerebral artery (or of the pia mater in the range of that vessel—its vascular expansion), but I submit that one particular form of epilepsy is. Perhaps a better expression would be epileptiform convulsions " (*London Hospital Reports*, 1864, p. 466). I now use, as stated, the term " epilepsy " for excessive, etc., discharges of any part of the cortex cerebri, and symptomatically for any symptoms thus caused. I do not make the above quotation for the purpose of claiming priority, as I find that the clinical facts of the varieties of epilepsy under remark were stated before I was born. I make the quotation because I am under the impression that it is useful for an investigator to show, as some evidence of his earnestness, that he is not putting forward hastily considered opinions. The following disposes of any priority I might have supposed myself to have. Charcot writes (*Revue Mensuelle de Médecine et de Chirurgie*, January 1877, p. 4) : " Enfin M. Hughlings Jackson s'est attaché depuis plusieurs années à démontrer que certaines lésions superficielles du cerveau peuvent determiner une forme spéciale d'épilepsie dont l'étude clinique avait été poussée fort loin déjà longtemps avant, en France, par Bravais (*Recherche sur les symptômes et le traitement de l'épilepsie hémiplégique*, 1827) dans une thèse très-remarquable qui dénote chez l'auteur une sûreté de jugement et une finesse d'observation peu communes."

[2] This principle is so important that I make here further remarks on its bearing on the representation of the special senses. Because I have said that deafness never results from disease of any kind in any part of either cerebral hemisphere *so far as I have observed*, it has been inferred that I do not believe the auditory nerves to be represented in the cerebrum. Nor in my experience has disease of any kind by *its mere destroying action* in any part of either cerebral hemisphere produced blindness or defect of sight. I say by its mere destroying action, as blindness often indeed occurs by an indirect process from disease of the cerebrum. Nevertheless I have not inferred that these nerves are unrepresented in the cerebrum. The fact is, I drew the very opposite inference from the absence of deafness and blindness from destroying lesions of the cerebrum. Thus (*Royal London Ophthalmic Hospital Reports*, 1865) I write : " This (the absence of deafness in disease of the brain) may be due in part to the wide connections which hearing probably has with mental functions. *Probably fibres from the auditory nerve through its nucleus spread more uniformly than fibres of the optic nerve to the cerebral convolutions*. There can, I suppose, be little doubt that the auditory nerve does send fibres to the hemispheres directly or commissurally."

In another part of the same paper I have written : ". . . One would not deny that the nerve fibres of each of the special senses spread, some more and some less, directly or commissurally, to every part (although more perhaps to some parts) of *their* periphery, *viz.* the convolutions of the cerebral hemispheres . . . it may be that the special senses are *represented widely in each cerebral hemisphere*, and thus that much even of both the hemispheres may be destroyed without affection of sight." The latter part of this quotation mentions expressly sight only, but implicitly all the special senses are spoken of.

I would not deny now, however, that sudden destruction to particular parts of the cerebral hemisphere may produce temporary blindness or deafness. Although I have no clinical evidence of it, I think it highly probable having regard to certain of Ferrier's experiments. It may be that I have not seen temporary blindness or deafness from sudden destruction of parts of the cerebral hemisphere because I have not seen cases of symmetrical destruction of those parts where the auditory and optic nerves are most specially represented.

[3] See Charcot, *Cerebral Localisation*, p. 152. He agrees with me as to the reasonableness of this figure of speech.

whole of the parts in the very same way ; that would be equivalent to no representation at all. The hypothesis is that the muscles of the arm, face, and leg are represented in every part of the corpus striatum, but in different combinations in each part.

Suppose the anterior units of the corpus striatum to represent movements of the arm *chiefly*, the middle units to represent those of the face *chiefly*, the posterior units to represent those of the leg *chiefly*, the hypothesis is, that each of these groups of units represents more nearly equally with the other two the more automatic movements of the eyes and head, and still more nearly equally the movements of the thorax, and still more nearly equally other movements to be spoken of later on in this article (p. 150). The ocular and head movements suffer in the Second Degree of Hemiplegia, because from the graver lesions too few units are left. I submit that this is a simpler hypothesis than that which supposes these additional symptoms to be owing to extension of damage from the corpus striatum to some other centre for the eye and head movements, or than that which attributes them to "shock." Fully believing that the eye and head movements will be somewhat more represented in some than in other units of the corpus striatum, the great matter is gravity of lesion—the number of units destroyed and the rapidity of their destruction. The more important element in chronic cases is the number of units destroyed.

This opinion as to the constitution of the corpus striatum agrees with the law of Dissolution (see p. 147), that there is from increasing gravity of lesions a twofold effect : (1) the most special or voluntary parts (arm, face, and leg) are more paralysed ; and (2) the farther the paralysis spreads in range to less special or more automatic parts (involves movements of eyes, head, etc.). The order of recovery confirms. The more automatic parts recover first ; the lateral deviations, except when a very large quantity of brain is destroyed, are transitory. Considering together the principle of Compensation and the law of Dissolution, it will be inferred that recovery follows not because other units take on duties they never had before ; but because these units having in health closely similar duties to those of the units destroyed, they can act nearly as well for the duties of both ; it is possible that their elements, cells and fibres, hypertrophy and perhaps increase in number, in order to perform more efficiently the extra work imposed on them.

The constitution of all nervous centres is supposed to be the same whatever their composition may be, that is, whatever parts of the body they may represent. It is just as the form of thought is always the same whatever may be the particular things thought about. The principle of Dissolution and the principle of Compensation, I suppose, hold for all nervous centres, as does also the principle of Loss of Control ; they are only different aspects of one thing. They are useful hypotheses for investigation.

In cases of post-epileptic hemiplegia, where the hemiplegia is of the second degree, the convulsion has been very extensive in range, and inferentially the discharge has been unusually excessive.

In a valuable paper in the *Journal of Mental Science*, January 1876, Dr. Julius Mickle records a case of post-epileptic hemiplegia in which conjugate deviation of the head and eyes was seen. He correctly quotes me ("Study of Convulsions," *St. Andrews Reports*, vol. iv, pp. 13, 169) as speaking doubtfully of the existence of conjugate deviation of the head and eyes in such cases.

But I have since that paper was written (1870) seen cases of post-epileptic hemiplegia with those deviations.[1]

Of these facts there can be no doubt whatever. That is to say, there is no doubt that hemiplegia of these two degrees follows a severe convulsion beginning in some peripheral part of the hemiplegic region, hand, face, or foot, in a patient who before that convulsion had no paralysis whatever.

I think it probable that there is sometimes, immediately after an unusually severe convulsion, and one which having begun unilaterally has *become* universal, a post-epileptic paralysis corresponding to what I believe is a third degree of, or rather a degree of paralysis *beyond*, hemiplegia. (See p. 103.) With paralysis of the side first convulsed there is, I think, probably paresis of the side secondly convulsed.[2] The facts of "descending wasting" show that the two sides of the body are represented in each of the corpora striata; the wasting often descends into each side of the cord, which shows that there are direct as well as decussating fibres. The conclusion from this is that the units of each of the corpora striata represent the whole of the muscles of the body, representing less those of the second than of the first side.

Respecting the principle of what was said (p. 148), the hypothesis is that the second side is still less specially represented in the units of the corpus striatum than even the movements of the head and eyes of the first side; there are fewer fibres more widely distributed, and thus it is only in gravest lesions that the second side is supposed to suffer. It can only be supposed to suffer transitorily after the severest epileptic discharges; the more automatic parts, those least and latest paralysed, recover soonest, as stated (p. 147).

Nothnagel, referring to Broadbent's hypothesis and to some previous statements of mine (*Lancet*, February 15, 1873), says, that I have *not proved* the existence of paresis of the second side; this is quite true, and as Nothnagel observes I have myself indicated those difficulties which are obvious. Let us consider the matter again after speaking of the convulsion which is supposed to correspond to the hypothetical paresis of the second side.[3]

On the doctrine of evolution the centres next higher (those in Hitzig and Ferrier's region) than the corpus striatum will each of them represent again, but in greater complexity and speciality, all the parts the corpus striatum (and doubtless centres still lower, geographically), has already represented. Yet each of the higher centres in Hitzig and Ferrier's region is supposed to represent more specially some particular part (face, arm, or leg), and each more generally all other parts, than they have been represented in the corpus striatum. We

[1] I may here mention that Dr. Mickle criticises an inference I drew as to the *modus operandi* of a meningeal hæmorrhage in causing unilateral convulsions. I thought then (*Medical Times and Gazette*, August 15, 1868, p. 179) that the convulsion depended on pressure on the otherwise healthy corpus striatum. I submit to the criticism. I should not nowadays draw such an inference.

[2] It is convenient in what follows to use the expressions "first side" and "second side." Thus, with reference to the right corpus striatum the left side of the body is the first side, the right side the second side. This is the physiological order of the representation of the two sides in the right corpus striatum.

[3] Nothnagel states that Broadbent believes the two halves of the body to be represented in each cerebral hemisphere. So far as I know Broadbent does not suppose, as I do, that muscles of the arms and legs are thus doubly represented. I make this remark, as I do not wish to impute to him views he may not share with me. I do not make the remark because I wish to claim any priority. I have written elsewhere (*Medical Press and Circular*, September 6, 1876): "I have carried the hypothesis farther than Broadbent, but, subject to his approval, I should say that I have added *nothing* to the *principle* of that hypothesis."

call these centres which are higher in degree of evolution than the corpus striatum, subordinate motor centres, because they are lower in evolution than the centres which are the substrata of consciousness. Let us call them middle centres. Each of these middle centres will re-represent movements of both sides of the body, because each of them represents the whole of the parts already represented in the corpus striatum.

If this be the constitution of the middle centres, there is, I submit, no difficulty in understanding how it is that in epileptic discharges of *one* of them, or discharge beginning in one of them, the convulsion after affecting one side of the body, the first side, the currents passing by the route of the decussating fibres, should become universal—that the spasm should "travel" to the other, the second, side of the body, the currents passing by the route of the direct fibres. It is fair to say that, so far as I know, I am alone in this opinion as to the mode of causation of convulsion of the second side. Nothnagel says that the convulsion of the second side may, in his opinion, be explained quite as well by the assumption of a secondary sympathy of the other cerebral hemisphere, or by a secondary affection of the pons or medulla oblongata.

It is important to note next that the two sets of wasted fibres "descend" into different columns of the cord; into the lateral column of the opposite side (first side), and into the anterior column of the same side (second side); the wasting in the lateral column affecting that part of it where there are most fibres of smallest diameter; the part of the anterior column being that where there are the thickest fibres of that column—the largest of all in the cord. This difference of necessity implies differences of *kind* of representation of the corresponding muscles of two sides of the body in each half of the brain if the fibres of the anterior column be the route of the current for the second side, for we cannot suppose the anterior columns to have just the same duty as the lateral columns.

We should expect, then, that when a fit begins in the hand of the first side, the spasm in the convulsion of the second side would invade the parts of that second side in a manner different from the invasion of the first side. There are, however, very few facts as to the mode of convulsion of the second side. My colleague, Dr. Gowers, has made some important observations on this matter. He writes (*Lancet*, November 6, 1875) of one case: "Invariably one arm (right) and both legs were convulsed, the other arm escaping entirely . . .[1] It is to be observed that in the right leg spasm of the extensors predominated, while in the left leg [second side] that of the flexors was distinctly greater than that of the extensors." The two legs, however, were convulsed simultaneously.

From a few observations, and from hypothetical considerations, I should expect that when a convulsion begins in the hand the spasm reaching the second side would affect first and most the parts affected last and least on the first side (head, eyes, leg, trunk first and limbs last). Hence, believing the paresis to be the counterpart of the spasm—not equal in range, however (see p. 147), I should not expect it to affect most those parts which on the undoubtedly paralysed side are most affected. I should expect it on each side to affect those parts most which have been first and most convulsed on that side. I do not pretend to have demonstrated that any paresis occurs on

[1] The part omitted in the quotation is: "May it be connected with the more frequent simultaneous use of the legs than of the arms?"

the second side; we should expect the paresis to be transitory. For if the law of recovery holds (see p. 149) here, any paresis there was would be transitory, and might disappear before the patient had regained full consciousness. (See p. 158, on loss of power during loss of consciousness and coma.)

I expect, then, that if there be paralysis of the second side it will be slight and transitory, and that it will not be of those parts *most* which are *most* affected in the paralysis of the first side.

That several of the above statements are hypothetical is no objection. Hypothesis is necessary in the investigation of complex and difficult subjects; an hypothesis is not a conclusion; it is only a provisional conclusion. But that my hypothesis that there is post-epileptic paresis of the second side is one about which I can only slightly indicate methods of investigation for proof or disproof, is almost an overwhelming objection. There is, however, I think, further, although indirect, evidence to be adduced.

It is convenient to adduce this evidence for another reason, *viz.* in order to enforce what was said (p. 139) as to the constitution of the substrata of consciousness—that they represent or re-represent the impressions and movements of the whole body. Surely this is evident *a priori*; since consciousness represents the whole subject,[1] must not its substrata represent the whole organism?

We shall approach the statement of this evidence by carrying still further the hypothesis of nervous evolution, and we shall see, I think, that the evidence when stated entirely agrees with this hypothesis, although it is quite independent of it. We continue to illustrate by the motor element only, except in a few preliminary remarks.

It is not of course supposed that the substrata of consciousness are motor only, nor that they are in but one side of the brain. It is supposed that each cerebral hemisphere represents the impressions and movements of the whole organism—the anterior part of each hemisphere being chiefly motor, the posterior chiefly sensory (see pp. 139–140). There is, I think, the broad distinction that the left posterior part and the right anterior part are the substrata of subject consciousness, that is to say, they represent the whole organism as it is affected by the environment—and that the right posterior and left anterior parts are the substrata of object consciousness, that is to say, they represent the whole organism as it reacts on the environment. Let us speak of sensations; we must not, however, narrow ourselves to the sensations of the special senses; there are what Lewes calls "systemic," and Bain "organic" sensations. A complete study of the senses under this enlarged definition would be a study of the whole body. All the senses are supposed to be sensori-motor; every sensation occurs during energising of sensori-motor arrangements. Still, as disease to some degree can separate the two elements (see p. 140) we shall speak of motor sensations and sensory sensations; these being brief expressions for "sensations occurring *during* energising of sensory and motor elements of nervous arrangements."

I suppose the organic sensory sensations from tissues, viscera, muscles, etc., to have first and most representation in the posterior part of the left

[1] We should say subject-object, for the correspondence of the organism with the environment is duplex. There are highest nervous arrangements by which we have received, and are continually receiving impressions from the environment (substrata of subject consciousness, chiefly sensory), and highest nervous arrangements by which we can and do react on the environment (substrata of object consciousness, chiefly motor).

cerebral hemisphere, and the visual, auditory, etc., sensory sensations the first and most representation in the posterior part of the right; again, that organic motor sensations would be first and most represented in the anterior part of the right; the visual motor sensations first and most in the anterior part of the left. This is equivalent to the statements already made as to seats of the substrata of subject and object consciousness.

Let us see how this hypothesis as to the particular constitution of the several divisions of the highest centres bears on the investigation of epileptic paroxysms. There are warnings by morbid development of sensations. When there are warnings of course the epileptic discharge does not begin in the very highest arrangements of the highest centres. But many of these warnings are very quickly followed by loss of consciousness, and thus loss of consciousness being almost the first thing, the discharge must begin in nervous arrangements which are next to the highest in the highest centres. At p. 137 we gave a rough list of warning sensations. There is the strange feeling at or near to the epigastrium so very common just before complete loss of consciousness; this is, I think, a development of highly complex systemic sensory sensations. There is eructation or nausea (physically incipient vomiting), a development of systemic motor sensations. Again we have the sensory sensation of colour, and the motor sensation of vertigo. It is important to note all warnings by different sensations, and with regard to accompanying physical manifestations. It is quite as important to note that a patient has the organic motor sensation of shivering as a warning of his paroxysm as that a patient has that of coloured vision. And in order to see whether or not different sensations have the order of degree of representation in the several parts of the cerebral hemisphere we have suggested we should note carefully the convulsion which follows each. Thus after any particular sensation warning do the two eyes turn to the right or to the left; does the convulsion begin in or preponderate on the right or left side? Such facts would tell us whether or not the sensation developed as a warning was owing to discharge of the right or left cerebral hemisphere. It is a strange thing that from epileptic discharges which we judge to begin nearly in the highest nervous arrangements of the highest cerebral centres we have sensations at both ends of the scale; we have the most special, as coloured vision,[1] and the least special, as shivering. The explanation is, I think, that the substrata of consciousness are (p. 152) duplex in function. All centres are bilateral, but the higher the centres, the less of a mere duplicate are they in function on the two sides; in the highest centres this difference in the doubles is carried to an extreme; the substrata of subject consciousness representing the organism as a whole, and as it suffers from the environment and the substrata of object consciousness representing the whole organism as reacting on the environment. The more quickly consciousness is lost after a warning, the more often is that warning low in the scale of sensations, "epigastric aura," etc.

[1] I believe, however, that the more special the sensation the more unilateral is the convulsion if there be one.

As stated on p. 139, I believe cases of migraine to be epilepsies (sensory epilepsies). Dr. Latham thinks the paroxysm in migraine to be owing to arterial contraction in the region of the posterior cerebral artery; Dr. Liveing that there is a "nerve storm" traversing the optic thalamus and other centres. I think the sensory symptoms of the paroxysm are owing to a "discharging lesion" of convolutions evolved out of the optic thalamus, *i.e.* of "sensory middle centres" analogous to the "motor middle centres" (see p. 151). I believe the headache and vomiting to be post-paroxysmal.

I do not mean that the above statements are true; they are only rough hypotheses for verification or disproof.

The occasional occurrence of coloured vision at the onset of some *right*-side beginning convulsive paroxysms (as was the case in Dr. Robertson's patient, p. 146) shows that these differences of the two sides of the brain are not so simple as they are here hypothetically stated. I have recorded a case of a patient who was subject to convulsion beginning in the right thumb, and who *at other times* had attacks of coloured vision (see p. 1). Still, I believe that most commonly warnings of coloured vision, noises in the ear, etc., are owing to discharging lesions in the right cerebral hemisphere.

Let us now consider the effects of epileptic discharge of motor elements of the substrata of consciousness; the discharging lesions being in but one side of the brain. We now apply the hypothesis of evolution to the highest centres, the substrata of consciousness, speaking only of the motor elements.

The very highest motor centres are supposed to be evolved out of the subordinate or middle cerebral centres in Hitzig and Ferrier's region, and perhaps out of still lower centres by fibres not passing through the central ganglia of the brain. Thus the highest centres differ from the middle centres only as the latter differ from their lower centres (corpus striatum, etc., see p. 150); the principle of difference being in each case a re-representation of the very same external parts, in more special and complex ways.[1] The corpus striatum represents movements of both sides of the body; these are re-represented in the middle cerebral motor centres, and they are re-re-represented in the highest cerebral motor centres—motor division of substrata of consciousness.

Thus units of these highest motor centres of each side of the brain represent the most special and most complex movements of the whole body, or rather of the body as a whole.[2]

It is not of course supposed that any unit represents the whole body—or a large part of the body—so that all the parts it represents are equally represented. The kind of representation is supposed to be analogous to the kind of representation attributed to middle centres in Hitzig and Ferrier's region. Each unit of the highest centre represents some part of the body very specially, and all other or very many other parts very generally, *i.e.* in common with, more equally with, many other units.

The units of the highest centres represent the whole body in innumerable different combinations of impressions and movements. "The seat of consciousness," Herbert Spencer says, "is that nervous centre to which the most heterogeneous impressions are brought," and I suppose that he would hold also that it is that centre from which impulses for the most heterogeneous movements depart. There is in the highest centres—the centres of centres—a most intricate and yet orderly space and time co-ordination. There is not only a representation of a great number of different movements of widely

[1] I say the *principle* of difference; there is, however, an obvious qualification. The higher a centre, not only the more complex is its re-representation of the parts lower centres have represented, but there is in many cases also an introduction of elements for new impressions and movements.

[2] An instance can be adduced showing that a very small part of the organism represents the whole organism, the sperm cell and germ cell; these united grow into a complete organism without any other help than the supply of warmth and nutrient material in a woman's womb. Were I to adopt any doctrine of genesis it would be that the germ and sperm cells are made up of detachments from the highest nervous centres.

separated parts of the body, but a representation of these at a great number of different intervals.

Thus far we have simply been carrying out the hypothesis of evolution. Now let us consider the experiments disease makes on these highest centres.

The epileptic discharge of many units of these highest centres puts in action both sides of the body ; that is to say, the convulsion in those cases in which there is loss of consciousness at the outset of the epileptic paroxysm is bilateral. However, it is not supposed that even in the very highest centres the movements of the two sides of the body are represented quite equally in each side of the brain. It is only supposed that the two sides are represented more nearly equally than in the middle centres. The bilateral convulsion, in cases beginning with loss of consciousness, commonly begins by turning of the eyes and head to one side, and the universal convulsion usually preponderates on one side. All that is said is that the two sides are more nearly equally convulsed in epileptic discharges of the highest centres than in discharges of middle centres. The several parts are convulsed more nearly contemporaneously. For, as stated, the innumerable different movements are represented in innumerable different intervals—so to speak, the time is divided into very numerous parts. Moreover, corresponding partly, I suppose, to differences in the sizes of the nerve cells, the epileptic discharges of the highest centres containing more small cells are more sudden and rapid, more " intense " (great quantity of energy liberated in a short time), than epileptic discharges of the subordinate or middle cerebral centres in Hitzig and Ferrier's region, where are many large cells. To resume, the convulsion is more quickly universal, the two sides of the body are more nearly equally and more nearly contemporaneously convulsed when part of the highest centres is discharged than when a middle or subordinate cerebral centre is discharged.

The convulsions from epileptic discharges of middle centres in Hitzig and Ferrier's region can now be more clearly compared with convulsions from discharges of the highest centres. I make this comparison because I have been misunderstood to believe that all epilepsies are owing to discharging lesions in Hitzig and Ferrier's region. I never believed the " genuine " epilepsy of authorities—that is, epilepsy beginning with loss of consciousness—to be owing to discharging lesions in this region. (See footnote, p. 148.) The following quotation, in which some verbal alterations are made, referring to the convulsions of " genuine " epilepsy and to unilaterally-beginning convulsions, shows that in 1870 I thought as I now think as to the differences betwixt the seat of the lesion in each :

" Those who say that the two classes differ ' only in degree ' make a remark the truth of which is admitted. In both there are occasional, excessive, and disorderly expenditure of *energy* on muscles, the discharge depending on instability of nervous tissue. But in what kind of degree do they differ ? Not merely in degree of more or less spasm—more or less instability of nervous tissue—but also *in degree of evolution*—of the nervous processes which are unstable. A convulsion which is *universal*, and in which the muscular regions affected are affected nearly contemporaneously, must depend on discharge of parts in which the nervous processes represent a more intricate co-ordination of *movements* in space and time than those parts represent which, when discharged, produce a convulsion, which begins in one limb and has a deliberate march. My speculation is, that the first class differs from the second in that convolutions at a greater physiological distance from the motor tract are discharged."[1]

It may, perhaps, be said that this hypothesis as to the constitution of the motor part of the substrata of consciousness is founded on the hypothesis stated (p. 152), where it was also said that an hypothesis is not a conclusion. But it was said, too, that an hypothesis is a provisional conclusion ; and it is quite legitimate to carry further, as we have done, the one stated, to see if it will explain the facts we observe. But the statements as to the constitution of the highest centres rests not on that hypothesis, but on quite another kind of evidence, which agrees with it. The paroxysms just spoken of are those which *begin with* loss of consciousness ; and this is equivalent to saying that the epileptic discharge begins in the highest centres. The effect of an epileptic discharging lesion there seated *is* convulsion of both sides of the body ; the two are more nearly equally and more nearly contemporaneously convulsed than when the discharging lesion is of middle or subordinate centres. The convulsions in " genuine " epilepsy may be looked on as experiments made by disease (using this expression metaphorically), which reveal to us the nature of the constitution of the highest centres (their motor elements). The evidence supplied by these cases is the " indirect evidence " spoken of at p. 152.

Of course there will be degrees betwixt the two classes of epilepsy. For among those epilepsies which are commonly classed as genuine epilepsy there are cases in which, whilst loss of consciousness is almost the first thing, there is yet some premonitory sensation (vertigo, shivering, creeping, etc.), showing that the discharge does not begin in the very highest arrangements of the highest centres, or consciousness would be lost at the very first. We should theoretically expect there to be *all* degrees betwixt the two great classes, and possibly there are. But it does not follow that there will occur at any rate *as numerous* intermediate degrees as are theoretically likely ; for we have to take note that some parts of the nervous system are more liable to *become diseased* than others are : it is evidently so as to clot or softening ; the peculiarities in the distribution of arteries account for the " seats of election " of these two morbid conditions even in details, as Duret has shown. It is, indeed, a very singular thing that there do occur the two groups of epilepsies with few intermediate cases showing in their paroxysms an intermediateness of degrees of bilaterality, and of degrees of contemporaneity of convulsion. I suppose these differences will be accounted for by differences in arterial distribution. But it may be asked, as was anticipated (p. 136), why is consciousness lost when there is a discharging lesion of but *one* part of *one* side of the brain ? Currents developed by discharging lesions will pass " laterally " as well as " downwards "—will pass to associated centres of the same rank, so to speak, as well as to lower centres.

The higher the centre the more numerous different impressions and movements it represents. But this is not all. Along with increasing division of labour there goes increasing co-operation of labourers ; increasing nervous differentiation is attended or is followed closely by more complete integration ; the higher the centre, the more " lateral " connections betwixt the nervous arrangements of the same hemisphere and of the two hemispheres. It is

[1] This paragraph is produced from the *Study of Convulsions*, 1870, with the alterations of " force " to " energy," " general " to " universal," and " muscles " to " movements," and with the intercalation of the word " physiological " in the last line but one (see p. 8, footnote).

evident *a priori* that the highest centres must be more integrated than the lower; their unity is chiefly the unity of co-operation; the unity of lower centres is more the unity of undifferentiation. Hence the units of the very highest centres which represent the most numerous different movements and impressions will have most interconnections. We see, indeed, in the scale of animal life that the corpus callosum is more and more developed the more independent are the movements of the arms: in the bird whose arms (wings) act equally in range and together in time there is no corpus callosum.

Thus the currents from a discharge in but one of the divisions of the highest nervous centres (see p. 155) will not only pass "downwards" but will pass "laterally" to other divisions of the highest centres with which the centre discharged is in physiological connection; thus the loss of consciousness from a local discharge is accounted for; the currents developed will affect the brain widely. In some cases (*le petit-mal*) of epileptic discharge of the very highest centres the "lateral" currents are chief; there is thoroughly complete loss of consciousness with little visible peripheral change; that is to say, little evidence of currents passing "downwards" (see p. 138); in some cases there is scarcely any, practically no, outward manifestations. When so the loss of consciousness is often most transitory. It is well known that some epileptics lose consciousness absolutely, and yet for so short a time that strangers sitting opposite them at dinner may notice no change. So much for local discharging lesions of the highest nervous centres.

It is otherwise with destroying lesions; it is very true that at the time the lesion is effected, if it be sudden, as hæmorrhage, there is "shock" doubtless from sudden development of widespreading currents by rapid tearing up of grey matter; these are effects of the mere act of destruction; there may even be convulsion. But from the mere absence of part of one of the highest divisions of the substrata of consciousness there is no *loss* of consciousness, for the part of the centre undamaged and the other divisions of the substrata of consciousness remain unaffected.[1]

In discharging lesions of the highest centres there are repeated discharges, and thus much of the brain will be disturbed again and again.

In this connection it is convenient to note that the epilepsies of which the discharging lesions are seated in the highest nervous arrangements are those which occur in asylums. Clinically speaking, asylum cases are most often those in which the paroxysms begin by loss of consciousness, which is equivalent to the anatomico-physiological statement that the discharge begins in the highest nervous centres. In equivalent clinical language we say that asylum cases of epilepsy are often those which begin without a warning. Crichton-Browne says (*West Riding Asylum Reports*, vol. iii, p. 160): "In lunatic asylum practice an aura is of rare occurrence in epilepsy." He says that, using the term "aura" in its widest sense to include "all prodromata, all symptoms, psychical, sensory, or motor, which immediately precede a paroxysm, an aura is rare in a lunatic hospital." He says, however, that the absence of aura may be owing to the fact that the patients are often far advanced in the disease when admitted; and again it may not be recognised by the patients because their feelings and intelligence are blunted. But in cases which occur in asylums there is sometimes an aura, but loss of consciousness soon follows; loss of consciousness *is almost* the first thing. Then the warnings are of a particular kind. They are

[1] For a long time; general cerebral atrophy follows on local damage to the brain.

frequently vertigo, epigastric sensations, or a universal creeping, tingling, or thrilling of the skin. On this matter I again quote Crichton-Browne. In a letter to me in reply to inquiries he says : " When auras are present in epileptic lunatics they are almost invariably general in character and consist in indescribable feelings in the head (vertigo) or abdomen, spreading thence over the body, or in universal creeping, tingling, or thrilling of the skin. Of course special warnings are occasionally encountered, but in a great majority of cases there is no warning of any kind." Thus the " auras " lunatic epileptics have are : (1) most frequently those which imply developments of the most highly representative of all movements (vertigo on its physical side is a discharge of ocular motor centres) ; and (2) those which there is good reason to believe imply developments of the most special of systemic sensations (the epigastric aura).

Again, the very cases in which the intellect is most rapidly affected are those in which there are very slight attacks beginning with or apparently constituted solely by loss of consciousness—*le vertige épileptique* and *le petit-mal* of the French. But this is not because the attacks are slight ; it is because the " disease " is of the very highest nervous arrangements in the whole nervous system, and of those which have the greatest integration, that is to say, of the substrata of consciousness. The following quotations are given to enforce this statement :

" The greatest injury to the intellect is not inflicted by the most frightful and frequent convulsions, nor when the mature and muscular man struggles like a chain-bound Hercules. Absence of mind, momentary obliviousness, vertiginous feelings, a pause, a stoppage, an intermission in consciousness, such as has been described as *le petit-mal*, as surely and swiftly produce enfeeblement. This was the conviction of Esquirol. It has been corroborated by many of equal discrimination " (" Epileptics : their Mental Condition," by W. A. F. Browne, *Journal of Mental Science*, October 1865).

" On a remarqué que l'absence, malgré sa légèreté apparente est la forme la plus redoutable au point de vue de l'altération des facultés intellectuelles " (Jaccoud, *Pathologie Interne*, p. 394).

Is there a condition after the convulsion from discharge beginning in the highest centres (the substrata of consciousness), that is to say, after the convulsion in those cases of epilepsy which *begin with* loss of consciousness, which compares with post-epileptic palsy of a limb ? I think there is a universal or widespread diminution of power corresponding to the universal convulsion. There is no local palsy anywhere demonstrable ; the loss of power is universally distributed, as the spasm in the convulsion was.

It may, however, be said that the universal loss or weakness of movement is simply owing to the patient being comatose—that it is apparent only. But what is it for a patient to be comatose ? Here, again, from another standpoint we must distinguish betwixt psychical and physical. First, then, for the psychical side of the condition. To be comatose is only a greater degree or greater depth of loss of consciousness, as this is only a greater degree of that slight defect permitting only slight confusion of thought (defect of consciousness). What are the physical states corresponding to these psychical losses ? Of course there must be negative states of nervous centres in these cases, as certainly as there are positive states during degrees of consciousness.

There is no such entity as consciousness ; in health we are from moment to moment differently conscious. Consciousness varies in kind and degree according as the parts of the brain in activity are different, and according to the degree of their activity ; and it varies in depth. Object consciousness is continually changing and varying ; subject consciousness is comparatively persistent and unvarying. The three degrees we have taken for illustration are of course arbitrary ; every physician knows that there occur all degrees, from the slightest and most transient defect of consciousness (attended by slight confusion of thought) to coma, and below this to death, psychical and physical. The patient who has slight defect of consciousness has lost the use of a part only of the very highest nervous arrangements ; the patient who has lost consciousness has lost more of them ; the patient who is comatose has lost still more. And as the highest nervous arrangements are only highly complex sensori-motor arrangements representing the whole organism, there are degrees of loss of power over the body corresponding to what are psychically degrees of affection of consciousness. In the case of a man who is comatose after an epileptic fit there will of course be more than this ; not only will the highest centres be exhausted, but more or less of many lower centres through which the currents developed have passed.

To say that a man staggers or lies motionless *because* he has lost consciousness or is comatose, is like saying that a man does not speak *because* he has lost the memory of words, which, at the best, is only repeating in technical terms that he does not speak ; it is like saying that a man does not move his arm *because* he has lost volition, which is only repeating in technical terms that he cannot move it. Nobody is any the wiser for these " explanations " ; they explain nothing at all ; they are attempts to explain physical states by mental states. They may be convenient empirically, but scientifically they are misleading.

Many talk as if a patient could lose consciousness without a loss of use of some parts of the nervous system ; or if they admit that there is loss of use of nervous arrangements along with loss (psychical) of consciousness, the inference from the statement of that admission often is that the nervous arrangements affected did not represent parts of the body, but are centres having nothing to do but to " play upon " the lower centres ; morphologically they are spoken of as part of the body, but physiologically they are spoken of as if they were as distinct from it as the most psychological of psychologists supposes mind to be independent of organisation. This view of the matter, indeed, only differs from that of those medical psychologists who speak of an immaterial mind influencing the body, in that the mind is considered to be solid. Those who take this view are not materialists in effect, nor psychologists either, but a little of both. On this view the centres for consciousness are not " evolved out of," but " placed upon," lower centres and " govern " them autocratically. There is no practical difference in a medical inquiry betwixt this view and that of those psychologists who speak of will, memory, etc., as " faculties " existing apart from physical organisation. On this metaphysico-materialistic view, which really ignores anatomy, substituting for it mere morphology, the centres for consciousness are not centres for receiving impressions, and giving out impulses for movements, but centres which " play upon " lower centres for movements autocratically. On this view, if the centres for consciousness could be sliced away without disturbing the rest of the organism, the physical operations of the body would be positively uninterfered with, although negatively there would be no " volitional impulses " sent down to put the body in this or that movement. Such is, indeed, the explanation actually given by some of the effects of removal of the cerebral hemispheres in certain lower animals. It removes the animal's mind, but does not affect its movements.

The view taken in this article is an anatomical one, *viz*. that the substrata of consciousness are sensori-motor arrangements re-representing all lower centres, and thus representing the whole organism. They govern it not autocratically, but *because* they represent it, and represent it in a far higher degree than an elected President represents a republican state. They *are* the organism in potentiality, giving out impulses to most heterogeneous movements, because they receive most heterogeneous impressions. On this hypothesis if they were sliced away there would be loss of innumerable highly complex and most special co-ordinations of the body as a whole, the lower co-ordinations being badly effected, not from want of autocratic governance, but from actual lack of the higher co-ordinations ; there would be a degree of paralysis universally distributed. Volitional impulses are in this view only the psychical side of activity of the very highest sensori-motor arrangements respecting the whole body. The animal who from lack of the experimentally removed cerebrum has no volition has lost those highest sensori-motor arrangements during activity of which automatic mental action breaks down into volitional action ; or, speaking of the physical side, where the most complex reflex action becomes imperfect and ceases.

The explanation here combated is a metaphysical one. It is a very common thing in medical writings to meet with pure metaphysics put forward as if they were something highly practical. Let me illustrate this statement by an example. In disease of the cerebellum a person is said to reel *because* he has lost the use of a co-ordinating centre. This need not be cavilled at. But then, unfortunately, the supposition often is that there *is* a co-ordinating centre which does not itself represent the most elaborate combinations of impressions and movements of the parts to be co-ordinated, but, as it were, stands outside or above the centres which are for impressions and movements and autocratically governs them, regulates them.

But the man who reels slightly from slight disease of the cerebellum does so because he has lost power over the muscles of his spine ; has actually *lost* the most special and most delicate nervous arrangements for balancing movements of the trunk, those which occur first in locomotion. Here again we see a duplex symptomatic condition (see footnotes on pp. 138 and 146). The movements the patient *does make* are owing to action of healthy centres ; the legs are doing their duty faithfully in running after the trunk to prop it up in its various over-inclinings. Not seeing that there are two elements (negative and positive) leads to the ignoring of the fact that the patient has *lost* something (negative) which is the indirect cause of the over-action of his legs (positive).

We must observe that in each of the three degrees of affection of consciousness (see p. 159) the condition is duplex. In the first degree (defect of consciousness) there is positively confusion of ideas, with the third there is positively conservation of such deeply automatic movements as those of respiration. For example, the confusion of ideas is owing to want of co-operation of those highest nervous arrangements whose loss is attended by the slight psychical affection we call defect of consciousness ; even confused ideation implies activity of nervous arrangements.

Here ends the general sketch, and here too must end my paper, although I have not yet adduced many important facts, which, I think, strongly support the statements made. In particular I have not stated the facts supplied by very limited palsies after very limited convulsions—as of an arm after convulsion of little more than that limb. The reader is asked to bear in mind that this is only part of a paper, and that therefore the argument is incomplete. The remainder of the paper will, if my engagements permit, be printed for private circulation with a reprint of the foregoing.

# ON THE SCIENTIFIC AND EMPIRICAL INVESTIGATION OF EPILEPSIES [1]

## I

### Part I—Introductory

So many books have been written on epilepsy that it may seem rash to add another; but, as I have studied epilepsy, epileptiform seizures, and many other diseases of the nervous system for some years with great care and labour, there is no impropriety in putting forward some of the conclusions I have arrived at. I have, however, already written so very many papers on the subject that what I am now about to write will, in essential matters (method and main conclusions), be a recapitulation. But this, assuming that what I have to say on epilepsy has any importance, is almost a sufficient reason for writing a *book* about it. The papers written during more than ten years are inconveniently scattered in volumes of Reports, in Journals, etc. Again, the work I have done on the subject is to be found in papers where many would never, from the titles of those papers, look for it. This has been the result of my way of investigating. I have studied epilepsy and epileptiform seizures on a novel method, and have written on it from widely different points of view. Besides studying in minute detail such cases as would ordinarily be called idiopathic, or true epilepsy, I have sought out for study simpler cases, or, let me say, until I give my definition of epilepsy, cases of epileptiform convulsion, and especially those complicated with other definite nervous symptoms. For I have long been convinced that "idiopathic epilepsy" is far too difficult a subject for precise investigation unless we approach its consideration from the basis supplied by the principles deduced from less complex kinds of cases. Hence the simpler cases of *partial* convulsion occurring with affections of the optic nerves, with hemiplegia, with disorders of speech, etc., have had particular interest for me. These "complicated" cases are really very much simpler than are cases of "idiopathic epilepsy." Thus it happens that perhaps the

[1] *Medical Press and Circular*, October 14, 1874, to December 13, 1876.

This and subsequent chapters to be published in this journal are the introductory chapters of a forthcoming work on epilepsy.

I must, to prevent misunderstanding, at once remark on one matter which will be considered more fully towards the end of this chapter, and at great length in future chapters. *Throughout this book the functions of the Cerebral Hemisphere are assumed to be the Co-ordination of Impressions and Movements.* The co-ordinations which the very highest centres in the hemispheres effect are only in great degree different from those of the lowest nervous centres. This does not exclude the other so-called "functions" of the cerebral hemisphere, "ideation," "consciousness," etc. Sensori-motor processes are the physical side of, or, as I prefer to say, form the anatomical substrata of, mental states. It is with these substrata only that we are directly concerned in an inquiry like the present.

For some years I have held the view above stated—*viz.* that the whole of the cerebrum is, like lower centres, made up of processes representing impressions and movements. I have stated it in innumerable places, especially with regard to Speech. I consider that this view accords with and is confirmed by the results of the now well-known experiments of Hitzig and Ferrier. With regard to Speech, Ferrier has recently, by independent investigation and from a different kind of evidence, come to conclusions essentially like mine.

most decided of my opinions are to be found expressed in papers, in the heading of which the word " epilepsy " or " epileptiform " does not occur, or in which it is mentioned only incidentally. I will illustrate this—in itself a very small matter—by references to several old papers, in order to show more clearly my manner of investigation, and to give an apology for the peculiar defects of it. Unless this work is a total failure the defects are partly counterbalanced by some advantages. A further reason for these references is that, as my method is unfamiliar, and as probably it may seem, to those who have worked at epilepsy under the accepted definition, vague and unreal, the extracts to be given will show that the opinions I have to express have, at any rate, not been formed hastily. On the contrary, there has been a very gradual development, and, of course, change of, opinion. Many expressions used in the extracts from former papers I should not use now.

In an article on " Loss of Speech " (*London Hospital Reports*, vol. i, 1864), after stating that we may investigate the relations of affections of speech to disease of one side of the brain in cases of unilateral convulsions (epileptiform seizures), as well as in cases of unilateral palsy (hemiplegia), I draw attention to the association of right-sided epileptiform seizures (without loss of consciousness) with temporary defect of speech. I then advance the hypothesis that these seizures depend on disease in the same region of the brain (that of the middle cerebral artery), as does permanent *loss* of speech with right hemiplegia. In other words, the Localisation is in the same region for both sets of symptoms. And I further suggest that the pathology of these cases of unilateral convulsion is a local change (in the vascular district mentioned), resulting from embolism, as the pathology of cases of loss of speech with hemiplegia often is. In one (to employ more recent terms) the embolic process has led to *destruction* (softening) of nervous matter ; in the other, to *instability* of grey matter.[1]

This, indeed, is almost the starting-point of my special investigations of epilepsy. Previously I had accepted what was then, and is still, the almost universal opinion that there is a grouping of symptoms presented paroxysmally, to be called epilepsy, or " idiopathic epilepsy," and that the morbid changes causing this clinical entity are in the medulla oblongata. But it occurred to me to study those simpler cases of convulsion (regardless whether they satisfied the definition of " true epilepsy " or not) which begin in, and chiefly affect, *one* side of the body, and to study them in comparison and contrast with a unilateral paralytic symptom (the common form of hemiplegia) which was *known* to be owing to disease of the corpus striatum. This comparison was made in a paper in the *Lancet*, February 16 and March 9, 1867—" Note on the Comparison and Contrast of Regional Palsy and Spasm " (see p. 5).

A case of paralysis of the face, arm, and leg, with turning of the head

[1] The following quotation may be given from the article mentioned in the text. I would remark before I give it that at the time I wrote I believed unilateral convulsion to be owing to discharge of the corpus striatum, and that the disease which led to that discharge lay in some part of the district of the middle cerebral artery, and I believed too the immediate cause of the discharge of the corpus striatum to be spasm of the arteries supplying that centre.

" We may investigate the subject in unilateral convulsion as well as in unilateral paralysis. There is sometimes temporary defect of speech with hemiplegic epilepsy, just as there is permanent defect of the faculty with decided hemiplegia. Now, I do not assert that epilepsy is due to disease of the middle cerebral artery, or of the pia-mater in the range of that vessel—its vascular expansion—but I submit that one particular form of epilepsy is. Perhaps a better expression would be epileptiform convulsion " (" Loss of Speech : its Association with Valvular Disease of the Heart, and with Hemiplegia on the Right Side—Defects of Smell—Defects of Speech in Chorea—Arterial Regions in Epilepsy "—*London Hospital Reports*, vol. i, 1864).

and two eyes from the side on which the limbs were paralysed, is compared with a case in which the face, arm, and leg were convulsed, and the head and two eyes drawn to the side convulsed; in the former there was disease of the corpus striatum (the thalamus was a little involved, too), and in the latter there was disease of convolutions near to the corpus striatum. One was supposed to be corpus striatum paralysis, the other corpus striatum convulsion. Hence, not only the conclusion that unilateral convulsions are owing to disease of one side of the brain, but that they are owing to disease of the brain in a particular vascular region (the region of the middle cerebral artery).

I ought here very prominently to acknowledge my great obligations to Dr. Broadbent's now well-known hypothesis as to the mode of connection of the bilaterally acting muscles with the corpora striata, by which he explains the escape of these muscles in hemiplegia. This hypothesis was of vast importance to me in working out the relations of hemiplegia to convulsions beginning unilaterally. In the paper referred to it was pointed out that Broadbent's hypothesis accounts not only for the escape of the bilaterally acting muscles in hemiplegia, but for their involvement in hemispasm. Broadbent's hypothesis is confirmed by Ferrier's researches.

Although the method just illustrated seems simple to me, I find it very difficult to convince other persons that it is simple. In spite of my reiterations that I am seeking the particular cerebral centres discharged in cases where any kind of grouping of symptoms is presented paroxysmally, I find that I often give the impression that I am working only to find the seat of but one grouping, *viz.* "epilepsy," as authorities define that disease,—that I am working only to find the seat of a disease in which there occurs paroxysmally loss or trouble of consciousness, with or without convulsion. A quotation from a more recent paper will show that my object has not been so limited (*St. Andrews Medical Graduates' Reports*, vol. iii, 1870) (see p. 8). After speaking of a case supposed to be carefully investigated on its own merits, I remark: "We *do not care* to say that a tumour of the brain (or minute changes near it) had 'caused epilepsy,' but that changes in a particular region of the nervous system—say in the region of the left middle cerebral artery—led to convulsions in which the spasm began in the right hand, spread to the arm, attacked next the face, then the leg, etc."

Dr. Eugène Dupuy, in his interesting monograph entitled *Examen de Quelques Points de la Physiologie du Cerveau*, says: "Before describing our researches apropos of Ferrier's experiments we will remark that the idea put forward by Wilks,[1] Hughlings Jackson,[2] and others, of localising epilepsy in the cortical layer of the brain is not new. It is to be found in the memoir of Boucher and Cazauvielh.[3] It will be shown further on that this theory is unsustainable."

[1] Wilks, *Guy's Hospital Reports*, vol. xii, 3rd series, 1866, p. 225. I will here quote part of what Dr. Wilks has written on the subject, to which Dr. Dupuy refers. I requote it from my article on "Convulsion," *Reynolds's System of Medicine*, vol. ii, 2nd ed. Wilks says ("Pathology of Nervous Diseases," *Guy's Hospital Reports*, 1866) that "the morbid conditions which we find to give rise to epileptiform convulsions are remarkably uniform. They all point to the presence of local irritation of the surface [of the brain]." Speaking of a case of epileptic convulsions in a patient who had tumour in the pons varolii—a case which had been supposed to confirm Schröder van der Kolk's "supposition that the cause of epilepsy is seated in this part"—he says: "I have no hesitation in saying that for one such case fifty might be found in which the marked changes producing these symptoms occupy the surface [of the brain]."

[2] Hughlings Jackson, *West Riding Lunatic Asylum Medical Reports*, vol. iii, p. 315 (see p. 90), and *Reynolds's System of Medicine*, article "Convulsion."

[3] Boucher et Cazauvielh, *Archives de Médecine*. Paris, 1825.

Whether the theory be sustainable or not I do not discuss for the present. I wish to point out that my aim has not been merely to find the seat of "epilepsy" in the sense in which that term is generally used. At first it was simply to localise the seat of one comparatively simple set of symptoms presented paroxysmally. It was in 1864 [1] to find the exact results of discharge of parts in a particular region of the brain, regardless whether the paroxysm caused by that discharge was genuinely epileptic or not. More recently, as will be seen, I have used the word "epilepsy" as a name for any set of symptoms, sensory or motor, dependent on abrupt and excessive cerebral discharges (paroxysmal discharges). The symptoms usually grouped under the name "epilepsy" constitute one, but only one, of many groupings of symptoms which I hope we shall be able to localise in different parts of the "cortical layer" of the brain.

The great object I have had in view, as the extracts show, has been to study the relations of epilepsy or epileptiform seizures to simpler diseases of the nervous system, and *through the latter to normal states*. For example, returning to an old illustration, paralysis of the face, arm, and leg (hemiplegia) points to destruction of or of part of the corpus striatum, and my inference is that mobile conditions of the face, arm, and leg (an epileptiform seizure in which these parts are convulsed, or irregular movements of them as in hemichorea) are owing to nervous discharges in the very same cerebral region—discharges of convolutions *near* to the corpus striatum. This is really the study of cases as *departures from healthy states*. For hemiplegia may, for this purpose, be properly regarded as an experiment made by disease revealing to us the external parts represented in the healthy corpus striatum. It shows that the corpus striatum contains nervous processes for the movements of the face, arm, and leg. The unilateral convulsion and the hemichorea are over-developments of such movements which are lost in the quasi-experiment of hemiplegia.

This is just the opposite of the ordinary method of investigating epilepsy and epileptiform seizures. The question commonly put about a case is solely "Is it a case of epilepsy?" or "Is it only an epileptiform seizure?" In other words, cases are often investigated solely in order to see if the symptoms reach or approach certain Clinical Entities, and not at all as they are signs of *departure* from health.

I may here quote again from an old paper already referred to (*Royal London Ophthalmic Hospital Reports*, 1866):

"We want positive information as to how a convulsion is a *departure* from health of muscles and muscular groups [2] and health of nervous organs and tissues, and not as to how far it *approaches* our idea of the almost metaphysical conception 'genuine' epilepsy. . . . There are to be found on record scarcely any positive statements of what has really happened in particular

[1] It would be only an exaggeration to say that at one time (1864 and some while after) I *did not care* about the seat of the lesion in cases of "genuine epilepsy." Writing about three years later (1867) in the paper on "Regional Palsy and Spasm," referred to in the text, I said: "But I fear *genuine epilepsy* is at present an *insoluble problem*. I would begin, as I have suggested, with a simpler kind of convulsion. I would try to find what condition of nervous matter in one part [of the nervous centres] permitted occasional spasm of the muscles which that part empowers; and I choose the corpus striatum, as we do know, from its frequent damage in hemiplegia, what muscular regions it governs."

[2] As will be seen in a later chapter (on Classification), I do not now object to clinical entities for practical purposes. I now admit that they are absolutely necessary. But I object just as strongly as ever I did to the claims of those investigations to be considered scientific whose aim is only to determine whether a case be or resemble one of "genuine epilepsy." Such investigations are very valuable, but they are empirical only.

convulsive paroxysms—a process which sometimes occurs under our very eyes. I am fully aware that there are admirable accounts of the worst fits as types, but some of these accounts are descriptions more of dramas of great human interest than calm and cold scientific observations in an orderly sequence of the outward phenomena of an inwardly suffering nervous system."

I have more to quote to the same effect regarding the localisation of one simple set of symptoms presented paroxysmally as an illustration of my method. In an article on " Defects of Sight," *Royal London Ophthalmic Hospital Reports*, vol. v, pt. 4, 1866, I found myself constantly obliged to speak of the investigations of Chronic Convulsive (Epileptiform) Seizures. For example, p. 268, when speaking of cases of optic neuritis, complicated with convulsions, beginning unilaterally, I urge the study of these mobile muscular disorders, regardless of the vested rights of clinical entities.

" Such a kind of work will be more hopeful than working at cases of amaurosis, as they are ' complicated ' by the entities ' epilepsy,' ' paralysis,' or ' chorea.' There are, very fortunately, cases in which the symptoms of unilateral muscular disorder refuse to be classed as either unilateral epileptiform seizures, or unilateral paralysis, or unilateral chorea. These cases are, I hold, of extreme value in leading to an organisation of our knowledge of altered physiological conditions higher than an arrangement of symptoms in groups, as epilepsy, chorea, etc. Ophthalmologists will be the last to purposely put amaurosis in association with the abstractions we call ' genuine epilepsy,' ' real chorea,' etc., when it is at all possible to avoid doing so."

As further references to past and scattered work on my subject, I may mention that in the article in the *Ophthalmic Hospital Reports*, already quoted from vol. v, pt. 4, 1866, the occurrence of temporary coloured vision, and of other temporary defects of sight in association with unilateral convulsion, is considered. In another article (vol. vi, pt. 1, April 2, 1868) is an expression of an opinion on that temporary loss of sight which I now call epileptiform amaurosis, and used to call epilepsy of the retina.[1]

A recent writer, after giving a very brief account of some of my opinions on epilepsies, concludes by saying that most physicians would not admit that the cases I speak of are really cases of epilepsy, because there is in many of them no loss nor trouble of consciousness. If he had said that I was not justified in using the word " epilepsy " in a new sense I could not have objected to his criticism as criticism. I repeat that epilepsy, as authorities define it, is but *one* of the grouping of symptoms which I believe to result from nervous discharges of parts of the cerebral hemisphere. It is but one of the group which I call epilepsies. Whether consciousness be lost or not, or whether it be lost early or late in an epilepsy, as I define epilepsy, depends on the seat of the " discharging lesion." Cases in which loss of consciousness is the first symptom are cases in which discharge *begins* in the highest centres (in the anatomical substrata of consciousness).

## PART II—SUMMARY

I shall be obliged, in carrying out the method above stated, to consider at length many subjects usually considered apart from epilepsy. I will here

[1] In passing, I would remark that those cases of migraine with temporary hemiopia and other visual troubles (recently well described by Latham and Liveing) are the most important cases of this class.

give a sketch of some of the more important of them. I do so chiefly because what has to come in the early chapters will involve anticipations of what has to be proved in later ones.

Before I go further I have certain obligations to acknowledge. I am under very heavy obligations to Herbert Spencer. I shall acknowledge these obligations in detail in later chapters. It will, however, be apparent in almost every part of the latter half of the present chapter that I am greatly indebted to him. Let me at once give a quotation from his *Psychology* with regard to evolution of nervous centres, a subject on which I have much to say: "In the functions of the successively higher vertebrate centres, reaching their climax in the human being, we see well exemplified the law of development of functions in general" (*First Principles*, p. ii, § 142). "This progress from co-ordinations that are small and simple to those that are larger and compound and to those that are still larger and doubly compound, is one of the best instances of that progressive integration of motions simultaneously becoming more heterogeneous and more definite which characterises evolution under all its forms" (*Principles of Psychology*, vol. i, p. 67).

I must mention very prominently Laycock's doctrine of the Reflex Function of the Brain. The following is a quotation from an article written by him thirty years ago. The first sentence of the quotation refers to a still earlier exposition of the doctrine in his treatise on the *Nervous Diseases of Women.* This book was published in 1840, and contains a chapter (p. 105) headed "The Instinctive Actions in Relation to Consciousness: the Brain subject to the Laws of Reflex Action."

"Four years have elapsed since I published my opinion, supported by such arguments as I could then state, that the *brain*, although the organ of consciousness, *is subject to the laws of reflex action, and that, in this respect, it does not differ from the other ganglia of the nervous system.* I was led to this opinion by the general principle that the ganglia within the cranium, being a continuation of the spinal cord, *must necessarily be regulated, as to their reaction on external agencies, by laws identical with those governing the spinal ganglia, and their analogues in the lower animals.* And I was confirmed in this opinion by finding, after the investigation and collocation of known facts, that observations and arguments like those satisfactorily adduced in proof of the existence of the reflex function of the spinal ganglia, may be brought forward in proof that the cerebral ganglia have similar endowments. In the present paper I propose to give these proofs connectedly" (*British and Foreign Medical Review*, vol. xix, January 1845, p. 298).

I have italicised some parts of this quotation which state clearly a principle I shall restate from a different standpoint when speaking of the relations of Psychology to the Anatomy and Physiology of the Nervous System.

It is scarcely necessary to point out that, like all other writers on epilepsy, I am in debt to Brown-Séquard.

To Dr. Ferrier I am very specially indebted. I shall have many opportunities of acknowledging my very great obligations to him. His well-known researches, and those of Hitzig to which he refers, are of inestimable value for clinical medicine, as well as for physiology.

To Prof. Bain I owe much. From him I derived the notion that the anatomical substrata of words are motor (articulatory) processes. (This, I must mention, is a much more limited view than he takes.) This hypothesis has been of very great importance to me, not only specially because it gives the best anatomico-physiological explanation of the phenomena of Aphasia *when all varieties of this affection are taken into consideration*, but because it helped me very much in endeavouring to show that the " organ of mind " contains processes representing movements, and that, therefore, there was nothing unreasonable in supposing that excessive discharge of convolutions should produce that clotted mass of movements which we call spasm.[1]

Not less are my obligations to Mr. Lewes. I shall have to refer to his writings in many parts of this book.

I now proceed to brief anticipatory statements of some of the topics to be discussed at length in later chapters.

The method of studying cases as departures from health obliges me to compare and contrast the effects of " destroying lesions " with those of " discharging lesions." I have incidentally illustrated this by the contrast and the comparison of hemiplegia and hemispasm for another purpose. I will now give another example. When I speak of *epileptiform* aphasia I must speak of aphasia caused by a permanent gross lesion. For, *after*, as well as *during*, certain epileptiform seizures, we find temporary defects of speech like those more permanent ones which so often result from embolism or thrombosis, or from clot. Sometimes there is hemiplegia with it—epileptic hemiplegia of Dr. Todd. It is unreasonable to study a suddenly occurring and transitory symptom without comparing it with what we have learned of the same symptom when permanent, which latter we can study with any degree of minuteness, and at our leisure.

Another matter closely connected with the subject just spoken of is that it is absolutely necessary to consider convulsion and other paroxysmal symptoms as " experiments[2] made by disease " which reveal the localisation of processes for different groupings of movements and impressions in different parts of the cerebral hemispheres. This is, so far as I know, quite unfamiliar, and, therefore, has an air of unreality. It requires a vast amount of time to observe cases of convulsion minutely enough for this purpose. Nothing in our clinical work demands so much patience. The results of the experiments of Fritsch, Hitzig, and Ferrier are infinitely more precise than those of the " experiments of disease," but the latter are nevertheless, I assert again, *absolutely necessary*, as they are the only experiments on the brain which can be observed for the localisation of movements in the case of man. For this purpose, since " destroying lesions " of much of the cerebral hemisphere produce no obvious or striking symptoms, we *are obliged* to study the effects of " discharging lesions " in these parts.

Epilepsy, like aphasia, has been studied with a psychological habit of mind, and, as I think this way of studying such a disease is unfruitful, I have to point out in detail the vast difference there is betwixt Psychology and the Anatomy and Physiology of the Nervous System. The confusion of the two, as I believe, is really one of the great hindrances to the acceptance of the view that the convolutions (parts of the " organ of mind ") represent movements. The notion

[1] I ought to mention that Dr. Bastian, a physician whose opinion on any such subject deserves the greatest respect, has vigorously and very ably combated Bain's opinion, and, at the same time, my explanation of the phenomena of aphasia founded on it (*Med. Chir. Revue*, January 1869).

[2] See " On Localisation of Movements in the Brain," *Lancet*, January 13, 1873. (See p. 63.)

seems to be that the " organ of mind " being for " ideation," cannot contain processes representing movements.

Admitting, as the whole educated world now does, that all mental states have parallel physical states, I think our direct concern as physiologists and physicians is with the latter only. Hence, I should not use such expressions as that hemiplegia is " owing to loss of volition," or that a person did not speak *because* he had lost the " memory of words." These are really little better than verbal propositions. I willingly plead guilty to having formerly used similar phrases open to the same criticism. I should also in an investigation like this, when possible, avoid such expressions as " centres of ideation," " emotional centres," etc., not because I dispute their correctness, but because our concern, as physicians, is with the anatomical substrata of ideas and emotions. Besides, the expressions objected to refer only to the material basis of mind. To give a material explanation of mental states, admitting its correctness so far as it goes, is not to give an anatomical explanation. Again, to say that the substrata of mind are made up of arrangements of cells and fibres or centres of cells and fibres, is to make a statement which is not disputed by educated people nowadays, but it is only a statement in morphology ; or rather, such expressions as " centres of ideation " are mixtures of morphological and psychological terms. They contain nothing anatomical or physiological. The anatomical substrata of ideas (of the more important, evidently) are sensori-motor processes. The whole of the central nervous system, cerebral hemisphere, spinal cord, etc., is made up of processes of differing degrees of complexity representing impressions and movements. There are, so far as I can judge, no other " materials " of which the " organ of mind " can be made up. As the quotation from Spencer implies, the very highest of all nervous centres are but complex rearrangements of lower centres, and these of still lower centres unto the lowest, which last *directly* represent impression and movements.

Perhaps one criticism on the above will be that I am confounding " mental " states with " physical states." A reader may perhaps suppose that I imagine processes for impressions and movements to become in the highest centres so fine that they " fine away " into mental states. I do not. To show what I really think, let me quote the words of Herbert Spencer :

" Though accumulated observations and experiments have led us by a very indirect series of inferences to the belief that mind and nervous action are the subjective and objective phases of the same thing, we remain utterly incapable of seeing and even of imagining how the two are related " (Spencer, *Principles of Psychology*, vol. i, p. 140). Elsewhere Mr. Spencer writes :

" See, then, our predicament. We can think of Matter only in terms of Mind. We can think of Mind only in terms of Matter. When we have pushed our explorations of the first to the uttermost limit, we are referred to the second for a final answer ; and when we have got the final answer of the second, we are referred back to the first for an interpretation of it. We find the value of $x$ in terms of $y$ ; then we find the value of $y$ in terms of $x$ ; and so on we may continue for ever without coming nearer to a solution " (*Principles of Psychology*, § 272).

To show my feeling on the matter, I will remark that I consider the confusion I have spoken of is really fostered by such classifications as those of aphasia which put together " ataxy of articulation " (physiological phraseology) and "loss of memory for words" (psychological phraseology) and imply nothing of the nature of the anatomical substrata of words.

How from or during the energising of sensori-motor processes, or of the highest of them, there arise mental states, is not our concern, not our direct concern at any rate, in such investigations as the present. Yet it is of no importance, for this investigation, what view of the connection of mind and matter we take. If any reader supposes mind to be a function of matter (thought, let us say, a secretion of brain), I should simply say to him that one does not concern one's self with *that* "function" in an anatomical and physiological inquiry, but with another function—*viz.* the energising of cells and fibres representing peripheral impressions and adjusted movements.

I make these last remarks because I think some people have the notion that to take a materialistic view is to take a "practical" view. But, as above stated, a merely material view is not an anatomical one. Admitting for the sake of argument that it is perfectly correct, so far as it goes, it has to go a stage further to be *anatomical*. I shall try to show later that under this supposed "practical" guise work has been done on the old-fashioned system. We judge people not by the names they use, but by their method. The old-fashioned method spoke of an immaterial mind. The very same method in a new dress still speaks of a brain as if it were a "solid mind" governing and acting on the body, and not as if it were simply the most developed part of the nervous system "regulated by laws identical with those governing the spinal ganglia" (*Laycock* requoted).

The first half of the compound word "sensori-motor" is not free from objection. The word "sensation" is often confusedly applied both to a physical state and to the mental state which occurs along with it (see Mill's *Logic*, vol. ii, p. 43); for example, it is used for colour (mental state) and for the molecular disturbances in the "optic nervous system" which occur therein whilst that mental state exists. It is used for pain, and for the associated disturbances in afferent nerves and centres. I think this confused use of the word leads to many misunderstandings. It makes it fallaciously easy to understand how it is that we have mental states from (or during) the energising of afferent nerves and centres, whilst no thought is given to the possibility that mental states arise during energising of efferent nerves and their centres. To give an example, it makes it seem easy to understand that energising of nervous processes representing retinal impressions should give us ideas of objects, whilst it leads to difficulty in accepting the opinion that energising of processes representing articulatory *movements* should give us ideas of words. The real fact is, that in neither case can we tell why during energising of cells and fibres we have ideas. The difficulty is just the same in the two cases, for mental states arise from or during *molecular movements* in nerve cells and fibres, and they arise, I submit, during molecular movements in nerve cells and fibres representing movements as well as during molecular movements in those representing impressions. "Sensations" in the sense of "mental states" arise, I submit, during energising of motor as well as of "sensory" nerve processes—with the "out-going" as well as with the "in-going" current. I should not dwell on this were it not that the distinction insisted on is of very direct importance. For example, I have to show that vertigo is essentially a motor symptom, and that the "sensation" of vertigo is no proof that vertigo is fundamentally an affair of "sensory" (afferent) nerves or centres.

Although I have, for convenience, spoken separately of afferent and efferent processes, and, if I may so speak of afferent and efferent centres, both are concerned together on the anatomical and physiological side of " ideation." The former are evidently concerned in *acquiring* ideas of the dynamical or secondary qualities of *objects*, the latter in *acquiring* ideas of the statical or primary. For example, in actually seeing objects, there is a strong discharge from periphery (retina) to centre, and from centre to periphery (ocular muscles).[1] There is not sensory action only, nor motor action only ; there is sensori-motor action. There is a similar process in having the ideas again. The faint and central discharges which occur in thinking of objects (recollecting, being conscious of, having an idea of, etc.) will be of nervous processes which are representatives of both[2] impressions and movements. For, in thinking of objects, there is not only a representation of surface (colour), but also of size and figure. In fact, the discharge will be of the very same series of nervous processes in presentation and representation ; in the latter the discharge is slight, and is limited to the centre, whilst in the former it is strong, and reaches from periphery to centre, and from centre to periphery. We shall see that in accordance with these views there occurs from the epileptic, what is not only a strong but an excessive discharge of " centres for ideas," brutal development of the two elements—crude impressions (clouds of colour appearing to the patient, for example) and that clotted mass of movements we call spasm.

As will be inferred, I adopt Bain's views on the " out-going " current. The facts of cases of vertigo, many ocular symptoms, but most strikingly the production of " ideal " movements by faradising stumps have led me to accept his opinion. I have in a former paper (in the 3rd vol. of the *West Riding Asylum Reports*,[3] p. 191) (see p. 85) spoken of the proof which such cases give that *central* excitations of processes representing movement suffice in internal speech and other mental operations. Remarks like these are foreign to the subject of epilepsy as that disease is usually studied, but not foreign to my view of it. For, as above stated, I believe epileptic paroxysms result from discharges of parts of the organ of mind, from discharge of parts containing anatomical substrata of ideas, into which substrata the element movement necessarily enters.

In order to obtain a realistic view of the symptom loss of consciousness, I have to speak in detail of the evolution of the higher nervous centres out of the lower. All nervous centres represent or re-represent impressions and movements. The highest centres are those which form the anatomical substrata of consciousness, and they differ from the lower centres in compound

[1] " The qualities of things admitted on all hands to be qualities of the external or object world—called the primary qualities—resistance and extension—are modes of our muscular energies ; the qualities that do not of themselves suggest externality or objectivity, the secondary qualities as heat, colour, etc., are our passive sensibilities, and do not contain muscular energy " (Note by Bain, p. 5, vol. i, of James Mill's *Analysis of the Human Mind*).

The ocular movements spoken of in the text are, strictly speaking, symbols of the tactual and locomotor movements that give us our ideas of the primary qualities.

[2] This statement embodies, I believe, Spencer's theory of the physical process which occurs during recollection (see *Principles of Psychology*, vol. i, pp. 124 and 456).

[3] I tried to show two things—(1) that energising of processes representing movements is a factor in the physical side of ideation (as, for example, in ideas of size and figure), and (2) that nascent excitation (excitation *limited* to the centre), or, otherwise expressed, a " motor impulse," suffices in memory, etc. For in the cases spoken of, notably in faradising stumps, we have ideas from excitation of motor centres when the current developed is physically debarred from reaching the muscles (*On Faradising Stumps*. See the masterly work of Weir Mitchell on *Injuries of Nerves*).

degree only. They represent over again, but in more numerous combinations, in greater complexity, speciality, and multiplicity of associations, the very same impressions and movements which the lower, and through them the lowest, centres represent. They represent the whole organism. They represent not only the impressions of the five senses, and the movements ordinarily so-called, but also organic or systemic sensations (Bain and Lewes) and movements of the heart, arteries, intestines, etc. "*The seat of consciousness is that nervous centre to which, mediately or immediately, the most heterogeneous impressions are brought.*"[1] The statement is not of the most *numerous* impressions, but most heterogeneous. To the seat or seats of consciousness, impressions of all orders are brought, and from it issue motor impulses of all orders.

Let us see how the paroxysms of certain cases of epilepsy corroborate this view—that the highest of the highest nervous centres re-represent the whole of the body. The cases I mean are those in which the symptom, loss of consciousness is the first event in the seizure (cases without a "warning"). Now, these are the cases in which the discharge begins in the very highest centres (in the substrata of consciousness). They are the cases which commonly go by the name of true or idiopathic epilepsy. To say of a paroxysm of epilepsy that it begins with loss of consciousness is a symptomatic expression; to say that the discharge begins in the very highest processes is the anatomico-physiological expression corresponding to it.

In those cases of epilepsy in which loss of consciousness is the *first* event in the paroxysm, the convulsion is universal, the two sides of the body are more nearly equally and more nearly contemporaneously convulsed; it is in these cases that there is, at the very first, much pallor of the face. I think these cases agree with the conclusion that the sensori-motor processes which form the anatomical substrata of consciousness are evolved out of, re-represent, and, so to speak, potentially contain, all other (lower) series of sensori-motor processes.[2] For a discharge beginning in these highest processes affects the whole body quickly, and affects the whole very nearly at the same time.

This realistic method of treating the symptom loss of consciousness is a matter of the utmost importance. We can, on this method, study the "mental" as well as the "physical" symptoms of epilepsy anatomically and physiologically, and free from that psychological bias which makes the symptom loss, or trouble of consciousness, an isolated phenomenon, with no relations to other nervous symptoms.

Here, reverting to a former topic, I may again draw attention to the importance of studying epilepsy by the aid of far simpler cases of nervous disease. I could not at an earlier stage give this illustration. From the facts of cases of cerebral hæmorrhage, cerebral tumour, etc., I have long since drawn the conclusion that the convolutions of the cerebral hemisphere represent not only ordinary movements and impressions, but the whole of the "vital" processes. In a paper in the *Medical Mirror*, October 1869, I write, except for a few verbal alterations, as follows: "We have now, then, to add to the constitution of the units of the cerebrum nerve fibres to the heart, vessels, and viscera, or rather

[1] Spencer, *Psychology*, vol. i, p. 105.

[2] It is most significant, whatever the explanation may be, that there are slight cases (*petit-mal*) in which, with merely transient loss of consciousness, there is deep pallor of the face, and a slight wave of universal movement. In such cases there is often a warning by a feeling mostly very disagreeable but not ordinary pain at the epigastrium. This feeling is, I believe, a development of systemic sensations.

probably to regions of the sympathetic system from which these parts are supplied. The inference we have now arrived at is that the units of the cerebral hemisphere (in the region of the corpus striatum, at least) represent potentially the whole processes of the body. If this be so we can understand how it happens that in cases of epilepsy (beginning by loss of consciousness, *i.e.* beginning in the highest nervous processes), besides obvious convulsion, we have premonitory shivering, pallor of face, and increased flow of saliva, and in some cases vomiting. Thus, too, we see how it is that emotional manifestations accompany intellectual phenomena. Emotional phenomena are wide and yet temporary bodily states, and we have seen that the heart, arteries, and viscera, as well as the large muscles of the body, are represented in the units of the cerebrum."

I must consider at some length another general principle—the principle of Compensation in nervous organs. This clears the superficial paradox stated in a former paragraph—*viz.* that destruction of parts in a certain region of the cerebrum produces no obvious or striking symptoms, notwithstanding that strong discharge of those parts produces exceeding violence of movement (convulsion).

The movements represented in the destroyed part are represented, although in somewhat different order, in neighbouring parts (the compensation is never absolute). Taken with the principle of evolution, the principle of compensation accounts, I consider, for the fact that fits, declared to be like the epileptic fits of man (and which I believe result from discharges of parts of the cerebrum), can result in lower animals from discharge of the pons varolii and medulla oblongata—can result, that is, when the cerebrum is taken away. For I shall try to show that, as I have already in principle said, when speaking of loss of consciousness, the cerebral hemisphere re-represents the very same external parts which the pons varolii, and all other lower centres represent, but more specially, in greater complexity, etc. In man re-representation or evolution is carried many stages further than in the brute : man has the large cerebral hemisphere ; the brute the large pons and medulla.

There is also to be considered the principle of Dissolution. As in evolution the development is from the general to the special, so in the opposite process of dissolution the *un*development is from the special to the general. Using psychological terms, and taking particular cases, we may illustrate by saying that the Insane Patient is one who is reduced to a more automatic condition of Mind, the Aphasic to a more automatic condition of Language, and the Hemiplegic Man to a more automatic condition of Voluntary Movement. If the reader bears in mind what was implicitly stated of evolution when the symptom loss of consciousness was considered (that there is a continuous transition from the lowest centres concerned in the most general or most automatic physical actions, through intermediate centres up to the highest centres concerned in the most special or most voluntary actions, that is, to the anatomical substrata of consciousness) he will see that the following statements on the conditions of the insane, the aphasic and the hemiplegic man are, although from a different standpoint, to the very same effect as the statements already made—that they are " reduced," etc. The insane man has lost the use of, or of some of, the most special of all nervous processes whatsoever ; he has, indeed, defect of consciousness. The aphasic man has lost the most special processes of the language series ; the hemiplegic man the most special processes for movement.

This principle will have to be expounded at length, because it enables us to understand the duplex condition in acute attacks of insanity occurring with epilepsy (epileptic mania) and also in insanity ordinarily so-called. I will speak briefly on it now. First let us recapitulate. The principle of evolution is that the higher centres are evolved out of the lower. The highest centres (the anatomical substrata of consciousness) are, as it were, the climax of the evolution, and re-represent *all* lower centres. In other words, they represent the whole organism (subject). It is only another mode of stating the same thing to say that they are the processes by which the organism, *as a whole*, is adjusted to its environment (object). There are after certain epileptic attacks Reductions to more general adjustments, corresponding to lower ranges of evolution—we may say there are lowerings of adjustment, owing to different depths of dissolution beginning in the highest centres.

This last way of stating the process of Dissolution is most convenient for our purpose. I will restate it with details. Considering the very highest of all nervous processes as those concerned in the most special adjustments of the organism as a whole to its environment (see quotation from Spencer in next footnote), and considering that these processes are evolved out of lower series of processes which represent more general adjustments, and these again out of still lower series representing adjustments still more general, and so on to the lowest series of nervous processes in the body—we can, I think, by taking note of the experiments of disease, show stages of lowering of adjustment as consequences of different depths of Dissolution beginning in the higher centres. Such lowering of adjustment is indeed but another aspect of Dissolution, and is equivalent to saying that the organism is reduced to a more automatic condition. On this way of putting it, it matters not whether consciousness is displayed or not during the play of the more general adjustments. The question is—" How is the Organism adjusted to its Environment ? " Let us now see how these principles apply to epileptic mania and to other conditions *following* severe epileptic discharges.

As before said, an epileptic maniac is one who has been reduced to a more automatic condition of mind. He is so reduced by loss of use of (exhaustion of) the highest centres, consequent on a strong nervous discharge beginning in them. But we shall see that there are, after different degrees of epileptic discharges beginning in the highest centres, *all* degrees of dissolution, or otherwise put, *all* degrees of lowering of adjustment [1] of the organism to its environment. Starting from a condition which is subjectively only slight confusion of thought, we can trace all gradations to deepest coma, in which last there remains only action, and that imperfect, of some of the most automatic of all processes, respiration and circulation. There is indeed sometimes a loss of all adjustment, which is death.

The condition of things in insanity differs only in degree from that in epileptic mania. The ordinary insane patient has *defect* of consciousness, analogous to the *loss* of consciousness of the epileptic maniac ; the " symptoms " of insanity are due to quasi-healthy actions of more automatic processes, as are also those of the epileptic maniac.

[1] " For since all modes of consciousness can be nothing else than incidents of the correspondence between the organism and its environment, they must all be different sides of, or different phases of, the co-ordinated groups of changes whereby internal relations are adjusted to external relations " (Spencer's *Psychology*, No. 25, p. 496).

Two things which should, I think, be considered separately, are often considered together under heredity. I have, then, to speak in two places of heredity. I have to show under pathology that there is hereditary transmission (1) of a tendency to diseases of tissues ; and in another place I have to urge that there is (2) transmission of imperfect organs. The " facts " of these hereditary transmissions are not, I consider, evidence that there is inherited a tendency to particular *diseases* or *symptoms*, such as chorea, epilepsy, insanity, etc. Let me show one kind of confusion. (I here speak of the " genuine epilepsy " of authorities.) If in an epileptic patient's family hemiplegia had been common, it would be no evidence whatever that a tendency to epilepsy was inherited (as a *nervous* disease I mean, of course), for the very simple reason that hemiplegia itself is not, strictly speaking, a nervous symptom. In the vast majority of cases it is an *arterial affair*. Hemiplegia mostly occurs because an artery breaks (hæmorrhage), or because an artery is blocked up (softening from thrombosis). Yet it is common to find such " facts " brought forward as proof of inheritance of *nervous* diseases, or of a tendency to them.

The neuroses in particular are mostly supposed to be hereditary directly, or by substitution. For the present I draw attention to the significant fact that *the pathology of these diseases, which are supposed to be pre-eminently hereditary*, is, according to most physicians, unknown. Under pathology I shall, I hope, show that in nearly all cases of " nervous " diseases or symptoms of which the pathology *is* known, morbid anatomy declares that the changes begin in non-nervous tissues. I confess that my impression is that this will be found to be the case with epilepsy and the allied neuroses. Indeed, I think there is already, to say the least, a strong case for the inference that one of them, chorea, is very often an arterial affair ; the discharging nerve tissue in this disease I believe becomes unstable from hyperæmia, a result of plugging of arteries.

Heredity with regard to the transmission of imperfect organs has to be considered in order to help to make clearer the nature of the symptoms of Epileptic Mania, and other forms of insanity. A man does not, according to my hypothesis, inherit insanity of any kind. The man whose insanity is said to have been transmitted is, I think, a person who inherits an imperfect nervous system, not imperfect in its tissues, but in relative development of its higher and lower centres. First, the higher, and metaphorically speaking, *controlling centres* are in him imperfectly developed, that is to say, psychologically speaking, the latest faculties acquired by the race are in him ill-developed. Secondly, the lower centres and corresponding lower faculties are in comparison over-developed.[1]

Such a man is more liable than another man to *become* insane, but not because he more than another man has any tendency to *disease of the tissues of the brain* (connective, arterial, or nervous), but because either any actual disease of the tissues of his brain, or general severe ill health, nay, even misery, etc., would

[1] I do not mean by " higher " faculties simply mind generally, or by " lower " the " passions and instincts." There are all gradations from instinctive actions, or even from the lowest and simplest reflex actions to the highest processes concerned in reasoning (see Spencer *passim*). Nor is the expression " emotional " limited, as it often is, to the common and superficial emotions. The highest faculties (those last acquired by the race) are the power of Abstract Reasoning (Intellectual) and the sentiment of Justice (Emotional) (Spencer). In cases of commencing disease of the brain, loss of power of connected thought on difficult and complex matters, with peevishness and selfishness, are owing to defects in these two highest faculties. These defects, when in slight degrees, are popularly called " alterations " of the disposition.

very easily impair, or put entirely out of use, the highest (controlling) nerve processes. On the principle of dissolution the highest of his nervous processes are those which will fail first, from causes affecting the whole brain. He is more easily than another man rendered insane by epileptic fits, because he can bear little damage of any sort to the highest parts of his nervous system. He is sometimes a man who would be easily excited (" maddened," his friends may say) by drink. (See Griesinger, *Syd. Society Transactions.*)

I do not believe that there is an insane neurosis interchangeable with epilepsy, chorea, or neuralgia. Insanity and such diseases as epilepsy and chorea are not fairly comparable. The *active* symptoms of insanity are not directly due to the *disease* of the brain or of any other part of the nervous system, as the symptoms chorea, convulsion, and spasm are. The " symptoms " of insanity are due to action of lower centres of the brain, which centres are healthy except for exaggerated action, consequent on loss or defect of the highest and controlling centres, the parts really *diseased.* The insane man is reduced to a more automatic condition of mind by loss of or defect in these highest and controlling centres, or, as we have otherwise expressed it, his adjustment is lowered. In the acute insanity of epileptic mania the " disease " is that the highest centres are temporarily and suddenly paralysed by a strong nervous discharge ; the mania, like the insanity, is owing to uncontrolled action of lower and more automatic [1] centres, which centres are not diseased.

I do not mean to imply that I can prove all these points satisfactorily. In particular, at present I have no satisfactory answer to the objection which is sure to be brought, *viz.* that epilepsy artificially induced in guinea-pigs (Brown-Séquard) is hereditary.

It will be granted that it is very difficult to show that such different lines of thought as those mentioned above harmonise. Evidently in writing the earlier chapters of this book I must anticipate conclusions to be reached in later ones. I have endeavoured to render my method less difficult to the reader by a free use of footnotes.

Such a way of handling a subject is, however, not favourable for clearness of exposition. It is far from easy to make plain the relations of things, some

[1] As will be inferred, I accept Laycock's doctrine on the Reflex Function of the Brain (*vide supra*). I accept also a principle formulated by Dr. Anstie, some years ago, that increased action of lower centres is due to loss of control by the higher, or, as I suppose we may say nowadays, to lack of inhibition (see his *Stimulants and Narcotics, passim*). The great differences betwixt epileptic mania and insanity ordinarily so-called are, I think, due to differences in the suddenness with which the highest processes are put wholly or partially *hors de combat.*

The following extract from the *Medical Times and Gazette*, July 9, 1873, referring to heredity, may help to make what I have said in the text clearer :

" The *facts* of ' transmission of disease ' are not denied, but a very different *interpretation* of them is suggested. There is now attending the out-patient room a boy who is manifestly the subject of congenital syphilis, and whose mind has failed several months. One sign of mental failure has been a magpie-like hiding of tools. It would be, Dr. Hughlings Jackson thinks, unmethodical to call this lad's mental condition ' Syphilitic Insanity '—obviously grotesque if, going into details, we should say that hiding his fellow-workmen's tools was a syphilitic symptom. The boy's father died insane in Colney Hatch. This boy has received as his father's share in his development not only a syphilitic taint, but a nervous system the higher division of which is easily ' reduced.' It *so happens* that the reducing agent has been in all probability syphilitic disease. The inheritance was not of insanity, but of a brain ready to fail on comparatively slight provocation of any kind—one probably easily upset by drink or excitement (easily excited, rather). No doubt anything which involved even slight damage to the cerebrum would in such a brain have ' caused ' insanity, from so-called ' alteration ' of disposition up to insanity as the term is commonly used."

of which have been almost universally considered separately from epilepsy. I have therefore for several years delayed the execution of this work; but the recent brilliant researches of Ferrier encourage me in the belief that a connected account of the work I have done on epilepsies may be acceptable. For he mentions that he undertook his experiments partly with the object of putting to "experimental proof" the views I have put forward on epilepsy.[1]

The value of Ferrier's researches as contributions to the anatomy and physiology of the nervous system could scarcely be overrated. But very naturally to me, a physician, their greatest value seems to be for the help they afford in the methodical investigation of that most inhuman of all diseases, epilepsy. It is a matter of great satisfaction to me to find that my views have passed well through the ordeal. Ferrier, speaking of his experiments, writes:

"The pathology of epileptiform convulsions, chorea, and epileptic hemiplegia, receive much light from the foregoing experiments. I regard them as an experimental confirmation of the views expressed by Dr. Hughlings Jackson. They are, as it were, an artificial reproduction of the clinical experiments performed by disease, and the conclusions which Dr. Jackson has arrived at from his observations of disease are in all essential particulars confirmed by the above experiments" (op. cit., p. 85).

In spite of the encouragement I have received from these researches, I feel that it requires more skill than I possess to make my subject clear to those who have long worked at epilepsy from a totally different point of view.

## II

## Definition

My definition of the word "epilepsy" has already been given by implication, but I must give it formally before I go further.

Epileptic discharges are occasional, abrupt, and excessive discharges of parts of the cerebral hemisphere (paroxysmal discharges).

Let me show another side of the definition. In each epilepsy there is an area of grey matter in some part of the cerebrum which is so abnormally nourished that it occasionally reaches very high tension and highly unstable equilibrium. It occasionally discharges, or it is discharged by some eccentric irritation or during some general bodily disturbance, as, for example, that attending fright.

After its discharge the portion of grey matter once more, by continuous nutrition, reaches high tension, and is again ready for discharge. It will be gathered that the "discharging lesion" is supposed to be a persistent and also a local lesion. For the definition I have given, it matters not as to the locality of the lesion, or, otherwise expressed, it matters not what particular symptoms result from the discharge; they may be sensory or motor—for example, they may be such as red vision[2] or convulsion. Difference in the phenomena

[1] "Experimental Researches on Cerebral Physiology and Pathology," by David Ferrier, M.A., M.D. (Edin.), M.R.C.P., *West Riding Lunatic Asylum Reports*, edited by Crichton Browne, M.D., F.R.C.P., vol. iii.

[2] We have already in Chap. I, pt. 2, p. 170, spoken of the double use of the word "sensation," and have insisted that sensations in the sense of "states of mind" occur during excitation of motor nerves and centres. The word "red" is really a name for a mental state. The proper comparison is not betwixt the sensation of redness (mental state) in an epileptic discharge and convulsion (physical state). This would be to compare two things which are utterly different.

depends on difference in the seat of the unstable grey matter. A list of epilepsies will be given further on. But it may now be mentioned that I believe epilepsies in which the phenomena are sensory, or in which strong development of sensation is the initial phenomenon, depend on discharges beginning in the posterior part of the brain ; whilst epilepsies in which development of movement is the chief and earliest thing depend on discharges beginning in the anterior part of the brain.[1]

Let us consider the subject from another point. We have, so far as is practicable, to study epilepsies as departures from healthy states. We must, then, give a brief sketch of healthy nervous discharges before we speak in more detail of epileptic discharges.

Where there is grey matter there discharge occurs during healthy functional exercise. This is a truism. If I move my arm there is of necessity an expenditure of force. This is not in muscles only, nor in nerves only. It must be in some nervous centre or centres. In the movement of any part, however limited, many muscles serve. Duchenne says that no man can move a muscle singly, except perhaps in the face. Evidently it follows from this fact that there is in every movement a discharge of a part where movements are co-ordinated. This is saying that the discharge is of a nervous centre, that is, of grey matter.

The above remarks on healthy nervous discharges do not refer only to what are arbitrarily distinguished as physical processes—to discharge of lower centres—they refer in principle to mental states also, or rather, of course, to their physical side. They apply to discharges of the highest centres. The nervous arrangements forming the substrata of mind are only in great degree different from the nervous arrangements of the pons or spinal cord. And when we think or speak, as well as when we walk, there are nervous discharges. I must, however, consider this matter in some detail, because I wish to show that epileptic discharges are discharges of parts of the chief organ of mind.

The anatomical unit of a nervous organ is not a cell or a fibre, or a compound of both. Such a compound is only the morphological unit. The anatomical unit *is a sensori-motor process.* It is not an afferent (sensory) process only, nor a motor process only, but these two put in a particular relation by cells of grey matter. It is just as the unit of speech is not a word, nor a series of words, but a proposition. The anatomical unit represents, either directly or indirectly, a peripheral impression associated with a muscular adjustment. The peripheral impression may be either on the surface of the body, or in its interior—epi-peripheral or ento-peripheral (Spencer). The surface impressions vary from those most general of mere contact of

The comparison, physiologically, would be betwixt abnormal excitations of optic centres and nerves and abnormal excitations of motor centres and nerves. We cannot observe the results of excitation of " sensory " nerves and centres. We have to rely on what the patient tells us, and, of course, he can only tell us of what occurs before he loses consciousness ; we can observe the results of excitation of motor centres and nerves after he has lost consciousness. The statements in the text and subsequent similar statements are, however, conventionally correct, and yet from a scientific point of view too absurd to be misleading.

[1] This is in accordance with an old conclusion that the anterior is the chiefly motor, and the posterior the chiefly sensory part of the cerebral hemisphere. I put forward this view some years ago, and it is a matter of satisfaction to me to find that it accords with certain of Ferrier's conclusions from his brilliant experiments. I shall have many times to refer to this topic, and will therefore give quotations bearing on it in an Appendix to this chapter.

ordinary objects with the ordinary surface of the body to those so special as retinal impressions. The impressions from the interior vary widely also. They are from muscles, viscera, etc., and form the chief part of what are called Systemic Sensations. The movements associated with these two classes of peripheral impressions vary similarly.

In the lower parts of the nervous system it is plain that surface impressions are put in relation with particular muscular adjustments by nerve centres. The units of composition of the lower centres are evidently sensori-motor processes. They represent impressions and movements *directly*. The experiments on the cord to prove reflex actions illustrate this well. What is, anatomically, a sensori-motor process is physiologically a reflex action necessarily implying central discharge. But I submit that the unit of composition of the very highest centres is the same. (See quotations from Laycock and Spencer, Chap. I, pt. 2, p. 167.) The highest centres can only re-represent the impressions and movements which the lower centres represent directly.

I will state the above in other words, already used. In the lower centres there is a direct adjustment of few and simple movements to few and simple peripheral impressions. In the very highest [1] centres there is an adjustment of exceedingly special movements (representing movements of the whole organism) to the most special of impressions from the environment.

So far for the anatomical units. Now for the physiology of them—that is, their conditions of discharge. There are discharges of the highest sensori-motor processes when we think, just as there are of lower processes when we walk. Let us take a convenient example of discharges occurring in mental operations. There is internal speech and external speech. There are central discharges when I speak internally, just as there are when I speak aloud. That in the former there are no outward effects makes no essential difference ; there is a central discharge in both cases, and of the same series of processes. It is absurd to suppose that different series of nervous processes are engaged when I say " gold is yellow " to myself and when I say it aloud. There is a difference in the strength, and consequently in the spreading, of the discharge. The discharge is slight, and limited to the centre when I speak internally ; it is stronger, and spreads from the centre first excited, to lower centres and to the muscles when I talk aloud. So far for healthy discharges.

Wherever there is nervous tissue disease may occur. Now, disease can lead to either of *two* kinds of changes in this tissue. It may lead either to destruction of function of nerve tissue, or to changes of instability of nerve tissue—either to an inability to discharge, or to an over-readiness to discharge. These are the two divisions of abnormal functional changes in nerve tissue, the simple and obvious ones, of " loss of function " and " over-function " ; there are destroying lesions and discharging lesions (instability). Every nervous

[1] Observe two differences of degree : In the ordinary reflex action the movement follows the afferent incitation with no, or with little, delay. In the highest centres, if my speculation as to the motor and sensory regions be correct (see footnote, p. 180, and Appendix No. 2), the movement will not be immediate. For the speculation assumes that there is in the highest centres wide geographical separation, and thus probably delay. Again, in the lowest reflex actions some particular movement is fatally necessary, and occurs rapidly after some particular impression. But in the highest centres it may be that there is not this absolute connection. The organisation is not complete. Thus, after seeing a red circle and a blue square we can think of a red square and of a blue circle. The sensory and motor elements which enter into the physical side of our perceptions of simple objects can be transposed. These statements appear to me to accord with certain views of Herbert Spencer. (See Appendix No. 1.)

symptom depends on one of these two abnormal functional states. The nervous changes in epilepsy, as I use the word, belong to the second division. There are in epilepsies abnormal discharges of areas of highly unstable grey matter. *These discharges are to be looked on as gross exaggerations of healthy nervous discharges*. Our next step, therefore, is to consider the differences betwixt healthy discharges of the sensori-motor processes of the brain and epileptic discharges of them. First let me make a brief re-statement.

I believe that epileptic discharges which result in spasm of muscles are excessive discharges beginning in convolutions—that is to say, that they are discharges beginning in parts of the chief organ of *mind*. I think, too, that discharges of the very same parts occur during healthy mentation.[1] Let us see how these two seemingly contradictory views really harmonise. Let us state a case. We have already spoken of internal and external speech we now take another series of nervous processes.

Suppose that a limited [2] part of the brain is the seat of visual ideas. The material basis of these ideas is, of course, made up of nerve cells and fibres. But this is, be it remarked, not a statement in either anatomy or physiology, and is of no use for our present purpose. The anatomical statement is, that the substrata of these ideas represent, or rather re-represent, retinal impressions and ocular movements. (Without an element of movement there would be no representation of size or figure.) They are fundamentally like the nervous arrangements for ordinary reflex action ; they are sensori-motor processes. We will call them retino-ocular processes. So far for anatomy. Now for physiology. The study of the degrees and conditions of excitation or discharge of nervous processes is a physiological study. We will first consider what occurs in health when we have visual ideas—that is, when we see or remember objects.

Most of our ideas are latent. The equivalent physiological statement is that the anatomical elements (sensori-motor processes) are unexcited. But we speak now of ideas actual and correspondingly of their anatomical substrata as being excited or discharged. Now, we have in health vivid ideas and faint ideas. We see objects and we can think of them afterwards. First for the vivid ideas. When we actually see and *recognise* external objects, we have *vivid* visual ideas. There is then strong excitation of the retina, thence to the highest centres in the cerebrum, and back to the ocular muscles. There is complete sensori-motor (let us say retino-ocular) action. If we *recognise* an object, the very highest centres must be engaged ; for recognition is, in common with classification, a modified form of reasoning (Spencer's *Psychology*, vol. ii, p. 127).[3] The process described is what is fundamental, however many intermediate centres we may like to suppose betwixt the afferent nerves (optic nerves and

[1] Since delirium, hallucinations, etc., are but caricatures of healthy mentation, we may put the statement in the text in another form which is nearly equivalent. A convulsion is, I think, as much a symptom of disease of the organ of mind as delirium is.

[2] This supposition is legitimate for mere illustration, although I do not believe in such narrow localisations ; and, as before stated, I think there is in the cerebral hemisphere a wider separation betwixt the motor and sensory elements of sensori-motor processes than in the lower centres ; the anatomical substrata of visual ideas must contain elements representing movements as well as impressions. As an illustration, the supposition in the text is convenient and legitimate.

The word " mentation," used in the text, was, I believe, introduced by Mr. Metcalfe Johnson.

[3] As before remarked, retinal impressions and ocular movements are signs of tactual impressions and movements and of locomotor movements. I may here reproduce a part of a paper, on " The Localisation of Movements in the Brain " (*Lancet*, February 15, 1873), bearing on the motor part of the mechanism of this symbolisation (see p. 75).

retina) and efferent nerves to the ocular muscles. Next for faint ideas. When we have faint visual ideas (think of objects when they are absent—" recollect " them, etc.) there is slight or nascent excitation (discharge) of those highest centres to which, when we actually saw the objects, the retinal impressions came, and from which the impulses to the ocular muscles departed. In other words, essentially the very same physiological process occurs in the two cases, and it occurs in the same anatomical series during thinking of or remembering objects as occurs during actually seeing them. I say essentially, as there are two differences of degree. In thinking of objects the central discharge is (1) slight, and (2) limited to the centre. In actually seeing them it is strong, and spreads from periphery to the centre and from centre to periphery.[1]

Now for the epileptic discharge. It must never be forgotten that it is an excessive discharge. Not only is it very much more excessive than the discharges which occur when we have faint mental states, but it is very much more excessive than those occurring in vivid mental states. Besides being excessive, it is of a limited part of the brain. It is rapid, and it is soon over. In such excessive discharges as the epileptic discharge of our supposed centre for visual ideas there could not be a development of ideas of objects either of such ideas as occur in health or of such as occur in delirium and insanity. We have, however, to do with what occurs physically. We have to do with epileptic discharges of those *sensori-motor processes* which are the anatomical side of ideation. There is in some cases of epilepsy evidence of excessive excitation of parts of the brain representing retinal impressions, as the patient has clouds of colour before his eyes. There often occurs also, as part of a larger fit, that clotted mass of movements of the ocular muscles which we call spasm (for example, strong lateral deviation of the eyes). In the first case there is, I believe, a sudden and excessive discharge of a limited part of the cerebral hemisphere, which contains crowds of the sensory element, and in the second of the motor element, in the highest processes of the series for visual ideas. The discharge in the epilepsy, being very strong, rapidly spreads down to the lower centres, and by these to the muscles, and thus produces innumerable ocular movements at once, or rather jams innumerable ocular movements into one stiff struggle.

The same reasoning applies, *mutatis mutandis*, to the discharge of the anatomical substrata of tactual ideas, the chief of which are impressions of surface of the fingers and adjusted movements of the hand. An epileptic discharge of the anatomical substrata of these ideas would produce numbness and spasm of the hand and arm.

Similarly, an epileptic discharge of the so-called centre for " memory of words " on the left side of the brain results, I consider, in convulsion of the articulatory muscles. For I believe, and have long urged, that the anatomical substrata of words are motor [2] (articulatory) processes. I should think, too, that an epileptic discharge of that part of the brain on the right side which corresponds to the supposed centre for words on the left would produce

[1] In the ideation of delirium the central discharges may be so strong that the patient believes he actually has snakes, etc., before him. In insanity, also, there is a similar exaggerated central action, but in both cases the discharge is, in comparison with the epileptic discharge, but a slight departure from health.

[2] I have urged this view for years. Until very recently I have been alone in that opinion, that is, amongst physicians in this country ; I am very glad, therefore, to find that Ferrier has quite independently reached a conclusion essentially similar.

an essentially similar convulsion ; for I believe that both sides of the brain are educated in words, but that the left is the leading [1] side.

That that which is commonly described as the epileptic paroxysm is the result of a discharge of some part of the nervous system is as certain as that paralysis is the result of destruction of function of some part of the nervous system ; the exaggerated movement of the convulsion could not result else. It is a truth, or truism. On the other hand, all abnormal nervous discharges are not epileptic discharges. There is, for instance, an almost continuous stream of discharges in tetanus, and there are rapidly succeeding discharges in chorea. The epileptic discharge comes on with more or less suddennes. The paroxysm is violent, and is soon over.

Briefly, the epileptic discharge differs from the other kinds of abnormal discharges above-mentioned in being paroxysmal. This is a fundamental difference never to be lost sight of. It is as important to note the *nature* of a nervous discharge as it is to note the external region on which the discharge works its effects. More will be said on this matter later on, under the head of co-ordination. But the difference may be briefly illustrated by saying that unilateral convulsion (cerebral discharge) differs from tetanus (cerebellar discharge) not only in that a different class [2] of muscles suffers, but in that in the former there is a paroxysmal, and in the latter a continuous, although remittent discharge.

I do not deny that any part of the nervous system which contains grey matter may become unstable, and may discharge abnormally. We shall have to note, however, that some parts of the nervous system are very much more liable to become diseased than other parts, and in the brain the region in the district of the middle cerebral artery suffers more often than other cerebral regions. Further, it is not certain that abrupt and paroxysmal discharges result from disease of the lower parts of the nervous system in man. There are, however, certain tetaniform symptoms in children occurring along with, if not dependent on, disease of the cerebellum, to be spoken of later on.

I may now give some examples of epilepsies in accordance with my novel definition of epilepsy. A paroxysm of red vision,[3] of strong smell in the nose, a paroxysm of vertigo, of spasm of certain parts of the body, tonic followed by clonic (of the hand and forearm, of the cheek, of the foot, of the whole of one side, going on or not into universal convulsion), of coloured vision, with other initial symptoms of an attack of migraine, are all epilepsies. So also is transient loss of consciousness, or loss of consciousness followed instantly by convulsion. In each of these cases there is an abrupt and excessive discharge. It is particularly to be observed that a convulsion in which consciousness is *not* affected is, under the novel definition, as much an epilepsy as one in which, as in slight *petit-mal*, consciousness alone is lost, there being, at any rate, no *observable* spasm. In the latter, as in the former, there is a sudden, excessive, and rapid discharge of nerve tissue. Since I believe that any part of the cerebral hemisphere may become the seat of a discharging lesion, there will be all kinds of phenomena produced ; and since there are supposed to be

[1] Here, again, I can adduce the independent confirmatory opinion of Ferrier. He calls the left the " driving " side.

[2] Or rather, perhaps, the muscles suffer in different order. In cerebral discharges the limbs suffer first and most ; in cerebellar discharges the trunk suffers first and most.

[3] See first footnote to this chapter, p. 177.

all degrees in the extent of the discharging lesion, the symptoms will vary in degree as well as in kind.

Perhaps the reader will miss one important set of symptoms from the list of epilepsies given.

Epileptic mania is usually, or often, spoken of as if it were owing to an *epileptic* discharge. An attack of mania is said to " replace " an attack of epilepsy. In agreement with this opinion I used to speak of short paroxysms of mania occurring in a person who at other times had convulsions as " epilepsies." I used to suppose that they directly resulted from such discharges as those which produce other paroxysms—convulsive paroxysms, for example—which I call epilepsies. I have for some years thought otherwise. There are discharges in epileptic mania, and they are abnormal, and they are of the organ of mind, but they are not epileptic (that is, not sudden, abrupt and excessive) discharges.

I have several reasons for change of opinion. There is in most cases of epileptic mania clear evidence that the mania occurs when the epileptic discharge is over—that is to say, that the maniacal action is post epileptic rather then epileptic. There are, however, cases in which there is no sign of an epileptic discharge (*i.e.* no outward sign) before the maniacal action begins, as in cases of so-called masked epilepsy. I do not, however, adopt the accepted explanation of these cases—that they " replace " an epileptic fit. I think the evidence is in favour of another hypothesis—*viz.* of a slight and unobserved fit. Let us consider, first, the cases of epileptic mania—I mean cases in which a prior fit is observed.

Epileptic mania occurs in those epilepsies where loss of consciousness is either the first, or nearly the first, thing in the paroxysm ; when there is " a warning," it is of a very general character. This is equivalent to saying that it occurs in those cases where the discharge begins in the very highest nervous processes. But it is found when the epileptic discharge is over, and the paroxysm has ceased. To explain the condition *after* the paroxysm, let us take a simpler case. Let us take a case where the discharge begins in a lower series of nervous processes—for example, in the corpus striatum, or rather in its adjacent convolutions. There is convulsion of the face, arm, and leg of the opposite side of the body, and possibly, if the discharge be excessive, universal convulsion. But after the discharge is over, there is, if the discharge has been unusually excessive, hemiplegia. This is, I consider, a sign to us that the corpus striatum has been put *hors de combat* by the violent discharge. We venture from these cases on the generalisation that " *Strong Epileptic Discharges Paralyse the Nervous Centre* (*or much of it*) *in which they begin or through which they spread.*"

Now we return to the cases where the discharge begins in the highest series, and apply the generalisation to them. There is loss of use of that series after a discharge beginning in it, when that discharge has been excessive. But obviously violent action (maniacal raving) could not result from this loss of use (a *paralytic* condition) of the highest centres. That accounts only for loss of consciousness (the highest centres which are now paralysed being the anatomical substrata of consciousness). That is only the patient's negative condition, and his condition is duplex. There is the positive element—the mania—to be accounted for. My opinion is that the mania is the result of over-action (morbidly increased discharge, but not epileptic discharge) of the processes just below those which have been put *hors de combat*. The patient is reduced to a more automatic condition of mind, or, as we have otherwise put it (Chap. I, pt. 2, p. 174), his " adjustment is lowered." But why *increased action* of the lower processes ? To lose consciousness is to lose control over the lower processes. This is a metaphorical expression. The physiological equivalent is to be given.

There is, after section of the spinal cord, increased reflex excitability of the segments below the injury. Now, of this Bernard says (*Leçons de Pathologie Expérimentale*, 1872, p. 205)—I draw especial attention to the words italicised : " Nous trouvons, dans ce phénomène, un fait pathologique qui mérite d'être sérieusement étudié, *d'autant plus qu'il est applicable au système nerveux dans toute son étendue*. Tout nerf séparé du centre dont il émane acquiert des propriétés spéciales, qui ne diffèrent cependant de celles dont il jouit à l'état normal que par un excès d'intensité."

The principle that we get over-action of lower centres from the mere removal of the higher centres has very important applications. It was distinctly formulated by the late Dr. Anstie some years ago. Thus, speaking of the effects of opium, he wrote : " The apparent exaltation of certain faculties should be ascribed rather to the removal of controlling influences than to the positive stimulation of the faculties themselves, or of the physical machinery by which they work " (*Stimulants and Narcotics*, p. 80).

Let us state another reason why the symptoms of mania cannot be produced by an epileptic discharge (I mean, of course, produced directly by that discharge ; they are, I think, as just stated, produced by it in a very indirect way). If the reader bears in mind what was said of the differences betwixt healthy and epileptic discharges, he will see that an epileptic discharge (*i.e.* a sudden and violent discharge) could not produce even that caricature of healthy action which is displayed in the doings of the epileptic maniac. This will be very plain if we take cases of elaborate mental automatism after very slight epileptic discharges. Thus, a man subject to epileptic attacks is found unconscious in the kitchen, mixing cocoa in a dirty gallipot (intended for the cat's food) with a mustard spoon. This was a very elaborate action, and that it was only a caricature of a normal action is plain, because it had just before been agreed on that his sister-in-law, who was on a visit, should have cocoa for her supper. It is impossible to believe that the cerebral discharges which produced such actions as the cocoa-mixing were like those discharges which produced convulsion. This patient was known to be the subject of slight attacks (*petit-mal*) and severe attacks (*grand-mal*). I believe that before the cocoa-mixing affair he had a slight attack of *petit-mal*—*i.e.* a slight discharge beginning in his very highest processes, which had left some of them *hors de combat*. Then, so to speak, " under this loss " (which, symptomatically, was loss of consciousness) automatic action went on. That action was, in this case, only a slight caricature of normal action. But after stronger discharges there is a deeper involvement of nervous processes (a deeper dissolution), and correspondingly a lower kind of automatic action—*e.g.* maniacal raving, etc. After very strong discharges there is coma, a condition lower than mania, for by the discharges which produce coma all processes serving in mind seem to be put *hors de combat*, and there is only left the lowest " physical " automatic action (respiratory, circulatory, etc.). But neither the mental automatism of mania nor the physical automatism in coma can reasonably be attributed to the direct effects of an epileptic discharge.

What I have just been saying is in principle simply the obverse of what was said when speaking (p. 180) of discharges of an hypothetical centre for visual ideas. It was pointed out that an epileptic discharge of those parts of the brain which are slightly discharged when we think of objects (or from somewhat increased discharge of which spectral images result) would not rouse ideas, but would cause simply clouds of colour and spasm of ocular muscles. The same principles apply to epileptic mania. An epileptic discharge could not produce actions so elaborate as maniacal action.

To recapitulate. In epilepsy there is, as in healthy operations, both so-called mental and physical, a nervous discharge. But the *epileptic* discharge is a very local discharge; it is a discharge of some highly unstable part of the cerebral [1] hemisphere; it is an abrupt and excessive discharge. This definition embodies the principle of the new method. It amounts to saying that the phenomena of epileptic paroxysms are considered as developments, although in a brutal way, of the functions of limited parts of the brain. Returning to an arbitrary example. Strong lateral deviation of the eyes and clouds of colour are supposed to be developments in a brutal way of the motor and sensory elements in the anatomical substrata of visual ideas. It is for this reason that I call the method Anatomical and Physiological. As I shall show at length later on, I have for some years considered different varieties of convulsions as results of experiments in anatomy and physiology revealing to us, although in the rough, the movements and impressions represented in different parts of the cerebral hemisphere; or, as I would otherwise put it, the localisation of the anatomical substrata of different classes of ideas, visual, tactual, etc. (See p. 180.)

Obviously the method differs both as a means of investigation and as a basis for classification from the accepted method. Premising that chronic cases are spoken of, the accepted method starts by establishing some clinical entity (grouping of symptoms)—epilepsy. And the question in a case is often only—"Does it satisfy the definition?" and not also—"How do the symptoms show a departure from health of some part of the nervous system?" The accepted definition of epilepsy is definition by type. The essential element in the accepted definition is loss of, or trouble of, consciousness, and this, for example, holds together the several varieties of epilepsy, vertigo, *petit-mal*, and *grand-mal*. It is sometimes said if there is no loss or defect of consciousness there is no epilepsy.

This absolute distinction into cases with, and cases without, loss or trouble of consciousness seems to me to be from a scientific point of view arbitrary.[2] It is an absolute distinction, not of anatomical or physiological, but of psychological parentage. Although it involves great recapitulation, I must consider the matter again in this place.

Loss of consciousness is not a symptom utterly different from other symptoms. It is not to be dismissed from analysis as a mysterious epiphenomenon or complication. Consciousness is mysterious, but *loss* of consciousness in cases of disease is to be considered on the same method as other nervous

[1] I wish particularly to mention now that I think *universal* convulsion with which there is loss of consciousness at or about the onset (cases of "idiopathic epilepsy" according to the accepted definition) depends on discharge of parts in *one* cerebral hemisphere. The reasons for this will be given later.

[2] In the next chapter I shall point out that clinical entities are necessary for practical purposes.

symptoms. Nor will it do merely to speak of consciousness as " a function " of the cerebral hemisphere. Of course, in a sense it is so ; but the expression is a vague one. For it is not a function in the same way as secretion of bile is a function of the liver. *Physiologically* the function of the cerebral hemisphere is, like that of the lower centres, to co-ordinate impressions and movements, or rather to reco-ordinate those impressions co-ordinated by lower centres. Consciousness has, of course, anatomical substrata, as much as speech or any other mental operation has. These substrata are sensori-motor processes. How that other so-called function consciousness arises during energising of these substrata is not our direct concern. Similarly we must not simply speak of *loss* of consciousness as being due to " loss of function of the cerebral hemisphere." It is true enough in a sense, but in that sense it is almost a barren truism. We have to consider in an inquiry like this the nature of the *anatomical* substrata which are implicated when consciousness ceases.

The sensori-motor processes concerned in consciousness are only in great degree different from those of lower centres. They are the *most* special of all special nervous processes—the series evolved out of all other (lower) series. *To lose consciousness is to lose the use of the most special of all nervous processes whatsoever*. Now, one of the many ways in which the use of them may be lost is by their being the seat of an epileptic discharge. It will be temporarily lost *during their discharge* (during their *excessive* excitation) as much as it is permanently lost when they are implicated by gross lesion. It is just as the use of an arm is lost during the severe spasm of its muscles as much as by palsy of its muscles.[1] So then, whether consciousness be lost or not in an epilepsy, as I define it, or whether it be lost first of all or later in the paroxysm, depends on the seat of the discharging lesion, and on how far the discharge spreads. If those parts of the brain, where the most special of all nervous processes lie, be *first* affected by the epileptic discharge, there is loss of consciousness first of all. If the discharge be slight there may be, as appears, loss of consciousness only. This is so in very slight cases of *petit-mal*. If strong, the discharge spreads from these very highest centres to lower centres, out of which these highest centres are evolved, and with which they are, therefore, continuous. The discharge widens as it spreads lower, and rapidly reaches the lowest centres and their muscles. There is loss of consciousness followed by convulsion. The accepted view makes the convulsion and the loss of consciousness to be two utterly different things depending on implication of two widely separate parts (medulla oblongata and cerebral hemisphere). This view, I believe, is partly owing to a psychological bias which, asserting that the brain is the organ of consciousness, finds it inconsistent with that assertion to speak of it also as an organ representing impressions and movements. On the view I take, discharges beginning in and spreading from the very highest centres (since they re-represent all that lower centres represent) will produce loss of consciousness, convulsion, and such symptoms as pallor of the face, passing urine in the fit, etc.

The view I have put forward will necessarily seem strange to those who are thinking of " Consciousness and Convulsion." They will see no possible

[1] We have also spoken of loss of consciousness as an after-effect of a strong discharge being due to exhaustion of a nervous tract consequent on excessive stimulation. This is so of the convulsed arm ; its use is often lost after the discharge as well as by being involved in spasm during the discharge.

relation betwixt the two things. Consciousness and convulsion *are* utterly different things. But then I am thinking only of loss of use of the *anatomical substrata* of consciousness. It is the excessive discharge of these (during which consciousness ceases) which is comparable with that discharge of lower centres which produces convulsion. The things to be compared are discharges of sensori-motor processes of different series. So far from comparing consciousness with convulsion, I should not compare it with anything whatever, except perhaps metaphorically. It is the metaphysico-materialistic method, erroneously called " practical," which leads to such comparisons and explanations.

So far for epilepsies in which discharges begin in the highest centres. If the epileptic discharge begins in a subordinate series of nervous processes—in a lower centre—loss of consciousness does not occur, or occurs later. It only occurs when the discharge spreads far. Let us take an example. In some cases of discharge of convolutions near to the corpus striatum, the convulsion begins in the hand, and if the discharge be severe it spreads gradually over the whole body. The inference is that there is internally a corresponding spreading of the discharge in the brain. In such cases consciousness is in most [1] cases not lost until, or just before, the leg on the side of the body first affected is reached by the spasm—that is, not until the central discharge has spread widely in the brain. Consciousness may be lost in such a case from one of two causes. It is lost either as soon as the most special of all processes *are reached* by the internal discharge which began in the subordinate series ; secondly, consciousness must be lost when a large quantity of a subordinate and yet important series of nervous processes is suddenly involved in the discharge.

The last remark is important. Let us state very generally what it involves. If a patient *suddenly* loses by any process the use of *any large part* of either of the two cerebral hemispheres he must lose consciousness. For since the highest processes are evolved out of, and are, as it were, *continuous with*, processes only in degree lower, and through these with still lower unto the lowest, they have no independent existence. Consciousness must be lost when any important although subordinate series is seriously involved.

Here it may be well to remark expressly that, although medical men speak *clinically* of loss of consciousness as if there were a well-defined entity called consciousness, there is probably not amongst educated persons any such belief. We must for clinical purposes have arbitrary standards (definitions by type). It is thus the universal custom for medical men to speak of " confusion," " stupor," " loss of consciousness," and " coma," although every medical man sees cases in which there are all conceivable degrees from slightest confusion of thought to deepest coma. Let me mention some slight degrees. Some patients will tell that in their fits they are not unconscious, but that they do not know where they are ; that they hear people talking, but do not know what they say. It is not at all uncommon for the patient to say that when in a fit he feels as if in a strange place—" in a strange country," one of my epileptic patients said.

It would be as absurd to judge of a medical man's opinions as to consciousness by the terms he uses for describing the states of his patients as it would

[1] Much depends on the rapidity of the discharge. I mean, for example, that consciousness is lost the sooner, the more rapidly, the spasm " runs up " the arm. If the spasm spreads slowly it may involve the whole of one side of the body without being attended by loss or even defect of consciousness.

be to judge of a botanist's opinion on biology by considering only the terms he used in speaking of plants in his kitchen garden. It must be admitted that the twofold use, the empirical and scientific, of terms leads to apparent contradiction in some of our medical phrases. Thus it is said "the patient was confused but was quite conscious." To be confused is to have defect of consciousness. Again, loss of consciousness is sometimes spoken of as being synonymous with coma.

It is clear, from what I have already said under Evolution, Chap. I, pt. 2, p. 171, that no abrupt limitation of consciousness is recognised in this book. Thus I have used the term "defect of consciousness" when speaking of insanity. To use the words of Herbert Spencer, "all gradations exist between wholly unconscious nervous actions and wholly conscious ones."

In an anatomico-physiological inquiry what we have to note is how the organism is adjusted to its environment. Thus we should say that the patient whose case was mentioned (p. 184) was only very slightly less specially adjusted to his environment than was normal to him. He went through "the form" of the cocoa-mixing, used implements of the right class, but not those exactly fitted for the purpose. In the case of the headless frog which rubs vinegar off its back with a hind leg, there is a degree of adjustment very like normal adjustment. Whether consciousness is displayed or not in such adjustments is not a physiological, but a psychological question.

Mr. G. H. Lewes believes that sensibility is a histologic property ; this is, he believes, a fundamental property of the ganglionic tissue. We ought, according to him, to consider the sensorium as having the same extension as the nervous centres. This view is not necessarily discrepant with the statement I have made about the anatomical substrata of consciousness (that they represent the whole organism). Mr. Lewes has made a remark which is at least parallel to that statement. He defines the common sensorium (*Physiology of Common Life*, vol. ii) as "*the sum of all the lower centres*, each centre being itself a small sensorium."

In the next chapter I shall show that, although from a *scientific* point of view the accepted distinction into cases of epilepsy without and cases with loss of consciousness is arbitrary, it does not follow that from a clinical point of view such arbitrary distinctions may be not only convenient, but essential. We must have arbitrary standards for practical purposes, as I have just been illustrating by terms used for degree of implication of consciousness.

## Appendix No. 1 to Chapter II

I here give a quotation from Mr. Herbert Spencer's *Psychology*, to which I have referred in Chap. II (p. 179), and to which I shall have to make frequent reference in later chapters. The quotation is full of matter of interest to medical men :

"Memory, reason, and feeling *simultaneously* arise as the *automatic* actions become complex, infrequent, and hesitating ; and will, arising *at the same time*, is necessitated by the same conditions. As the advance from the simple and indissolubly coherent psychical changes to the psychical changes that are involved and dissolubly coherent is itself the commencement of memory, reason, and feeling ; so, too, is it in itself the commencement of will. On passing *from compound reflex actions* to those actions so highly compounded as to be imperfectly reflex—on passing from the organically determined psychical changes which take place with extreme *rapidity* to the psychical changes which, not being organically determined, take place *with some deliberation, and therefore consciously, we pass to a kind of mental action, which is one of memory, reason, feeling, or will, according to the side of it we look at.*

"Of this we may be certain, even in anticipation of any special synthesis. For since all modes of consciousness can be nothing else than incidents of the correspondence between the organism and its environment, they must be all different sides of, or different places of, the co-ordinated groups of changes whereby internal relations are adjusted to external relations. Between the reception of certain impressions and the performance of certain appropriate motions there is some inner connection. If the inner connection is organised, the action is of the reflex order, either simple or compound; and none of the phenomena of consciousness proper exist. If the inner connection is not [1] organised, then the psychical changes which come between the impressions and motions are conscious ones; *the entire action must have all the essential elements of a conscious action—must simultaneously exhibit memory, reason, feeling, and will;* for there can be no conscious adjustment of an inner to an outer relation without all these being involved." [2]

## Appendix No. 2

I find that I have already given a quotation on the motor and sensory regions of the brain in this journal, January 28, 1874. The following quotation is from an abstract of my second Gulstonian Lecture (*British Medical Journal*, March 6, 1869):

"He does not think it, *a priori*, likely that the optic nerve, any more than the radial nerve, would be represented in any *one* part of either or of both the cerebral hemispheres, but in every part of each of them; and, excepting to an inconsiderable extent, only indirectly. Taking illustrations from disease, the kind of 'sensation disorders' we should expect from disease of the cerebral hemisphere would be spectral illusions—a disorderly reproduction of *very complex impressions* which differ from defects of sight as a mistake in a word does from a cramp in the tongue. On this higher level, however, there will doubtless be some kind of localisation, and its most general character may be inferred. Since—as Lockhart Clarke has pointed out—the structure of the anterior convolutions does differ from the posterior, they must serve differently in mind.

"*Facts seem to show that the fore part of the brain serves in the motor aspect of mind, and we may fairly speculate that the posterior serves in the sensory.*"

This speculation seems to me to accord with one of Ferrier's conclusions from his masterly experiments. The following is a quotation from a summary of his most recent researches (*Medical Record*, March 18, 1874): "The whole brain is considered as divided into a sensory and motor region, corresponding to their anatomical relation to the optic thalami and corpora striata and the motor and sensory tracts."

[1] See footnote [1], p. 179.

[2] Spencer's *Psychology*, vol. i, p. 496. (No italics in original.)

## III

### On Classification and on Methods of Investigation

It has been said that we can best judge of a person's character by what he finds laughable. No doubt we may best judge of a man's intellect by his classifications, for, as Spencer says (*Psychology*, §§ 309–16), classification is really a process of reasoning. When, he says, we think of the objects compared, we classify; when we think of the relations betwixt them, we reason. From a person's classifications we judge of his "form of mind." We may adapt and apply Spencer's statements thus: In investigating cases of nervous disease, we are really classifying them or their symptoms. From all points of view classification is of vast importance. I shall, therefore, consider it in its most general bearings, as well as specially for the present subject of epilepsies.

When, in the first chapter, I spoke of the anatomical and physiological investigation of epilepsies, I mentioned that we require clinical entities for practical purposes. This admission was certainly contrary to the spirit of the quotations contained in that chapter. In short, since the papers quoted from were written, I have modified my opinion so far as to hold that we require two kinds of classification. I believe I have been much influenced in this matter by Dr. Moxon. The following quotation is from an article by him:

"When we are dealing with the public or social functions of names we must keep in view the distinction between a science nomenclature and an *art* nomenclature. The aim of a science is the increasing and unlimited knowledge of the things it concerns itself with; a science seeks out and names with no other object than to know. The scope of any art is, on the contrary, limited and prescribed; it has its proper sphere of work and it must borrow from the nomenclature of the sciences which it rests upon such names only as are useful for its practical purposes. Two opposite principles, then, must govern the construction of a nomenclature for use in an art such as that of medicine. These principles are:

"First, that every subject which it is important that the followers of the art should be able to mutually recognise, or to communicate to each other, should be embodied in a distinct and suitable name.

"Second, that names should not be introduced into the nomenclature of the art except on account of their applications to subjects of practical importance in the purposes of the art.

"Another and a very obvious principle is, that the names adopted should be so far carefully chosen that they may not contradict or misrepresent the actual facts of the subjects to which they are applied" (Dr. Moxon, "On the Necessity for a Clinical Nomenclature of Disease," *Guy's Hospital Reports*, vol. xv, p. 482).

We are in medical art and science, as in other arts and sciences, obliged to make arbitrary divisions where there are no clear divisions in Nature. Thus, at the close of the last chapter, I spoke of the arbitrary standards medical men make for describing cases in which there are different degrees of affection of consciousness ("confusion," "stupor," "loss of consciousness," and "coma"). There really occur all shades of affection of consciousness (see p. 187, and also further in this chapter). But such arbitrary divisions as those just mentioned are absolutely necessary for clinical purposes. Let me give another illustration; I have a double purpose in giving it.

There are from lesions of different degrees of gravity in and of the cerebral hemisphere, near to the corpus striatum, all degrees of defect of language, from a slight ataxy of articulation to a state in which there is loss of all power of expression, whether active (intellectual), or passive (emotional). For this reason I have strenuously objected to the abrupt divisions made by nosologists. The divisions usually made are exceedingly abrupt, passing from physiology into psychology at a bound (ataxy of articulation—anatomico-physiological phraseology—and " loss of memory for words "—psychological phraseology). But I found that I was making arbitrary divisions too. I found myself speaking of " an ordinary specimen of *loss* of speech." Whilst as strongly as ever I believe that from different degrees of damage of the left corpus striatum and adjacent cerebral hemisphere there result all degrees of defect, from a slight ataxy of articulation to entire loss of power of expression, I admit that we must have arbitrary divisions of affections of language for clinical purposes. For all that, I insist that the classification of defects of language on a mixed method of physiology and psychology is an illegitimate one. To remark on this point is my chief reason for giving the illustration. Where the expression " loss of memory for words " would be used I should say there is " defect of speech," or that the patient " makes mistakes in words." These simpler expressions are really quite as definite, though they sound less definite; they have no technical ring. It may be said that they amount to the same thing. Practically they do not; they have no psychological associations. The expression " loss of *memory* for words " takes the symptom out of the category of such other nervous symptoms, as hemiplegia. For there is no conceivable community betwixt loss of " memory " and loss or defect of " movement,"—betwixt " loss of memory for words " and ataxy of articulation—not enough in common as a basis for the widest contrast.

I must, indeed, at the beginning of a chapter on Classification, urge strongly that we are to rid ourselves as much as possible of psychological bias in what is an anatomical and physiological inquiry. I do not mean that we have no concern at all with psychology. On the contrary, it is perfectly obvious that it is impossible for us to *begin* to study the anatomical *substrata* of mind without prior psychological analysis.

On this matter I will quote Mill: " And even if that hypothesis [phrenological] were true, psychological observation would still be necessary; for how is it possible to ascertain the correspondence between two things by observation of only one of them? To establish a relation between mental functions and cerebral conformations requires not only a parallel system of observations applied to each, but (as M. Comte himself, with some inconsistency, acknowledges) an analysis of the mental faculties. . . ." (Mill, on *Comte and Positivism*, p. 66).

But I urge again that our concern with states of mind is indirect. We start with the assumption that all mental states have material bases, and our direct concern in such an inquiry as this is with the latter only. Clearness on this matter is of very great importance for our subject, and of immense importance when speaking of classifications and methods of investigation of diseases of the higher nervous centres.

There are two ways of investigating diseases, and two kinds of classification corresponding thereto, the empirical and the scientific. The former is to be illustrated by the way in which a gardener classifies plants, the latter by the way in which a botanist classifies them.

The former is, strictly speaking, only an arrangement. The gardener arranges his plants as they are fit for food, for ornament, etc. One of his classifications of ornamental plants is into trees, shrubs, and flowers. His object is the direct application of knowledge to utilitarian purposes. It is, so to speak, practical. The other kind of classification (the classification properly so-called) is rather for the better organisation of existing knowledge, and for discovering the relations of new facts ; its principles are methodical guides to further investigation. It is of great utilitarian value, but not directly.

The difference here is plain, because the gardener and the botanist are different persons. But in our profession, the same person has to classify for the organisation and advancement of his knowledge, and to make an arrangement for direct utilitarian purposes of daily life. The reader will now see that there was no cynicism intended in the illustration just given. We require two classifications, or rather an arrangement and a classification. An arrangement corresponding with that of the gardener is essential for the practice of our profession. It is a technical or artificial classification. A scientific classification is necessary for the organisation and development of our knowledge of disease. It is a natural classification, and is thus a means of investigation.

We require for practical purposes types as foundations for arrangement.[1]

On this subject I shall quote largely from Handfield Jones (see Appendix). We require clinical entities, such as locomotor ataxy and idiopathic epilepsy. As the matter is one of exceeding great importance, I will illustrate the two kinds of classification, or, what is fundamentally the same thing, the two methods of investigation, by several examples. Some of them are purposely taken from cases of other nervous diseases or symptoms than those resulting from epileptic discharges.

In a case of disorderly walking we endeavour to determine whether the gait resemble that which authorities have described as the gait of typical Locomotor Ataxy, or that of typical Cerebellar Reel. We might conclude from examination of a case as follows : This patient has tumour of the cerebellum, because (besides having severe pain in the head and double optic neuritis), whenever he walks, he walks with his legs apart, and reels from side to side or from back to front—walks as if drunk ; he has no ear disease. This is the empirical or clinical study. Scientifically, we seek to know in what way the patient's walk differs from healthy walking. To say that it is a difficulty in co-ordinating the movements of locomotion is a merely verbal explanation ; it is objectionable as an explanation. But clinically, as distinguishing the motor symptoms from paraplegia, the nomenclature is useful. The " explanation " is given in the untechnical statement that " the patient reels." The scientific investigation would demand prior knowledge of the play of the muscles of the trunk and legs in the various positions of healthy walking. It is a study of symptoms and diseases as they show departures from healthy states ; this is

[1] " By a type, Whewell meant a well-selected average member of a class, removed alike from all extremes, a concrete embodiment of the class, to be used for purposes of identification in preference to any verbal definition. The motive was the existence of *anomalous* members of many groups in Natural History " (Bain's *Logic,* Induction, p. 191).

only another way of saying that it is a study of cases as anatomical and physiological experiments on the nervous system. The reel would be—this is my belief—found to be a departure from healthy walking on account of feebleness of movements of those muscles which brace up the spinal column. Assuming the correctness of this explanation, we can make the more scientific use of the case. We see more clearly the affinities of the reel; we see that being, dependent [1] on palsy it is far more like hemiplegia than, for example, like chorea. In fact, the hemiplegic man has lost a certain number of "co-ordinations of movements" of his face, arm, and leg of one side. The patient who reels from disease of the cerebellum has lost a certain number of "co-ordinations of movements" of his spine, and later on in the disease, of his legs. On the empirical or clinical view, this is not manifest; indeed, the reel and chorea are often spoken of as if they were similar disorders of co-ordination. Their resemblances are most superficial; they are fundamentally different, not only in the very superficial way that they are affections of different regions of the body, but in that the central changes in one are those of loss of function (a palsy), and in the other those of over-function (owing to a "discharging lesion"). Thus considered, the case can be compared with tetanus, just as a case of hemiplegia can be compared with a case of hemispasm. In tetanus there is a discharge first and most upon those muscles which serve first and most in locomotion, that is, upon the muscles of the spine and legs and upper parts of arms—that is, upon those muscles which are first and most affected in the cerebellar reel.

Let me now illustrate the differences by taking a series of symptoms belonging to our subject. I believe that epileptic vertigo, epileptic *petit-mal*, and epileptic *grand-mal* are, *when regarded from an anatomical and physiological point of view*, simply differing degrees, that is to say, that they depend on different strengths of discharge, beginning in and spreading from the same parts of the brain. The discharge in each begins in the very highest centres of the cerebral hemispheres, that is to say, in the anatomical substrata of consciousness. If it be very slight there is vertigo only, if stronger there is loss of consciousness, and if very strong there is convulsion also. This is the scientific classification and method of investigation.[2]

The relations betwixt loss of consciousness and convulsion have already been spoken of implicitly in Chap. I, pt. 2, pp. 172 and 173, and explicitly in Chap. II, p. 186. We now speak more in detail, and take into consideration the third symptom—vertigo. Vertigo, like convulsion, is a *motor symptom*, and since in *petit-mal* there is loss of consciousness, the statement that there are degrees betwixt epileptic vertigo, *petit-mal*, and *grand-mal* may seem at first glance strange. Let us consider the question raised.

A word, says Lewes, is not only a symbol of a thing, it is also a centre of association. The expression "loss of consciousness" has evidently very strong psychological and very slender physiological associations; what it automatically arouses are chiefly thoughts about "memory," "volition," "will," etc. Thus, there is a feeling that comparisons such as the one spoken

[1] I say "dependent on," as no doubt there is a compound effect from the spinal paresis, just as there is from paresis of anocular nerve. (See footnote later, on Vertigo.)

[2] As will be pointed out later on, authorities declare that, to use the words of Niemeyer, "there are many intermediate stages between epileptic vertigo, the *petit-mal*, and complete epilepsy." But the assertion in the text is that they are different degrees depending on discharges of different strengths beginning in the same part.

of are comparisons attempted betwixt mental states and physical states. But the associations which the expression " loss of consciousness " should arouse in an inquiry like this are thoughts of *other* nervous *symptoms*, which thoughts would lead to such comparisons as those of morbid conditions of the *material basis* of consciousness with those conditions of inferior centres which cause other nervous symptoms. We have to deal with loss of consciousness as a symptom due to implication of nervous centres which are, except in degree, just like other nervous centres. The centres which are the anatomical substrata of consciousness also represent impressions and movements, or rather, they re-represent in greater complexity, etc., the impressions and movements represented in *all* lower centres, being evolved out of those centres. They thus represent the whole organism, and represent it as a whole in adjustment to its environment. On this basis the comparison is legitimate. Physiologically, *loss* of consciousness is a loss of adjustment of the organism *as a whole* to its environment, being a loss of use of the nervous processes by which that adjustment is made. Vertigo is a defect in that adjustment ; it is a motor symptom. It is in this way that we trace its relations through loss of consciousness to convulsion.

If we consider the facts of the vertigo attending palsy of the ocular motor nerves, we see plainly that it is a *motor* symptom.[1] It is, however, sometimes spoken of as a sensory symptom, because a " sensation " attends it. It is one of those disorders of co-ordination which has a subjective side. But the " sensation " in this case is a state of mind (see Chap. I, pt. 2, p. 170), and states of mind may arise during energising of motor as well as of sensory nerves and centres. Our direct concern is with the physical process which goes on in the nervous system whilst the " mental state " which is a feeling of vertigo continues ; it is the physical process which is a disorder of motion—actual or nascent. There is as much difference betwixt the sensation or feeling the giddy man has and the physiological process which goes on in his nervous system as there is betwixt pain and the changes in the sensory (afferent) nerve which exist whilst the pain lasts, or as there is betwixt the colour red and the change in the optic nervous system associated with it.

Hitzig's researches on galvanising the cerebral hemisphere in man (the electrodes being applied to the outside of the head) show clearly, I think, that vertigo is on its physiological side a motor symptom. An account of these experiments is to be found in the third edition of Althaus's *Medical Electricity*, p. 141, from which I borrow the facts below given. Hitzig distinguishes three degrees of vertigo : a slight current produces no outward effects, but there is a feeling of uncertainty as regards the position of one's body, or of external things ; in the second there is no outward effect, but there is a feeling of move-

[1] The giddiness is not due to double vision, as is often supposed. It is owing (1) to erroneous estimation of the position of external objects, or, speaking technically, to " erroneous projection," and (2) to over-action of associated muscles. In this principle we have the full explanation of the cerebellar reel, the ataxic stagger, and some other " disorders of co-ordination," dependent, as I believe, on palsies or paresis of motor nerves and centres.

It may seem that I am trying to prove in the text that partial loss of consciousness is a state of mind—*i.e.* that partial *loss* of consciousness is a state of consciousness. There is really in what we call defect of consciousness a double state ; the " mental state " may be *partly* due to over-action of subordinate centres, from loss of control, by defect in their highest nervous centres. I shall consider this principle, already several times referred to, later on. There is a duality in the anatomical substrata of consciousness ; *diminished* " object consciousness " is, I think, constantly attended by *increased* " subject consciousness."

ment; in the third degree the patient actually does turn. These experiments, taken with clinical facts, show that epileptic vertigo is on its anatomical and physiological (or objective) side a *unilateral* disorder of motion; or, otherwise expressed, that it is a particular defect in the adjustment of the organism as a whole to its environment. In the first and even second degrees of "galvanic giddiness" there is only faint excitation of those centres which, when strongly excited (third degree), cause actual movement.[1] So in calling "galvanic" or epileptic vertigo a unilateral disorder of motion one means that it is essentially so; there is nascent or incipient movement in the slighter discharges, and actual movement in stronger discharges.

Vertigo, a motor symptom, has a subjective side in the feeling, or "sensation," of confusion. This is really a *defect of consciousness*. *Loss* of consciousness in the stronger discharge occurring in cases of *petit-mal* is on its physiological side a *loss* of adjustment to the environment.

I nevertheless, in spite of these fundamental resemblances, consider that some such arrangement as that into the three clinical entities is necessary for practical purposes. Our patients consult us for symptoms. A man comes to us for vertigo, and we have to *find out* whether it is epileptic vertigo or not. For this purpose the empirical classification or arrangement is the best. For example, a patient having an attack of vertigo, it is important first to consider it as vertigo simply, in order to ascertain whether in its superficial features and circumstances it corresponds to epileptic, to aural, or to so-called stomachic vertigo. We thus identify it, and can afterwards trace its fundamental associations. Again, if a patient temporarily loses consciousness, we have a similar investigation to find out whether it be *petit-mal* or ordinary fainting. Thirdly, if there be convulsion, we try to determine whether there be apoplexy, uræmia, tumour, etc. It may be well to illustrate this point at more length. Let us take a really difficult case. We will not suppose that a man comes telling us he *is subject to convulsive seizures*, but that a patient is brought by the police to our hospital for a fit which happened in the street. We should take note of the prominent facts, of the convulsion, with loss of consciousness, followed by coma, and with bitten tongue. We should in our minds make a rapid clinical arrangement of the conditions under which such convulsions occur. If the convulsion had been universal, and if there were no paralysis after it, we could not tell (I mean from the condition of the patient) whether there was uræmia, cerebral hæmorrhage, or tumour. For the epileptic fit (I now mean the *grand-mal* of authorities) may not differ from the convulsion in some cases of uræmia, in some cases of cerebral hæmorrhage, and in some cases of intra-cranial tumour. If from the patient's age, and from an examination of his eyes, arteries, urine, etc., we could eliminate uræmia, cerebral hæmorrhage, and tumour, we should in all probability be right in saying there was epilepsy *grand-mal*.[2]

I will now take an example more striking than any. There is, I consider, an essentially similar functional condition of nervous tissue in epileptic mania,

[1] Excitation of motor centres suffices to give us ideas of movements, even when the motor organs have been removed. (See footnote [1], Chap. I, pt. 2, p. 171, and Weir Mitchell on "Faradising Stumps," op. cit.)

[2] The diagnosis is really more difficult, but the above will suffice for illustration. Of course, if we had a history of fits, occurring now and then for months or years, or if we waited until the patient recovered consciousness completely, we should practically have the diagnosis made for us. If the fits were one-sided the difficulty would be a little less.

in epileptic aphasia, and in epileptic hemiplegia. As I have already, for another purpose, spoken of epileptic mania (Chap. II, p. 183), and have at the same time spoken of epileptic hemiplegia, I must speak briefly here. In each of the three there is temporary exhaustion of a nervous tract after, and as the result of, an excessive nervous (*i.e.* epileptic) discharge. In the first instance that tract consists of processes underlying consciousness, in the second of processes of the speech series, and in the third of processes for movements of the limbs, etc. (the corpus striatum).[1]

But clinically, the cases are extremely different, especially the condition of the extremes, that of the epileptic maniac and of the hemiplegic man. It would be absurd to put the man who is raving and the man who is hemiplegic in the same ward for care simply because from a scientific standpoint they are fundamentally alike. They would require different kinds of supervision. It would be absurd also to treat them in the same way; one patient would require to be put to sleep, the other would not. That each was suffering from an essentially similar morbid functional state (exhaustion of part of his brain, the consequence of a strong nervous discharge) makes no difference for empirical or practical arrangements. It would be as absurd to consider the two cases as alike for practical purposes as it would be for a gardener to put his plants together, not as fruit trees, ornamental shrubs, etc., but according to the division Rosaceæ, Cruciferæ, etc. So much for the clinical investigation and arrangement. Now for the other side—for the value of the scientific investigation and classification. I do not see how we are to understand the very complex problem of epileptic mania until we have studied it in relation with the simpler one of epileptic aphasia, and the still simpler one of epileptic hemiplegia. We must make a comparative study of them, and to do this we must reduce the cases to their lowest terms. We must, in other words, classify them on a fundamental basis, as depending on exhaustion of nervous tracts, that is, as after-effects of epileptic discharges. It is as justifiable for scientific classification of our cases of disease to underrate superficial differences when we can trace fundamental resemblances as it is for the botanist to put together a lily, a tulip, an onion, and the asparagus plant, or for a zoologist to classify a whale, a bat, a hedgehog, and an elephant as mammals.

I think a good illustration of the two kinds of classification and methods of investigation may be taken from insanity. I have the less hesitation in giving it, as when I come to speak at length on epileptic mania, I shall have to speak generally of insanity. It is a part of my subject, for epileptic mania is acute temporary insanity.

There are very many classifications of insanity, and this is good evidence of the difficulty in dealing with the complex problems the cases present. For my part, I think we should have arrangements of cases of insanity for practical purposes, and a classification on some natural system for the purpose of increasing our knowledge of "diseases of the mind." The arrangements,

[1] The nomenclature here is confusing. The mania in epileptic mania is not the analogue of the epileptic aphasia or epileptic hemiplegia. There is a duplex condition in each. Loss of consciousness in the epileptic maniac is the analogue of the loss of speech and of the hemiplegia. These are the three negative elements. Now for the three corresponding positive elements. The mania is the positive element in the first. The positive elements in the other two (the analogues of the mania) are conservation of the more automatic factors in language (smiling, laughing, etc.) and conservation of all movements more automatic than those of the face, arm, and leg.

entirely artificial, would only be provisional. They would in asylum practice start with the very general definition of a lunatic as a person who requires restraint on account of mental disorder. The arrangements would vary very widely as the cases were considered from a pathological or therapeutical point of view, or as the patients required different degrees and kinds of supervision. If a certain kind of insanity were often found along with phthisis, this would be a good reason for making a group "phthisical insanity" for treatment, and also for the accumulation of otherwise unrelated facts bearing on pathology. If the patient were suicidal, there would be very good reason for taking that to be the leading feature of this case for certain practical purposes. Then the grouping epileptic[1] insanity is a very useful one. But for increasing our knowledge of insanity and, indirectly, of mental operations in health, these practical arrangements alone will not suffice. We require also a theoretical arrangement, or rather a classification properly so-called—in fact, a classification on a natural system.

Cases of insanity should, I think, be classified and investigated on the basis supplied by the doctrine of evolution of nervous centres. We shall have enormous help in the work Spencer has done in his *Psychology*. We have already explained that we use the term Dissolution as the opposite of Evolution. Insanity is dissolution beginning in the highest nervous processes. The highest processes form the anatomical substrata of consciousness. In insanity there is partial or total loss of use of the highest processes, the symptom being loss or "defect" of consciousness. Metaphorically speaking, the disease is of the controlling processes. These are negative statements. There is, stated from the positive side, reduction to a more automatic condition of mind, or, physiologically stated, a "lowering of adjustment." (See Chap. II, pt. 2, p. 174.) The elements of the duplex condition, dissolution and automatic action, are in inverse proportion. The "shallower" the dissolution, the higher and more special (more nearly normal) is the automatic mental action permitted; the deeper the dissolution, the more general is the automatic action. The ravings, grotesque actions, visual and auditory hallucinations, etc., are due to action of centres which, except for over-excitement from loss of control, are healthy.

The varieties of insanity would be explained (1) by the depth of the reduction or dissolution; (2) by the rapidity of the reduction; (3) by the kind of brain in which the reduction occurs; and (4) by the influence of external circumstances and internal bodily states on the patient who is reduced. These factors will vary in relative amount infinitely. Insanity is a function of four variables.

Moreover, of course, what we here call the scientific investigation of insanity is really an experimental investigation of mind; and in this regard the slightest departures from a person's standard of mental health are to be studied, and not only the cases of patients who require to be kept in asylums; indeed, the slighter cases (*e.g.* the cocoa-mixing affair—see p. 184) are the more important in the scientific investigation. For whilst in studying evolution we study from the general to the special, it is easiest to study in the reverse way the effects of dissolution. For example, the more special (the more nearly normal) the

[1] We have, of course, to distinguish betwixt (1) transient mania following an epileptic paroxysm, (2) the more lengthy mental infirmity after a succession of attacks, (3) the persistent deterioration which is a gradual result of seizures often repeated for months and years.

mental automatism after an epileptic discharge is, the easier is it understood. The cocoa-mixing automatism is a more valuable experiment on mind than is a case of epileptic mania.

Although for convenience we used above the conventionally correct expression investigation of " diseases of the mind," we mean, of course, as has been also explicitly stated, investigation of those diseases which begin in the *highest centres of the nervous system.* We have to do with changes in nerve cells and fibres making up sensori-motor processes, which are not mind, but only the substrata of mind. Strictly speaking, it is as erroneous to say that the insane patient has disease of the *mind* as to say that a patient the subject of simple and incipient optic atrophy who cannot see red has " disease of colour." It is exceedingly important to get rid of the psychological implication which the convenient expression " disease of the mind " has. Our concern with mind is indirect. Now, in an anatomico-physiological inquiry on the principle of evolution we do not make any abrupt limit to nervous processes serving in mind. We look on the whole nervous system as made up of processes for the co-ordination of impressions and movements. Why, during the energising of some of the highest and most special of these, mental states arise, we do not inquire. In dissolution there are all gradations traceable as a consequence of disease (for example, exhaustion after epileptic discharges) beginning in the highest centres, from such slight " depths " of dissolution as those which permitted actions so nearly normal as the cocoa-mixing affair (see p. 184), to dissolution so deep as coma, in which there is no evidence of mentation, and but the most general and most automatic physical action. For, I repeat, in an anatomico-physiological inquiry the question is not the psychological one—Is consciousness displayed ? but, How is the organism adjusted to its environment ? We have to trace all degrees of defective adjustment corresponding to different depths of dissolution. In the cocoa-mixing affair the adjustment was almost as special as is normal ; in mania where the dissolution is deeper it is far more general ; and in deepest coma the adjustment is of the most general character compatible with life.

Epileptic mania is acute temporary insanity, but in insanity ordinarily so-called there is clinically an essentially similar double state. There is *defect* of consciousness analogous to *loss* of consciousness, and there is slightly increased automatic action analogous to the raving. The difference in degree depends, I believe, on the second variable (*vide supra*), on the difference in the rapidity with which the dissolution is effected (control removed). Dissolution is effected with extreme rapidity by an epileptic discharge, whereas in insanity ordinarily so-called the morbid process removing or impairing control is usually very slow indeed.

That the insane patient has defect of consciousness cannot, I think, be doubted ; for example, in a patient who has illusions or delusions (positive or active element) there is really, I uphold, a negative or passive element—affection of consciousness. The cases are, however, always spoken of from the positive element only. The negative is the more important medically. The patient who has a delusion has it for the same reason that the dreamer has delusions. There is in each loss of ability to correct automatically arising mental states (which are very active) by objective states, because, since the processes serving in the latter are implicated, clear objective states are not possible. Speaking technically, the judgment is defective. The nervous processes implicated are those which form the anatomical substrata of consciousness, or, otherwise expressed, those by which the organism, *as a whole*, is adjusted to its environment. There is in insanity a less special, or, otherwise put, more general adjustment. The man who in hospital imagines himself to be at his home has defect of consciousness, and, as a consequence, also lowering of adjustment; his automatically arising states are not corrected by objective states. He is in a dream from which awakening is sometimes not possible. There are degrees from the very slightest and most temporary departures from healthy mental states to dementia, which, so far as it shows implication of processes serving in mind, is the analogue of coma.[1]

It is of much importance to my argument in many parts of this book to show that defect of consciousness is, on its anatomico-physiological side, defective correspondence with the environment. I would refer the reader to the quotation from Spencer in the first Appendix to the last chapter (p. 188). I now give a further quotation from his *Psychology* on what takes place in healthy mentation:

" . . . We pass into the domain of psychology the moment we inquire how there comes to exist within the organism a relation between *a* and *b* that in some way or other corresponds to the relation between A and B [in the environment]. Psychology is exclusively concerned with this connection between (A B) and (*a b*)—has to investigate its nature, its origin, its meaning, etc.

" A moment's introspection will now make it clear to the reader that he cannot frame any psychological conception without thus looking at internal coexistences and sequences. If he studies the simplest act of perception, as that of localising a touch in some part of his skin, the indispensable terms of his inquiry are—on the one hand, a thing (1) and a position (2), both of which he regards as objective; and on the other hand a sensation (3), and a state of consciousness constituting his apprehension of position (4), both of which he regards as subjective. Again, to cite an example from the opposite extreme, if he takes for his problem one of his involved sentiments, as that of justice, he cannot represent to himself this sentiment, or give any meaning to its name, without calling to mind actions and relations supposed to exist in the environment; neither this nor any other emotion can be aroused in consciousness even vaguely without positing something beyond consciousness to which it refers. And when, instead of studying psychology subjectively, he studies it objectively in the acts of other beings, he similarly finds himself incapable of stirring a step without thinking of inner correlations in their references to outer correlations " (*Principles of Psychology*, vol. i, p. 133).

After these digressions, purposely made in order to show principles of classification, which are to be applied so far as possible to all kinds of cases of nervous disease, I return to Epilepsies.

I admit two classifications to the Empirical Classification, or rather Arrangement of Varieties of Epilepsies, and of Epileptiform Convulsions would be—

### Empirical Arrangement

#### A. Epilepsy Proper

(1) Vertigo.
(2) *Petit-mal.*
(3) *Grand-mal.*

[1] No doubt these degrees are (like increasing degrees of hemiplegia) " compound degrees." The more the special processes are affected, the wider is the implication of the more automatic.

B. Epileptiform, or Epileptoid

(1) Convulsions beginning unilaterally.
(2) Unilateral Dysæsthesia (migraine).
(3) Epileptiform Amaurosis, etc.

Plainly enough, such an arrangement goes by what is most superficial or striking. The advantages of it are obvious. It facilitates identification and the application of knowledge to utilitarian purposes. But it must not be trusted as a natural classification. However much it may be further elaborated, it can make not even an approach to a scientific classification. No amount of refined subdivision starting from a definition which makes loss of consciousness a symptom *sui generis* would make the arrangement a natural classification, for there would never be points of contact with other classes of nervous diseases or symptoms. No common principle underlies it. It is a great misfortune when a student takes such an arrangement, founded obviously on superficial differences and resemblances, as a natural system, and endeavours *only* to see if a given case approach nearest this or that entity. The clinical divisions are avowedly artificial. Authorities are fully agreed on this point. As regards the clinical divisions of the symptoms of epilepsy (of what, in the arrangement, is called epilepsy proper), there are very many intermediate degrees traceable. On this point authorities agree—they agree, that is to say, as to the clinical facts.[1] There are, clinically, degrees traceable from a slight and transient loss of consciousness,[2] which, to give an example, simply permits the hand to fall in raising a fork to the mouth, the mouthful being the very next moment safely delivered, to severe universal convulsions, with loss of consciousness, followed by deep coma. So far, I speak of different cases. The same patient may have seizures of different degrees, sometimes *petit-mal* and sometimes *grand-mal*. Again, a patient, after being for months subject to *petit-mal*, or even to slight vertigo, becomes subject to the *grand-mal*, or to both ; and in many cases of patients who suffer both there is clear proof that the *petit-mal* is an abortive fit—*i.e.* the initial stage of the *grand-mal*. In these cases the *petit-mal* merges into the *grand-mal*. Then, although we have illustrated by *loss* of consciousness, there are really in slight attacks of epileptic vertigo, or *petit-mal*, all degrees of affection of consciousness. It is not very uncommon for a patient to have for months sudden and short queer feelings at the epigastrium, and a little confusion of thought, which conditions later on he recognises as being just the same as the initial symptoms of his attacks of *petit-mal* and

[1] They do not admit that they are degrees in the sense which I hold them to be—*viz.* as being due to discharges of different degrees beginning in (see Chap. II, p. 187) the highest centres of the cerebral hemispheres.

Let me state the differences categorically. The reader is reminded that the epilepsy of authorities (" idiopathic epilepsy ") is spoken of.

The accepted opinion is that two different and distant parts (the medulla oblongata and the cerebral hemisphere) are concerned in the epileptic paroxysm. I think but *one* part, the cerebral hemisphere, is concerned, and that of this only the highest centres are the seat of the discharging lesion. (The discharge, of course, spreads through lower centres.)

The accepted view assumes two different processes—(1) a *discharge* of the medulla oblongata, and (2) a *contraction of the arteries* of the brain. Correspondingly there are, according to it, two essentially different states—(1) passive, in the cerebral hemisphere, and (2) active, in the medulla oblongata. I think there is but *one* process in the paroxysm, an active one—that is, a discharge beginning in the highest processes of the cerebral hemisphere. Consciousness will be lost during the excessive excitation of these processes.

[2] Loss of adjustment, etc.

of *grand-mal*. As mentioned (Chap. II, p. 187), a patient may tell us that he is confused only, and will say that he hears people talking, but does not know what they say. This is only defect of consciousness. Again, we see, as has been repeatedly stated, that there are all degrees of automatism *after* different degrees of epileptic seizures, and this is indirect evidence of all degrees or depths of implication of the anatomical substrata of consciousness.

If we take cases of what are called " epileptiform " seizures, we find all degrees even in the same patient—we find, for example, attacks of convulsion of the arm without a trace of affection of consciousness ; and again, attacks in which he loses consciousness, and is deeply comatose when the fit is over. There are, indeed, all degrees of discharges, from those causing twitching of the index-finger to those causing universal convulsion. Similarly, there are very numerous degrees of paralysis after convulsion of different degrees of violence, from numbness of a hand to hemiplegia with lateral deviation of the eyes.

However convenient the empirical division may be *clinically*, and I admit its convenience, the division is not an anatomico-physiological one ; it is, I think, of psychological parentage.

So, in admitting the necessity for clinical purposes of an arrangement of varieties of epilepsy, I urge that in a scientific classification we must start from a more fundamental basis. The one I suggest is that there is in each epilepsy a sudden and violent discharge, and that those varieties called by authorities genuine epilepsy are explainable on the supposition of a discharge beginning in the highest series of nervous processes. Other seizures begin in series of a lower range of evolution (subordinate series)—for example, convulsions beginning in hand, face, foot, etc.

In this book I deal chiefly with the Scientific Investigation of epilepsy, but I must frequently speak of the Empirical Investigation : it will be absolutely necessary to do so. What I hope I shall not do is to mix the two classifications.

The reader who does not make allowances for the distinctions I have made may give reasons for rejecting my method altogether, but if he does reject it he can scarcely be considered a fair critic of details. A botanist would not think a gardener ignorant because he put together his plants as they were of use for eating or for ornament and a gardener would not think a botanist ignorant because he classified plants regardless of their being herbs, trees, or shrubs. Let me state the method anew.

In the Scientific Investigation of a case in which there is loss of consciousness, vertigo, convulsion, or *any symptom whatever presented paroxysmally*, the endeavour is not to determine if there be any approach to or departure from any clinical standard—to, or from, what has been described as genuine epilepsy for example. There being occasionally a paroxysmal presentation of symptoms (see List, p. 182), an internal and local discharging lesion is inferred. Since any part of the convolutional surface of the brain may become unstable—may become the seat of a " discharging lesion "—there will be many varieties [1] of epilepsy. Since the size of the discharging lesion will vary, and as probably the grey matter affected differs in degree of instability, there will be seizures

[1] It does not follow that there will be as many practically as are theoretically possible ; for some parts of the brain are more often damaged than other parts—the Sylvian region, for example ; this is a consequence of arterial arrangements. When I come to speak of pathology I shall consider this subject, and especially with regard to embolism and thrombosis, as possible pathological processes in inducing local " discharging lesions."

not only of all kinds, but of all degrees. Not only will the paroxysms of different patients differ in that, as, for an example, the paroxysms in one affect first the leg—in another, first the arm, but there will be such differences as that of two fits beginning in the hand : one is limited to the arm, and the other spreads all over the body.

We must, however, even in the Scientific Classification and Investigation, make arbitrary divisions—for instance, we shall speak of three degrees of convulsions beginning unilaterally ; we shall be obliged to do so. All classifications in all sciences make distinctions more exact and abrupt than any that exist in nature.

It may seem to the reader that this is returning to the old method. In the first place, the new method takes count of all kinds of paroxysmal discharges, even such as " subjective " sensations of smell. And in speaking of degrees we do so only for the sake of exposition. In actual practice we encounter all conceivable degrees. And this method necessitates a precise study of what occurs in the paroxysm in each case on its own merits, regardless whether it approaches any arbitrary standard, and equally regardless whether it be one of the degrees spoken of for clearness of exposition in the Scientific Investigation. It necessitates also a very careful localisation of the changes discoverable post-mortem ; for, as stated, every epileptic paroxysm is considered as a brutal development of the function of some part of the brain.

The researches of Hitzig and Ferrier will help this investigation to an extent difficult to over-estimate ; for I most willingly admit that the method I uphold has made very little way. From their researches we shall learn where to look for the minute changes which constitute the discharging lesions in different epilepsies. Whatever interpretation may be put on their facts, there is no doubt, at any rate, that irritation of different parts of the surface of the brain leads to different classes of movements. Correspondingly, there is no doubt that at least some epilepsies beginning by movements in different parts of the body depend on " disease " of different parts of the surface of the cerebral hemisphere.

## Appendix to Chapter III

The following is the quotation referred to at p. 192 :

" Let us first consider the *range* of the term [epilepsy], let us see what disorders are properly ranked under this head. It is no easy matter to do this exactly and correctly ; we may err in two ways : on the one hand, by too closely restricting our conception of the disease to its more classical types, and so leaving out of count and consideration a great number of more or less closely allied derangements ; and the other, by too great laxity in the use of the term, leading us to overlook important distinguishing circumstances. We shall best meet this difficulty, I think, by referring to the principle so well laid down by Whewell (*Philos. of Ind. Sc.*, vol. i, p. 494). This is that Natural groups are determined not by Definition, but by Type ; not by a boundary line without, but by a central point within ; not by what they strictly include, but by what they eminently include ; by an example, not by a precept. ' A type,' he proceeds, ' is an example of any class, for instance, a species of a genus which is considered as eminently possessing the characters of the class. All the species which have a greater affinity with this type-species than with any others form the genus, and are ranged about it, deviating from it in various directions and different degrees. Thus, a genus may consist of several species which approach very near the type, and of which the claim to a place with it is obvious ; while there may be other species which straggle further from this central knot and which yet are clearly more connected with it than with any other. And even if there should be some species of which the place is dubious, and which appear to be equally bound to two generic types, it is easily seen that this would not destroy the reality of the generic groups any more than the scattered trees of the intervening plain prevent our speaking intelligibly of the distinct forests of two separate hills.' To apply this to the case before us. It appears to me that, taking the convulsive form in its entirety, for *the type*, it shades off on one side by the *petit-mal* into mere vertigo, on another, into hysteria and choreic convulsion, on a third, into delirium, catalepsy, and somnambulism, on a fourth, into neuralgia. Convulsion and unconsciousness, recurring more or less frequently, are the grand features of epilepsy, but the former symptom we know may be often absent, and though the latter, in a greater or less degree, is much more constant, it is occasionally much attenuated or awanting. I make this statement on the authority of Trousseau and Sieveking, which my own experience tends to confirm. When the intervals are very long, several years for instance, the character of recurrence loses most of its value. This character is further weakened by the circumstance that the intervals are by no means always free from various morbid phenomena, similar in kind, but less in degree than those which constitute the paroxysm. Thus, the convulsive fits may come to be few and far between, but attacks of giddiness may be pretty frequent, and of somewhat long duration, and these mark the persistence of the disorder almost as much as the fits. Viewing this malady from its *phenomenal* side, I can only express my entire concurrence with what my friend, Dr. Sieveking, has said—" That several of the diseases that are commonly regarded as residing mainly in the nervous system merge into one another, and that the boundaries by which they would appear to be circumscribed by nosologists are by no means so uniformly to be traced " (Dr. Handfield Jones on *Functional Nervous Disorders*, art. " Epilepsy," p. 285).

## IV

### General Remarks on the Causes of Epilepsies

Epilepsy, or rather Epilepsies, have been defined as depending on abnormal conditions of nerve tissue. Such permanent alterations occur in the nutrition of areas of grey matter in the cerebral hemispheres that it becomes highly unstable. The sign of this instability is an occasional excessive discharge. In short, there is a permanent " discharging lesion " in each epilepsy.

That there is a " discharging lesion " in those cases of epilepsy where there is convulsion is evident, for there does occur now and then a paroxysm which gives proof of there being an internal, sudden, excessive, and rapid discharge of nerve tissue. In cases of *petit-mal*, in which loss or trouble of consciousness is the chief and almost sole observable thing, there is in the pallor of the face evidence of strong discharge ; for there is great arterial contraction.

The reader will bear in mind that I believe that in cases of *petit-mal*, as well as in cases of convulsion (*grand-mal*), the discharging lesion is of some part of the cerebral hemisphere. The accepted view is that in both cases the discharge *begins in* the medulla oblongata. Indeed, what is essential to my definition of an epilepsy is that there be a sudden excessive and violent discharge of nervous tissue. Affection of consciousness is not essential. I have repeatedly spoken of loss or trouble of consciousness in epilepsies. It is a matter of such vast importance that I must speak of it again and again. The absolute distinction into cases with and cases without loss of consciousness is only to be justified on the score of practical convenience. It is an empirical and not a scientific distinction. It is not a distinction analogous to that made by a botanist, but analogous to one made by a gardener. It has no anatomical or physiological warrant. It is a distinction of psychological parentage. Consciousness is often spoken of as if it were an entity. It is also spoken of as if it were a "function" of the nervous system or of some part of it. Suppose it *is* a "function" of the nervous system, we have, at any rate, to distinguish this function from that other function—*viz.* energising of nervous arrangements representing impressions and movements. It is with the latter only that we have to do as medical men; it is on an anatomical basis only that we can trace relations betwixt cases in which consciousness is lost and cases of convulsion, paralysis, etc.

In whatever way an epileptic seizure may begin (in the thumb, in the great toe, by what is subjectively coloured vision, sensation of smell, etc.), consciousness will be lost *if the discharge be strong enough*. The stronger it is the further it will spread in the brain.[1] In the cases mentioned (where the earliest signs of the discharge are spasm of the hand, or of the foot, etc.) the discharge begins in some subordinate centre. Seizures beginning with loss of consciousness (cases without "a warning") are those in which the discharge begins in the highest of all nervous processes of the cerebral hemisphere—that is to say, in nervous processes evolved out of all lower subordinate centres.

Even the empirical distinction should really be into cases in which consciousness is lost first, very early, late, or not at all. Those cases in which it is not lost at all are cases in which the discharge, beginning in a subordinate centre, is slight, as shown either (1) by the fact that the part of the body affected is limited, or (2) by the fact that although a considerable part is affected, it is slowly affected. Much depends on the rapidity of the discharge. How arbitrary the distinction is must force itself on the notice of the most superficial observer; for of any case in which there are convulsions without loss of consciousness we should mostly be right in saying that some day or other the patient would have one with loss of consciousness—*i.e.* there would occur a discharge a little stronger, which would therefore spread more widely in the brain.

The one thing common in the many superficially different seizures which I (see p. 182) call epilepsies is the unstable condition of grey matter; in other terms, there is a "discharging lesion" in every epilepsy. This is the *functional* affection in epilepsy. The next point is as to the seat of this functional affection. Grey matter may be unstable in many different parts of the cerebral hemisphere (organ damaged); hence many differences in the symptoms from cerebral discharges. There is a third inquiry. The pathological

[1] As I have several times suggested, I think there is a twofold spreading. The part which is morbid (unstable) discharges, and this discharge, if strong, (1) unlocks lower and subordinate centres (discharges them), (2) and also discharges associated and, so to speak, collateral centres. I believe the second process is by the intermediation of arteries; the suddenly induced contraction of the artery discharges the cells of grey matter it supplies. There are two kinds of Co-ordination: there is Melody of Movement as well as Harmony of Movement. The arteries, I think, regulate the former, which is time Co-ordination.

processes (alterations of nutrition) by which grey matter can be rendered unstable are no doubt numerous.

Let me again remind the reader that for epilepsy, as I define it, loss or trouble of consciousness is not essential. What is essential is a sudden, abrupt and paroxysmal discharge. What I am now about to urge of a case in which there is loss of consciousness applies in principle to other epilepsies in which there is none. Without intending to make an abrupt limit, we may, for simplicity of illustration, say that in some paroxysms of *petit-mal* there is loss of consciousness only. In such a case we have just as much as in any other variety of epilepsy (in one, for example, in which the symptom is convulsion of the arm) to (1) search for the seat of the lesion, the substrata of consciousness ; we have to discuss (2) the abnormality in the function of these substrata (strong discharge of these substrata during which consciousness is lost) ; and (3) to consider evidence bearing on the disorder of the nutritive process by which cells and fibres of these substrata get into such a state of unstability that they occasionally discharge strongly.

That loss of consciousness, a negative symptom, should be ascribed to an active process (discharge) seems, at first glance, unlikely. We see, however, that patients lose the use of an arm during the stage of tonic spasm of it as much as they do in paralysis of it. I think, then, that consciousness may be lost during the *excessive discharge* of the anatomical substrata of consciousness.

Besides other reasons for ascribing loss of consciousness from an epileptic discharge, the discharge is rapid. Time is required for consciousness. On this matter I will quote Spencer, *Psychology*, vol. i, p. 107 :

" A subjective state becomes recognisable as such, only when it has an appreciable duration : it must fill some space in the series of states, otherwise it is not known as present. This general truth harmonises with a general truth before pointed out respecting nervous action, as well as with the above interpretation.

" The observed fact that time is taken in the transit of a nerve wave is not to the point ; for this transit has no concomitant subjective state. But the inferred fact that the change set up in a nerve centre must take time, and a more considerable time (§ 35), is relevant ; for what is objectively a change in a superior nerve centre is subjectively a feeling, and the duration of it under the one aspect measures the duration of it under the other."

During *the excessive and rapid discharge* of the anatomical substrata of consciousness we could not expect that conscious states would appear ; on the contrary, we should, *a priori*, expect loss of consciousness.

To speak of the anatomy, physiology, and pathology of the symptom loss of consciousness may seem strange ; but we have already explained that the anatomical substrata of consciousness are only highly compound sensori-motor processes fundamentally like those of lower centres, differing in being the most special and complex of all. They have, then, their anatomy, their physiology, and their pathology.[1]

Recapitulating, but putting the facts in slightly differing order, we have to

[1] Moreover, the anatomico-physiological statement is not loss of consciousness, but, as previously explained, loss of the correspondence of the organism as a whole, with its environment. When we come to anatomy we shall point out that there is not one seat of this correspondence, for consciousness is a varying quantity—that is, we are from moment to moment differently conscious, we are continually changing correspondence with our environment.

study the anatomy, the physiology,[1] and the pathology of epilepsies, or rather of each epilepsy; or, stating the facts in a more abstract form, and in the reverse order, we have to study the abnormalities in the absorption, in the expenditure, and in the transfer of force in cases of epilepsy. It is an anatomical inquiry to search for the seat of lesions. It is a physiological inquiry to note how the function of nervous matter is affected. It is a pathological inquiry to trace the morbid nutritive processes by which local changes of instability are brought about.

The above shows in chief part how we use the word "cause." We must use it, however, not in a threefold, but in a fourfold sense. The fourth group of so-called causes is for the conditions which determine individual paroxysms, but more particularly the first paroxysm in a case. We shall have a separate chapter for these so-called causes. But for the present we speak only of causes with reference to the three lines of investigation—Organ, Function, Nutrition. The word "cause" is frequently used by medical men for any one of the three. It is used for the seat of the lesion (organ). Thus hemiplegia is said to be "caused by" disease of the corpus striatum. It is used for the functional nature of the lesion, as when it is said that epilepsy is "caused by" increased excitability of the medulla oblongata. It is used for the pathological process (alteration of nutrition), as when it is said that loss of speech is "caused by" "softening," the result of embolism. But properly we have, in each case of nervous disease, before our conception of it is anything like complete, to find the seat of the lesion (anatomy), the functional nature of the change (physiology), and the derangement of the nutritive process (pathology). In other words, our classification aims to be threefold, as our method of investigation should be. The principles apply to all cases of nervous disease. I will now, therefore, on the principle of studying first the simplest problems, give the order of the three lines of investigation of a case of hemiplegia of the common from—we will suppose of the left side. Such a case is far simpler than is a case of convulsion. Indeed, our knowledge of the "causes" of the latter is much too imperfect for clear illustration. As illustration only is intended, a mere sketch will suffice.

*Anatomical Investigation* (Organ Damaged—Seat of Lesion—Localisation, etc.).—We find that the face, tongue, arm, and leg are affected on one side. This points to the organ damaged, which is the corpus striatum.

This kind of evidence points to nothing more. It tells us only that the corpus striatum is damaged, but tells us nothing as to the functional nature of the lesion, nor as to the pathological process by which it is brought about.

*Physiological Investigation* (Affection of Function—"Destroying" or "Discharging" Lesion).—We find that the parts affected are paralysed. We can now say that the functional affection of the corpus striatum is loss of function—that nerve fibres are destroyed.

It will, I fear, seem mere affectation to give this separately, as when we saw that the patient's face, arm, and leg were affected we saw that they were *paralysed*. But from this very simple case I wish to illustrate a method; I wish to show that it is the regional affection in epilepsies, chorea, etc., which localises, regardless of the *state of the muscles* in that region.

*Pathological Investigation* (Alteration of Nutrition).—On inquiry we

[1] Of course we mean by physiology, in this application, abnormal function, and correspondingly for the other terms.

discover that the palsy came on suddenly, and that there was deep coma. Further, we examine the patient and conclude that he has chronic renal disease, atheromatous arteries, and hypertrophy of the left ventricle of the heart. We now say that the loss of function was the result of breaking up of fibres and cells by irruption of blood.

Here, again, it may seem simply tiresome to separate the functional affection from the pathology. It may be needless for practical purposes in cases like that furnishing the simple illustration now before us ; but I think there are few things in neuro-pathology more unfortunate than the confusion of the physiology of epilepsies with their pathology. For example, the statement that the medulla oblongata is over-excitable is a physiological statement. By what pathological process did that excitability result ? is a question in pathology. This is a *very distinct* question.

In so simple a case our investigation and classification are complete. Such a case is indeed so simple that it seems, as we have said, mere pedantry to write out three stages in diagnosis. But in methodical investigation we must do it ; we must separately consider the two things, muscular *region* affected and the *condition* of the muscles affected. Again, we must not mix our physiology and pathology.

When we pass from palsies to mobile affections resulting from nervous discharges, and particularly to the effects of the paroxysmal discharges in epilepsies, we cannot accomplish this threefold classification. We can often only be certain of the second—the nature of the functional affection. If we take cases with convulsions, we can be certain of that—we are sure that nerve tissue is unstable. The fact that certain parts of the body are occasionally put in excessive action is as certain a warrant for the conclusion that a certain area of nerve tissue is unstable as paralysis is for the conclusion that the function of some area of nerve tissue is destroyed. But as to the organ damaged, we can, in most cases, say nothing with certainty. It is only a speculation to say that the organ or part affected in the epilepsy of authorities is the medulla oblongata. I hold the counter-speculation that the cerebral hemisphere is the part in which the discharging lesion lies, in the epilepsy of authorities (which is one epilepsy in my classification). But assuming that there is a localised state of instability in the medulla oblongata, we cannot in most cases trace, except roughly, any links in the pathological process by which that localised discharging lesion resulted.

The method is of great value in keeping up expectation. The causes of epilepsy are wide of the mark unless they bear on one of the three (organ, function, nutrition). If we are told that a patient's epilepsy has been " caused " by anxiety or fright, we gladly accept the important fact that the first epileptic paroxysm was preceded by fright. But the paroxysms continuing to occur, we still ask—Where is the discharging lesion in this case ? If it be replied, " In the medulla oblongata," we may, for the sake of putting a further necessary question, provisionally accept this, and next ask—" By what pathological process does fright lead to such instability of nerve tissue in the medulla oblongata, that it occasionally discharges excessively ? Of course I do not expect that those who declare the medulla oblongata to be the unstable part which discharges in epilepsy should have answers to such questions. I simply wish to point out what the questions really are.

## V

## Physiology of Epilepsy

Physiology has to do with the dynamics of the nervous system, with the conditions for and modes of activity (discharge) of arrangements of nerve cells and fibres. It deals with the function of nerve tissue. The function of nerve tissue in health is to store up and to expend force. This twofold definition is true of all organic matter, but it is strikingly true of nerve tissue. Nerve tissue, by continuous nutrition, stores up force, and in healthy operations gives it out (" discharges ") on certain definite provocations. This applies to nervous processes of all nervous centres, to those of the spinal cord, ciliary ganglion, and to the highest processes of the cerebral hemisphere.

In every movement, and also in every thought, there is a central nervous discharge.[1]

In this book the word " physiological " is used for the two *abnormalities* in this healthy function of nerve tissue—*viz.* for loss of its function and for over-function. These are our two classes of functional changes already referred to in Chap. IV. In the first class of functional changes nerve tissue is frequently actually destroyed, as when it is broken up by a clot ; but at any rate its function is lost, it cannot discharge at all. In the second class nerve tissue is unstable, it discharges too much ; moreover, it discharges on slight provocation. The nerve tissue is of high tension, and also of very unstable equilibrium, or shortly, it is unstable.

There are what I call " destroying lesions " and " discharging lesions." It matters nothing for the definition *how* the destruction or the instability be brought about—by what abnormal nutritive processes. These are important questions in pathology, not questions in physiology at all. Let us first illustrate the difference betwixt physiology and pathology by a case of loss of function, as this is the simpler of the two classes. Destruction (or more generally speaking, destruction of function) of nerve tissue may be the result of softening from blocking of an artery, of tearing up by blood clot, of slow wasting (as in spinal amaurosis). Then it must not be forgotten that it may be the result of a strong discharge, as in cases of paralysis [2] after convulsion (epileptic hemiplegia, for example) ; here there is loss of function from exhaustion of nerve tissue.

Next as to over-function, or instability. It may, I believe, be produced by hyperæmia consequent on blocking of vessels, by the irritation of tumours, and doubtless in many other ways. I repeat, the mode of production of functional changes is a question in pathology. The most striking case, showing the difference betwixt physiology and pathology, is tumour with convulsion. No one can suppose that a tumour discharges. When we say that a tumour " causes " convulsion, the only meaning the expression can have is that the tumour *leads to* instability of grey matter, which forms part of sensori-motor

[1] The movement and thought are not of course the things comparable. In both there is discharge of nervous processes, and in all centres the nervous processes represent impressions and movements. The comparison is betwixt energising of centres of higher and lower degrees of evolution. It is betwixt active states of nervous processes which form the anatomical substrata of mind, and active states of nervous processes of other and lower centres which (that is, as commonly supposed) have no mental side.

[2] As implied in the text, one does not mean necessarily either *physical* destruction of fibres and cells, or *permanent* loss of function of them ; what is essential is loss of function, however caused.

processes representing movements. The discharge causing the convulsion is of this unstable grey matter.

We shall see in the next chapter that there are good grounds for the belief, that whilst loss and excess of function depend on abnormalities of nerve tissue, the pathological processes by which those abnormalities are caused *begin* in the non-nervous elements of nervous organs.

We have, of course, in a work on epilepsy, to do more particularly with the second division of functional changes—with instability permitting abnormal nervous discharges. I must, however, say, explicitly as well as implicitly, before I go farther, that I do not use the word " functional " in senses in which it is frequently used.

The word " functional " is sometimes used as a name for " minute " changes, or for those the existence of which we can only infer because nervous symptoms are present, but which we do not expect to discover post-mortem. For instance, it is said that epilepsy and chorea are functional diseases, it being meant that the changes on which the symptoms in these two affections depend are so slight that they do not involve actual alterations of structure. It is thus a term for the neuroses. The neuroses are often spoken of as " functional diseases." This is, I think, an inconvenient way of using the word. The real meaning in this application is little more than that the morbid changes in the nervous organs are as yet undiscovered. In the second class of what I shall call functional changes—instability—the changes are slight, *i.e.* not easily discoverable post-mortem, if at all; but their slightness is no essential part of the definition to be given. What is essential is that the changes are of over-function (instability), or in other words, " discharging lesions." Again, it has been pointed out that the first class of changes *may be* minute or undiscoverable, as for example, when temporary hemiplegia results from temporary exhaustion of nerve fibres by the strong discharge in a convulsion. But the essential matter here also is that there is loss of function, not that there is slightness of change.

The term " functional " is often used more loosely still. Thus, when a patient has a transient and imperfect paralysis—for instance, slight hemiplegia, lasting a day or two, or a few hours only—the internal changes on which it depends may be declared to be functional, *i.e.* in the sense of slight change, *simply because the external symptom presented was a slight and transitory one*. There are several reasons why this error should be pointed out, for an error it most decidedly is. The slightness and transientness of a paralytic symptom depend on the slight *extent* of lesions of nervous organs, not on slight *degree* of change. If there be a very limited lesion, even if nerve tissue be actually destroyed, smashed up by clot, for example, the patient will recover quickly ; and his recovery does not always follow, if indeed it ever does, because the damage to the motor tract is repaired. It is often irreparable. He recovers simply because he has lost only a *small quantity* of that tract. For it is manifest to those who make post-mortem examinations that recovery from paralysis occurs where a part of the motor tract is *permanently wanting*. They find gaps in the motor tract of those who died free from obvious [1] paralysis. The recognition of this fact is important in many ways for a clear knowledge of epilepsy.

[1] Nor will this be strange to those clinical observers who *do not* make post-mortem examinations if they consider the facts bearing on the plan of structure of nervous organs, and that when recovery follows in a case of paralysis it observes a particular order—it is from that of the more automatic parts to that of the most voluntary.

Recoverability from paralysis is chiefly a question of the *size* of the lesion—I mean of the quantity of nerve tissue destroyed. As lesions differ in size in all degrees—there are, for example, lesions produced by clots from the size of a pea to that of a hen's egg—there are all degrees of paralysis, and many degrees of recoverability. There is no need to explain a transient paralysis by a slightly altered *state* of nerve tissue. As a mere matter of fact, transientness of paralysis cannot be taken as evidence that nervous *structure* has not been permanently destroyed, and here I mean destroyed physically, broken up.[1]

That parts of the cerebral hemisphere may be destroyed when there are no obvious or striking symptoms has long been well known. But it is so of the motor tract also. I shall have again to insist on this class of facts. They are of very great importance. They are most striking as illustrating what I call the principle of Compensation (see Chap. I, pt. 2, p. 173, and later on in this chapter, p. 215).

The distinction of functional changes in two divisions is at the very bottom of methodical classification of nervous diseases ; it is so important that I here give a striking illustration of a way in which confusion results from ignoring it.

The term " disorder of co-ordination " is frequently used ; but it is applied to diseases which are fundamentally different ; for example, it is applied to chorea and to locomotor ataxy. Of course, both these *are* disorders of co-ordination ; but the term is used without qualification, and this leads to the two different, indeed opposite, states being considered as alike in their physiological or functional causation. Chorea and locomotor ataxy are not only unlike in that different parts of the body are affected, but unlike in the functional affection. In the former there is " over-function " ; in the latter there is loss of function. In view of the active motor disorder of the ataxic patient, the statement that there is loss of function of the nervous centres for locomotion seems, at first glance, absurd. But is there not wasting of nerve fibres in the posterior column of the cord ? And what could this " cause " ? It would " cause " nothing active. It could not " cause " the disorderly gait—in fact, it could " cause " nothing. The disorder of co-ordination in locomotor ataxy and in some other affections is owing to a double difficulty consequent on *loss* of function of nerve tissue ; there is really paralysis. There is (1) over-estimate of a movement intended to be executed by the centre diseased, but not accomplished, and (2) by healthy centres, increased action of associated movements in accordance with the over-estimate. But in chorea there are morbid discharges ; there is the very opposite condition of nerve tissue—*viz.* that of over-function. So, then, in the one disorder of co-ordination there is a destroying lesion (loss of function) ; in the other disorder of co-ordination, a discharging lesion (over-function). The explanation given of the disorder of co-ordination in locomotor ataxy applies *mutatis mutandis* to the reel from disease of the cerebellum.[2]

We must now consider the healthy function of the two elements of nerve tissue in order to have clear ideas of the two abnormalities of function we are

[1] Paralysis after convulsion is often transitory, and is so because the nerve tissue affected is only exhausted, not broken up. But here, again, mistakes are made. It is sometimes said of such cases, " There can be no organic disease, because the paralysis passed off very rapidly." Now, as a mere matter of fact, these are the very cases in many of which one would really expect to find a tumour. It is true that the tumour acts very indirectly in causing paralysis. The tumour leads to instability of grey matter. There is a violent discharge through the corpus striatum, which causes convulsion. After the convulsion there is hemiplegia as a result of exhaustion of the corpus striatum by the violent discharge.

[2] *Lancet*, January 30, 1875.

speaking about. There are ganglion cells and nerve fibres. The cells store up force and discharge. The nerve fibres carry the current, and provoke discharge.[1] Correspondingly there are such symptoms as palsy and anæsthesia from destruction of fibres, and there are spasm, neuralgia, etc., from instability of cells.[2] We shall see in the chapter on Pathology that there are notable differences in the blood supply of grey and white matter—differences in their vascular condition corresponding to differences in their function. It is obvious enough that this separation of duty is to some extent artificial, for the cell is not only a mass of " explosive " matter, but also a connecting link betwixt nerves. It is not only a generator, but a conductor of nerve force. As Spencer says, the " centres in which molecular motion is liberated are also the centres in which it is co-ordinated." Similarly, as the axis cylinder of the nerve is composed of matter similar to that of the cell, we may suppose that it also stores up and expends force. It must perhaps, therefore, be admitted that instability of the axis cylinders of fibres will produce some over-function, and that destruction of the cells will produce some loss of function. But it is not likely that instability of the axis cylinder would produce such excessive discharges as occur in convulsion, chorea, and neuralgia, and it is not likely that destruction of grey matter, unless very widespread, would produce such paralysis as occurs in hemiplegia.[3]

The distinction we have made, that loss of function is an affection of fibres and over-function of cells, is not absolutely correct ; but it represents extreme degrees of difference, and may be taken as sufficiently correct for practical purposes.

I confess that I used to consider the two functional states of nerve tissue to be degrees of but one condition. I now see that this was a great blunder ; they are diametrically opposite states. One reason I had for erroneously thinking so was that paralysis is frequently associated with convulsion. This association must have arrested the attention of every clinical observer. I will state some of the facts of it. Hemiplegia is not unfrequently found after convulsions beginning on one side of the body ; it is the epileptic hemiplegia of Dr. Todd. (I now explain this remarkable sequence, as I have many times said, by the supposition that the paralysis depends on exhaustion of the corpus striatum *by the strong discharge* of convolutions in the fit.) But far more remarkable, there is occasionally hemiplegia (usually imperfect hemiplegia *before* the first convulsion. When the attack is on, we see that those very parts which have been *paralysed* are those which are first and most *convulsed*. This puzzles some students. They think it impossible that paralysed parts should

[1] Of course such expressions as " store up force," " carry the current," etc., are used conventionally. I have no theory as to " nerve force," or force of any kind.

[2] Let us give examples from particular motor symptoms. In the first division there is hemiplegia, reeling gait (from disease of the cerebellum causing paresis of the muscles of the spine), locomotor ataxy, loss of consciousness (or defect of consciousness in chronic insanity, for example), etc. In the second division there is hemichorea, hemispasm, and, as I would call them, hemikineses generally, tetanus (due to discharge of those processes in the cerebellum which, in the reeling gait, are paralysed or paresed). In every member of each division the condition of nerve tissue is the same.

[3] We have already spoken of certain disorders of co-ordination (the cerebellar reel and the erratic gait of locomotor ataxy), which, being erroneously compared to chorea, may be erroneously supposed to depend on discharging lesions. They are really palsies, and depend on destroying lesions. But such disorders as the agitation in paralysis agitans, the tremor of sclerosis, and the irregular movements of the arms and hands of some ataxic patients, and some cases of chorea-like movements after hemiplegia are really, I think, essentially palsies too.

be the very ones which are " picked out " for spasm ; and in trying to " remember " on which side a patient was convulsed, a student will occasionally really *infer* the side convulsed, as is shown by his saying, for example, " It *must* have been his left side, *because his right side was paralysed*." Were he to trust inferences, a good clinician would draw the very opposite conclusion.

I used, as above mentioned, to explain the association of palsy and spasm by the notion that the condition of nerve tissue which caused the paralysis was a more extreme degree of the same condition as that which caused the spasm. Now I think the two conditions are opposite. A satisfactory explanation can be given of the co-existence of palsy and spasm—I mean of parts permanently paralysed, being subject to occasional spasm.

Anticipating the chapter on the Principle of Compensation, I will now try to explain how it is that symptoms of loss of function and of over-function of the same *external* part can co-exist. Some parts of the nervous centre concerned have lost function, whilst other parts of the same centre have over-function. Unfortunately, a further digression is required to make this statement clear. We have to answer the following question : How can loss of function of *one* part of the corpus striatum cause palsy of muscles of *one* side of the body, whilst over-function of *another* part of the same nervous centre is causing a mobile condition of *the very same muscles* ? Putting the question more concretely—How is it that destruction of one part of the centre causes permanent paralysis of the face, arm, and leg, whilst instability of another part of that [1] centre causes occasional convulsion of the paralysed face, arm, and leg ? The reply is—(1st) That the corpus striatum does not, as the question assumes, represent the *muscles* of the face, arm, and leg, but *movements* of these parts in which movements the muscles serve in all degrees and combinations ; speaking metaphorically, it represents, not notes, but chords. (2nd) That *each* part of the corpus striatum contains nervous processes for movements of the *whole* of the face, arm, and leg. This second remark needs amplification and illustration.

Suppose the corpus striatum be divided into three parts from front to back, A, B, C. Symbolising the parts of the external region as $x$, $y$, and $z$, we say that A represents [2] them as $x^3, y^2, z$, B as $x^2, y^3, z$, C as $x, y^2, z^3$. Each third represents the whole region, but represents it differently. So, then, if A be destroyed, the face, arm, and leg are weakened ; if B be destroyed, the face, arm, and leg are weakened ; if C be destroyed, the face, arm, and leg are weakened.[3] From destruction of a third there is only weakening, because the remaining two-thirds represent the same muscles, although they represent different movements of them.[4]

[1] I believe the correct statement is that the convulsion results from discharge of convolutions near to the corpus striatum, the current developed *passing through* the corpus striatum. But for purposes of illustration the statement in the text suffices.

[2] Of course the representation is infinitely more complex ; and of course I am not bound by the mere words of an illustration chosen for its simplicity, as, for example, when I speak of destruction of one-third of the corpus striatum causing only weakness of the external parts.

[3] If a very small part were destroyed, there would be no permanent palsy, because the undamaged remainder of the centre would suffice for the movements which should be represented by the part destroyed. Hence the use of the word " compensation." The compensation is never absolute.

[4] Here, again, the illustration is not to be taken literally ; it is only an illustration. There are, no doubt, all shades of highly compound movements represented in the corpus striatum and thalamus opticus, from such as those in which the arm is much used and the leg scarcely at all, to movements in which the leg is very much used and the arm scarcely at all.

There is not absolute paralysis of part of the external region from lesion of any one of the three; for example, not paralysis of the face only when A is destroyed, nor of the arm only when B is destroyed, nor of the leg only when C is destroyed. From partial destruction of the centre there is not "paralysis of parts" of the region, but "partial paralysis" throughout the region. We infer, then, that each of the three divisions A, B, C contains movements for the whole region. Or leaving this clumsy and yet convenient illustration, we may say that the corpus striatum is a mass of nerve units, a mass of little corpora striata, each one of which represents movements of the whole region, the face, arm, and leg. We thus understand that loss of function of a certain number of these units may be causing partial palsy of the face, arm, and leg, whilst occasional discharge of other unstable units may cause abnormal movements of the very same external parts.

As I have stated in Chap. II, on Definition (p. 177), the discharging lesion in every epilepsy is supposed to be a *permanent* lesion; there is grey matter, which, since it is permanently under conditions of abnormal nutrition, is permanently abnormal in function. This permanent abnormality is, however, varying; the grey matter *occasionally* reaches high tension, and therefore *occasionally* discharges (or is discharged). There are waves of stability and instability in the "discharging lesion."[1]

It is not difficult to understand that from a *permanent* abnormality of nutrition of a part there can result *occasional* disorderly exhibition of function of that part. The process in epilepsies roughly corresponds to what is supposed to occur normally in the ganglia of the heart. There is here, it seems to me, only a particular application of a certain physiological principle long since put forward by Paget. Thus, I quote from Baker's edition (seventh) of Dr. Kirkes' *Physiology* (p. 141): "Why these nervous centres [nervous ganglia of the heart] should issue impulses for rhythmic rather than for continuous action, is still a debatable point. The most philosophical interpretation yet given of it, and of rhythmic processes in general, is that by Mr. Paget, who regards them as dependent on rhythmic nutrition—*i.e.* on a method of nutrition in which the acting parts are *gradually raised* with time-regulated progress to a certain state of *instability of composition*, which then issues in the discharge of their functions,

[1] It follows from this that the first fit is supposed to be a discharge of a part which has for some time before been in a state of malnutrition; and a still further inference is, that such "causes" of epilepsies as fright are only determining causes of the *first* explosion. Many of the "premonitory symptoms" of a first attack are probably results of slight discharges. They are miniature fits. I think, too, that very slight discharges are causes of irritability and distress to epileptics. Their general nervous tension is high. I once congratulated a mother on the fact that her son had not had a severe fit. She, however, regretted it, saying that the severe fit "cleared his system," while the slight fits rendered him, from their frequency, unable to go to business. Medically speaking, I think it better that a patient should have many slight fits than that he should have one violent seizure. Indeed, were it possible to frequently discharge the area of unstable grey matter, it would, I think, be good practice to do so. The object would be to discharge it when its tension was small and its potential energy little. When tension is high and the potential energy great, discharge of the morbid part leads, I think, to discharges of lower and healthy centres, and thus to stoppage of respiration and other disastrous effects; slight discharges would not, I think, discharge, or would not discharge many, healthy centres. The statement that cases of epilepsy in which mental infirmity follows are the very cases in which there are slight fits is not an argument against such a procedure. For really the fact is that mental infirmity follows in cases where the discharge begins in the highest nervous processes—that is to say, the true relation is with the important seat of the discharge, not so much with the slightness of the discharge and consequent slightness of the fits. In those epilepsies where the discharge begins in the very highest nervous processes mental infirmity follows, *because* they are the highest.

*e.g.* of nerve force in the case of the cardiac ganglia, by which force the muscular walls are excited to contraction. . . . *All organic processes* seem to be regulated with exact observance of time ; and *rhythmic nutrition and action*, as exhibited in the action of the heart, are but well-marked examples of such chronometric arrangements." (No italics in original.)

Schrœder van der Kolk writes, as his fourth conclusion on epilepsy, that " the special seat and starting-point of these convulsive movements is situated in the ganglionic cells of the medulla oblongata, which, as reflex ganglia, possess the peculiar property that, when once brought into an excited condition, they may more or less suddenly discharge themselves and communicate their influence to different nervous filaments. After their discharge a certain time is required to bring them to their former degree of excitability, and to render them capable of fresh discharges, just as we see to be the case with electric batteries, or in the phenomena of an electrical fish." [1]

I use the word " instability " for the condition of the grey matter in the discharging lesion " ; it includes two things —(1) high tension (much potential energy), and (2) unstable equilibrium (readiness for discharge, conversion of potential to actual energy). The higher the tension the more unstable the equilibrium. " Speaking generally," says Spencer (*First Principles*, p. 293), " stable compounds contain comparatively little molecular motion, and in proportion as the contained molecular motion is great the instability is great."

It may, however, be asked—How is it that with a permanent local lesion of the brain there are not permanent local symptoms—symptoms in the intervals of the discharge ? If a discharge of a particular part of the brain produces severe movement—say of the arm—how is it that the patient can move his arm well in the intervals of the paroxysm ? For a part of the brain representing movements of that limb continues " diseased " [2] at all times, and when the patient is at his best.

For this amounts to saying that the patient can move his arm apparently well when a part of the brain which represents movements of that arm is " diseased." This is indeed the case. We have so far used the general term " diseased," but we will use a more precise expression.

A part of the brain may be altogether *destroyed* without causing any obvious symptoms ; but discharge of that part would cause severe symptoms. Supposing the part of the brain to represent movements of the arm, that part may be lost without causing loss of movement of the limb (palsy) ; but a strong discharge of it would cause violent movement of the limb (spasm).

The reason why the patient does not suffer paralysis from lack of the part destroyed is that the movements it should represent are also represented in neighbouring parts. Let us consider this point.

We supposed (see p. 212) the corpus striatum to be divided into three parts, each third representing muscles of the face, arm, and leg. Each third, however, represents all these muscles, but each represents them in a different

[1] *Sydenham Soc. Trans.*, p. 283.

[2] I have several times spoken of paralysis of a part after a convulsion in which that part had been first and most involved. I am, however, correct when using in the text for some cases the expression " use his arm well in the intervals," because in many cases there is no obvious palsy after the seizure, and when there is it is transitory. Besides, I think when there is palsy that palsy is not due to morbid condition of the area of grey matter, which is unstable. It is owing to exhaustion of nerve fibre of some subordinate centre, consequent on discharge of that unstable grey matter.

combination; we symbolised the several representations[1] as $x^3, y^2, z$; $x^2, y^2, z$; $x, y^2, z^3$. The convolutions near to this centre are evolved out of it—that is, they re-represent in more numerous and more intimate combinations the muscles which are already represented more simply in the corpus striatum. So we may suppose that the muscles of the face, arm, and leg, which are all represented in each of three places in the corpus striatum, are all represented in each of nine places in the next range of evolution—that is, in the convolutions. Thus limited destruction in this higher range will have less effect than an equal quantity of destruction of the corpus striatum. Suppose that a patient should lose from a certain sized lesion of the lower centre (corpus striatum) one-third of the power he should have over the muscles of the face, arm, and leg, he would on the principle of evolution lose only one-ninth of his power over these muscles if a lesion of the same size occurred in our next stage of evolution—that is, in convolutions evolved out of the corpus striatum.

We have here another illustration of the principle of Compensation. But next comes the question. Admitting that the patient could do *without* part of a motor nervous centre, how is it that from *discharge of* such part, when it is not destroyed, but unstable, he suffers not only spasm, but *very severe* spasm? If loss of the part causes practically no loss of function at all, why should discharge of the part lead not only to function, but to exceedingly great function?

The paradox is explained by the principle of Evolution, many times adverted to in these chapters. Let me make a general statement.[2]

The process of evolution results in such a kind of representation of muscles that the higher the centre the less effect does a given quantity of destruction of part of it produce, and the *more* effect does discharge of an equal quantity of it produce. The reason is that the process of evolution is such a one that it results in a multiplication both of fibres and of ganglion cells from the lower to the higher centre. Of course the more fibres in a centre there are representing an external region, the less paralysis must result from destruction of a part of that centre; and equally obvious is it that the more ganglion cells there are, the greater external effect (convulsion) must be produced by discharge of a part of that centre. Briefly, the higher the centre the more tolerable is a given quantity of destruction, and the more intolerable a given quantity of instability. The most striking case is that if a part of the *very highest* centres be removed, there may be no obvious symptom; whereas discharge beginning in them will put instantly in action all the muscles of the body.

" The conclusion I have arrived at from the study of cases of disease is, that the higher centres are evolved *out of* the lower. The higher centre re-represents more specially the impressions and movements already represented generally in the one below it. The co-ordinations are continually being reco-ordinated; for example, those of the pons and medulla are reco-ordinated in the cerebrum. There are in the lower centres sensori-motor processes for very *general* purposes, but in *their* higher representatives for the more special. A rude symbolisation would be to suppose the pons Varolii to represent the simpler sensori-motor processes of the cord raised to the ' fifth

[1] The reader must never forget that the " organ of mind," like lower centres, is supposed to represent impressions and movements.

[2] In an Appendix to this chapter I give quotations from former papers, which show that I have long held the views here stated as to compensation in nervous organs. I am anxious to show that they are not opinions hastily formed.

power,' and the cerebral hemispheres these processes suddenly raised again, let us say, to the 'fiftieth power.'"

The following quotations from Spencer's *Psychology*, vol. i, bear closely on the increase of "explosive" material during increasing complexity of nervous centres (no italics in original):

"Meanwhile these centres in which molecular motion is liberated are also the centres in which it is co-ordinated; and the successively higher and larger centres which evolve successively larger quantities of molecular motion, are also centres in which successively more complex co-ordinations are effected, *whence follows the general result that along with each further development of the nervous system, enabling it to make all parts of the body work together more efficiently in simultaneous and successive actions, there goes an increased power of evolving the energy required for such larger aggregates of actions*" (op cit., p. 67).

"Each vesicle, or each portion of grey matter that establishes a continuity between the central termini of fibres, is not *merely a connecting* link; it is *also* a *reservoir* of molecular motion, which it gives out when disturbed. Hence, if the composition of nerve is determined as above indicated, it follows that in *proportion to the number, extensiveness, and complexity of the relations*, simultaneous and successive, that are formed among different parts of the organism, will be the *quantity* of molecular motion which the nerve centres are capable of disengaging.

". . . the *quantity* of molecular motion evolved in the nervous centres will become great in proportion as the nervous relations increase in *integration and heterogeneity*" (*Spencer*, op. cit., p. 35).

I think the statement in the following quotation, although to the same effect as the two above, is better suited for my purpose:

". . . this establishment of more numerous, more involved, and more varied relations among the parts of the organism, implies not simply this grouping of fibres and this arrangement of centres, but also a multiplication of the nerve corpuscles, or portions of grey matter, occupying their centres. And we found it to follow that where the compound relations formed are among many points, or where the points are to be combined in many orders, or both, great accumulations of grey matter are needed: an important corollary being that the quantity of this matter capable of giving out much motion increases in proportion as the combinations to be formed become large and heterogeneous" (*Spencer*, op. cit., p. 45).

Hence, in the convolutions there is not only great complexity of representation of movements and impressions, but, *as a consequence of this*, there is a large quantity of explosive material.

Let us consider the process with some artificial illustrations. Suppose that a nervous centre, which we will name the first centre, represents three [1] different movements of the muscles of the same external part. The next higher centre which is evolved out of the first—we call it the second centre—

[1] Of course the numbers given here are quite arbitrary. Moreover, the illustration is inadequate in other ways. It is only to be taken as an illustration for a limited purpose. The higher centre is not simply an evolution out of *one* lower, but sometimes out of several lower. The highest nervous processes (the anatomical substrata of consciousness) are evolved out of *all* lower centres. Thus the highest nervous processes represent innumerable and widely separated movements; hence the discharge of them produces universal symptoms nearly *simultaneously*. Moreover, the highest nervous processes represent movements with innumer-

will, we suppose, represent nine different movements of the external part; the third centre will represent eighty-one different movements, and so on. The higher centre re-represents more elaborately what the lower centre has represented. At length each part of the highest centres of all will fully represent innumerable different movements of just the same muscles represented by very simple movements in the lowest centre. Now, of course, however little the difference may at length become in the movements as they are greatly multiplied, the nervous process for each one of them requires new fibres and requires separate ganglion cells. We have both more conductors and more generators of nerve force. Differentiation of Function implies Differentiation of Structure. Hence, as stated, the higher the centre is in evolution, in other words, the greater the number of different movements the centre represents, the greater the multiplication of both cells and fibres.

Putting this in another way, we say that the number of cells and fibres in a centre does not vary simply with the size and power of the muscles themselves, but also with the number of different movements of the muscles.

Spencer has pointed out that the size of an animal's nervous system varies not only with the size of the animal, but with the complexity of its movements. He writes:

" But after all modifying causes have been allowed for, there remain substantially intact the fundamental relations set forth—namely, that wherever much motion is evolved, a relatively large nervous system exists; that wherever the motion evolved, though not great in quantity, *is heterogeneous in kind*, a relatively large nervous system exists, and that wherever the evolved motion is both great in quantity and heterogeneous in kind, the largest nervous systems exist " (Herbert Spencer, *Principles of Psychology*, p. 13).

## VI

### The Pathology of Epilepsies

The expression Pathology of Nervous Diseases is used for the abnormal processes of nutrition which lead to either of the two abnormal functional states of nervous tissue spoken of under the head of Physiology. I must speak at length on the relations of physiology and pathology.

It is a matter of exceeding great importance not to confound the physiology with the pathology of epilepsies. It is true that I am not using the words " physiological " and " pathological " in their popular significations, but I must refer to the definitions I have given of them. As before said, I mean by the physiology of a case of nervous disease the departure from the healthy *function* of nerve tissue. That function is to store up and to expend force. There are two modifications of the function—one is loss of function. In cases of epilepsy (as also in chorea, tetanus, etc.) there is the opposite condition of over-function. There is an exaggeration of the function of nerve tissue, especially of that of the nerve cell. The nerve cell in health stores up force and discharges on moderate

able intervals; hence discharge of them produces the universal symptoms nearly *contemporaneously*. It may be said that " simultaneous " and " contemporaneous " mean the same thing. It is convenient to use the two terms, because the highest centres are evolved out of lower centres which represent movements which are not simultaneous, and which occur at different times. The process by which it finally results that the highest nervous processes represent (1) the whole organism and represent its parts (2) simultaneously and (3) contemporaneously is a gradual one.

provocation, but in epilepsy and in the other neuroses mentioned the cells (that is, the cells in some part) store up large quantities and discharge abundantly on very slight provocation : there is what I call increased instability, or shortly, instability, or what is otherwise spoken of as increased excitability. This is the physiology, abnormal physiology of course. In the last chapter we were concerned with this class of functional changes, *however produced* ; in this chapter we are concerned with their mode of production. This is a purely pathological question ; it is a problem in disordered nutrition.

In health nerve tissue is nourished—stores up force—and when unstable it is over-nourished. It plainly must be over-nourished, or it could not over-expend. The area of grey matter unstable in every epilepsy is limited. There is a local " discharging lesion " of some part of the cerebral hemisphere. So we say there is local over-nutrition of grey matter. The question in pathology of a case of epilepsy can now be put more definitely. From what pathological process does the *local* instability result ? Or, in other words, how is the local increase of nutrition caused ? This, be it observed, is equally a question for those who consider it proved that epilepsy depends on instability (increased excitability) of the medulla oblongata. Difference of opinion as to the *seat* of the nerve tissue unstable makes no difference in the most general question above put. Supposing for a moment that we were convinced that the medulla oblongata *is* the part which discharges in epilepsy, this is physiological, not pathological knowledge. We still have to seek the pathological processes by which nerve tissue in the medulla oblongata *becomes* so unstable that there is every now and then, during a period of months and years, an occasional violent discharge. The " causes of epilepsy " are wide of the mark if they do not bear on this question. Facts as to most so-called " causes " of epilepsy are simply materials towards obtaining a knowledge of causation. Often they are merely " exciting causes," or causes determining the first discharge of areas of grey matter, which, before that first discharge, had been slowly getting into a state of instability, that is, into a readiness for discharge on any kind of provocation. In this chapter, however, it is a matter of secondary moment, that is, so far as broad principles are concerned, *where* the unstable grey matter may be. For we are not now concerned with some clinical entity and with the causes of that entity. We rigidly narrow the inquiry to this point, by what pathological processes does grey matter anywhere become unstable ? It does not matter for this inquiry whether the discharge of the part which has become unstable causes sudden and transitory loss of consciousness or causes sudden and transitory spasm of the great toe. And although we speak of instability in epilepsy, the principles will apply to instability in chorea, tetanus, etc.

The confusion of the two things physiology and pathology under one (pathology) leads to confusion in considering " causes." Thus, for example, we hear it epigrammatically said that chorea is " only a symptom," and may depend on many causes. This is possibly true of pathological causation ; in other words, it may be granted that various abnormal nutritive processes *may lead* to that functional change in grey matter which, when established, admits occasional excessive discharge. But physiologically, that is to say, from the point of view of Function, there is but one cause of chorea—*viz.* instability of nerve tissue. Similarly of any epilepsy, there is but one " cause " physiologically speaking—*viz.* instability of grey matter, but an unknown number of causes if we mean pathological processes leading to that instability.[1]

I confess I find it difficult to make the distinction betwixt the physiology and the pathology of cases of nervous disease clear to many people, and especially with regard to epilepsies and other mobile nervous disorders. A visible, especially a coarse, alteration in the nervous system, is sometimes spoken of as a " cause " of convulsion. The rudest part of a pathological process, for example, a tumour, which only *leads* to instability (physiological abnormality), is spoken of as " the disease " without any qualification. And it seems to many easy to " understand " that a tumour in the left side of the brain can " cause " convulsion of the opposite side of the body, but when nothing is *discovered* post-mortem they are not convinced that any local disease exists. This is not always owing to carefulness from *scientific* scepticism, for the strangest " causes " of such seizures are easily admitted, such as fright, dyspepsia, anxiety, and the like.

A little thought would show two things—first, that local symptoms of necessity imply local disease ; and second, that the state of nervous organs or tissues on which a discharge directly depends (the " discharging lesion") is not likely to be easily discovered ; for the discharge in convulsion is only an excessive exaggeration of the normal function of the cells and fibres. What we should have to discover is the difference betwixt cells which discharge excessively and those which discharge normally—not a likely thing to be easily discovered. In some cases of epilepsy we sometimes do not trace even roughly the pathology of the discharging lesion ; we may discover no alteration post-mortem of any sort. When we do see a coarse change (tumour, let us suppose) we do not trace the steps by which that coarse change led to the instability of cells of grey matter which the convulsion obliges us to infer to exist. The tumour is not the discharging lesion ; it is a " foreign body " which leads to these changes in grey matter which constitute the discharging lesion.

Let me observe again, that as regards demonstration of local changes in any epilepsy, those who hold the accepted views are in no better case ; for I am

[1] I will here remark on the difference of the two things by quoting from an article on Hemichorea which I published in the *Edinburgh Medical Journal*, October 1868 :

" ' Just as loss of function—for instance, palsy—follows destruction of nerve tissue, *however produced*—by clot, by tumour, by injury, etc.—so *disorder* of function—(discharge) for instance, chorea or spasm—results from instability of nerve tissue, *however produced*—by mechanically produced anæmia [hyperæmia, I now think], and, as I think, by embolism.'

One reason for quoting *that* article is to correct a misapprehension under which most of those labour who have criticised my opinions on the pathology of chorea. The remarks quoted in the text, taken with the statement of the second division of my hypothesis on an earlier page of the article quoted from—' That this local instability is *frequently* brought about,' etc.—show that I have not undertaken to defend the doctrine that embolism is the *sole* cause of chorea (cause of the instability of nerve tissue in chorea). The fault, however, is my own ; I freely admit this. By a clerical error which I ought to have corrected, I am made, in the ' Mirror ' of the *Lancet*, November 26, 1864, p. 606, to say ' limited *to* softening ' of the brain, instead of ' limited softening ' of the brain. I have, however, corrected it by implication. In a report of the Obstetrical Society (*Medical Times and Gazette*, August 1, 1868) I say : " This instability, although *frequently* the result of anæmia [hyperæmia, I now think] from blocking, *might doubtless be induced in other ways*, as in the choreiform movements which sometimes occur during recovery from epileptic hemiplegia, the secondary results of coarse disease of a cerebral hemisphere.' In the *London Hospital Reports*, vol. i, 1864, p. 459, I write : ' I think, from many circumstances, that embolism is a *frequent* cause of chorea.' I believe, however, that embolism (or blocking of arteries by some process) is *almost* the sole cause of chorea. Nay, speaking in the very strictest sense, I do not believe that two *different* pathological processes would damage an organ in absolutely the same way ; from two pathological processes leading to instability of convolutions near to the corpus striatum, I should expect slight, even if insignificant differences.

now speaking of cases in which no lesion is found in any part of the encephalon, as is commonly the case in the epilepsy of authorities. Who has, in any case of "idiopathic epilepsy," traced the pathological process by which the medulla oblongata becomes so unstable that it, or some part of it, occasionally discharges ?

A moment's thought will show that when there are visible changes (in the case of tumour for example) we do not really discover the *discharging* lesion ; the discharge is not of the tumour, it is of the grey matter irritated by the tumour. Let me quote authorities on this point :

"The structural diseases which are found in association with convulsions are not the immediate, but the remote causes of the latter. 'They act by inducing those interstitial changes which are the proximate cause' (*Liverpool Medico-Chir. Journal*, January 1, 1858, p. 9), and it is because this relation has been misunderstood that so much confusion has existed in cerebral pathology" (Reynolds on Epilepsy).

The following extract is from the general summary of Kussmaul and Tenner on *Epileptiform Convulsions from Hæmorrhage*, p. 107 :

"Circumscribed anatomical alterations of the brain or alterations of protracted duration cannot be regarded as the proximate cause of epileptic attacks, but may cause epileptic *affections* (dispose to epilepsy).

"Pathological anatomy cannot give any explanation as to the nature of epilepsy."

The following is from p. 87 of the same work :

"All these different facts furnish sufficient grounds for asserting that it is only microscopic alterations of the brain that can be the cause of epileptic affections. Tubercle of the brain, cicatrix of the brain, of the spinal cord, or of a cutaneous nerve, are therefore in an exactly similar way to be regarded only *as remote causes* of epilepsy, and should visible alterations occur in the brain or other parts of the body during eclampsia and epilepsy, they must be regarded as nothing else than *predisposing* influences."

Here is a further quotation to the same effect. The authors speak, I suppose, of naked-eye appearance :

"Thirdly, *it can be no visible alteration of the brain, anatomically demonstrable, that can act as the proximate cause of an epileptic attack*" (p. 86).

The question in pathology in a case of convulsions with tumour of the brain is, How did the irritation of a tumour lead to the "discharging lesion" which, whether we discover it post-mortem or not, the localised convulsion declares to have existed during life ?

No doubt the primary pathological changes which lead to the one physiological condition of instability of the grey matter are numerous. Tumour and other coarse disease is but one cause of instability. It is scarcely likely that we should easily discover abnormality in the cells of the grey matter which discharge, and that excessively—which function strongly, too strongly. In the other classes of functional lesion (destroying lesion) we often do discover a change, or rather we find absence (destruction) of nerve tissue. Let me therefore illustrate the distinction I make by the simple case of a pathological process producing the physiological abnormality *loss* of function, taking cases in which function is lost by a very gross lesion. We shall take a motor symptom for simplicity of illustration ; we are indeed repeating part of an old illustration.

Just as convulsion points *only* to the abnormal physiological state of instability, so paralysis points only to the abnormal physiological state of loss of function. It points to no pathological process in particular. Thus there is hemiplegia of exactly the same kind from clot, softening, or a tumour affecting the corpus striatum. Hence the hemiplegia is not a symptom of cerebral hæmorrhage or of softening ; it is a symptom resulting from loss of function (destruction) of the corpus striatum by these or any other pathological processes. It is a symptom of the abnormal physiological condition of loss of function of the corpus striatum.[1] I have here illustrated by gross changes, which destroy the corpus striatum physically ; but when speaking of the " after-effects " of strong epileptic discharges I have suggested that the corpus striatum is left temporarily *hors de combat* after strong nervous discharges. If this hypothesis be correct, we see that a similar physiological or functional state (loss of function) is produced by pathological processes so different as clot,[2] softening, tumour, and epileptic discharge. A simple illustration was taken purposely. What follows is another illustration to the same effect ; it is not so simple, but is of direct importance for our subject. There is a confusion of physiology and pathology in discussions on the nature of the symptom loss of consciousness. To lose consciousness is to lose the use of the highest of all sensori-motor arrangements, or to lose the use of any large part of either cerebral hemisphere (the highest processes being *evolved out* of those next lower, and so on to the lowest). I have used the general expression " loss of use " because the nervous processes underlying consciousness may be put out of use or may lose their function by very different *pathological* processes. We have already pointed out that consciousness is lost *during* excessive discharge of the highest processes, and also that it remains lost *after* an excessive discharge (the highest processes being exhausted by that discharge). It is extremely important, with regard to loss of consciousness, that the physiological condition be not confounded with the pathological process. Just as hemiplegia may be caused by anything which puts a subordinate series of sensori-motor processes, those in the corpus striatum, *hors de combat* (clot, softening, tumour, strong epileptic discharge), so loss of consciousness may be caused by anything which puts the highest nervous processes *hors de combat* (clot, softening, severe squeezing by tumour, and epileptic discharge). Whether, in a case of cerebral hæmorrhage, the loss of consciousness be due to shock, to squeezing, or to arterial anæmia, is a question in pathology. The physiology of loss of consciousness is clear. It is loss of *use of* the highest of all nervous processes—those evolved out of all lower nervous centres.

Once more let me remark that I do not use the word " consciousness " as the name for some entity that must be either lost or not lost. I mention this because the expressions one must use may seem to have that implication. There

[1] Mr. Square, of Plymouth, has mentioned to me a case in which hemiplegia and aphasia followed accidental injury to the brain by the tooth of a rake. It is from a scientific point of view as absurd to say that hemiplegia is " a symptom of cerebral hæmorrhage " as it would be to say that the hemiplegia and aphasia of Mr. Square's patient were " symptoms of rake-tooth." The clot does just what the rake-tooth did, and is equally extra-nervous.

[2] It will be pointed out, however, that there is a difference in the gravity of the symptoms produced by action of the various pathological processes depending on difference in the suddenness with which they destroy. This principle is especially important with regard to loss of consciousness. Moreover, different pathological processes are associated with particular symptoms. For example, embolism, when it leads to *defect* of speech, very often produces that particular defect which is in psychological language called loss of " memory for words." Then clot, when it produces only *defect* of speech, produces that particular defect which is called ataxy of articulation. The reason is that these two different pathological processes do not affect the very same parts of the region of the corpus striatum.

may be slight affections of consciousness, a slight confusion of thought, and from this there are all degrees down to deepest coma.

We may certainly affirm two things of the nerve tissue which is the seat of discharge in the epileptic paroxysm : (1) It is a minute change. Good evidence of this is found in the fact that the condition has not been discovered. It has not been discovered in the medulla oblongata by those who consider the changes of epilepsy to be seated there. We have already seen that the discovery of gross alterations is not the discovery of the very changes on which the discharge depends, is not the discovery of the alteration in grey matter which renders it unstable. It is not an alteration likely to be easily discovered.[1] " Experience teaches us," Niemeyer says, " that the lesions from which abnormally active impulses proceed are insusceptible of anatomical demonstration."

Another affirmation is that, (2) as previously remarked, the nutrition of grey matter which over-expends will be increased, for so far as there is over-function, so far must there be over-nutrition. " The proximate cause of convulsion is an abnormal increase in the nutritive changes of the nervous centres " (Reynolds on Epilepsy).

Here, when speaking of abnormal nutrition, we may conveniently state further facts which support the views (see p. 211) as to the difference of function, or degrees of difference of function, betwixt nerve fibres and cells. We speak for the moment of conditions of healthy nutrition. Grey matter is the nervous element which is most vascular ; white matter is comparatively little vascular : and it is to be observed that there is not only the difference that white matter has comparatively few vessels, and grey matter many, but that the cells of the grey matter lie close to their capillaries, whereas the axis cylinder of the fibre is separated by the white substance. The inference is that the grey matter not only gets more blood, but that it is more immediately dependent upon nutritive supply. The bearing of this on our immediate subject is, that when both the cell and the fibre are subjected to the same conditions of altered vascularity, the cell will be more affected than the fibre. That this is so, is shown, too, by the greater prevalence of convulsive diseases in young children ; greater instability of nerve tissue is here seen to go with more abundant supply of blood. There is an exception proving this rule. Dr. Eustace Smith points out that convulsions do not so often occur in feeble as in robust children. The dependence of the nerve cells on a continuous supply of blood is shown by the facts of certain recent experiments (Hitzig and Ferrier). It used to be said that the brain was not excitable ; the fact is that some parts of it are, but that they may soon lose excitability. The highest centres are furthest from the heart, and will soonest lose their blood supply. Again, the dependence of the brain on blood is seen in another way ; in the case of an animal bleeding very rapidly to death, convulsions ensue. Eustace Smith's observation is in harmony with Kusmaull and Tenner's observation that bleeding feeble animals to death does not produce convulsions.

It is no contradiction to the statement that the nerve cells require much blood —that *suddenly* produced anæmia by *rapidly* bleeding an animal to death produces convulsions ; this is simply the cause of the *paroxysm*, the cause of

[1] Healthy nervous discharges occurring when we are acting or thinking may be likened to playing the chords of an overture with proper emphasis and at the right intervals over a considerable period of time ; the epileptic discharge is analogous to playing all the notes of several pages of that overture in a few seconds.

the excessive discharge of nerve cells. For *slow* bleeding to death does not cause convulsions. It is not from want of blood, but from *sudden change* in the conditions of the grey matter, that the discharge results. It is quite evident that all that is required to upset the equilibrium of a nerve, and inferentially of a nerve cell, is a sudden shock of almost any kind.[1]

The question now is—How is the nutrition of the nerve cell so altered that there results a mere exaltation of its normal function ?

I confess that in most cases we cannot tell how this increased nutrition is brought about. We are certain that it exists. But I would repeat that this is a difficulty to all of us. Whether we take the accepted view, or any novel view, we can rarely answer the question—" *By what pathological process did nerve tissue become unstable in this case ?* " We do not take refuge in an obscure use of the word " cause." Vividly realising such sequences as fright and convulsion, we do not, nevertheless, consider that there is an explanation of the central question in such sequence. We do not make the audacious statement—" Fright is one cause of epilepsy." And if, for the sake of argument, we admitted it to be true, the question would still come—" How did fright lead to instability of nerve cells ? " It is repeated that such so-called causes of epilepsy are wide of the mark if they do not bear on the question just put.

We have, however, to seek answers to three questions—(1) What is the *general* nature of the altered nutrition of the nerve cell ? (2) In what tissues which make up a nervous organ does the pathological process begin which leads to this over-nutrition ; does it begin in the nerve tissue or in some subordinate tissue ? (3) How do the changes beginning in tissues of nervous organs lead to the increased nutrition of the nerve cells ?

(1) *What is the general nature of the altered nutrition ?* —At one time, following Radcliffe, Handfield Jones, and Anstie, I considered that the nutrition of nerve tissue was *imperfect* in unstable nerve tissue. In a certain sense I think so still. There are, I submit, two ways in which nutrition may be imperfect—in quantity and in quality. I believe that nerve tissue in " discharging lesions " is over-nourished in the former sense, and worse nourished in the latter. Recently, indeed, I have been led to think that the view I now hold is, in some respects, simply a modification of the one the above-named physicians have long taught. I say this, however, to acknowledge an obligation. The reader will, of course, judge of the views of these physicians from what they have written themselves, and hold me responsible for what I now write.

In order to make my meaning clearer, I will take chemical illustrations and use chemical nomenclature. Two bodies may be of the same constitution, but yet of very different composition ; for example, the constitution of acetic acid and of the chloracetic acids is the same, but they differ in composition,

[1] It is well put by Dr. Gamgee in an interesting popular lecture :

" If we isolate a nerve going to a muscle and subject it to a succession of little blows, each blow will originate changes in the nerve, which, being propagated to the muscle, induce contraction. If the blows follow one another with only a moderate rapidity, the muscle shortens, and immediately thereafter becomes elongated ; whilst if the blows follow one another with great rapidity, say forty or fifty times in a second, the muscle is shortened and remains shortened during the whole time that the nerve is excited by the blows. Instead of exciting the nerve by blows, we might employ electricity. If, for example, we pass a single induction shock through a nerve, we shall produce a single muscular contraction ; if we pass a series of rapidly succeeding shocks, we observe the persistent form of contraction, such as is produced by a succession of blows. By bringing heated bodies near a nerve, or some chemical compounds, as solution of common salt, in contact with a nerve, we can similarly induce contraction in the muscle or muscles to which it is distributed."

as in the latter hydrogen has been replaced by chlorine. The "structure," however, is unaltered. By certain substitutions some compounds are rendered explosive (gun-cotton), and some drugs have their therapeutical power altered by substitition (strychnia and methyl-strychnia).

I believe, then, that the highly unstable grey matter of disease (in a "discharging lesion") differs in composition, but not in constitution, from the comparatively stable grey matter of health. The alteration in composition is, of course, such that the nervous substance formed is more explosive.

We must suppose that there is some order in this substitution-nutrition; it plainly is in the direction of explosiveness or instability. The following is a speculation as to the kind of alteration of composition:

One important component of nervous matter is phosphorus. This substance belongs to the chemical class of triads of which other members are nitrogen and arsenic. My speculation is that in the abnormal nutritive process producing unstable nervous matter the phosphorus ingredient is replaced wholly or partly by its chemical congener—nitrogen. There is a "substitution compound." The replacement probably occurs in different degrees, as it does in the three differing chloracetic acids. If nitrogen be substituted, as supposed, we can easily understand that the substance produced would be more explosive. For nitrogen enters into nearly all unstable compounds. The supposed value of arsenic [1] in certain nervous affections is in this view significant; it is another member of the group of triads.

The nutrition is therefore supposed to be defective not in quantity, but in quality in those functional alterations of grey matter which I call "discharging lesions." It is hasty nutrition. There is more force and less stability. The following quotation from Beale's third Lumleian Lecture is important as regards the general truth in this special case:

"As it were between the two extremes, are forms of bioplasm that grow and deteriorate, but still live for years under adverse circumstances, the structures formed never attaining a state of vigour, but still being formed and acting in an imperfect way, and perhaps for a long period of time. The weak, succulent, too quickly developed vegetation of our fern cases is an example; and the soft rickety tissues of some of our weak, flabby, over-fed, town-bred, highly precocious children supply a very painful instance of too quick formation and growth. In such cases the bioplasm has grown too fast, and tissue has been formed too quickly. Time has not been allowed for its condensation and strength, and for the acquisition of resisting and lasting properties. But is it not a mistake to point to such cases as examples of diminished *vital action*? (The italics in what follows are mine.) *It seems to me that life has been carried on too fast and not too slowly. Too much pabulum has been taken up—not too little. Too much heat, too much food, favour a quick, rank, succulent, spongy sort*

[1] The following is an old speculation on the action of remedies:

"How substances practically foreign to the organism act in disease is an important problem, and we should investigate their action more generally from the part salts, minerals, etc., play in healthy changes of nutrition, in building structure and developing function. The chlorides, the iodides, and the bromides are very strikingly homologous in their chemical and physical properties, and I cannot but think the efficacy of the two latter is due to their replacing as it were with greater energy, the commoner chloride. The fact that large quantities of the chlorides are present in active changes of tissue—the healthy development of cartilage, or the uproar of those changes which are rapid and extreme enough to be called inflammatory—is a very significant one") From note on "Substitution Nutrition," in a paper on "Defects of Sight in Diseases of the Nervous System," *Ophthalmic Hospital Reports,* 1866, vol. v, part iv, p. 291.

*of development, inducing the formation of soft bones and weak imperfectly acting tissues which are likely soon to deteriorate.*"

I think this speculation that the unstable grey matter is over-azotised has a practical bearing on the dietetic treatment of epileptics. I advise epileptics not to eat much meat (not much nitrogenised food). I was, however, led to advise my epileptic patients not to eat much meat, not by the speculation just mentioned, but by the following remarks of Dr. Haughton :

" The hunted deer will outrun the leopard in a fair and open chase, because the force supplied to its muscles by the *vegetable* food is capable of being given out *continuously for a long period of time* ; but in a sudden rush at a near distance the leopard will infallibly overtake the deer, because its *flesh* food stores up in the blood a reserve of force capable of being given out *instantaneously* in the form of exceedingly *rapid* muscular actions."[1]

Of course, this quotation bears very generally. It shows, I submit, that highly nitrogenised tissue is less durable and more easily and rapidly decomposable.

As the two following quotations show, there is no novelty on my part in the dietetic advice above given. Speaking of the treatment of epilepsy in children, Dr. West says :

" The diet should be mild, nutritious, but usually unstimulating, and, as a general rule, should include meat comparatively seldom, and in small quantities. I have certainly seen epileptic fits increased in frequency and severity by an abundant meat diet, and diminished in both respects when a diet chiefly of milk and vegetables was adopted " (West, *Diseases of Children*, 6th edition).

Dr. West adds in a footnote (op. cit.) " My attention was first drawn to the importance of abstinence from a meat diet in epileptics by Dr. Maxwell, formerly resident physician to the Asylum for Idiots. This caution, too, gains still greater weight from the testimony of Dr. Jackson, of Boston, in America, who, in his *Letters to a Young Physician*, 12mo, Boston, U.S., 1855, p. 67, insists very strongly on its importance."

Dr. Ireland writes, in a very valuable paper on Idiocy :

" Where improvement follows treatment, I am disposed to attribute it as much to diet as to medicine. Benefit is sometimes derived from excluding flesh meat from the dietary of epileptics, a piece of advice which I got long ago from Trousseau on his visits to the Hôtel-Dieu, and which has been lately repeated by Dr. Hughlings Jackson. It is likely that the gymnastic training given by us is also of advantage in treating epilepsy " (Ireland, *Edinburgh Medical Journal*, January 1874).

I think a great part of the " weakness " and languor of some of those persons who suffer what is popularly called " nervous debility," and who are often hypochondriacal, is explainable on the supposition that their nervous tissue is over-nourished in quantity, and yet so imperfectly nourished in quality that it is explosive ; or, let us use, in this simple and not uncommon condition of ill health, the expression more irritable nervous matter. They often keep up this irritability by frequent eating and drinking. They feel languid and yet excitable, unable to rest, and yet unfit for sustained exertion ; and thus they try to keep themselves up by alcohol and strong food. My colleague, Dr. Andrew Clark, insists that the most successful treatment of such persons is putting them on a very simple unstimulating diet, alcohol in particular being forbidden.

[1] *Address on the Relation of Food to Work*, p. 28. No italics in original.

My speculation is that the good results of this treatment are partly owing to the formation of less explosive or less irritable nervous substance—one of a *more normally stable composition*. The excitability of these patients reminds one of the fact that the nerves of a weak animal are found, experimentally, to conduct with greater velocity than those of a healthy one.

Professor Rutherford (*Lancet*, March 4, 1871) says : " A weak state of the nerve increases the velocity. It is quite easy to perform the experiment which I have shown you if you take well-nourished frogs which have just come from their native resorts ; but when you have to deal with frogs which are weak from insufficient nourishment, you will find how difficult it is to get a result such as that obtained by us to-day. The velocity is so great in this case that it may be scarcely measurable.

. . . . . . .

" Electricity, temperature, deficient nutrition, all affect nerve conductivity in the same way as they affect nerve excitability. Further investigation is needed ere we decide as to whether these properties of a nerve are always similarly affected."

We obtain illustrations of the principle mentioned from the study of the coarser morbid processes of the body. During that uproarious " growth " of parts in inflammation there is a production of numerous cells which decompose early ; they are unstable cells. This is seen also in syphilitic and other growths ; there is a production of many young cells which soon die.[1]

As regards treatment of changes of instability, we are in a different position from that we stand in with regard to changes of loss of function. Nutrition in unstable grey matter is going on indeed too fast, and it may be interfered with for good. To take a particular case :

We can do some good for epilepsy, however long the disease may have lasted ; for the grey matter which discharges is still part of the body, is nourished with it, and takes even too large a share in function (coarse brutish function). We can interfere in changes that *are going on*. The bromide, we must suppose, by some process leads to the formation of nervous matter of more stable composition. Indeed, some believe that in healthy people it leads to anæsthesia. Similarly iodides, I imagine, cure syphilitic ulcers, etc., by ensuring the production of more stable cells than the normal haloids (the chlorides of sodium or potassium) can do.

The above seems to me to harmonise with certain other speculations on the *pathology* of discharging lesions in some cases to be afterwards mentioned—as to their production by hyperæmia consequent on embolism and thrombosis.

[1] Anstie, speaking of the changes produced by such a lesion as that induced in cartilage by drawing a thread through it, writes :

" In the immediate neighbourhood of the damaged part all the cells are enlarged, indicating a distinctly increased nutrition of them. If now we inquire what is the result of a higher degree of irritation, such as that which is present in the case of so-called ' ulceration ' of articular cartilage, we find that a greatly increased *proliferation* of the cells is the characteristic feature of the process in parts which are strongly affected, the formative activity being indicated by the presence of mother-cells, which are crowded with numerous contained cells, probably representing successive generations, or more often with nucleoli. And in the parts which actually border on the focus of irritation, we perceive unmistakable evidence that the exuberant formative process is attended with contemporaneous *degeneration*. The inference would seem plain that the agency which produces all this mischief is a debilitating, devitalising one, and that all this ill-timed and hasty excess of nutrition and formation is but the result of a shock to the vital condition of the part, of which the highest expression is seen in the positive degradation of the new-formed matter, in the most strongly affected localities, from the very moment of its generation " (*Stimulants and Narcotics*, p. 101).

Before passing to the next topic I give the following quotation from Spencer bearing on nitrogenised substances and explosiveness.

Speaking of "the combinations into which nitrogen enters," he says: "These have the two characters of being specially unstable, and of containing specially great quantities of motion. A recently ascertained peculiarity of nitrogen is, that instead of giving out heat when it combines with other elements, it absorbs heat. That is to say, besides carrying with it into the liquid or solid compound it forms, the motion which previously constituted it a gas, it takes up additional motion; and when the other element with which it unites is gaseous, the molecular motion proper to this, also, is locked up in the compound. Now these nitrogen-compounds are unusually prone to decomposition; and the decompositions of many of them take place with extreme violence. All our explosive substances are nitrogenous—the most terribly destructive of them all, chloride of nitrogen, being one which contains the immense quantity of motion proper to its component gases, plus a certain further quantity of motion."

I suppose, too, that the more nitrogenised a body is the more *rapidly* will it decompose or explode. Professor Jellett (Address at Belfast Meeting of the British Association, *Nature* report, August 20, 1874) says, ". . . chemists now speak as familiarly of the *velocity* of chemical reactions as engineers do of the velocity of a cannon ball." Increased velocity of the discharge of the unstable cell is very important as regards abnormal nervous discharges (discharge is the result of chemical decomposition), the *intensity* of the current will be greater, and thus it will be more likely to overcome the resistance of lower centres. (The occurrence of explosion of a nerve cell depends not only on the degree of tension reached, but on the amount of resistance by the parts which have to "carry" the current.) The following quotation illustrates the above remarks:

"Mr. Watts has appropriately likened the manner in which the term 'intensity' is used with regard to electricity, to the way in which the term 'temperature' is applied with respect to heat. Thus, a pint of water at 100° C. produces many effects which a gallon of water at 50° cannot produce; for instance, it will cause alcohol to boil, and fat to melt, although the quantity of heat in the pint, as measured by the quantity of ice which it will melt, is actually less than that contained in the gallon" (Althaus' *Medical Electricity*, 3rd ed., p. 11).

The next question is, "In what tissue of a nervous organ does the pathological process begin which leads to instability of the nerve cells?"

This is the question in each case of epilepsy. If answered in any case we are far from being able to say how the change, when begun and established, leads to instability of the nervous tissue. Thus, in a convulsion "caused by" syphiloma of the brain, we know that the change constituting syphiloma begins in the connective tissue. But how the syphiloma formed by that growth of connective tissue acts on the grey matter about it ("irritates" it) so as to produce changes of instability we know not, any more than we know how any other kind of foreign body acts in their production. Before we speak further we must consider the several materials which make up nervous organs.

We must always, in investigating any class of nervous diseases, bear most vividly in mind that the ingredients of a nervous organ are only in part nervous.

This great truth must not become a truism. Besides nerve fibres and cells, the peculiar and leading constituents, there are arteries, capillaries, veins, and some connective tissue. There are, in short, several tissues, the arteries and veins being reckoned as "compound tissues." The "compound tissues," we may suppose, enter into the composition of organs as simple tissues do, just as we may say, for illustration's sake, the compound element ethyl enters into ethylamine as a single element in replacing an equivalent of hydrogen in ammonia.

Nervous organs, like all other organs, are made up of materials which exist in different combination in other parts of the body. The non-nervous elements are those which are usually attacked first; the nervous elements suffer secondarily. There are, indeed, very few "diseases of the nervous system" if by that expression pathological processes *beginning in nervous tissue* be meant. I must speak at length on this principle, and that, too, with regard to nervous diseases in general.

Pathological processes beginning in non-nervous tissues damage nervous organs. Some tissues in an organ are more liable to *become* diseased than are the other ingredients of the same organ when all are subjected to apparently the same evil influences. This statement is in accordance with what Beale says (*Life, Matter, and Mind*, p. 154): "The connective tissues, fibrous tissues, capillaries, arteries, and veins being involved before the nerve elements are attacked, *and of these the lowest as regards function suffer before those which are concerned in the most exalted nervous actions.*"[1] The distinction is a matter of extreme importance, both as regards diagnosis and treatment. For example, all discoverable syphilitic affections of the nervous system are plainly owing to faults in connective tissue, over-vegetation of it, and the nervous symptoms result because nerve fibres and cells are squeezed, softened, etc.; they suffer secondarily. Then all intra-cranial tumours, excepting perhaps the *true* neuroma of Virchow, are extra-nervous; so are cerebral abscesses, all kinds of meningitis (traumatic and tubercular), hydatid cysts, etc. I may here quote an old statement of this principle from a lecture I delivered at the London Hospital:

"Never forget that every organ is made up of constituents which exist more or less in the greater part of the body. We have in nervous masses, nerve cells and fibres, blood vessels, and also connective tissue. So, too, we find

[1] This is a very striking remark, and the principle involved in it is of great practical importance. I therefore give the following further quotation from Beale's work. (No italics in original.)

"And I may further remark that different forms of germinal matter in all parts of the organism suffer *in inflammation* in different degrees and in different *order*. Generally, those which are of least importance, and which, as regards their *formative* capacity, are lowest in the scale, are the first to suffer. The germinal matter of epithelium and connective tissue are soon affected; that of capillaries, including the white blood corpuscles, follow next in order; then that of fibrous tissue, cartilage, and bone, the germinal matter of muscular-fibre cells of the small arteries and veins; while that belonging to the voluntary muscles, that of the peripheral nerve organs, and the peripheral ramification of the nerve is the last to be involved. In like manner, the germinal matter of the *several* tissues *entering into* the formation of the great central nerve organs is affected *in different order*—the connective tissues, fibrous tissues, capillaries, arteries, and veins being involved before the nerve elements are attacked, *and of these* the *lowest* as regards *function* suffer before those which are concerned in the most *exalted* nerve actions. These last seem to be preserved from damage for a long while, but when at last they become involved death succeeds before time has elapsed for any great degree of morbid change to have taken place; while in other cases the germinal matter with the tissue may have completely degenerated without the death of the individual having been occasioned.

"The living matter concerned in mental operations is that which is last formed, and is probably the highest condition which living matter has yet assumed" (pp. 152–3).

*that diseases of the nervous system are not always diseases of nervous tissue*, but often of other tissues which enter into the composition of nervous organs—of blood vessels, connective tissue, etc.

. . . . . . .

" It may seem contradictory to say that I have no experience of syphilitic diseases of nervous matter, when in the next breath I speak of syphilitic epilepsy and syphilitic paralysis. But you will readily see that it is really important to know whether the epilepsy be due (directly or indirectly) to disease of the connective tissue in or on the nervous masses, or to some change in the nerve fibres or nerve cells themselves. We cannot set to work to treat an *organ* like the corpus striatum, but we may prescribe for a patient who has syphilitic disease of connective tissue, wherever it may be. Now syphilitic ' deposit ' in the pia mater is essentially the same as a node of the tibia, or a cellular node of the skin, or of the spleen or liver, and it requires the same treatment as these. I cannot too much impress on you that we ought above all things, in brain disease, to study diseases of tissues. It is of infinitely more importance than to know the exact organ of the brain damaged ; for instance, to know that there is lymph effused in the pia mater, than that the attendant epilepsy, the disorder of function of part of the brain, has certain physiological peculiarities. Indeed, for my part, I fear we are too late, for cure at least, when the epilepsy is well established. Then, the tissue changes in the pia mater have settled down, the brain is damaged, and its functions will continue to be disordered more or less in spite of what we can do. It is in the stage of inflammation, when, as I have before said, the patient comes with pain on one side of the head, that we may help, not when he is ' well ' of this, and a few months afterwards comes for epileptiform seizures affecting the opposite side of the body. It is when the pia mater is in a condition analogous to acute iritis, and not in one analogous to occluded pupil from bygone inflammation of the iris " (*London Hospital Reports*, vol. i, 1864, p. 153).

Rindfleisch speaks more strongly, as I should do now : " One of the most striking features in the pathological histology of the nervous system is the trifling and always passive share taken by the proper nervous elements in all those changes which affect the brain, spinal cord, or peripheral nerves. As every effort has been made to refer the diseases of the nervous system, and particularly psychical disorders and other essential neuroses, to morbid changes in the ganglion cells and nerve fibres, we may with perfect confidence, supported by the negative result of all such investigations, maintain the thesis, that the causes, perhaps of all (?) diseases of the nervous system, are to be sought in anatomical lesions of the non-nervous elements " (*Morbid Anatomy of the Nervous System*, p. 297).

A more useful illustration of the non-nervous origin of nervous symptoms than that from syphilitic disease of the brain will be that supplied by cases of the most important of all nervous symptoms—hemiplegia. The commonest causes of this paralysis are hæmorrhage and softening from thrombosis. Now plainly, the disease here is not strictly a nervous one. The pathology in such cases is arterial disease ; a diseased artery has broken or has become blocked up. The nervous tissue is not *in fault* ; a nervous organ *suffers* because one of its arteries is faulty. He who limits his attention to the paralysis and to the localisation of the changes producing it—who limits his attention to the nervous system—may be a good anatomist and physiologist ; but he is not a good clinical pathologist. The clinical pathologist examines the heart, the arteries, and the urine, and seeks far and wide for facts in the medical history to ascertain (1) why the patient comes to have *bad arteries*, hypertrophied heart, and renal disease, and then (2) why his arteries rupture or get blocked up. He seeks also, of course, to know why they so often rupture or get blocked in the corpus striatum, etc., in particular.

Obviously, when the hemiplegia is very slight and transitory, the important matter is, not to dwell with exaggeration on the nervous symptoms, but to inquire into the patient's bodily state in order to arrest further degradation of tissues, and to make the patient live a life suitable to his degenerate state.

As a pathological study, the common run of cases of hemiplegia from cerebral hæmorrhage are of just the same significance as cases of epistaxis ; it is just as necessary to examine the arteries, heart, and urine in nasal as in cerebral hæmorrhage. It is in both cases a question of bad arteries, their mode of production and the causes of their rupture. Nasal, retinal, and cerebral hæmorrhages are pathologically identical things.

Here, then, in hemiplegia, is a striking instance of a nervous symptom having what is essentially a non-nervous pathology.

To the list of nervous symptoms depending on non-nervous pathological changes we have to add apoplexy, hemiplegia, and aphasia from cerebral hæmorrhage or from softening of the brain.

These matters have a very important bearing on heredity of nervous diseases, and this point can be discussed here without real digression from our present topic (see also p. 175). I do not myself believe that nervous diseases or symptoms are transmitted. I believe that a person is born with (1) a tendency to changes in systems of tissue, and (2) that an inferior brain is transmitted.[1] I see no evidence that the frequent occurrence of such nervous " diseases " as hemiplegia, softening of the brain, apoplexy, etc., show a transmission of a nervous tendency. For these are not, strictly speaking, nervous diseases at all—that is, the pathological change is not primarily nervous. The evidence is all the other way. So far as I have ever heard, there is no such thing as hemiplegia beginning in nervous tissue. It is, as aforesaid, nearly always due to disease of the arteries of nervous organs. There is no such disease as softening of the brain beginning in nervous tissue. It is nearly always due to disease of the arteries of nervous organs. It is useless for the support of an opinion that some patient's epilepsy is here-

[1] I have already spoken (see p. 175) of the transmission of insanity, stating my disbelief that it consists in a transfer of any pathological change or tendency thereto. To inherit insanity is, I think, to inherit an imperfectly developed *organ*—a brain easily affected temporarily by alcohol, by an epileptiform discharge, or, indeed, by any general state of ill health. It is not, I think, to inherit any neurosis, nor any excitable condition of nerve cell or fibre, nor any tendency to pathological change. Such a brain is easily affected, because it has a slighter development of the higher in comparison with the lower nervous arrangements. On the principle of Dissolution, the higher processes fail first, and in these cases there is little to fail. Similarly, I think, a person's predisposition to phthisis (I do not mean tuberculosis) lies in the fact that he has small lungs, and so for other organs ; the organ is not necessarily small in volume, but has a too small number of functional elements. It is one easily over-worked. Similarly, no one inherits " asthenopia " ; he inherits a hypermetropic eyeball.

I do not believe that epilepsy and insanity have anything physiologically or pathologically in common. I should not call insanity or hysteria neuroses. Epilepsy often causes insanity, especially in those whose brain is imperfectly developed, but only, I think, as alcohol does, by damaging the brain. The cases of epilepsy in which mental infirmity follows are those in which the discharge begins in the very highest nervous arrangements—cases without " a warning " or with a vague and general one.

ditary to point to the fact that many of the ancestors of the patient had died of "disease of the brain," for the disease of the brain in most of them would not have been really of *nervous* origin. I may here quote a report of remarks made by me at the Harveian Society (*British Medical Journal*, November 24, 1866, p. 587):

"A child's father died hemiplegic, and the child's mother had epileptiform seizures. The father's paralysis would be due most likely to disease in the brain, such as tearing up by effusion of blood of a nervous organ, usually the corpus striatum, and not to primary changes beginning in nerve tissue itself; for hemiplegia was nearly always due to cerebral hæmorrhage. The mother's fits might have followed syphilitic disease of the brain's membranes. Then their child, if it became hemiplegic or epileptic, could not be said to have inherited a tendency to either of these symptoms, although it might be born with a tendency to degeneration of tissues forming part of the vascular system, or with a syphilitic taint, which taint so often induced or allowed disorderly growth in a low vegetal tissue forming part of very different organs. Whilst it was not rare for grandfather, father and son to suffer hemiplegia from cerebral hæmorrhage, the grandson could scarcely be said to have inherited this kind of paralysis but rather to be born with his family's tendency to wide degenerative changes, of which disease of the blood vessels was nearly always one part, and the changes of chronic Bright's disease very often another."

For simplicity we have illustrated chiefly by cases of paralysis, because it is obvious that they are in most cases due to gross lesions of non-nervous origin, or, to speak with the strictness necessary for method, the functional abnormality in nervous tissue on which they depend is evidently produced by pathological processes beginning in non-nervous tissues. I cannot show that the same principle applies to the so-called neuroses—chorea, epilepsy, etc. But, then, we must never lose sight of the very significant fact that the pathology of these diseases is, according to most physicians, unknown. This is to be borne in mind when we speak on the hereditariness of this class of disease. We cannot say that they are hereditary (as *nervous* diseases, I mean), because we do not know that they are really of nervous origin (begin in nervous tissue). If my hypothesis (after Kirkes) of the pathology of chorea be correct, this disease is not hereditary as a nervous disease, because the changes in it are not strictly of nervous origin; the nerve tissue suffers secondarily from occlusion of arteries.

I am anxious to state prominently that there is one fact against the doctrine I here put forward which is a very powerful one. I am trying to show that *diseases* like epilepsy are not hereditary. But Brown-Séquard finds that epilepsy artificially produced in guinea-pigs is hereditary. I most willingly admit that this is a most damaging fact to my hypothesis above stated.

What I wish to urge is that we should investigate the pathology of all the neuroses in the same style as we do cases of paralysis. If a man has the common form of hemiplegia, we say that in his case nerve tissue is destroyed in the corpus striatum; then we make an altogether new inquiry to find out the pathological process by which this destruction was effected. We consider all the possible causes by which the several tissues which make up that organ may fail. Similarly, if we determine that there is a "discharging lesion" (let us suppose of the medulla oblongata) we ought to make a special inquiry as to the pathological process which caused it. In what tissue does it begin? We have few clues at present. We must inquire into all sources of ill health. And in seeking the indirect evidence of hereditary transmission we should not limit ourselves to inquiry about " nervous diseases " in a patient's family ; for most of these " nervous diseases " are not of nervous origin—are not really nervous diseases at all. The fact that apoplexy, cerebral softening, hemiplegia, loss of speech, and such symptoms, have occurred in the family of a patient the subject of a neurosis epilepsy, for example, is a very important one. I rate its importance as high as anyone can do. But the importance can only be that it shows the patient inherits a tendency to *arterial* changes. Such symptoms *cannot* show that he has a tendency to *nervous* disease. For with very rare exceptions all the symptoms mentioned are unquestionably dependent on changes beginning in arteries. That the patient's father had after middle age epistaxis or retinal hæmorrhage would be just as significant as if he had had hemiplegia, for all these are arterial affairs. I confess I think it will turn out that the pathology of the neuroses is in most cases owing to arterial disease. I would urge at any rate that in all the neuroses we should inquire carefully for history of rheumatism, gout, etc., as well as for a history of " nervous diseases."

Whilst expressing my opinion (which is only an hypothesis, *as is the opinion to the contrary*) that epilepsy, whether we use that term in the sense in which authorities use it, or in the sense in which I have used it in these chapters, is not hereditary *as a nervous* disease, I am not denying that it may be hereditary in the indirect way in which hemiplegia may be said to be hereditary.

The next question is, *How do changes beginning in non-nervous elements damage nervous tissue so as to cause " discharging lesion " ?* Obviously in many cases we can only speculate on this matter, for of many cases it is clearly but an hypothesis that the change does begin in non-nervous tissues. I would remark to those who think that in some cases, as in genuine epilepsy of authorities, the pathological process begins in the nervous elements, that that is an hypothesis too. But referring to that (see p. 229), I would repeat that, of nervous diseases o*f which the pathology is known*, there are very few, and possibly *none* in which the pathological change *begins* in the nervous elements of the nervous organ affected.

The pathological processes which lead to the one condition of grey matter, instability are no doubt numerous. I can only speak with any degree of confidence of two processes which I believe to start in the non-nervous elements of nervous organs.

1. Occlusion of vessels (embolism and thrombosis).
2. The " irritation " of coarse disease.

1. *Occlusion of vessels.*—The reader will bear in mind that we are seeking the causes of instability, not the cause of some clinical entity. Thus the remarks apply to the production of changes of instability in general. I will, then, speak first of an hypothesis as to the mode of production of instability in chorea.

The following is, with a few verbal alterations, from a paper I contributed to the *Medical Times and Gazette*, March 6, 1869. It applies equally well, I think, to instability in some cases of epilepsy. When I first put forward my speculation on the pathology of chorea I did not know that blocking of arteries most often caused hyperæmia. I used to say it caused anæmia. In the paper from which the following is a quotation I made the necessary correction.

" If arteries be plugged, it seems certain that the nutrition of parts they supply will be *imperfect* ; still, it does not follow that it will be *decreased*. For, according to certain physiological experiments, it seems that plugging of a small artery does *not* always cause *anæmia* of the capillary region to which the vessel should deliver arterial blood. On the contrary, it may cause *congestion*, and may even lead to extravasation. I must, for the facts and arguments of this question, refer the reader to MM. Prévost and Cotard's work, *Études physiologiques et pathologiques sur le Ramollissement cérébral* (Paris, 1866), and especially to a section (p. 38), ' De la congestion qui accompagne infarctus.' I will only quote the last of the three conclusions from their experiments (italicising some words) : ' Consécutivement aux *oblitérations artériales* il se produit habituellement de *l'hyperémie* et de la tuméfaction,' etc. Dr. Ivan Poumeau has also published very interesting statements on the effects of plugging of vessels (*Du Rôle de l'Inflammation dans le Ramollissement cérébral*, 1866).

. . . . . . .

" As it seems to me, the local increase in quantity of blood . . . has an important bearing on the production of chorea *and other symptoms implying increased expenditure of force*. If it be venous we may suppose that although nutrition may be carried on faster, it will lead to *more imperfect* and more easily decomposable nervous matter, or if we suppose the nerve force is supplied from the blood to the nervous structures in the same way as recent investigators believe force is supplied to the muscles, the increase in the quantity of blood is still significant when associated with increased expenditure of force. I suppose we may fairly say that the general character of blood, which is stagnant or slowly changed, will be venous rather than arterial."

Since this was written Cohnheim's researches have appeared. He thinks as Virchow does, that the hyperæmia and extravasation in the infarction results from venous reflux.

This speculation seems to me to accord with the speculation given (see p. 222) as to the alteration in composition of nervous matter in " discharging lesions." From such a morbid stagnation of blood as embolism causes we should expect a greater quantity of nutrition, but one of a more general character, of worse quality. I suppose a tissue of more nitrogenous and less phosphorised composition. And it harmonises too with the dietetic treatment of epilepsy adopted by James Jackson, West, Trousseau, and Ireland.[1]

Let me now speak on conditions for embolism in association with convulsion. Some clinical facts are, I think, indirectly, evidence in favour of the production of local instability by occlusion of vessels.

It is not very uncommon to find when a patient has recovered or is recovering from hemiplegia, the result of embolism of the middle cerebral artery, or of some branch of this vessel, that he is attacked by convulsion beginning in some part of the paralysed region, almost always, I believe, the face or the hand. I have not, however, yet made a post-mortem examination on a patient whom I knew to have had fits *of this kind* after supposed embolism. It will be safer, then, to say that such seizures occur in patients who have recovered partially, or seemingly entirely, from hemiplegia occurring with heart disease, or with the parturient state. And as I have made no post-mortem examination in any

[1] In the just issued fifth volume of Crichton Browne's *West Riding Asylum Reports*, there appears a most valuable paper by Dr. Merson on " The Influence of Diet in Epilepsy." I shall refer to and quote from that article in an Appendix to this Chapter.

such case I will not relate any cases in illustration. I have recorded several cases of the kind in a paper on "Loss of Speech," in the first volume of the *London Hospital Reports*, 1864.[1]

Dr. John W. Ogle and Dr. Murchison have drawn attention to the fact that aneurisms of the larger cerebral vessels have been found in patients who have been subject to "epilepsy," that is, to chronic convulsive seizures before the fatal one due to rupture of the aneurism. Mr. Callender (*St. Bartholomew's Hospital Reports*, vol. iii, 1867, p. 426) has made the very important observation that "the epileptic attacks belong to aneurism of the middle cerebral artery." I have, in vol. vii of the *London Hospital Reports* above referred to, spoken of the significance of the fact of aneurism of the middle cerebral artery being attended by fits. But I know of no case on record *in which the particular kind of fit associated with aneurism of that vessel has been described*. I surmise that in these cases the convulsion begins on one side, but I have, I repeat, no facts on the matter.

I do not think as I then did (1864) that in cases of embolism the *persistent* condition of nerve tissue on which the fits depend results from *diminished* supply of blood to healthy nerve tissue in this vascular region. Plugging of small branches of the middle cerebral artery would lead to congestion, and thus to over-nutrition, and consequent instability of the convolutions (and possibly of the grey matter of the corpus striatum).

*Venous Thrombosis.*—There are cases of disease of the ear (attended by discharge) with which epileptic or epileptiform convulsions occur. I believe the accepted explanation is that these seizures are due to reflex action, the results of irritation starting from the ear. My speculation is that the local instability on which they depend is the result of local hyperæmia from infarction of cerebral veins ; it is, I suppose, a result of a minor degree of the same process as that which sometimes leads to cerebral abscess. I do not enter into this matter here. I may refer to remarks on the subject—*British Medical Journal*, June 26, 1869, p. 591, and to the *Medical Times and Gazette*, January 6, 1872 ; in the latter there is adduced evidence that venous thrombosis causes instability and indirect evidence that disease of the ear may be the origin of such thrombosis.

*Coarse Disease.*—By coarse disease I mean such disease as tumour (including syphilitic growths and masses of tubercle), cysts, abscesses, etc. All these are "foreign bodies."

This subject is far too extensive for full treatment here. I must, then, speak categorically. Any one of these foreign bodies may be latent ; for as we have seen, much of the brain may be destroyed when there are no symptoms of any kind. They often do not produce symptoms of importance by their direct action, *i.e.* because they destroy so much either by involving a part in their growth or by squeezing other parts. There is another way in which they can act. They are sources of irritation,[2] and thus, I suppose, cause a local encepha-

[1] I think it very likely that in some cases of convulsion after embolism we should find post-mortem aneurism of a branch of the middle cerebral artery. The autopsies I have had in cases of death by rupture of aneurisms of large cerebral vessels tend to confirm the view Dr. John W. Ogle has put forward as to the causation of aneurism by embolism. For facts in support of this view see Dr. Church's admirable paper, "Contributions to Cerebral Pathology," *St. Bartholomew's Hospital Reports*, 1869.

[2] Dr. Burdon Sanderson, in his first "Lectures on Inflammation" (see Abstract, *Lancet*, January 8, 1876), writes : ". . . ; such words as 'irritation' must be got rid of—words which, in their original meaning, assume a property of irritability, and we must substitute for it the phrase 'injury of tissue.'"

litis. Speaking otherwise I would say that they produce instability of grey matter about them by irritation. The chief symptoms of the instability they produce are headache, optic neuritis, vomiting, and convulsion.

*Eccentric Irritations.*—There is yet another way in which it is believed by most physicians that local instability may be developed—*viz.* by eccentric irritations. The case of tetanus is very striking.

We have to distinguish betwixt irritations discharging nerve tissue already unstable, and irritations causing that instability. It may be, however, that we have here only two degrees of one thing. What Reynolds says strikes me as most to the point. He writes : " The general mode in which an eccentric irritation passes over into convulsion is the same in each instance—*viz.* by inducing the peculiar organic condition upon which the paroxysm depends. An impression made upon an afferent nerve determines, not only in it, but in the centre to which it is attached, an interstitial change ; and this latter is the cause or essential condition of a motor impulse, which is transmitted along a motor nerve to the contractile fibres of the muscles or the vessels. In such conversion of impression into motion, we have the simplest idea of a ' reflex ' action " Reynolds' (*Epilepsy*, page 18).

This subject always makes me recall cases mentioned by Sir James Paget in a lecture he delivered many years ago—neuralgia set up by injury persisting when the nerve to the injured part was divided. It seemed as if the local injury to the nerve had led to permanent changes of instability in some connected part of the sensory centres, for the patient continued to feel pain in the injured part when it was quite anæsthetic from surgical division of the nerve trunk supplying it.[1]

Eccentric irritations will have to be considered more carefully later on. It is a matter of great importance, as everyone acquainted with Brown-Séquard's researches knows.

## Appendix I

Although I speak in the text, as is the custom, of the body as if it were made up of tissues, I think the expression is not a correct one. I no more believe it to be a scientifically adequate expression to say that the body is made up of tissues than to say that a language is made up of words. Language is made up of propositions in which words are arranged in a particular order of interdependence ; I believe that an organ is made of tissues arranged in a particular order of interdependence. Using the chemical terms composition and constitution, we may say that an organ is composed of tissues, but is constituted by particular arrangements of tissues. Thus, a piece of brain is composed of connective tissue, arteries, capillaries, and veins, as well as of nerve cells and fibres. The functional unit (the nervous organ in miniature) is, however, constituted by the particular relation which its components have. The nervous is the leading tissue, subordinate to it is a circulatory system (artery, capillaries, and veins), and probably there is a nervous system by which, according to requirements of the leading element, the arterial tonus in increased slightly, or the artery is strongly contracted. Perhaps there is inhibitory action. Lionel Beale writes of the frog :

" If a small artery be brought into focus and the tip of one of the toes be very

[1] If so, it is but a caricature of the process by which such changes are established in nervous centres by outward objects as enable us to see the objects ideally during subsequent excitations limited to these altered centres.

lightly touched, the artery is seen to contract immediately, and somewhat irregularly, in different parts of its course. Sometimes a few blood corpuscles are firmly compressed, and for several seconds the vessel remains so strongly contracted that not a corpuscle passes along it. By performing this instructive experiment the observer may realise the effects of the wonderful contractile power of the coats of the smaller arteries, and demonstrate conclusively that the afferent nerve fibres distributed to the skin of the foot generally, influence the nerve centres from which the nerves ramifying amongst the muscular fibres of the arterial coats take their rise. This is a beautiful instance of reflex nervous action affecting the vessels" (*How to Work with the Microscope*, fourth ed. p. 135. See also Beale's *Croonian Lecture*, 1865).

Beale writes also (op. cit.): "In many instances ganglia are seen in connection with the nerves ramifying amongst the muscular fibre cells encircling the vessels. I have seen such upon the vessels of all the viscera and those of the palate of the frog: they are to be detected on the iliac arteries in considerable number. The results of Mr. Lister's experiments render it probable that ganglia exist in connection with the arteries of the limbs."

My hypothesis is that in every nervous action there is a physical change not only in the nerve cells of the nervous unit, but in its arterial system. In some cases where the functional exercise of the leading element is excessive, there results, we may suppose, loss of "tonus" in the over-tasked arterial system. It becomes exhausted: an illustration is that from over-use of hypermetropic eyes there ensues great redness, and even some swelling of the optic disks.

I think that on this principle we may account for the origination of some degenerations—atrophy of optic nerve, chronic Bright's disease.

I submit that degeneration is not the first thing. It is plainly not so in degenerations of arteries. There is here a prior active stage called endarteritis.

Before degeneration sets in there is, I submit, as an indirect consequence of *over-use* of the leading elements (nerve cells, gland cells, etc.), a stage of arterial relaxation permitting increased quantity of blood and yet less change of blood. This is a circumstance unfavourable for the proper nutrition of the tissues of leading function (nervous, gland cells, etc.), and comparatively favourable for the proper nutrition of the tissues of subordinate function (connective tissue). The leading elements will be over-fed and yet worse fed, and thus will easily degenerate (slowly "decompose"). We see how there results degeneration of nerve elements and increase of connective tissue. In the optic atrophy of so-called tobacco amaurosis there is increased redness of the disks before atrophy sets in. The pains of locomotor ataxy are, I think, the signs of active changes, which lead to further degeneration. Pathological changes causing pains cannot be merely degenerative.

Of course, widespread arterial relaxation is produced in other ways, by the ingestion of alcohol for example. Local capillary repletion is produced by embolism or thrombosis of arteries.

This hypothesis as to "functional units" brings nearly into one the two hypotheses (see p. 175) that the hereditariness of disease is (1) a tendency to disease of particular tissues, and (2) of an inheritance of imperfectly developed organs. An ill-developed organ is, in the case of an organ like the kidney, one which has few "functional units," in the case of the brain, where the units differ, one in which the most special units are few. The inheritance of a tendency to phthisis is, I think, not an inheritance of a tendency to any kind of tissue change, but an inheritance of small lungs ; the smallness of the lungs being inferable from the size and the expiratory form of the chest. The small organs are organs easily overworked, there is less reserve.

## Appendix II

Dr. Merson writes (op. cit., p. 233) : " Another way in which the nutrition of the brain may be influenced through the food is by the effect of the latter on the circulation, and the general nutritive activity of the system. Dr. Parkes has proved that the power of the heart's action is capable of being diminished by a reduction of the nitrogenous principles of the food, especially if the voluntary muscles are kept in active exercise. A man was fed for five days on a diet of non-nitrogenous matter, consisting of fat and starch alone. It was found that the voluntary muscles, excited by the will, could act with as much force as ever, although starved of nitrogenous matter ; but it was not so with the involuntary muscles. The heart soon began to suffer in nutrition, and its force, as shown by the sphygmograph, was reduced nearly one-half. ' I draw the conclusion from this experiment,' says Dr. Parkes, ' that if the nitrogen is cut off and the voluntary muscles are kept in their usual action, they do not fail ; but that the power of the heart may be thus reduced if it be desired to do so.' In other words, the food the heart requires is attracted from it by more potent actions. Here, then, we possess a power of affecting the action of the heart if it be needed. *The same remarks will, of course, apply to the muscular tissue throughout the circulatory system.*"

These statements, especially the concluding sentence which I have italicised, are very important. I had overlooked the facts Dr. Merson mentions.

Dr. Merson concludes, as regards his experiments : " On a review of the whole evidence furnished by these observations, I think, after making due allowance for all circumstances likely to tell in the opposite direction, that there are fair grounds for the conclusion that a farinaceous diet is likely to be more useful in the treatment of epilepsy than a nitrogenous ; but in order to get satisfactory results, observations would have to be extended over a longer period than was at my disposal in the present instance. I hope, however, to continue these observations, and at some future time may record the results of my further experience " (Merson, op. cit.).

Dr. Merson does not, however, find that the administration of phosphorus is of value, as according to my speculations it should be. I should, however, like much to hear of observations by Dr. Merson on the use of arsenic instead of phosphorus. It is one of the congeners of phosphorus. I have suggested (see footnote, p. 224) that the therapeutical value of the iodide of potassium is due to its replacing its congener, the commoner, and as I suppose, less potent haloid, the chloride. I believe there is a substitution nutrition. Similarly it may be that arsenic will replace the phosphorus, and lead to nervous tissue of more stable constitutions.

The central nervous system and the superficial layer of the skin have one embryological origin. It is well known that arsenic is a valuable remedy in certain skin diseases. Dr. Broadbent, who believes that substances which have a chemical relationship may have allied therapeutical powers, has, in illustration of his doctrine, suggested the use of phosphorus in certain skin diseases.

## VII

### Anatomy[1]

Anatomy is concerned with the Statics of the Nervous System. The nervous system is a representing system. A knowledge of the anatomy of any section of it is a knowledge of the parts of the body which that section represents and of the degree of complexity with which it represents those parts. Now the only things it can represent are Impressions and Movements.

The word " impression " thus used is obviously an awkward one ; I do not know what other word to use. I mean, of course, an alteration effected at the origin of an afferent nerve producing activity in a nervous centre because the nerve fibre is connected with that centre ; the principle of action is the same if the impression leads by the intermediation of one or more lower centres to an active state in the very highest centres. I use the word because it implies nothing, at least I intend it to imply nothing, as to sensation in the sense of mental state. It is a name for an active physical state only. Whether the change at the origin of an afferent nerve leads to further physical changes attended by a conscious state (that is, to a sensation) or not depends partly on the height of the centre which the current developed reaches and partly perhaps on the *amount* of disturbance it provokes there. Nerves from all parts of the body (from the tissues generally and viscera, not from the surface only) are included among afferent nerves ; and among efferent nerves are included those which pass from the central nervous system to all parts of the body, not those which pass to muscles only. The expression " disturbance or excitation at the periphery " would perhaps be better than " impression " in the case of the afferent nerves arising in tissues and serving in the systemic sensations, as the word " impression " seems to imply some outward object acting ; but it is convenient to make the one word " impression " do for all. Then all efferent nerves do not provoke movements, some stop movement, are inhibitory. The inhibition of movements is represented in nervous centres. Again, some efferent nerves pass to the penetralia of glands and provoke secretion.[2]

It is plain enough that the lower nervous centres represent impressions and movements. But the very highest nervous centres can only be highly complex sensori-motor arrangements.[3] There is nothing else that they can be. The highest centres *re*-represent the impressions and movements already represented in all lower centres, and represent very largely the most special of all bodily impressions and movements, those of the eyes,[4] the hands, etc. Thus they

[1] I should say that all that may appear to be of importance in this chapter is little more than a reflection of certain of Herbert Spencer's psychological teachings, or an application of them to cases of nervous disease, were it not for the fear that I might be guilty of the offence of distorting his doctrines or misapplying them.

[2] " . . . we shall be considerably helped by thinking of the afferent nerves as *recipio-motor* and the efferent nerves as dirigo-motor ; while we think of the nervous centres as composed of libero-motor elements along with elements that perform both the other functions " (Spencer, *Psychology*, i, 49).

[3] It is supposed that they are not only complex in the sense that they represent innumerable different combinations of impressions and movements, but that they represent the combinations in innumerable different intervals.

[4] In former chapters I illustrated the proposition that the unit of composition of the highest parts of the nervous system is sensori-*motor* by the case of the substrata of vision. But in an article, *Medical Times and Gazette*, August 7, 1875, I tried to show that the auditory nerves also have direct association with movement. An hypothesis there stated is that the cochlear division of the auditory nerve is afferent to the heart and arterial system ; whilst the tripartite

represent the whole organism. This is saying that the definition we started the chapter by giving applies to those centres which are in activity whilst we have mental states quite as much as it applies to the lower centres, during energising of which centres there is commonly supposed to be no attendant mental state.[1] To find the anatomy of any nervous centre whatever (" mental " or " physical ") is to find what parts of the rest of the body are represented in it. Let us take a simple example. Our anatomical knowledge of some particular segment of the frog's spinal cord is derived from such facts as that an irritation within a particular area of its skin develops currents which, being transmitted to that segment, discharge its grey matter ; this discharge by connected nerve fibres next develops movements in such and such muscular regions. What are physiologically reflex actions are anatomically sensori-motor arrangements.[2] The same is true of the centres which are the substrata of mental states in man.[3] Let us return to an old illustration. When we see a brick it is plain that a certain part of the surface (the retina) is impressed, and equally plain that there are associated movements of the ocular muscles ; the sensory element is the peripheral part of the mechanism for colour of the object (surface), the motor element for its shape and size (extension). And, of course, as we are conscious of the brick[4] (only a technical way of saying *we* see it), the disturbance of the retinal impression effects ultimately an active change in the highest centres, which provokes impulses carried by motor fibres to the ocular muscles. The arrangement is here as it is in the cord, sensori-motor, but one infinitely more complex and special than our sketch implies it to be. But we can think of the brick when it is removed. Now when we do so we of necessity think of it as in the environment, and therefore the substratum of the visual idea of the brick can only be made up of elements which represent a past experience of seeing it in the environment. All we could learn of the brick when we first did see it—

division for the three semicircular canals is afferent to centres for movements which are leading in locomotion. The nerve we call auditory might with propriety be called affero-cardiac and affero-locomotor. Associated with these movements the auditory nerve serves in the estimation of intervals (time) as the eye does in extension (space). I suppose also that systemic sensations have their motor congeners in movements of the skin, intestines, arteries, etc.—that there are systemic sensori-motor processes.

[1] I say " is commonly supposed," but it seems to me more and more evident that we must accept Lewes's doctrine—that a " sensibility " attends energising of all centres. The reader will note, however, that there is nothing in the text to imply that when the nervous centres have reached an exceeding complexity of structure any kind of physical states *becomes* any kind of mental states, but simply that as centres become exceedingly complex a mental state *attends activity of them*—is parallel with their activity. This is the most commonly received doctrine. Mr. Lewes, on the contrary, thinks " that the neural process and the feeling are one and the same process under different aspects."

[2] But such facts as that the cord has certain sized and certain shaped columns of white matter and certain shaped areas of grey matter are facts of morphology. So, too, are facts as to the course of fibres and arrangements of cells disclosed by microscopical examination The latter is not Minute Anatomy, but Minute Morphology ; and however minute it becomes it does not turn into physiology. It is only when the shapes of cells and course of fibres, etc., are shown to be subservient to the reception or conduction of particular impressions and to the development of related movements that morphology ceases or rises into anatomy.

[3] There is reflex action here, too, but it is imperfect reflex action ; reflex action " breaks down " in the very highest centres.

[4] It is understood, of course, that no idea can occur singly ; it can exist only as one of a class. " To say what a thing is is to say what it is like " (Spencer). Moreover, a visual idea, as do other ideas, requires translation into a tactual idea before its meaning can be fully known (Spencer). I have suggested that there is evidence of the mechanism for the physical side of the process of translation in certain cases of hemiplegia of extensive range. Bur for purposes of limited illustration we consider the idea and its physical substratum as occurring singly. Indeed, what we speak of in the text as a " correspondence " is betwixt the organism *as a whole* and some part of the environment.

we speak of what occurred physically at the periphery—was from the impression it made on some part of the surface of our bodies (the retina) and from our reacting movements (ocular) upon it. The nervous arrangement concerned in this actual experience and partly developed by it, or, let us say modified[1] by it, remains as the physical substratum of all we can ever after know of the brick in its absence. It represents an adjustment betwixt the organism and the environment. After seeing the brick the modification (or, we might say, education) in a certain nervous arrangement is an actual part of our body. But the excitation or discharge of this modified nervous arrangement having ceased with the removal of the brick, the idea becomes latent; the adjustment is potential. For when at any time afterwards the mere central parts of that arrangement are re-excited even but *slightly*, an idea or vision of the brick is roused, although in a faint form; and as there is a more limited (only a central) excitation, the idea is less vividly referred to the environment.[2]

What we have been saying is equivalent to repeating that the substrata of consciousness represent impressions and movements. For the highest nervous arrangements are the substrata of consciousness. We have been speaking of a particular state of consciousness arising during either a strong or a slight excitation (corresponding to "vivid" and "faint" ideation) of a limited part of the substrata of consciousness—that part which represented certain retinal impressions and adapted ocular movements. It is understood, of course, that it is the particular arrangement and the definite association of these nerve fibres and cells answering to impressions and movements which constitute the substrata. We have to discover the nature of these arrangements. For a mere number of recipio-motor, libero-motor, and dirigo-motor elements only form the "empirical" formulæ, not the "rational" formulæ of the substrata of mental states.

Let us state the principle involved in our definition more generally as a sort of recapitulation.

Everybody believes that our ideas are acquired by experience, or rather, that experience is an essential factor. This is admitted by those who hold that we have innate forms of thought, whether they admit the Spencerian doctrine that our forms of thought are inherited experiences of things or believe that they are innate in the old sense of the word. In other words, ideas are acquired during the correspondences betwixt the organism and its environment—the innate forms are then developed and filled up. The sensori-motor arrangements we have been speaking of constitute the inherited mechanism by which these correspondences can be effected; the mechanism itself being

[1] What the exact nature of the structural modification may be we do not know. Huxley ("On the Hypothesis that Animals are Automata," *Fortnightly Review*, November 1874, p. 563) says: "I do not know that any modern theory of the physical conditions of memory differs essentially from these [Haller and Hartley], which are all children—*mutatis mutandis*—of the Cartesian doctrine. Physiology is at present incompetent to say anything positively about the matter or to go further than the expression of the high probability that every molecular change which gives rise to a state of consciousness leaves a more or less persistent structural modification, through which the same molecular change may be regenerated by other agencies than the cause which first produced it."

[2] Or, using popular expressions, we "think of the brick," "are conscious of it," "see the object ideally," etc. That excitation limited to central nervous arrangements will suffice in ideation is proved by such facts as that when the eyeballs are atrophied the patient still dreams of objects he formerly saw. Occasionally the irritation of the stumps of the optic nerves provoke, even during waking hours, not merely "sparks and colours," but definite spectral visions of persons and things. Indeed, the annoyance from this is one reason assigned by Graefe for the operation of section of the optic nerves of atrophied eyeballs.

perfected during the process. It is only stating this principle most simply (with regard to the highest mental processes at least) to say that ideas are acquired during contact of objects with particular parts of the surface of our bodies, and during the reaction of parts of our bodies on the objects.[1]

So far we have illustrated by sensori-motor processes representing surface impressions and corresponding motor reactions of the surface. But we have many times insisted that the units of the substrata of consciousness represent the whole body : they represent the tissues (including the skin *as a tissue*), the viscera, the intestines, heart, arteries, etc., that is to say, they receive afferent nerves concerned in systemic[2] (Lewes) or organic (Bain) sensations, and they send out also fibres for the corresponding organic or systemic movements. That these are represented in the very highest nervous arrangements disease shows. And we should infer such representation *a priori* from the constant accompaniment of intellectual by emotional states. For evidently these systemic sensations and movements are concerned during emotional states. The nerves *from* the skin, viscera, etc., and nerves *to* the heart, arteries, intestines, etc., are only, of course, the raw material of the substrata of emotional states ; it is their particular arrangements which constitute the substrata of emotional states. They, too, are sensori-motor, and no doubt in the highest centres sensori-motor arrangements of exceeding great complexity.[3]

The systemic sensori-motor arrangements cannot be said in any ordinary use of the expression " to represent adjustments betwixt the organism and its environment." They represent adjustments of parts of the organism to one another. The best examples of these adjustments are those furnished by the innervation of the circulation ; these adjustments are very intricate. But since on Spencer's doctrine of nervous evolution all our nervous arrangements are the sum of the residua of ancestral correspondences betwixt the series of organisms and their environments, the systemic sensori-motor arrangements would in a sense come under the definition. We shall, however, say that they represent parts of the organism in adjustment to one another.

In saying that the substrata of consciousness represent or re-represent the whole organism, it is not meant that there is a dead uniformity of representation of all parts of the body in these highest nervous centres. Whilst they represent impressions and movements of all orders, the most special of the impressions and movements (those of the eyes, head, and hand) will have the leading representation. There will be innumerable degrees of subordination down to representation of the most automatic of all movements and the most organic of all sensations (those of the tissues, muscles, viscera, etc.).

In speaking so far of the substrata of consciousness we have ignored the fact that they are in several parts of the cerebrum. We spoke of the substrata of consciousness as being the highest nervous arrangements. Yet to avoid misinterpretation we pointed out explicitly some time back that we do not really suppose there to be one fixed seat of consciousness. Now, if the expression may be permitted, we shall speak of several highest nervous arrangements.

[1] Of course the word " contact " is used here in an unusually extended sense, not for tactual impressions only, but for aural and retinal.

[2] The systemic sensations are numerous. Those from the tissues might be called " common systemic sensations " ; those from the viscera, " special systemic sensations " ; whilst hunger and thirst deserve the name of " compound systemic sensations."

[3] " [Emotions] are of far more involved natures than sensations, and imply the co-operation of extremely intricate nervous structures " (Spencer, *Pyschology*, vol. i, p. 122).

Consciousness is not an unvarying independent entity. Consciousness arises during activity of *some* of those of our highest nervous arrangements by which the correspondence of the organism with its environment is being effected. Our present consciousness is our now mental state ; it is such or such according to the kind of correspondence now being effected. As this correspondence is continually changing, the nervous arrangements concerned are continually different. Our present consciousness is, psychologically speaking, the present relation betwixt the subject and the object, or, anatomico-physiologically speaking, it arises during the present adjustment of the organism to its environment. It is an anatomical problem to discover where in the nervous system those nervous arrangements lie which are in leading activity, whilst we are conscious thus or thus. The steps are—(1) What is the adjustment, and what parts of the surface or periphery are concerned in it ? In visual ideation the adjustment is retino-ocular, the retina and ocular muscles being the parts of the periphery concerned in it. The further question is—(2) Where are the highest nervous centres representing those parts of the body ? I do not ask the reader to take the answers I am about to give as facts, but as *admittedly imperfect* hypotheses. When we think of the brick as coloured, the *leading* activity is of nervous arrangements in the right posterior lobe. This is intended to mean that it is of a part where retinal impressions are most represented in complex combinations and definite associations. When we think chiefly of extension (the shape and size) of the brick, the *leading* activity will be in the left anterior lobe—that is, in a part where certain ocular movements have the leading representation. What is quite certain is that, as from moment to moment we are differently conscious—that is, are conscious of different kinds of things, the nervous substrata in activity cannot be the very same at each moment. There is as certainly a localisation in some part of the nervous system of arrangements concerned in each particular state of consciousness as there is a localisation of movements of the hand, or of the face, or of the foot. I do not mean, of course, that we have yet been able to localise in the former as we have in the latter, nor that the localisation is equally definite in the two. When we think of one object, as a rose, the substrata excited will not be just the same as those excited when we think of another object, as a brick.

The excitations above spoken of are healthy nervous discharges. Metaphorically speaking, they cause development of the rational formulæ of the nervous system, and correspondingly of clear and definite mental states ; and as the excitations occur at certain intervals they are in orderly sequence. But from the excessive and sudden discharge of these substrata in an epileptic fit there only occurs the crudest mental states (clouds of colour), and not movements of the eyes (nascent or actual), but spasm of the ocular muscles ; there is a *sudden excessive* development of innumerable nervous arrangements all at once. The spasm and crude sensations (or rather the implied excessive excitations of sensory nervous centres) as it were present us with crude heaps of the raw material of these substrata, not even in the rough order of their empirical formulæ.

Now for another qualification. When we either actually see or only think of a rose we have a state of consciousness of a thing particularly coloured and extended. There is then, we suppose, activity of certain elements of the substrata of consciousness which lie in the right posterior and left anterior lobe. But we seem to have two mental states together or in reversible succession ;

we seem as if we had not only an idea of the rose, but *we* seem to know that *we* have it. We seem to remember the rose as if we had a general consciousness in addition to and yet distinct from another more special consciousness, a sort of " faculty " of remembering the rose. Similarly for other so-called faculties, especially the will. Let us state an hypothesis explanatory of this feeling. It is that the substrata of consciousness are double, as we might infer from the physical duality and separateness of the highest nervous centres. The more correct expression is that there are two extremes. At the one extreme the substrata serve in subject consciousness.[1] But it is convenient to use the word "double." We have already spoken of the substrata of object consciousness. But we shall now consider the relations of the two. We speak first of the substrata of subject consciousness.

Subject consciousness is first in all mentation. This half of the double substrata is made up of nervous arrangements representing the parts of the whole organism *in relation to one another*. Here their representation is in the order from the most general (systemic or organic) movements and most general (organic or systemic) sensations up to the most special movements and most special sensations. By this half of the substrata impressions from the environment are received ; it is the passive half ; the chiefly sensory half. We say chiefly, for there must be a motor element too, or there could be no notion of the locality of an impression. Sensory action is first and most ; the sequent movement represented in these substrata simply serves in the physical process during which the part of the surface of the body acted upon is registered in subconsciousness ; it does not give a notion of externality or of the thing acting. In any impression received, affection of what is called the systemic sensations will be first ; there is first, that is to say, a most general sensation[2] representing the organism as a whole as being affected before there can be the sensation that it is being particularly affected here or there ; this process is usually unconscious or subconscious, unless the local impression be excessive. When it is excessive (when there is the psychological state of pain) the impression in many parts of the body, if not in every part, *does disturb the whole system*, causes pallor, faintness, and sickness, develops systemic sensori-motor processes. This is very important, for the implication is that in the slightest local impressions the whole organism becomes affected in the sense that the highest nervous arrangements *representing the organism as a whole* are disturbed.[3]

The activity of the substrata of subject consciousness in health is not attended by what is commonly called full consciousness. They form the anatomical side of what is a continued under-consciousness (persistence of consciousness) and are those most concerned in the wide bodily states which are

[1] Subject consciousness is not commonly spoken of as consciousness ; it is a subconsciousness bordering on unconsciousness.

[2] The term " sensation " is very awkward here ; it is meant that there is a contribution to a state of subconsciousness, bordering on consciousness. Lewes's doctrine that sensibility attends activity of all nervous centres would save us from the awkwardness of using expressions which are strictly equivalent to the contradiction of " unconscious sensations."

[3] " Ludwig has found that irritation of a sensory nerve has a double effect—(1) it causes the vessels of the part to which it is distributed to dilate ; (2) it causes the vessels in other parts of the body to contract, so that the general blood pressure is raised " (Lauder Brunton, *St. Bartholomew's Hospital Reports*, 1875). This shows that a local irritation, when excessive, affects the whole organism. It is believed, however, by physiologists, that the irritation is conveyed only so far as the vaso-motor centre—that is, only as far as the medulla oblongata.

the physical side of emotions.[1] These substrata are in constant slight action and in but slightly varying action. They rise in activity before that of those nervous arrangements which constitute the second half of the double begins.

The second half of the substrata of consciousness represents the physical side of object consciousness—consciousness commonly so-called. These nervous arrangements represent parts of the body in the order from the most special and voluntary movements and sensations to the most automatic and general movements and sensations. So that these like the last represent the whole organism, but in the reverse order ; they represent the body in the order of its power of reacting on the environment, not in its possibilities of being acted on. This is the chiefly movement half. Movement here comes first.[2] The sense of resistance is first and ever present in this half as the systemic sensations are in the other half. There is first in the former, that is to say, the sensation of the organism as being impeded here or there, as in the latter, of the organism as being affected thus or thus. They are the arrangements by which some part of the organism (already represented as a whole by the substrata of subject consciousness) is reacting on its environment ; the reaction varying much from moment to moment. In conscious states it is not simply that an impression received from the environment develops this reaction ; the impression received affects the whole organism, and it is this which leads to the reaction. These substrata serve in what is called perception as distinguished from sensation. To perceive a thing is *to refer it to the environment* or to some part of the body.[3]

This division into substrata of object and substrata of subject consciousness appears to me to correspond anatomico-physiologically with the psychological distinctions betwixt subject and object made by Spencer and with that by Bain betwixt[4] object and subject consciousness.

[1] *Emotion* is the most general feeling ; we are always in some state of feeling, just as much as we are always alive. What are commonly called emotions, meaning particular emotions, are variations of this constant state. The physical process underlying emotion involves the whole organism, and each particular emotion is, so to speak, a special attitude of it. When this or that particular emotion predominates these or those parts of the body have the leading excitement or depression. *Sensation* is a less general feeling ; its physical process involves much of the organism, but some part of it especially. Perception is least general, most special, and the physical process in it involves some part of the body, and is mainly the reacting of some part definitely *after* a local impression which has but faint if any attendant sensation. So there are gradations of feeling from those forming part of subject consciousness only to those rising into object consciousness ; there is in this ascending series of mental states diminishing consciousness of the organism and increasing consciousness of the environment.

[2] It is not meant that movement begins here without prior excitation from some afferent nerve or nerve centre corresponding to afferent nerves.

[3] Obviously, even by this definition sensation and perception are not abruptly separated. A local pain *as a pain* is an affection of subject consciousness. A sudden and severe pain anywhere, or in many places, at any rate (*i.e.* the nervous change underlying the pain), affects the whole organism ; it evidently leads to changes in the circulation of the whole body. To know that the pain is in this or in that part of the body is an affair of object consciousness, and implies local movement, actual or nascent, of some part of the body. At least the principle is the same ; although we cannot say that the part of the body in pain is part of the environment. It is a part which for the time is considered as separate from the rest of the organism by a high degree of local independence of feeling. Moreover, the particular emotions, those which vary from the common feeling, are known as emotions by being referred to the environment ; we attribute modesty to the daisy, just as we attribute redness to a brick.

[4] Bain gives several distinctions (*Emotions and Will*, 3rd ed., p. 575 *et seq.*). I do not follow Bain's order in the subjoined. (1) " The feeling of expended muscular energy as against sensations wholly passive." This nearly agrees with the distinction into *chiefly* motor and *chiefly* sensory elements of the two substrata. (2) " The contrast between Indifferent Feeling and pleasure or pain fuses itself with the object and subject contrast." Thus it seems to me to

If the substrata of consciousness be double their duality is but an illustration on the highest level of the duality of nervous arrangements in general. The unit of action of the nervous system is double the unit of constitution; it is " a molecule of two atoms." The lower centres are double, and so are the centres of centres—those which sum up and potentially contain all lower centres. But the noteworthy thing is that in the highest parts of the nervous system the two halves of the double unit are not *mere* duplicates as they are in the lower centres. One half acts before the other, and acts differently.

We have already suggested that certain regions of the cerebrum are concerned in object consciousness, which we then spoke of as " consciousness " only—the right posterior and the left anterior lobe. We have next to speak of the seat of the substrata of the corresponding subject consciousness. We believe they are the right anterior lobe and left posterior lobe. By these nervous arrangements we learn how and where our organism is affected, as by the corresponding object consciousness we learn what and where the thing in the environment is which affects us.

What has just been said is but repeating in a more general way what I have said in the paper on the " Nature of the Duality of the Brain," January, etc., 1874. For to speak is to be conscious in words; to perceive is to be conscious in objects. But such full consciousness arises out of, and is posterior to, the corresponding under-consciousness called subject consciousness. For example, the automatic and unconscious (or subconscious) reproduction of words and images of things precedes, I there argued, that reproduction of them which is attended by full consciousness.

The above view is not parallel to the view popularly taken that we have a consciousness apart from, and as it were served by quasi-independent faculties of " volition," " memory," etc., and also sometimes governed by them. On the contrary, these so-called faculties are only different sides of constantly varying states of object consciousness which *arise out of prior states of subconsciousness or unconsciousness*, directly out of subconsciousness. It is supposed that there is a constant play betwixt the two—an unceasing rhythm. Spencer writes : " It seems to me that the consciousness of self and the consciousness of not-self are the elements of an unceasing rhythm in consciousness—a perpetual alternation ordinarily so rapid as to escape observation, though occasionally so much retarded as to be observable. Like the divergence already set forth (§353) from Sir W. Hamilton's interpretation of the antagonism between Sensation and Perception is the divergence that arises here; this second divergence being in truth a corollary from the first. Just as before we saw that Sensation and Perception respectively dominate in consciousness with degrees of strength that vary inversely, thus excluding one another with varying degrees of stringency; so here we shall see that the consciousness of self and the consciousness of not-self are ever tending each to exclude the other but each failing to do this for more than an instant, save in those exceptional cases where it is raised to extreme vividness " (Spencer's *Psychology*, vol. ii, p. 438).

accord with the two orders in which I suppose the sensation to be represented in the substrata. (3) " The contrast of intellect and feeling coincides to a very large extent with the contrast of object and subject." (4) " Definite feelings connected with definite movements; feelings independent of our movements (subject)." This nearly coincides. (5) " Experience common to all (object), as against experience special to each (subject)." This last is a very important distinction, and again, there is a harmony.

This doctrine is supported, I think, by facts which we shall adduce later when speaking of the After-effects of Excessive Nervous Discharges. We shall see that exhaustion produced by these discharges and also in other ways of a higher centre allows the one next lower, the one next least automatic, to *spring into activity*. The substrata of object consciousness are the higher of the two substrata. With exhaustion of the substrata of object consciousness there goes increased activity, or let us say excitement, of the substrata of subject consciousness. The exhaustion may be only very slight, as in the " brilliancy " of the mentally over-fatigued, which brilliancy is owing to an excitement of the substrata of subject consciousness *permitted by* slight and partial exhaustion of the substrata of object consciousness—there is metaphorically speaking loss of control. The " rhythm," unceasing in health, is stopped by disease, or goes on at a lower level, because the use of one half, always first the object half, is temporarily lost, or is impaired. Let us take a very simple illustration. In a delirious hospital patient there is a loss or defect of object consciousness from exhaustion of its substrata. The facts proving this assertion are that the patient does not know where he is ; does not know any persons or objects rightly. But there is increase of his subject consciousness, for he believes that the ward is the place most familiar to him—the place where he works, or his home, and he takes the nurse for his wife, and a boy patient for his nephew. He is, in short, to borrow both ideas and words from Bain, defective with regard to " experiences common to all (object) " and exalted " with regard to experiences special to each (subject)."

Although we speak of the correspondence betwixt the organism and the environment, what occurs anatomically and physiologically is a rhythm betwixt the two sides of the brain (or betwixt two differing units of one side) ; one representing the organism as it is acted on in this or that part, the other as reacting on this or that thing in the environment. This is evidently all that can occur when we are thinking about the action of absent persons in places at a distance. To perceive a brick is to refer it to the environment ; we so refer it just as certainly when we think of the brick as when we see it. But it is equally certain that when we have the fullest object consciousness, when we see a brick before us, what we are concerned with (as anatomists and physiologists) is a state of our own organisation—specially a state of our own nervous system produced in some unknown way by the brick acting on us and by our reacting on it. As repeatedly insisted on, the only difference betwixt seeing the brick and thinking of it is a difference of degree. To perceive a thing is, we repeat, to refer it to the environment ; we do this just as certainly when we think of the brick as when we see it. The former is commonly called an idea, the latter a perception. But an idea is only a faint external perception, and an external perception is only a vivid idea. In the former the externality also is faint, in the latter strong. For in the former the environment itself is faint, in the latter vivid. In no case can we think of a thing except as in the environment ; our idea of justice is an attributing a certain feeling we have to some person or persons. In thinking of an object there is of course the difference that the environment is, to speak shortly, " remembered," or constructed. This difference of mere degree sinks into insignificance before that difference implied by the rhythm of subject and object consciousness, and illustrated by the unconscious and automatic reproduction of images of objects *before* that perception which is a conscious and voluntary reproduction of them.

Just as localisation of ideas, or rather of the substrata of ideas, means anatomically localisation of certain highly complex and special nervous arrangements representing particular impressions and movements, so localisation of symptoms in epilepsies means the same. A convulsion from disease of the brain is a *brutal* development of the function of the substrata of some ideas. We have to bear in mind that the discharging lesions in epilepsy are not only local, but that their discharges being very strong lead to excessive developments of the functions of that part of the brain which they happen to involve ; the discharges of health lead to sensori-motor actions ; the discharges of epilepsy not only develop the functions of a part brutally, but develop nearly solely the functions of that one part ; there may occur motor symptoms almost only and sensory symptoms almost only.

Thus convulsion of the hands may represent a violently active state of the motor elements only in the substrata of tactual ideas ; convulsion of the tongue, palate, lips, etc., of the substrata of words. In some cases of migraine we have the corresponding sensory elements. Let me take a parallel case from physiological experiment. It is well known that irritation of definite areas of the skin of a headless frog provokes an excitation of the nerve cells in some part of the cord by which certain related movements are developed. This, however, is not the illustration. To give a case analogous to that of convulsion in man we must suppose the frog to be strychnised ; then the cells in the animal's cord are raised to a degree of instability analogous to that of the cells of the cortex in a discharging lesion in the epilepsy of man. They discharge strongly, rapidly, and many of them at once. From this results a convulsion (in the frog, tetanus), that is, a sudden, rapid, and brutal development of numerous movements.

In the brutal discharges of epilepsies we have no mental states except the crudest, as of clouds of colour, numbness of the hands, etc. Let us speak of epileptic discharges beginning in the substrata of consciousness, and also try to show that the epileptic paroxysms dependent on discharges of these substrata differ according to the part of the substrata excited. We speak of the genuine epilepsy of authorities.

The paroxysm may begin by loss of consciousness, the patient having not the least precursory sensation. When this is so, we have no help from him towards localising the discharging lesion in any part of the substrata of consciousness. But sometimes the loss of consciousness is preceded by some crude sensation. It is very often a feeling referred to the epigastrium, and this is, I think, a coarse development of certain systemic sensations, that is, of sensations leading in subject consciousness, or it may be coloured vision, that is, a sensation leading in object consciousness. Now we speak of movements : these we can see ourselves, or infer them by their effects. A paroxysm sometimes begins by pallor of face, that is, by coarse development of movements leading in subject consciousness. There are the movements corresponding to systemic sensations. Then there is often a brutal development of movements of the eyes (spasm of the ocular muscles), that is, a development of movements leading in object consciousness. These are the motor correlative symptoms of coloured vision.

Different modes of beginning of epileptiform paroxysms necessarily point to differently seated discharging lesions. That we may be quite unable to declare exactly where the discharging lesion is in any of the instances just alluded to does not invalidate this very general remark. We may at any rate say that the paroxysms spoken of begin by discharges in the very highest nervous arrangements, for loss of consciousness occurs almost instantly after the warnings spoken of. But we spoke of " several highest." There are the highest centres concerned during subject consciousness (left posterior lobe being sensory, and right anterior lobe motor), and there are the highest centres concerned during object consciousness (right posterior lobe sensory, left anterior lobe leading motor).

We begin with sensations. The left posterior lobe is the lobe where the substrata represent sensations in the order from the most general (systemic) to the most special (sight) ; the right posterior lobe where sensations are represented in the reverse order. They correspond respectively to the order of representation of sensory elements in subject and object consciousness. Hence a fit beginning by coloured vision I think most often depends on a discharge beginning in the right posterior lobe, whereas discharge beginning in the left posterior lobe should most often produce first such brutal development of sensation as that feeling referred to the epigastrium by many epileptics. I suppose this is a brutal development of certain systemic sensations. It accords with this opinion that there is often a deep emotional state, " a fear," " sensation of horror," etc., attending the epigastric feeling.

I do not pretend to know that there are these particular local differences in representation. I am only certain that there are the several kinds of fits, and thus that the discharges must be differently seated. I certainly do not pretend to know that there is such an abrupt separation of duties betwixt the two posterior lobes as the above illustrations imply. For several reasons I believe there is less difference betwixt their sensory functions than there is betwixt the motor functions of the twin anterior lobes. Again, the discharging lesions may be in any one of numerous parts of either of the posterior lobes, so that different sensations may be developed ; some epileptic seizures begin by an " aura " of noise. I nevertheless consider that some hypothesis is necessary in guiding investigation in these most difficult cases of epilepsy, and I submit the above.

We now speak of the *first* effects of epileptic discharge of the anterior lobes. They are chiefly turning of the eyes and head ; if the head and eyes turn to the left there will be discharge of the right cerebral hemisphere ; if to the right, of the left cerebral hemisphere. Vertigo in epileptics is on its physical side a motor symptom ; even when unattended by outward movements it implies nascent movement of certain parts of the body, and this depends on slighter epileptic discharge of those parts of the anterior lobe than those discharges which make them actually move.[1]

There are often organic motor symptoms, as contraction of the arteries, especially of the face. We should theoretically expect that there would be also slowing or stopping of the heart from excitation of nervous arrangements representing the quasi-motor fibres which inhibit the heart. There *is* stoppage of the pulse at the onset of some paroxysms of epilepsy.[2]

[1] From theoretical considerations I think it most likely that discharges of the right anterior lobe should cause nascent or actual movement (turning) of the whole body, and thus the sensation of the body itself moving, and that if the discharge of the left anterior lobe caused vertigo, it would be from nascent or actual movement of the eyes, and thus there would be the sensation of outward things moving.

[2] One would not expect the systemic movements to be so specially represented as the higher movements, those of the eyes and hand, and not so separate from their corresponding

I should imagine that nerves for the arteries (systemic and pulmonary) would be more represented in the right side of the brain, and the inhibitory fibres of the heart more on the left side. In the lower animals the right pneumogastric has, according to Arloing and Tripier, more to do with the heart, the left more with respiration. In some animals the reverse obtains, as regards the splanchnics. The section of the right causes comparatively little sinking of arterial pressure. These peripheral differences, one must suppose, imply differences of representation in the highest centres. One would expect *a priori* the inhibition of the heart to be most specially represented in the leading motor side (left anterior lobe or left hemisphere generally). I here add a quotation from Brunton bearing on the representation of the systemic sensori-motor processes concerned in vomiting in centres so high as the corpus striatum and optic thalamus :

" Budge states that the cerebral centre for the movements of the stomach is the *right* corpus striatum and optic thalamus, especially the latter. Irritation of these parts causes the stomach to move, while irritation of the corresponding parts on the left side of the brain has no action whatever. From this observation we are led to suspect that when any irritation exists in the right cerebral hemisphere it will occasion vomiting more readily than irritation in the left cerebral hemisphere, and according to Budge, this is actually the case " (Lauder Brunton, *Practitioner*, December 1874). Dr. Brunton refers to an experiment by Gee on a dog (*Clinical Society Transactions*, 1860). Gee injected a large dose of apomorphia (two grains) into a dog. The dog vomited, and in two or three minutes began to course round the room in which the experiment was performed in a curiously persistent methodical manner. Brunton (op. cit.) says : " This effect of apomorphia points to an action of the drug on the nervous centres, and is all the more interesting when we remember that Budge placed the cerebral centre for the stomach in the *right* thalamus opticus."

The first thing we do in the scientific investigation of a case of epilepsy is, as in a case of palsy, to localise the lesion—to seek the organ damaged. In no case of nervous disease of any kind is there any *rational* clue to the seat of the internal lesion other than that furnished by observing the external symptoms. The principle, which seems, and indeed I think is, a mere truism, is not fully acted on in practice. It is carried to its logical conclusion in cases of paralysis of muscles, but not in cases of mobile affection of muscles, chorea, convulsion, etc. Most careful attempts are made to describe the regions affected in palsies. But there is little, if any, attempt made to note the regions affected in cases of chorea and convulsion. We are told that disease of the surface of the brain " causes epilepsy," but we are often not told what regions of the body are first in spasm in the paroxysm, or that one side is convulsed, or convulsed first and most. No one could imagine that there was any other way of finding out the seat of the internal lesion in a case of paralysis than by studying care-

sensations (systemic sensations). For example, the connection betwixt sensory nerves from the intestines and their corresponding motor nerves would be more closely organised and also more organised in the lower centres. Then, on the contrary, as regards the most special sensations and movements, one would, I think (considering our power of forming new or " ideal " combinations out of our actual experiences), expect them to be represented more widely apart and less certainly connected. But in the most special sense the separation would not be absolute. Thus in some cases of migraine there is not only a development of colour, but a zigzag outline ; this, I presume, implies an excitation of motor elements—of such elements as in health serve in the " insect " vision of giving us ideas of roughness, small patterns, etc.

fully the external region paralysed. If the face, arm, and leg are paralysed on the left side, the arm suffering much more than the leg, we can infer that the lesion is in the right corpus striatum. If the face is paralysed on the right side, and the arm and leg on the left, we declare the lesion to be on the right side of the pons Varolii. And if we were asked to declare the seat of a lesion when told simply that the patient " was paralysed," we should think the question a strange one and reply that we could not tell. But no such minute work is attempted in cases of convulsion. It does not appear to most people at all a strange thing to be asked, " Where is the seat of epilepsy ? " For " epilepsy " is to them an entity, and it appears a fair question to ask where is the seat of the change causing it. It is often taken as proved that the seat of the discharging lesion in general convulsion is the medulla oblongata. But this assumption, granting for the moment its correctness, is no justification for the neglect of a minute study of the paroxysm. Those who hold " orthodox " opinions on epilepsy admit that the paroxysms differ in different patients. If so, different parts of the medulla oblongata must be discharged. Here I give authority for the double statement that fits differ in different patients, and yet that the fits in the same patient are very much alike.

Voisin[1] writes : "Axenfield a faut remarquer que les attaques se reproduisent le plus souvent avec une uniformité absolue, avec leurs auras, leurs caractères propres et leurs complications. Il s'établit une sorte d'habitude d'après laquelle tel individu sentira toujours la même aura, poussera toujours un cri et le même cri, tombera sur le même point du corps, le front l'occiput se blessera de la même façon, présentera les mêmes mouvements convulsifs, se mordra la langue au même point, se luxera toujours une même épaule, sera toujours pris de délire après l'attaque."

This being so, those who hold that the medulla oblongata is the part of the nervous system which discharges in the epileptic fit have, as much as others, to note *paroxysms* with great care, in order to find out how it is that in one patient there are fits of a certain kind, and in another of another kind. If, then, epilepsy *is* a disease of the medulla oblongata, differing fits in two patients must depend on discharge of different parts of the medulla oblongata, however much the seizures in the two patients may agree in the most fundamental characteristics required by the ordinary definition of epilepsy.

The following quotation from Falret, *État Mal des Épileptiques*, is given to show that epileptic paroxysms differ, and yet that in the same patient they are uniform. I draw particular attention to the parts italicised. It is true that the quotation refers chiefly to the mode of onset, but this is the most important matter in localisation. The part first convulsed, for example, is the part which has the leading representation in the centre discharged. Falret is speaking, too, of mental symptoms, but the principle is the same. A fit which always begins by the same " remembrance " is evidence of a *local* discharge as much as is a fit which always begins by colour vision. I do not think, however, that these intellectual auræ are symptoms of the same kind as coloured vision, or local spasm, as I shall try to show at length later on.

Falret remarks first, however, that the convulsive attacks of epilepsy must often occur suddenly without being announced by any symptom " soit physique soit moral." This is what one would expect of cases of epilepsy in

[1] *Nouveau Dictionnaire de Médecine et de Chirurgie Pratiques*, p. 959, art. " Épilepsie." This is an article of great value.

asylums ; for a fit to begin without a warning is for the fit to begin with loss of consciousness, that is, for the discharge to be of the very highest nervous arrangements. Theoretically, we should expect that the epileptic patients who are most likely to become insane would be those who have discharging lesions in the very highest nervous arrangements.

Crichton Browne (*West Riding Asylum Reports*, vol. iii, p. 160) says : " In lunatic asylum practice an aura is of rare occurrence in epilepsy." This may, however, be, as he points out, in part because epileptic lunatics are epileptics far advanced in their disease, and thus are unable to describe their symptoms exactly. The following is the quotation from Falret :

" Independently of these precursory symptoms, which may occur at a distance greater or less from the epileptic attack, there are other more immediate intellectual premonitory symptoms, a kind of intellectual aura, which precede the convulsive attack only by some minutes, and which constitute in some kind the first symptom of it. One sees, for example, some epileptics in whom the same idea, the same remembrance, or the same hallucination occurs spontaneously at the moment of commencement, and infallibly precedes its appearance. The patient sees flames, circles of fire, frequently the colour red or purple, a spectre, or a phantom ; he hears the noises of clocks or a determined voice which pronounces always one word ; sometimes he has finally a certain smell. *These ideas, these remembrances, these false sensations, which differ singularly in different patients, are generally reproduced with remarkable uniformity in the same patient at each new attack*."[1]

It is true that the study of the region affected in cases of palsy is easy ; we can do it quietly, whereas in the simplest epilepsies, those with convulsion, the motor affection is so sudden and so quickly over, that we may be tempted to deal in generalities, and especially to give a pictorial rather than a scientific description. But the work must be done. If we could safely omit it clinically, we could not physiologically. We must describe the paroxysms not only on a method analogous to that in which a gardener would describe a plant, but also in the deeper way in which a botanist would describe a plant ; we must observe analytically, *i.e.*, the relations of the several phenomena to one another, both in co-existence and in succession. To observe an epileptic paroxysm with a gardener-like mind would be to dwell most on the struggling, the foaming, the staring eyes, and the tongue-biting ; to describe it with a botanist-like mind would be to note where the first symptom showed itself, how the spasm spread, when consciousness was lost, etc. Both kinds of observation are essential, one for empirical, and one for scientific diagnosis.

In localising we shall not specially concern ourselves with the *condition* of the muscles in the range affected by convulsion. The *condition* of muscles tells us plainly what the functional nature of a lesion is—whether it be a destroying lesion or a discharging lesion. It is the regional affection which localises. It matters little for purposes of localisation *how* the muscles in any region are affected. Thus paralysis of the face, arm, and leg (hemiplegia), irregular movements of the face, arm, and leg (hemichorea), occasional spasm of the

[1] Falret continues : " It is curious to add that very often this remembrance, this idea, this image is the reproduction of the idea or sensation which provoked in the patient the first epileptic attack. Many among them, in fact, become epileptic after some strong moral emotion or profound terror, and see in their mind or under their eyes at each fresh attack the painful circumstances of the frightful scene which produced the disease in them the first time." These facts will be referred to later on.

face, arm, and leg (hemispasm), all point to lesions of the same cerebral region, although to different kinds of lesions of that cerebral region. We say that hemiplegia and hemispasm both depend on lesion of the same cerebral region, because the muscles affected are the same. We say, too, that the functional nature of the lesion in each is different, because in the hemiplegia, since the muscles are palsied, nerve tissue is destroyed, whilst in the hemispasm, since the muscles are in occasional spasm, that nerve tissue cannot be destroyed, but is unstable, and discharges occasionally.[1]

Very likely it will be denied that there can be a local lesion in many cases of epilepsy—for example, in those cases of convulsion with loss of consciousness, which are called genuine epilepsy by authorities. In these cases there is often a universal affection—convulsion all over the body. It seems at first glance unlikely that this should depend on a local discharging lesion in but one side of the brain. However, I believe it does ; I believe there is limited instability of some part of but one cerebral hemisphere in these cases. The evidence will be given when speaking of convulsion beginning locally and becoming universal. Again, there is often loss of consciousness at the onset, and it seems at first glance unlikely that a *local* discharge in but one of two cerebral hemispheres should cause this symptom—cause it as the very first thing, I mean. This will have to be considered later ; we have already replied indirectly to the objection in speaking of the different seats of varying consciousness. That pallor of the face should occur in these cases seems to me explicable by the fact, if I may call it one, that the vaso-motor system is represented in the cerebrum ; thus the arterial muscular coat suffers, as do the large muscles. For the present we shall take into consideration the simplest cases, those in which the external symptoms are partial, that is, cases in which some part only of the body is affected.

Of these cases we may say that the very fact that the movements are local (one-sided) shows there to be an internal local lesion. Local symptoms must of necessity depend on local lesions. If it were not so, all that has been written by all observers on localisation would be sheer nonsense. It is no answer to this remark to point out that a local symptom has been very transitory, or to say that there is only " functional " change in any sense of the word " functional." The point of first importance in localisation is not the degree of the symptom, but obviously its localness. And as to slightness of charge, if we were to hold some such vague hypothesis as that epilepsy or convulsion depends on a " polarisation of the molecules of nervous matter," then in a case of hemispasm there is *local* polarisation in nerve cells so long as the symptom continues to be presented. Or if we were to return to the oldest hypothesis—that there is Satanic possession—then in local seizures the possession must be of some part of the nervous system.

What is said of motor discharge applies also to sensory discharges. A fit which *begins* with coloured vision must depend on a discharge of a different part from one which begins by a sensation of smell or of sound, however much the seizures may resemble one another in their progress after the warning.

[1] I do not say that the *condition* of the muscles is of no value in localising. In a certain sense it is of very great value, as I shall point out later on. The region affected, however, is the most decisive evidence as to the seat of the lesion. I shall try to show that in discharges of the highest centres there is greater intensity of current from their discharge (greater quantity of nerve force in a given time), whilst in subordinate centres there is greater quantity of force from their discharge, and that this difference accords with the morphological difference, the sizes of the nerve cells. Thus from the kind of spasm we shall learn something as to the seat of the discharge.

We cannot now localise in many cases, but there is one thing we can do now—we can observe external symptoms in *an orderly manner*. It is just what we do in cases of palsy. We describe minutely the range of the palsy and minutely the degree in which the several paralysed parts suffer.

Of course the investigation does not end in the study of the parts affected in the paroxysm. We have already spoken at length on the pathology of such cases. We must, however, study the external symptoms carefully. It is not of much value nowadays to say that a tumour of the brain in the region of the middle cerebral artery produced convulsion (or epilepsy or an epileptiform seizure) unless we know what kind of convulsion it was, any more than it is of much value nowadays to say that a tumour of the corpus striatum produced paralysis unless we know what sort of paralysis there was.

It is believed, as aforesaid, that the discharging lesion of every epilepsy is a local one, and that on the beginning of the discharge depend the first symptoms of the paroxysm. Some of the further symptoms probably depend on discharge of healthy nerve tissue ; the unstable part gives rise to strong currents, which not only pass direct to muscles, but to lower healthy centres, and also probably by the intermediation of arterial contraction to neighbouring healthy centres and discharge them.

There seems to be great inconsistency in the commonly received or commonly acted upon principles of localisation. No one would think of denying permanent and complete hemiplegia to be the result of a local lesion, but when the case is a mobile affection of the very same muscles it is denied in effect, or rather it is ignored. The reason probably is that in the intervals of his fits the patient is apparently quite well. As has been several times stated, the principles of compensation and of dissolution fully explain the seeming discrepancy. If the patient's fits are local, frequently recur, and are always similarly localised, it is surely a necessary inference that there is some local disease in his nervous system.

It is equally obvious that if in two cases two different external parts are affected, in each there is a differently placed internal local lesion. It is no answer to this to bring evidence to show that most careful investigations have discovered no lesions post-mortem in such cases. This is very true indeed, but it is no objection to the method as method. Suppose a patient has occasionally a sudden stench in his nose, followed by loss of consciousness for a short time, we may not be able to declare where the lesion is. But it is still certain that there is a local lesion in some part of the nervous system, because a certain part of the body is affected (sensation locally referred). It is just as certain after a careful post-mortem examination which discloses no traces of local lesion. What is uncertain is the particular locality. To deny that partial external symptoms imply internal local lesions is to deny that there is any kind of organisation in the nervous system. If local external symptoms do not imply corresponding local internal lesions, it is, I repeat, sheer nonsense to attempt studying the localisation of nervous disease at all.

The minute study of epileptic or epileptiform convulsions has met with very little favour. We have, it is true, many descriptions of the "epileptic" paroxysm, but we have very few reports which give an exact description both of the muscles most convulsed, and of the order in which they are convulsed. And I know of few attempts to give an account of the whole of the phenomena which occur in the *simplest* cases of convulsions. The object seems often to be, from a very general view of the phenomena—such as the universality of convulsion, tongue-biting, loss of consciousness, etc.—to be able to say only whether the paroxysm be an epileptic one or not—whether it be epileptic or epileptiform. Thus we hear the diagnosis of cerebral hæmorrhage negatived because the patient had a fit of an " epileptic character." Yet the convulsion from cerebral hæmorrhage may be just like convulsion from many other causes, or it may be safer to say it has not been shown to be different. In all severe convulsions the patient may bite his tongue.[1]

Of course convulsions from a clot in one side of the brain, due to sudden breaking up of grey matter, or to irritation by the suddenly intruding foreign body, are utterly different, *pathologically*, from chronic cases of epilepsy ; but they have their counterparts anatomically.

I have no doubt that to some these remarks will be mere truisms. But I know well that by others the principle will be denied, and by many it is ignored. It seems to me to be denied in effect by those who attribute local seizures to very general conditions as their sole causes. This is not at all uncommon. For example, cases of convulsion beginning in one hand, affecting the face, arm, and leg of but one side, are attributed to fright, and we even hear of emotional hemiplegia. Almost always there is only evidence of sequence. No one of course denies that fright produces certain severe nervous symptoms ; but where is the evidence that it produces any local nervous symptom ? and where is the evidence that it is in cases of epilepsy more than an exciting cause of the discharge of some part of the nervous system already unstable ? The principle is ignored by those who do not attempt to study regional spasm in as realistic a way as they do regional palsy. But these may ignore it for the intelligible reason that it is not practicable, or that, if practicable, it is a kind of work not worth doing.

It must be particularly borne in mind that there are all degrees of seizures, or, as we may say, all degrees of discharge. When the discharge is slight and limited we have a development only of the most special movements and impressions represented in the part unstable. Thus there may be spasm of the index-finger only, red vision only, subjective sensation of smell only, or a feeling at the epigastrium which is, I think, a crude development of certain systemic sensations. For these the word " aura " is often used as synonymous with warning and sometimes there is the warning only—the fit is abortive. These are developments of what is *most* represented in the part discharged. Similarly there may be loss of consciousness. This, and even only defect of consciousness (confusion of thought), stands in the same category as the earliest symptom developed.[2] What I wish now to assert is that a so-called aura is not a fit of a

[1] Under Diagnosis Jaccoud says, in his article on Epilepsy : " A ne considérer que l'attaque elle-même, l'épilepsie ne diffère pas de l'ECLAMPSIE ; mais cette dernière, qui est un *symptôme*, et non pas une *maladie*, est caracterisée par la répétition des accès coup sur coup, par la rapidité de la terminaison, mortelle ou favorable, et par les conditions étiologiques spéciales qui lui donnent naissance (puerpéralité, urémie, intoxication saturnine ; chez les enfants, dentition, irritation intestinale). LES TUMEURS CEREBRALES, et plus généralement les lesions de l'encéphale, provoquent souvent, par l'action directe ou à distance qu'elles exercent sur la bulbe, des convulsions dites *épileptiformes* ; la similitude de ces accès et de ceux de l'épilepsie légitime peut être absolument complète, c'est donc dans la situation de malade pendant l'intervalle des attaques que doivent être cherchés les caractères différentiels."

[2] Of course, strictly, the comparison is not that affection of consciousness in discharge of the highest nervous arrangements is analogous to spasm of the hand from discharge of a subordinate series ; the comparison is betwixt the earliest movements (for we can here learn nothing about sensation) developed in those excessive discharges of the highest nerve centres during which consciousness ceases and the spasm of the hand.

different kind from one which goes on to universal convulsion. It is an aborted paroxysm. Loss of consciousness, however, is not commonly called a warning, nor of course could it be one to the patient. It is not here a word and a blow, but a blow first, and only. Instead, then, of aura or warning, we shall use the expression first symptom, including in that both what the patient can tell us and what we see. Spasm of the index-finger, subjective sensation of smell, loss of consciousness, are all due to the beginning of a discharge leading to development in a brutal form of the impressions and movements most represented in the unstable discharging part.

A paroxysm of spasm of the hand (tonic followed by clonic) is not, then, a *different* kind of fit from one which, beginning also in the hand, spreads all over the body. It is a fit of slighter degree. The proof is that patients who have partial fits often have also fits which, beginning like the partial ones do, become universal. Again, there are all degrees from epileptic vertigo through *petit-mal* to *grand-mal*; but they are not different kinds of fits. They are, however, not differences of simple degree, but of compound degree.

Another thing to be carefully noted in paroxysms of convulsions is the march of the spasm. A patient may have convulsion varying in degree from that slight degree in which the index-finger and thumb only are convulsed to universal convulsion. We have to note how it *becomes* universal. Let us take an arbitrary limit for illustration. We will suppose we witness a paroxysm in which the convulsion affects the whole of one side of the body, that of course in which the spasm begins. It most often begins in the hand; and we will suppose we witness such a case. We have to note how one part of the arm after another is affected; at what stage the face is affected; how the spasm spreads over it; if the spasm goes up or down the leg, and so on. We should then be able to say not only that the part discharged represented the index-finger and thumb, but that it (and other centres of grey matter directly controlled by it) represented certain other movements in subordination to the movements of these digits and in a particular order of subordination.

## VIII

### Recapitulation—The Method Exemplified

We have in each case of epilepsy three lines of investigation: Physiological, which deals with abnormal Function of nerve tissue; Anatomical, which deals with abnormalities of particular Structures (organs); and Pathological, which deals with abnormalities of Nutrition. Or, putting these in their most abstract form and in reverse order, we have to study defects in the Absorption, in the Distribution, and in the Expenditure of nerve force. The threefold method of investigation will now be exemplified.

1. *Physiology.*—We assume that there is a permanent local "discharging lesion" in every epilepsy. The "discharging lesion" is a permanent instability of grey matter; this unstable grey matter occasionally discharges and the discharge produces effects in, or referred to, the periphery of the body.

2. *Anatomical.*—I try, in *each* case where there is a paroxysmal presentation of symptoms, to find the seat of the "discharging lesion" corresponding to them. In any case—let us suppose, however, it is one of convulsion—the question is not "Is it a case of epilepsy?" but "Where is the unstable grey matter which permits the occasional excessive discharge on muscles in this

case ?" "Of the function of which part of the cerebral hemisphere is the convulsion the brutal development ?" Let us put this in another way. If we were present at an autopsy disclosing local gross disease of the cerebral cortex in one who had died subject to convulsions, the question would *not* be "Were the fits which this local disease produce epileptic ?" but "What symptoms resulted from the sudden discharge of unstable grey matter near the gross lesion in this case ?" If it be replied that the seizures were like those of the "genuine epilepsy" of authorities, we do not consider the reply sufficiently definite, and repeat the question. For paroxysms of "genuine epilepsy" differ, and therefore the seats of the discharging lesions *must* differ. If it be true that epilepsy is owing to disease of the medulla oblongata, different parts of the medulla must be diseased in cases where the paroxysms differ.

3. *Pathological.*—The question in pathology is not "What causes epilepsy ?" but "What pathological processes lead to local 'discharging lesions'?" "What is the nature of the abnormal nutritive process by which the cells of grey matter become over-nourished and thus unstable ?" Inquiries as to the so-called "causes" of epilepsy are wide of the mark if they do not bear directly on this question. I do not mean that empirical inquiries as to what are called "causes" of the supposed entity "genuine epilepsy" are not valuable; but I think they are only valuable as heaps of unassorted material towards determining the real direct pathology of "discharging lesion." Many of these "causes" are simply things determining the first discharge of grey matter already unstable.

It is in accordance with scientific method to study first the simplest problems. No one with any great scientific feeling would study defects of speech before he had studied hemiplegia, or "diseases of the mind" before he had studied the coarser and simpler diseases of the nervous system. Similarly it would be contrary to scientific method to study first the complex, suddenly-occurring and transitory paroxysms of "genuine epilepsy" before studying those simpler cases of epilepsy which are commonly called "epileptiform seizures."

As we have seen, there are within the limits of my definition of epilepsy all kinds and degrees of phenomena in the paroxysms resulting from "discharging lesions" of numerous different parts of the brain. Any part of the cerebral cortex may become unstable—either its sensory or its motor region. The motor phenomena, for obvious reasons, are more easily studied. Our illustration must, then, be an epilepsy in which convulsion is the chief thing. But there are varieties of these. I have paid most attention to those cases of convulsion which begin deliberately in some part of one side of the body, in the hand for example. These are of all convulsive seizures the simplest; they are far more easily studied than cases of "genuine epilepsy." In many cases of "genuine epilepsy" there is no warning or there is but a vague one; the convulsion is usually universal, nearly equal on the two sides of the body, and the spasm of different parts is more nearly contemporaneous. Moreover the fit comes on suddenly and is rapidly over. On the other hand, convulsions beginning unilaterally are opposite in all these respects and are the very simplest epilepsies we can study: let me state the reasons categorically.

1st. Because, since the spasm begins long before the patient loses consciousness and because it sets in slowly, he can tell us much about his seizure. We can thus learn upon what muscular region the first discharge is, if we can learn no more. In some cases of limited convulsion there is neither loss nor defect of consciousness. In the convulsion of " genuine epilepsy " we learn from the patient or from his friends very little more than that there was much struggling, tongue-biting, and other facts which are not of great use in an inquiry like ours.

2nd. Because, since the spasm is often deliberate, we can ourselves when luckily present at a paroxysm note the place of onset and watch the march of the spasm. We learn what parts it affects first and most, how far it spreads, and in what order. In " genuine epilepsy " the spasm is so sudden, so rapidly universal, and so soon over that it is difficult to observe the details of what takes place.

3rd. Because unilateral convulsion not unfrequently leaves a temporary hemiplegia which writes down, so to speak, the parts which in the paroxysm were first and most affected. This of itself is strong, indeed I think conclusive evidence as to the position of the discharging lesion.

4th. Because it has frequently the very definite temporary complication of affection of speech (aphasia), or of optic neuritis (with or without amaurosis). When there is optic neuritis we can infer so much of the pathology of the case as that the " discharging lesion " is the result of the irritation of coarse disease of some kind (" injury " by coarse disease), or, as it is commonly expressed, we can say that there is organic disease.

5th. Because, since it is the form of epilepsy which depends most frequently on organic disease, we may obtain post-mortem disproof or verification of the diagnosis of locality we made during life. We can from the position of the coarse disease infer the seat of the minute changes of instability which constituted the discharging lesion.

6th.—From these cases we learn how arbitrary the distinction is into cases with, and cases without, loss of consciousness, for in convulsions beginning unilaterally there may or may not be affection of consciousness ; all depends on the severity of the discharge, on how far it spreads, and on the rapidity of the discharge.

This kind of convulsion I have named variously Unilateral Convulsion, Hemiplegic Epilepsy, Corpus Striatum Epilepsy, and Convulsion beginning Unilaterally. I am not enamoured of any of these terms. Corpus striatum epilepsy seems to me useful as bringing into prominence the analogies betwixt these convulsions and varieties of hemiplegia. " Convulsion beginning unilaterally " is a term not strictly defensible, as the convulsion in the epilepsy of authorities often begins by preponderance of movement on one side. It is, however, the one least open to objection.

The reader is again reminded that I consider the " genuine epilepsy " of authorities to be but one epilepsy in my definition. It differs from convulsion beginning unilaterally simply in difference in the seat of the " discharging lesion." In it the grey matter unstable is that of sensori-motor arrangements which are the highest of all—the series of series ; in the convulsion beginning unilaterally those of a subordinate series are unstable. This is the reason why, in the former, loss of consciousness is the first or nearly the first thing in the paroxysm, and that in the latter it is a later event. Those who say that the two differ " only in degree " make a remark the truth of which is admitted. In both there are occasional excessive and disorderly expenditures of force on muscles, the discharge depending on instability of nervous tissue. *But in what kind of degree do they differ ?* Not merely in degree of more or less spasm—

more or less instability of nervous tissue—but also in degree of evolution of the nervous arrangements which are unstable. A convulsion which is universal and in which the muscular regions affected are affected nearly contemporaneously, must depend on excessive discharge of parts in which the nervous arrangements represent a *more intricate* co-ordination of movements in space and in time than those parts represent, excessive discharge of which produce a convulsion which begins in one limb and has a deliberate march all over the body. My speculation is that the first kind of convulsion differs from the second in that convolutions at a greater distance from the motor tract—that is, nervous centres of a higher degree of evolution—are discharged.

Let me state some of the differences betwixt " genuine epilepsy " and convulsions beginning unilaterally, in tabular form. In either case there may be a partial fit, or in other words there may be a slight and limited discharge. Thus there may be only vertigo and confusion of thought in the former, and in the latter numbness of the hand and spasm of the thumb and index-finger. But we shall take for comparison cases in which the fits are severe and the convulsions universal.

| *Genuine Epilepsy of Authorities.* | *Unilaterally beginning Convulsion.* |
|---|---|
| 1. No warning or a transient one. | A warning deliberate and local. |
| 2. Consciousness lost very early. | Consciousness lost late. |
| 3. Spasm often universal. | Spasm often limited. |
| 4. Spasm *begins* nearly contemporaneously—on two sides of body, *i.e.* is nearly universal at once. | Spasm *not* contemporaneous on two sides of body, *i.e. becomes* universal by degrees. |
| 5. Spasm nearly equal on the two sides. | Spasm very unequal on two sides. |
| 6. March of spasm rapid and quickly over (currents of " great intensity "). | March of spasm deliberate and lengthy. (Currents of great quantity.) |

Unless we have well studied the phenomena of discharges of subordinate centres we are not properly prepared for the study of the phenomena resulting from discharge of the highest centres—the centres evolved out of the subordinate centres—that is to say, cases of the " genuine epilepsy " of the authorities.[1]

From a simple case of the group of unilaterally beginning convulsion I can illustrate the three lines of investigation of an epilepsy. The investigation is to be on the same style as that of a case of paralysis. In the paralysis, as well as in the convulsion, there is a physiological, an anatomical, and a pathological inquiry. We can, indeed, compare and contrast a case of hemispasm with one of hemiplegia. We speak of the common form of hemiplegia, that so often caused by destruction of the corpus striatum by clot or softening.

*Physiology.*—In each we begin by determining the physiology of the case, *i.e.* the functional condition of nerve tissue. In hemiplegia nerve tissue is destroyed, in hemispasm there is clear evidence of instability, for there is every

[1] Cases of migraine are the sensory analogues of the unilaterally beginning convulsion. The cases of " genuine epilepsy " of authorities which begin by " subjective " sensations stand, I suppose, in the same relation to them as the cases of genuine epilepsy which begin by " subjective " movements do to the unilaterally beginning convulsion.

now and then a discharge. In one there is loss of function; in the other there is over-function. Thus the first step—the physiological—is easy in each case.

*Anatomy.*—As the epileptic discharge results in convulsion of the very same parts as are paralysed in the hemiplegia, and as we know that this paralytic symptom is due to destruction of, or of part of, the corpus striatum, I conclude that the discharge is of convolutions in the region of the corpus striatum.

Before we can with confidence point to the particular parts of the convolutional region which is unstable, we must have more autopsies in well-observed cases. Hitzig and Ferrier's work is, however, what will be of most use in these investigations.

*Pathology.*—The third step is the pathology. Just as in hemiplegia, so in this case; we have to find the pathological process which *leads* to the physiological or functional change. In hemiplegia the question is, " By what pathological process was the *destruction* of the nerve fibres and cells of the corpus striatum produced ? " In the epilepsy, " By what pathological process did the instability of the grey matter of the convolutions result ? "

In the former case our task is comparatively easy. If the hemiplegic patient be past middle age; if he have Bright's disease, rigid arteries, and hypertrophy of the left ventricle, and if his paralysis came on with deep loss of consciousness, we say the destruction of the corpus striatum is by clot. If he have no Bright's disease, and if the paralysis comes on deliberately, for example in a quarter of an hour, without any loss of consciousness, we say there is local softening from thrombosis of an atheromatous artery. (It is needless to give further illustrations.) In the case of hemispasm our task is far more difficult. We ask, first, " Is the local instability the result of a ' coarse ' change, such as tumour, or not ? " If there be severe pain, vomiting, and double optic neuritis, we say there is " coarse disease." We have then to ask, " Is this coarse disease glioma, syphilis, abscess ? " The differential diagnosis cannot be entered on here. Let us suppose we can only conclude that there is a coarse change of some kind. In such cases the inference is that the neighbouring grey matter has become unstable by the irritation of the coarse disease. If, however, we find no evidence of the existence of coarse disease we mostly do not trace the pathological process.[1] We often do not even at post-mortem examinations. We discover neither local disease of the cerebral hemisphere nor disease of the medulla oblongata. We often discover no local abnormality in any part of the nervous system.

This method, which from long working at seems to me to be simple, will appear just the contrary to those who have worked in a diametrically opposite way. It will seem more simple to first determine by general evidence whether a case be one of " genuine epilepsy " or not—whether it does or does not conform to some authoritative definition. Next, supposing the diagnosis to be that it *is* a case of " genuine epilepsy," to investigate its causes—the causes of some entity, " the causes of epilepsy." As has been said, the method I have been illustrating cannot be fully carried out in most cases, but it can be carried out as far as the orthodox plan can. The orthodox teaching assumes not only the physiology, but the anatomy. That is to say, it assumes that it is proved not only that epilepsy depends on increased excitability, but also that the part

[1] Inquiry for conditions allowing embolism and thrombosis (including venous thrombosis resulting from aural disease) should be made. (See Chap. vi.)

over-excitable is the medulla oblongata. As to pathology, the orthodox opinion is certainly in no better case. We all fail in tracing the steps of the abnormal nutritive process by which grey matter anywhere (whether in the medulla or brain) becomes unstable so that it discharges occasionally. When we do discover a gross lesion or local change post-mortem, we do not even then find out *how* any part of the cerebrum or the medulla oblongata has become unstable as a consequence of that disease. It is, I suppose, the consequence of an inflammation excited by the gross lesion.

## IX

### Unilaterally Beginning Convulsion

In the last chapter we spoke of unilaterally beginning convulsion merely in order to illustrate the method of investigation of epilepsies in general. We now consider this class of cases in detail.

They are in our definition of the term Epilepsies. They are, I consider, the results of discharging lesions beginning in subordinate nervous centres—*viz.* in the convolutions which are near to the corpus striatum. They are, as has been repeatedly stated, the mobile counterparts of cases of that unilateral paralysis which depends on " destroying lesion " of the corpus striatum. The rule is that these fits begin in those *parts* which *suffer most* in cases of hemiplegia—(1) hand, (2) face, or tongue, or both, (3) foot. This is an illustration of the law of dissolution. For both in hemiplegia and in these convulsions the parts which suffer first and most are those which have the most varied uses—that is, parts in the order above given. The seizures which begin in the hand are the mobile counterparts of those cases of hemiplegia in which the arm suffers more than the leg. These are the commonest cases of hemiplegia and of unilaterally beginning convulsion. The fits which begin in the face are the analogues of those cases of hemiplegia in which there is a complication of aphasia. (In the convulsion there is stoppage of speech at the onset, and speech may be left temporarily impaired when the discharge is over.) This is the next commonest corresponding pair of cases. Fits which begin in the foot are the analogues of those cases of hemiplegia where the paralysis affects the leg most. This pair is least common.

We see that the order of *frequency* in which parts suffer also illustrates the law of dissolution. Fits beginning in the hand are commonest; next in frequency are those which begin in the face or tongue, and rarest are those which begin in the foot. The law is exemplified in details. When the fit begins in the hand, the index-finger and thumb are usually the digits first seized; when in the face, the side of the cheek is first in spasm; when in the foot, almost invariably the great toe. These facts are very significant.

It is very interesting that Ferrier's independent researches confirm the general principle regarding the modes of onset of these convulsions so far as experiments on lower animals can be supposed to be comparable with the experiments disease makes on man. (The parts which have the most varied uses will not be the same in each animal.)

The following general remarks will show how the mode of onset of convulsive seizures illustrates the law of dissolution:

In this group of fits the spasm " prefers," so to speak, to begin in those parts which have the more voluntary uses; in other words, in those parts which have the more leading, independent, separate, and varied movements; in other words still, in those parts the movements of which are last acquired (" educated "). In strict physiological definition, a voluntary part—the hand, for example—is one which has the greater number of *different* movements at the greater number of *different* intervals;[1] shortly, the more " varied " uses. An automatic part—the chest, for example—is one which has the greater number of more nearly like movements at the greater number of more nearly equal intervals; shortly, the more " similar " uses.

That convulsions which begin in the hand begin in most cases in the thumb and index-finger—in the most " voluntary " parts of the whole body—is a very significant thing. The thumb and index-finger are the most voluntary or specialised parts of the body; they have the most varied uses. The thumb in man has a distinct flexor longus pollicis. In the *Anthropomorpha*, Huxley (" The Anatomy of Vertebrate Animals ") says: " The *flexor pollicis* is more or less closely connected with the *flexor communis perforans* or with that part of the muscle which goes to the index digit." On the intellectual importance of this muscle Duchenne insists strongly. " En somme, ces faits cliniques demontrent que le long fléchisseur du pouce est l'un des muscles qui sont essentiellement destiné, chez l'homme, aux usages manuels les plus delicats; à tenir et à conduire la plume, le crayon, le pinceau, l'aiguille, etc.; qu'il aide, en un mot, à l'exécution des travaux manuels qui sont à la hauteur de son intelligence supérieure " (*Physiology of Movements*, p. 251). And in his work on *Electrisation* he says that when the small muscles of the thenar eminence are atrophied, the hand loses its distinctive human character and approaches that of the monkey. The thumb in the monkey is less specialised than in man. If, then, we discover in a monkey the homologue of the centre discharged in man causing fits beginning in the thumb and index-finger, we shall expect from *its* discharge a fit of a less special kind; for example, not a fit beginning in the animal's pollex, but more likely one beginning in the whole of its five comparatively little differentiated digits at once, if not in the whole arm.

It is not supposed that there are abrupt demarcations betwixt the two kinds of movements. Movements of the shoulder (intermediate betwixt the arm and the thorax) may be considered as " voluntary " when compared with those of the chest, and automatic when compared with those of the forearm; they are more " varied " than the movements of the chest, and more " similar " than those of the forearm.

An automatic part may possibly be more *often* in movement than a voluntary part, and thus it may in a sense be said to have more movements. But we are speaking of numerous *different* movements. The numerous movements of an automatic part are often but repetitions of one kind of movement in different degrees, or the persistence of one movement, or of several allied movements. Thus, the muscles of the spine are always in action except in sleep (I am not here referring to mere tone of muscles). But the movements of these muscles when most varied, as in walking, are comparatively little varied; in standing or in sitting there is scarcely any variation in their action; there is little more than one continuous " tetanoid " contraction. Moreover, what is just as important, when in their most varied action there are fewer distinct intervals; indeed, the movements glide into one another. But there are parts which have

[1] It will be seen that the definition takes count of what I have called Time Co-ordination. There is a melody of movement as well as a harmony of movement.

fewer variations in their movements than even the muscles of the back. Indeed, the ciliary muscle has but one kind of movement, although an infinite number of degrees of that movement.[1]

It is, however, granted that convulsion may begin in any part of the region which is paralysed in hemiplegia, for example, in the shoulder, thigh, etc. I speak in this chapter of the cases which are most common. It is a very important matter in the physiology of epilepsies that the spasm "prefers" the parts which have the most varied uses. We saw (see p. 216) that the parts whose muscles are represented in the greater number of *different* movements would be represented by the greater *quantity* of grey matter.

Spencer has pointed out that the quantity of grey matter in an animal's nervous system varies not so much with the size of its muscles as with the complexity of its movements; or we may put the principle in more detail, that the quantity of grey matter varies not so much with the size of the muscles of a part as with the number of different movements of that part. Thus the small muscles of the hand will be represented by much more grey matter in the highest centres than will be the large muscles of the upper arm, because they serve in more numerous different movements. It is equally obvious that the larger quantity of grey matter representing numerous *different* movements must be made up of a great number of separate parts. Each movement, so far as it differs from all others, must have so far special representation in the nervous centre. Greater differentiation of function implies greater physical separation. There must be separate representation, however little different the movement may be from other movements, and however much of it may be a reco-ordination of other movements. So far as there is a degree of independence of movement, so far must there be a degree of separateness of representation of that movement by distinct cells in the nervous centres.[2] And yet, of course, the separa-

[1] I requote the following from an article I published in *British Medical Journal*, May 10, 1873:

"The significance of the fact, that the hand is the part in which convulsions, beginning unilaterally, most often start; that the arm suffers first, or most, or both, in the greater number of motor affections from brain disease (hemiplegia, chorea, paralysis agitans), will be better realised after reading Herbert Spencer's remarks on tactual organs, in chap. viii, vol. i, p. 359 of his *Psychology* (second edition), from which I give these extracts.

"He points out and shows the significance of the 'striking instances which the animal kingdom presents of unusual sagacity co-existing with unusual development of organs, which, by the help of complex muscular arrangements, give complex tactual impressions.' After remarking, that it will perhaps be difficult to understand why *touch*, the simplest and earliest sense, should in its higher forms be more than any other sense associated with the advance of intelligence, he says: 'The explanation lies in the fact that tactual impressions are those into which all other impressions have to be translated before their meanings can be known.' Of the human hand: 'All that we need here notice is, the extent to which, in the human race, a perfect tactual apparatus subserves the highest processes of the intellect. I do not mean merely that the tangible attributes of things have been rendered completely cognisable by the complex and versatile adjustments of the human hands, and that the accompanying manipulative powers have made possible those populous societies in which alone a wide intelligence can be evolved. I mean that the *most far-reaching cognitions, and inferences the most remote from perception*, have their roots in the definitely combined impressions which *the human hands* can conceive.' [No italics in original.]

"The study of cases of disease of the nervous system appears to me to supply continual illustrations of the correctness of many of Spencer's deductions."

In an article, *Lancet*, February 15, 1873, p. 75, also I referred to the above remarks by Spencer, and pointed out that cases of hemiplegia and unilateral convulsion with lateral deviation of the eyes show us part of the physical process for the "translation" of visual ideas into tactual ones. I there also refer to the corresponding sensory symptoms, hemiopia and hemianæsthesia.

[2] It seems to me to accord with this that the highest centres (anterior and posterior lobes) have smallest cells. Hitzig and Ferrier's points of excitation, that is to say, the subordinate motor centres, have many very large cells. I should, for theoretical reasons, expect that of the subordinate centres, those which represent movements in small muscles (eyes, face, and hands)

tion is not isolation ; on the contrary, the greater the differentiation, the more complete the integration of the separate elements, for they have to act together or in succession.

Each of these varieties of fits beginning unilaterally depends, I believe, on discharge of the nervous arrangements of some particular series. The mode of onset gives us a clue to the series. Thus, those convulsions which begin in the hand are supposed to depend on a discharge beginning in parts of the cerebrum where the hand is largely represented in movements to which other movements (those of the arms, eyes, and leg) are sequent and subordinate. It is probably a discharge of the motor element in the substrata of tactual ideas. Convulsions which begin in the side of the mouth or tongue probably depend on discharges of centres which are the substrata of words. Again, in fits beginning in the foot the internal part discharged contains nervous arrangements for certain movements of the foot and lower limb, to which certain other movements (those of the upper limb) are sequent and subordinate. In *this* series the foot has the leading representation. Hence the remark that the mode of onset is the most important matter in the paroxysm for our consideration. *It points to the part of the brain which discharges, or where the discharge begins.* The leading movements are developed first. As is thus implied, I do not believe that nervous centres represent limited regions of muscles, nor even isolated groups of movements. There are parts where, for example, the ocular, manual, and pedal movements have the *leading* representation. This statement implies the further belief that any part, especially such a one as the hand, is represented in innumerable places. Hence " compensation " (never absolute) in " destroying lesions." The seizure may be limited or universal ; there are all degrees of range. But it is to be observed that when universal it becomes universal ; the spasm is not at once contemporaneous ; it is a sequence. It begins in a certain part in each patient, with rare exceptions, in the same part, and *spreads* over the body. Probably in no case of convulsions, even in those of " genuine epilepsy," is the convulsion ever universal in the sense that the whole of the muscles of the two sides of the body are convulsed absolutely equally and quite contemporaneously. In those cases of epilepsy where the spasm is nearly universal and contemporaneous, there is some part which suffers somewhat sooner, as well as some part (one side) which suffers somewhat more. Indeed, it follows from the doctrines of evolution that there may be all degrees of difference, from cases in which the spasm begins very locally, very deliberately, and spreads very gradually, to cases in which the discharge is sudden and nearly universal at once. In the former there is discharge of lower, in the latter of highest centres.[1]

The reader will note that there are two *kinds* of difference here spoken of—(1) that convulsions depending on discharge of lower centres will begin deliberately in parts and spread to other parts, whilst the convulsions from discharges of higher centres will be more nearly universal at once ; (2) the discharge in the

will have cells comparatively small—smaller than the cells superintending movements of the large muscles of the limbs, but not so small as the cells of the very highest centres. As previously suggested it is probable that instability of numerous small cells will produce currents of greater " intensity " than instability of the same quantity of grey matter in few large cells ; or it may be more correct to say that when small and large cells are subjected to the same abnormal nutrition the small cells sooner become unstable.

[1] We have, however, to bear in mind that certain regions of the nervous system are more liable to damage than others, and it is significant that, as a matter of fact, there are two large groups of cases with few intermediate cases.

former will be slower than in the latter; it will be of less "intensity." In what follows we limit ourselves to the unilaterally beginning seizures.

A patient may have attacks of spasm limited to the hand, or even to one finger, or to the arm. A patient may have spasm of one side of the face only, or spasm of one foot or of one toe. It not unfrequently happens that the patient has limited fits before he has his first one becoming universal. Both the limited fits and those becoming universal begin in the same part. The patient who has been long subject to fits may have on one occasion a partial fit, and on another a universal seizure. Thus, suppose the fit to begin in the right index-finger and thumb, there may be one day twitching almost limited to these digits, another day the arm may be in spasm, on another occasion the whole of the right side is seized, on another occasion the spasm may spread to the left side—the patient becomes universally convulsed. Hence, then, we have to speak not only of ranges of the spasm, but of the order in which parts are involved in any range—sequence of spasm. In observing a paroxysm we have to note both with care.

Let us take in illustration a case in which the spasm begins in the hand: (*a*) We note the complete range of the convulsion; for example, we may have to say "the spasm involved the arm, face, and leg of the right side; (*b*) we note the order in which it "went over" the parts of that range; as, for example, we may have to say, "it began in the hand, passed up the arm, attacked next the face, passed down the leg." We shall afterwards point out that this sequence is a compound sequence, although, for convenience, it is here spoken of as if it were simple.

We shall speak of range first. We have above admitted that there are all degrees of range, from spasm so local as twitching of one finger to universal convulsion. But we shall make three degrees of range. They are entirely arbitrary and yet convenient:

1st. The spasm affects the most voluntary muscles of one side—face, arm, and leg. This is the analogue of the first degree of hemiplegia. It will be convenient to call the side first affected the "first side." But there is the discrepancy that some muscles of the trunk are convulsed on both sides.

2nd. It affects the most voluntary and other muscles more automatic. This is the analogue of the second degree of hemiplegia.

3rd. It effects all these and the unilateral muscles of the other side of the body (we call this the "second side"). This is the analogue of the third degree of, or rather degree of paralysis beyond, hemiplegia.

There are not only three degrees, but also several varieties of hemiplegia. We speak of degrees of that kind of hemiplegia only in which the arm suffers more than the leg; these three degrees from destroying lesions of different degrees of gravity of the corpus striatum correspond to the three degrees of convulsion.

*First Degree* [1]

| *Corpus Striatum Palsy.* | *Corpus Striatum Epilepsy.* |
|---|---|
| Right side of face paralysed. | Mouth drawn to right. |
| Right arm paralysed. | Right arm convulsed. |
| Right leg paralysed. | Right leg convulsed. |
| | Chest fixed on both sides. |

[1] I have never, in a case of convulsion affecting one side, made trustworthy observations on the tongue and palate.

The muscles of the chest in this degree of convulsion are involved on both sides, that is, they are involved on both sides when the unilateral muscles are involved but on one side. Yet, in cases of the first degree of hemiplegia, they are not involved. Here is a discrepancy to be carefully considered.[1]

The difficulty is cleared by what is known as Broadbent's Hypothesis. Broadbent supposes that the muscles acting bilaterally are represented in each side of even the highest division of the motor tract. Let us take the extreme case of the intercostal muscles to illustrate his hypothesis. He supposes that the nucleus in the cord, for these muscles on one side, is united by a commissure with the nucleus for the fellow-muscles of the other side; thus the two nuclei become in effect a single nucleus—a "unified double," I will call it. By fibres from each corpus striatum to each nucleus, both nuclei are put under the control of each side of the brain. This hypothesis explains satisfactorily how it happens that the intercostal muscles on *both* sides can escape in destroying lesions of one of the corpora striata notwithstanding that they are or rather were represented in the centre destroyed. Let us suppose that part of the left corpus is destroyed; no palsy of either side of the chest results; this is because the fibres which pass from the other—the right—corpus striatum are intact, and can act not only on their own nucleus in the cord, but by commissural fibres on the twin nucleus. Now let us speak of the *discharge* of the convolutions near to the corpus striatum, practically for our present illustration of a discharge of that centre itself. Broadbent's hypothesis is in entire accord with the fact that the bilateral muscles are put in action on *both* sides. The current from the discharged corpus striatum will discharge the nucleus of its own (opposite) side, and by the commissure the twin nucleus. The discharge will therefore put the intercostal muscles in action on both sides.

There are certain objections to this hypothesis. In the first place it may be denied that the intercostal muscles escape paralysis on the side hemiplegic from destroying lesion of the corpus striatum. To this objection it might be replied that authorities differ as to the fact, so that there is no appeal to them. Nevertheless, I am prepared to grant that in large lesions, and very soon after the attack in small lesions, the chest on that side on which the face, arm, and leg are paralysed may expand less than the other. But it is quite certain that the muscles are but slightly affected—so little, I repeat, that some authorities deny that they suffer at all.

After all the principle of the hypothesis remains intact. Subject to the correction of its distinguished propounder, I would say that its principle is "that the more muscles are bilateral in their action, the more equally are the muscles of both sides represented in each side of the brain." At any rate this is what

[1] I use the expressions "unilateral" and "bilateral" here for the *action* of the muscles. The muscles of the arm, leg, and some of those of the face can be used independently of their fellows of the other side of the body. Perhaps in strictness we ought to admit that the movements of parts which are most independent in their action are not absolutely so. But, for our present purpose, this would be hypercriticism; they can be used differently from their fellows on the other side. Other muscles, as those of the chest, must move with their fellows of the other side; they are bilateral *in their action* or very nearly so. There are no abrupt demarcations betwixt the two classes of movements. From the most independently unilateral movements of the hand to the necessarily bilateral movements of the chest there are intermediate degrees, as we have remarked.

The expressions "unilateral of one side" and "bilateral of both sides" are not tautological, since they are abbreviations of the expressions "muscles of one side which can act independently of their fellows on the other side," and "muscles which must act with their fellows on the other side."

I think. I have carried the hypothesis further than Broadbent, but, again subject to his approval, I should say that I have added nothing to the principle of that hypothesis. Were it proved that Broadbent's opinion as to the particular mechanism by which bilateral action is ensured is wrong, the principle of his hypothesis would remain.

I have been, from the first moment when I heard Broadbent's hypothesis stated, strongly impressed with its great value. I published cases confirmatory of it, *Lancet*, vol. i, 1867 (" The Regional Study of Palsy and Spasm "), and *Medical Times and Gazette*, August 15, 1868 (" Case of Corpus Striatum Epilepsy (Hemispasm ").[1]

We now come to the second pair of correlated symptoms.

### *Second Degree*

A graver lesion of the corpus striatum produces the paralytic symptoms named in the next list, and there is a further degree of convulsion which corresponds. As we are now speaking only of range, as distinct from sequence, we give the symptoms in order from above downwards in the body.

| *Corpus Striatum Palsy.* | *Corpus Striatum Epilepsy* |
|---|---|
| Head turns to left. | Head drawn to right. |
| Two eyes turn to left. | Two eyes drawn to right. |
| Face turns to left. | Face drawn to right. |
| Chest muscles slower and weaker. | Chest muscles in spasm. |
| Trunk muscles weaker on right. | Trunk muscles in spasm on right. (?) |
| Arm and leg paralysed on right. | Arm and leg in spasm on right. |

### *Third Degree*

In the third degree of unilaterally beginning convulsions the spasm becomes universal. Both sides of the body are affected. I believe that this results from a discharging lesion in but one cerebral hemisphere, as do the first and second degree—that it is the result of a severer discharge. But it will be asked, Where are the paralytic symptoms from destroying lesion on *one* side of the brain which pair off with the spasms of the " second " side in the third degree of convulsions ? The spasm after affecting the unilateral muscles of the right side affects next those of the *left*. What in—or of course beyond—hemiplegia corresponds to the spasm of the left, the second, side ? There is, I think, a third degree of hemiplegia in which the whole of the muscles of the body are

[1] I think the hypothesis is valuable in many ways. I still think of it as I did (*Medical Times and Gazette*, August 15, 1868), when I wrote " Remarks on Broadbent's Hypothesis : Broadbent's hypothesis, *mutatis mutandis*, helps us towards a clearer idea of the most general nature of the defects of intellectual expression, and strikingly to the explanation of the involuntary utterances of those patients who cannot speak voluntarily. The fact that patients who cannot speak voluntarily can utter words involuntarily shows that there are sensori-motor processes for words *somewhere* in their brains. And just as " innate " bilateral movements are represented in each of the corpora striata, so acquired processes, when they have become automatic, may also be represented doubly. . . . Moreover, it will be found, I think, that cases of double hemiplegia confirm Broadbent's hypothesis. With regard to this, however, I will content myself by urging those who observe defective bilateral movements with hemiplegia—particularly difficulty in swallowing—to inquire carefully if the patient has not been previously paralysed on the other side. Again, at an autopsy on a patient known to have been paralysed of *but one side*, and who had had difficulty in swallowing, we should search *both* sides of the brain for evidences of disease. For it is a fact that much of the motor tract may be *destroyed* without the production of hemiplegia, or, at all events, without permanent hemiplegia."

affected. Of course the word "*hemi*plegia" is now a misnomer; it is a degree of paralysis beyond hemiplegia. The expression "beyond hemiplegia" is used because the paralysis results from a lesion graver than—but in the same place as—those which produce the first and second degrees of hemiplegia.

Immediately after a very grave [1] lesion of one side of the brain there is universal powerlessness. I believe this to be two-sided paralysis. Let us continue to suppose the side of the brain damaged to be the right. It presents no difficulty, of course, that the left side of the body should be paralysed from a right-sided cerebral lesion; but I think the lesion paralyses the other side of the body also—*i.e.* the unilateral muscles on the side of the cerebral lesion. There is not only a "decussating" paralysis, but also, I think, a "direct" one.

Let us glance at some facts supplied by experimentation on different animals which have different movements. We have seen that in man the bilateral muscles suffer less from a destroying lesion of one side of the brain than do the unilateral, although both are or were represented in the part destroyed. Let us consider the movements of a dog's limbs. The movements of these limbs, even of the anterior, are chiefly alternate, *i.e.* their action is intermediate betwixt unilateral and bilateral action. He can, it is true, use one fore-leg at a time, but only in a few closely similar motions (although for many purposes). The movements of a dog's limbs approach in character those of the bilaterally acting chest muscles in man. Any lesion of *one* side of this animal's brain produces not hemiplegia, but weakness more on one side, but yet of both sides. This shows that in the dog the unilateral muscles of both sides are more nearly equally represented in each side of its brain. Let us now take the case of the bird. This animal's chief movements (of its wings) are quite equal and quite synchronous on the two sides. Here we find that lesion of one cerebral hemisphere produces no one-sided effect. Its chief movements and the representation of them are in the same case as those of man's most bilateral movements; the wing movements of both sides will be represented equally in each corpus striatum.

When we come to man we should expect that the difference of representation should be carried to an extreme. Thus, except from the gravest one-sided lesions, we do not find that there is any obvious paralysis of the muscles of the second side of the body. Nevertheless, there is proof that the unilateral muscles of both sides are represented in each corpus striatum. The proof is given by cases of Wallerian wasting. Thus, after old lesions of the right corpus striatum, there is "descending wasting" of fibres. We trace wasted fibres through the right crus, right side of pons and medulla, and thence into the *left* side of the cord. All this is simple, and corresponds with the left hemiplegia. But we trace also a band of wasted fibres into the same (the right) side of the cord. Thus, from disease of but one side of the brain, the fact that convulsion, although beginning unilaterally, becomes universal, is in accord with anatomical facts.

We shall have more to say on this when speaking of the sequence of spasm. So far we have spoken only of range of spasm. Under sequence we shall consider the further differences.

[We should here speak of aphasia attending epileptic discharges of the

[1] I use the word "grave" as inclusive of two factors, "(1) extent of lesion and (2) rapidity of lesion." They vary in relative amount in different kinds of pathological changes. This matter will be considered at length later on.

centres for speech ; but it is convenient to consider it when discussing the after-effects of strong epileptic discharges.]

## X

### Sequence of Spasm Unilaterally Beginning in Convulsions

In the cases we have been considering there are all ranges of spasm, from such as twitching of a digit to a seizure in which the whole body becomes convulsed. The spasm of the several parts is in these cases a very distinct sequence. It "goes up" the arm to the side of the face, then down the leg, affects the bilateral muscles, and finally the unilateral muscles of the other side. *It is to be noted, however, that the sequence is compound.*

In each differently beginning convulsion there are no doubt different directions of spreading throughout the body after the involvement of the part in which the spasm begins. To take the case of the limbs. A fit beginning in the hand goes *up* the arm and *down* the leg. A fit beginning in the foot goes up the leg and down the arm.[1] In cases where the spasm starts in the side of the face, it usually, I believe, goes down the arm ; I have few facts on this matter.

I limit what I have to say of sequence to those cases in which the spasm starts in one hand. I am sorry that I have but little to say. The spasm as a rule begins in the index-finger and thumb ; it next attacks the other fingers, then the arm.[2] The spasm next involves the face, and nearly at the same time goes down the leg (so far our first degree, see p. 264). Then the eyes and head turn, the body twists to the side affected ; the chest muscles become fixed (second degree, p. 266). Lastly, the unilateral muscles of the other side become involved (third degree, p. 266).

The following is extracted from papers I published, *Medical Times and Gazette*, December 19, 1868. Both range and sequence are spoken of, and the figures are intended to illustrate that the sequence of spasm is compound : thus the figure 3 in each of the three following sentences points out that to the best of my power of observation the upper arm, the eyelid, and the thigh of the right side were in spasm at the same time. It is important to note these associations, as doubtless they imply associations of movement represented in the centres discharged.

#### *Unilateral Muscles of Right Side*

*Arm.*—(1) Thumb and index-finger, (2) whole of fingers and forearm, (3) upper arm.

*Face.*—(3) Cheek drawn up, (3) closed, (4) both eyes to right, (5) head to the right.

*Leg.*—(3) Thigh, (4) leg.

Sometimes the leg is affected before the face.

[1] However, in several cases the patients have told me that the spasm, after affecting the leg, affects next the hand and goes *up* the arm.

[2] There are obviously many sequences in the arm (as a patient says, "it twists about all manner of ways"), but they cannot be easily analysed. The presumption is, that the sequence in the arm (and in the whole body) will be different as the exact part of the hand first seized differs. The hand, the most important part of the body (see p. 260), will be represented in many places. A fit beginning in the little finger would depend on discharge of a different centre from that discharged in a fit beginning in the thumb, although the whole hand will, I suppose, be represented in each of the centres and in many others.

*Bilateral Muscles*

(3) The occipito-frontalis. (4) I think the next thing is that the two buccinators, the orbicularis oris, the right zygomatici, and depressor anguli oris, are contending. The appearance is an ovoid mouth drawn to the right, the large end of the ovoid being to the right. The lower jaw is drawn down. Next, the two masseters and temporals are acting, and bring the jaws together. (5) The thoracic and abdominal muscles are involved, the inspirations becoming snatched ; the chest rocks, and in the severest cases breathing seems to stop for an appreciable time at the height of a full inspiration.

*Unilateral Muscles of the Left Side*

The unilateral muscles of the opposite side commence to move when the chest begins to be decidedly involved. First the head becomes straight, both eyes look forward, and then the head and eyes turn to the left, and the left arm and leg are in a spasm.

I must say again what I said when the above was written :

" It is most important to observe convulsive paroxysms minutely, but it is obviously difficult to observe them precisely. It must be understood that the foregoing only purports to give what is, to the best of my belief, the *usual* sequence in *one* variety of those convulsions which begin unilaterally. I never forgo an opportunity of watching patients in fits, but the opportunities are rare, and the observations are painfully difficult to make. I dare not therefore imply that the above is in all respects an accurate representation. Moreover, the description is admittedly incomplete." [1]

What we shall chiefly consider now is the order of representation of the movements of the left, the second side which, as aforesaid, we believe to be represented in the left side of the brain by non-decussating fibres (see p. 267). We shall do this mainly by speaking of the difference in the convulsions on the right (first) and left (second) side, which imply differences in the representation of the same muscles (fellow-muscles) of the two sides in the left side of the brain. The convulsions of course only give us a very general knowledge of the order of representation of movements. In saying (p. 267) that the unilateral muscles of both sides have a double representation (a representation on each side of the brain), we did not imply that they were represented alike. We suggested that the representation becomes more unequal and more different the higher the class of animal, or rather significantly, the less bilateral and synchronous became the movements of the limbs of the two sides of its body. There are unfortunately few facts supplied by the observation of convulsive seizures which bear on the matter, that is, there are few precise observations on the convulsions of the second side. Let us note some ways in which convulsion of the second side differs from the convulsion of the first side. It will not be forgotten that we are speaking of convulsions which have begun deliberately in one hand.

1. The convulsion is later.
2. It is less severe.
3. The parts are convulsed more nearly contemporaneously.
4. It is more quickly over.
5. The spasm is more tonic. (?)

[1] The fit is supposed to begin on the right side of the body, the discharging lesion being in the left side of the brain.

All these differences are important. But there are others more important to note. We have to note the *sequence* of spasm in the several parts of this second side. There are very few observations, indeed, on this matter.

There is strong *a priori* warrant for the assumption that the movements of the second side are represented in different order from those of the first side, and therefore that in epileptic discharges of the centres representing them the spasms will present a different sequence. That warrant is that in the descending atrophy to which we have referred in the last chapter (p. 267), whilst the wasting is of the fibres in the lateral column of the side opposite the half of the brain (motor tract) injured—that on the same half is in the anterior column. Thus the inference is warrantable that the two sets of fibres are for different kinds of movements of the two sides.[1] But if they do represent different kinds of *movements*, it does not follow that they do not pass to the same, *i.e.* fellow-muscles ; for muscles are represented in the nervous centres as movements. We may suppose, for example, that in the left half of the brain the muscles of the right side of the body are represented in one order (from voluntary to automatic ?) and those of the left side of the body in the inverse order (from automatic to voluntary ?), or, in chemical metaphor, the two sets of movements have the same *composition* but a different *constitution*, or again, that the two are isomeric or metameric. Once more considering the muscles as notes, we may say that there are two different tunes formed[2] from the corresponding notes.

To demonstrate this difference of representation the mode of invasion of the second side must be carefully watched in cases of convulsions. We have—taking a case in which the fit *begins* in one hand, say the right—to observe whether the left leg or the left arm is the part of the second side first *reached* by the spasm. And in each limb we have to note whether the spasm begins in the upper or lower part. But there is another thing to be observed—*viz.* whether spasm of the extensor or of the flexor muscles preponderates. For example, if, in the case of the arm (we still speak of the second side), the arm is first raised and then the fingers extended, or the reverse. These remarks are a reproduction from a paper in the *Lancet* (since reprinted as No. 1 of *Clinical*

[1] Since, as this evidence seems to show, each side of the body sends fibres to, or receives fibres from, both sides of the brain, we are led to think of the arrangement in the optic commissure. We have, however to add inter-cerebral fibres (cerebral commissures) analogous to the inter-retinal, and we have to add the commissures of the cord analogous (?) to the fibres which pass from one optic track to the other. The arrangement of fibres in the optic commissure, so far (Beale says) from being peculiar to the optic nerves, is found in every part of the body to which nerve fibres are distributed. These facts and inferences point to the conclusion—which *a priori* is likely—that the whole of the nervous system and its parts are developed on the same fundamental plan (*Medical Times and Gazette*, October 23, 1869).

A difference, however, has to be pointed out. In the central nervous arrangement in each hemisphere the muscles of the limbs of the two sides of the body are represented in *different* order ; the diagram of chiasma of the fibres for the limbs must be represented on a plane surface.

[2] I quote the following from an article I published in *Medical Times and Gazette*, January 29, 1872 :

" In describing the spread of the spasm the muscles in action were named, but it is better to speak of movements of the parts. The fit is a discharge of a centre which does not represent muscles directly, but which represents them indirectly as movements. There is, however, from the distribution of nerves to muscles by anatomically recognisable nerve trunks up to the centre, a gradually increasing complexity—an increasing harmony. Hilton's observations show that even in the ultimates of the body there is incipient co-ordination—incipient harmony. No doubt the very muscles represent in the *most general* form the method of co-ordination of the highest centres. But in noting what takes place in a fit, it is better not to speak of the muscles, but to put down what movements take place. When this is done we can afterwards consider the play of the several muscles we suppose to have been directly concerned."

*and Physiological Researches on the Nervous System*, February 15, 1873. (See p. 74.) I wrote then, " I have, I regret to say, no useful observations on the order of spreading of spasm on the *left* side. [The fit is supposed to have begun in the right hand.] As I think it very important to make observations thereon, I will write down certain questions.

1. Does the spasm of the left side begin in the leg ?
2. Does it go *down or up* these limbs ?
3. Does it affect the extensors more than the flexors, or vice versa ?
4. Is the spasm more tonic than on the other side ? "

I have since had few answers to these questions. Before they were made I published the case of a boy whose fits began in his two outer (ulnar) fingers of the left side, and who said that *once* the arm of the right side was slightly involved, and that it began to be involved in its upper part (*Medical Times and Gazette*). In another case, in which I saw many convulsions beginning in and passing up the right hand, the left side was reached by the spasm. My friend, Mr. Mercier, watched the left arm. The spasm passed *down* this limb.

Some highly important remarks on the sequence of spasm are made by Dr. Gowers in a paper on a case of convulsion, published in the *Lancet* of November 6, 1875. Among many other observations of scientific and practical value Dr. Gowers draws attention to the following points : " Invariably one arm [right] and both legs were convulsed, the other arm escaping entirely. May it be connected with the more frequent simultaneous use of the legs than of the arms ? It is to be observed that, in the right leg, spasm of the extensors predominated ; while in the left leg, that of the flexors was distinctly greater than that of the extensors."

In order to facilitate the comprehension of what has been said let us consider certain healthy movements which seem to me to be in ranges and sequences like the movements developed in that variety of convulsion which begins in one hand and *becomes* universal. I allude to what is technically called effort, and in particular, to effort in lifting weights with one hand. Ignoring for convenience the possibility that any effort in lifting even a small weight requires a new equilibration of all the muscles of the body, we shall note only the striking sequences of movement in lifting weights made gradually heavier. The words of our description will imply that there are distinct intervals in the movements as they spread ; really they glide into one another as the weight becomes heavier.

If we lift a slight weight with the right hand we use only the muscles of the hand and forearm ; if it be made gradually heavier, we bring into play those of the shoulder, next those of the right side of the spine, leg, then of the jaws and chest. At a certain stage the muscles of the opposite side of the body come into play. I should perhaps say at an uncertain stage, as the sequence is much more involved than I describe it. Speaking, however, of the second side only.[1] What must happen first is stiffening of the muscles of the left side of the spine, next stiffening of the upper part of the left leg, next that limb is lifted off the ground in extension and away from the body, and a little in advance of it.

[1] Everybody recognises simple degrees, as from lighter to heavier, but scarcely any attention is given to that what I have called compound degrees. Anyone might admit or easily understand that intellect varies directly with mass of brain, or with complexity of brain, or with a symmetry of the two hemispheres. But that it varies not according to degree of any one of them, but in a compound degree of the three factors is an hypothesis which would strike many as being not simply complex but as being confused. It may be untrue, but it is not confused.

Then the arm is raised, the forearm being in extension ; the hand is extended, the fingers being straightened out. (This is an amplification of a paragraph from the paper already referred to (see p. 74).

This spreading shows well also the compound sequence.[1] The heavier the weight, not only the more the arm is used, but the further does movement spread to automatic parts.

Another thing we see here is that the muscles of the same name on the two sides of the body are not constant congeners. The muscles of the upper arm are in the above instance of effort congeners of those of the upper part of the opposite leg. Probably the flexors of one side are in many actions the congeners of the extensors of the other side. It is so in the case of the muscles of the two eyes. The inferior oblique of one eye is the congener of the superior rectus of the other eye for lateral movement of the two eyes.[2]

Another thing to be noted is the kind of spasm in the different sequences. My own belief is that the further the range the more tonic, the less clonic, the spasm. In other words, the spasm of the more automatic parts is chiefly tonic. The correct expression is " discharge of parts representing more automatic and subordinate movements." The epileptic discharge of such centres, I suppose, produces tonic spasm. The relations betwixt tonic and clonic spasm is one of degree, for at the onest of all convulsions there is tonic spasm, which breaks down into clonic spasm, and, as above implied, the sooner the more voluntary is the part affected by the spasm. The following quotation from an article (*Medical Times and Gazette*, January 27, 1872) bears on these matters. The occurrence of tonic, soon followed by clonic spasm in the most limited convulsions shows that obstructed respiration and circulation of badly aerated blood is not necessary for the production of either.

" Just as there is an increasing harmony of movement from the muscles to the highest nerve centres, so, no doubt, there is an increasing melody. Harmony of movements is space co-ordination—the co-ordination of simultaneous movements ; melody of movements is time co-ordination—the co-ordination of movements in succession. The latter is scarcely traceable, however ; but we are warranted in assuming that from the (nearly) equal and simple intervals of respiratory movements to the most unequal and intricate intervals of movements represented in the highest centres, there is a gradually increasing melody. The two kinds of co-ordination are inseparable in health, and in disease we have to note abnormal conditions of both ; we have to observe not only the region affected by convulsive movements, but the intervals betwixt movements. As we observe that increase in range is from the voluntary to the automatic, it seems probable that, at the same time, the intervals of the movements developed become shorter. It is very difficult to note the latter in cases of convulsion ordinarily so-called. But, using the word ' convulsion ' in an unusually extended sense, we observe that the convulsions from disease of the cerebral hemisphere are chiefly clonic ; and that the convulsions of tetanus, which affects more automatic movements (those represented in the cerebellum ?) are chiefly tonic. In tonic spasm the intervals are so short that the very ' idea ' of

[1] So in the convulsions the sequence is compound ; as the most voluntary parts are more in spasm, the further does the spasm spread to automatic parts.

[2] There must be automatic action before there is voluntary action. The chest must be fixed before the arm can use it as a fixed point. There is a prior wave of equilibration from automatic to voluntary although the general form of the entire sequence seems to be from the voluntary to the automatic, and in this way we have stated it.

succession is lost; the intervals are indeed bridged over, and there is, in a sense, no apparent movement—as the humming-top, when in excessively rapid rotation, seems still."

I would in this connection remark that the study of "circus movement," and "rotations" from experimental injury of different parts of the encephalon, is of importance in helping one to methods of precise investigations of convulsions.

Before leaving the subject of sequence of spasm I would urge again the importance of studying all varieties of one-sided mobile disorders in relation to one another. To all those depending on abnormal discharges I have given the name of Hemikineses. I say *all*, because I have been misunderstood to mean by that term only one variety—the Athetosis of Hammond. I quote the following from a paper I published (*West Riding Asylum Reports*, vol. iii, "Localisation of Movements in Cerebral Hemispheres," see p. 79):

"To give examples of the relations of different symptoms: there are several *mobile* counterparts of hemiplegia. There is hemichorea, there are certain cases of hemispasm, and there is what I may call hemi-contracture, a mixture of palsy and spasm. I call these one-sided mobile symptoms 'Hemikineses.' I believe that each of them depends on disease of the same *internal* region as does hemiplegia—the region of the corpus striatum. For the same *external* region is affected in each. To obtain a knowledge of the movements represented in the cerebral district mentioned, we have to study each one of these symptoms carefully. As some evidence that this method of study is practically useful, I may adduce Dr. Radcliffe's testimony. In his article on Chorea,[1] after stating the reasons I have advanced for the localisation of the changes producing chorea in convolutions near to the corpus striatum, he writes, 'For most assuredly the difficulties which beset any attempt to localise the choreic lesion in the nerve centres are not a little simplified by thus insisting upon the clinical relations between hemichorea and hemiplegia, as a ground for believing that the region of the corpus striatum is the part affected in both disorders.'"

I may here mention that I do not include among Hemikineses paralysis agitans, or the tremor sometimes attending unilateral dysæsthesia; these are, I consider, owing to destructive lesions, and differ from chorea *toto cœlo*. The same remark applies to the tremor of disseminated sclerosis.

(*No continuation of this paper can be traced, although it is marked "to be continued" in M. P. and C. Dec.* 13, 1876.—Ed.)

[1] Reynolds's *System*, 2nd ed., vol. ii, p. 199. (Passage not in first edition.)

# INTELLECTUAL WARNINGS OF EPILEPTIC SEIZURES[1]

Referring to the second of the two important cases of epilepsy reported by Dr. Joseph Coats in a recent number of the *British Medical Journal*, Dr. Hughlings Jackson said that he believed the " thought " which that patient had was subsequent to a very slight discharge of the very highest cerebral centres. It is not very uncommon for epileptics to have vague and yet exceedingly elaborate mental states at the onset of epileptic seizures, or rather, Dr. Hughlings Jackson thinks, just after the very earliest part of the discharge. For, as stated in the last note, he believes that *all* elaborate, although morbid, mental states arise during activity of all centres which are healthy, except for " loss of control." The epileptic discharge places the highest or controlling centres *hors de combat*. Moreover, they will be equally *hors de combat during excessive discharges*, as when left exhausted by that excessive discharge. Some illustrations are taken from Dr. Hughlings Jackson's case-books. The elaborate mental state, or so-called intellectual aura, is always the same, or essentially the same, in each case. " Old scenes revert." " I feel in some strange place " (a boy expressed it—" in a strange country "). " A dreamy state." " A panorama of something familiar and yet strange." " If I were walking along and had a fit, I should think ' Oh, I saw that before ! ' " Such a feeling of " reminiscence " is not very uncommon. Another patient, trying to explain the feeling he had at the onset of a fit, put it thus : " If I were to have a fit, and see that fender, I should say, ' Dear me, I saw that fender before ! ' " It is well known that such sensations of " reminiscence " are not uncommon in healthy people, or in trivial disorders of health. Some healthy people occasionally have the *feeling* that they had seen something exactly like what they were then seeing, although *at the same time* they *believe* that they could not possibly have seen it before. But we have been adducing instances of these feelings in epileptics—in patients who have them often and have them as premonitory symptoms of their paroxysms. An educated patient has called the condition one of " double consciousness," which Dr. Hughlings Jackson believes is a perfectly accurate account. There is, he thinks, diminished object consciousness, with increased subject consciousness, a revelation of the normal duality of all healthy mental action.

Feelings like the above are sometimes called " intellectual auræ." Dr. Hughlings Jackson thinks they are not comparable to ordinary warnings ; they are not, he thinks, the result of the epileptic discharge of the highest centre, but are owing to over-activity of next lower centres, as yet untouched by the discharge. It is very common—indeed, he thinks it is the rule—for patients who have these so-called intellectual warnings to have slight abortive attacks stopping short at them—to have the so-called intellectual aura only. And here is a practical point—*viz.* that these " abortive " seizures are sometimes early in the case the sole ones. If a man has these vague " reminiscences " or " reveries " frequently and suddenly, we should inquire of him and his friends

[1] *Medical Times and Gazette*, December 23, 1876, p. 702.

for vertigo, for sudden "epigastric sensation," for transient pallor of the face, etc., preceding them or perhaps apparently accompanying them. These physical symptoms are signs of involvement of the higher centres, permitting activity of those next lower. And if we hear of these physical states we should expect that serious epileptic seizure will occur. When, however, they herald a severe fit, the epileptic discharge spreads to the lower centres, the over-activity of which produces the "intellectual aura," and renders all mental action impossible. There are convulsion and coma.

Lower than these in degree of elaborateness are much more definite mental states, as seeing spectral faces at or directly after the onset of the paroxysm.

# LECTURES ON THE DIAGNOSIS OF EPILEPSY

*Delivered before the Harveian Society* [1]

## Lecture I

Mr. President, Gentlemen,—The first thing I have to do is to thank you most heartily for the great honour you have conferred on me in asking me to give these lectures, and the next is to assure you that the task is in all ways a most pleasant one.

The subject I have chosen is the Clinical Investigation of Epilepsy. Epilepsy will be considered chiefly with regard to diagnosis. Such a subject is, however, far too wide. I must, therefore, omit large parts of it. To show more definitely how I shall handle my subject, some preliminary remarks on classification generally may be made.

There are two kinds of classification of diseases—one scientific, generally called theoretical, for the advancement of knowledge ; one empirical or clinical, for practice. In the scientific or theoretical, so far as is possible, we classify diseases as they are *departures from healthy states*—as they show abnormalities of structure, function, and nutrition. Empirically or practically, we classify them as *they approach certain types*. We will first consider the scientific classification of epilepsy, or rather of epilepsies.

Scientifically, I should consider epilepsies on the hypothesis that the paroxysm of each is dependent on a sudden temporary excessive discharge of some highly unstable region of the cerebral cortex. There is, in other words, in each epilepsy a " discharging lesion " of some region of the cortex cerebri. The discharging lesion is nothing more than a group of cells whose instability is raised far above normal. This is considering an epileptic fit as being a development of the impressions and movements represented in some unstable region, and in other regions secondarily discharged ; but yet, since the discharges are excessive, an excessive and, so to speak, brutal development of them. Thus epilepsies are, scientifically regarded, departures from normal states by excess. As implied, the " discharging lesion " is supposed to be local. The discharge of the highly unstable cells constituting it (the primary discharge) leads to secondary discharge of healthy cells in other centres (collateral or lower) with which there is anatomical connection by fibres, the degree and width of the secondary discharges varying according both as the force of the currents developed by the primary discharge and the resistance opposed by fibres and by cells of the healthy centres vary. We must not forget the resistance offered to local discharges in our consideration of their effects. The " discharging lesion " may be likened to a fulminate which overcomes the resistance of less unstable compounds.[2]

It is in the study of epilepsies as departures from normal states that the

[1] *Medical Times and Gazette*, 1879.

[2] The importance of considering resistances in our estimation of the consequences of nervous discharges in diseases of man, and in the abnormal physiological conditions induced in animals by some drugs, was, I believe, first stated in a methodical way by Sydney Ringer.

researches of Hitzig and Ferrier have enormous value. Whatever interpretations psychologists and physiologists may give of them, the *medical* value of these researches is incontestable. By galvanic or faradic excitations of the cortex cerebri in dogs, convulsive seizures can be produced which are as closely like epileptiform seizures in man from disease in the same cerebral region as we could expect, considering the difference of the natural movements of the two animals.

I would take this opportunity of very strongly urging the importance of Ferrier's investigations of the sensory region of the brain. His conclusions harmonise so well with clinical observations that I think they are of inestimable value in giving method to our investigations. It is quite certain that there are paroxysms consisting chiefly of sensory symptoms, which pair off with, and are strictly analogous to, unilaterally beginning convulsions. At any rate, Ferrier has, I think, given a new starting-point for the methodical, the scientific investigation of a most important class of paroxysmal affections which are, in a scientific regard, epilepsies. There are also cases of epilepsy in which, although the paroxysms are for the most part motor (ordinary epileptic convulsions), the " warning " of the fit is by some crude sensation—*e.g.* by " noise in the ear," or by some " taste " (this is very rare indeed), or by " coloured vision," or by a " strong smell in the nose." In each patient the " warning " is always the same crude sensation ; and very often he has, besides severe fits heralded by his crude sensation, slight paroxysms consisting of little more than that " warning."

Since the cerebral cortex is part of the chief organ of mind, the tacit assumption in the above statements is that the whole of the chief organ of mind (the cerebrum) is, like all other nervous centres, made up of nervous arrangements representing impressions and movements. Another way of stating this is to say that not only have the so-called motor and sensory regions this kind of constitution, but the rest of the brain also has it. It is not said that mind, but that *the organ of mind*, is so constituted.[1] This is a necessary outcome of the doctrine of evolution.

There are numerous epilepsies under the definition that any epilepsy is, on its anatomical side, a " discharging lesion " of some region of the cortex cerebri. The kind of paroxysm differs according to the particular region of the cortex affected ; and since many regions, if not any region, of it may be affected, the number of different epilepsies, scientifically regarded, is great. There are some, as migraine, of which the phenomena are chiefly sensory ; others of which the phenomena are chiefly motor. In some, loss of consciousness is first of all or early in the paroxysm ; in others, it occurs late in it, or not at all. Besides, there are degrees of paroxysms of each kind, depending on the degree of the discharge of this or that part of the cortex and on how much resistance it can overcome.

Before leaving this part of my subject dealing with classification—only another name for scientific investigation—it must be remarked that the scientific investigation of epilepsy owes very much to Broadbent. For my part I think his hypothesis as to the mode of representation of certain movements of the

[1] It is with considerable satisfaction that I read the following in a recent paper : " It is impossible to conceive of what other materials the ' organ of mind ' can be composed than of processes representing both movements and impressions " (W. J. Dodd, *Journal of Anatomy and Physiology*, vol. xii, p. 462). The article from which the quotation is taken is a valuable contribution to the methodical study of the organisation of the cerebral centres.

two sides of the body in each half of the brain is essential to the full interpretation of all kinds of severe epileptic seizures.

The above-described scientific or theoretical classification, whilst of value in extending and simplifying our knowledge, is worthless for practical purposes. It would, I think, include migraine. To arrange migraine along with ordinary epileptic seizures—with cases of loss of consciousness and convulsion—for practical purposes, would be as absurd as a scientific zoological classification would be for fishermen, hunters, and graziers. Whilst scientifically migraine [1] is, I think, to be classed with epilepsies, provisionally, at least, as being dependent on a " discharging lesion " of some part of the cortex cerebri—probably of some part in Ferrier's sensory region—it would be as absurd to classify it along with ordinary cases of epilepsy for practical purposes as to classify whales with other mammals for purposes of practical life. A whale is in law a fish ; in zoology it is a mammal.[2]

We have first to find out that our patient's seizures are epileptic—by no means an easy thing when they are very slight and transitory. We have to consider individual cases as each is presented to us. A patient does not come complaining of a " discharging lesion " of some part of his cerebral cortex ; but tells us that he has " had a bad fit," or that he " occasionally loses himself for a moment," and so forth. For practical purposes we require quite a different classification from the scientific one—or rather, we must have a mere arrangement ; we must have types, not definitions, and consider cases presented as they approach this or that type.

In saying the foregoing, I am only repeating what Handfield Jones said long ago about the classification of epilepsy, and am using similar expressions. As Moxon insists (*Guy's Hospital Reports*, vol. xv), we must have a clinical nomenclature. The clinical or empirical types are only the most frequently occurring cases ; there is, really, no such thing as " genuine " or " real " epilepsy, or " epilepsy proper," except in this arbitrary sense.

I trust I shall not be supposed to underrate the scientific study of disease in advocating the separate clinical study of it for practical purposes. It is not likely that I shall fall under this imputation, since I am following in the path of one [3] of the most scientifically minded men in our profession. A man who really dislikes scientific study, or, as he may say, hypothesis or theory, not merely professes a dislike in order to bring his practical ability into relief, is a one-sided man quite as much as those who do not, or rather cannot, care for music, or poetry, or art.

[1] Dr. Latham thinks that the paroxysm of migraine is owing to arterial contraction in the region of the posterior cerebral ; Dr. Liveing that there is in the paroxysm a " nerve storm " traversing the optic thalamus and other centres.

[2] Griesinger classifies migraine and some other periodical seizures under the term " epileptoid."

[3] Moxon states (Introductory Address, Guy's Hospital, session 1868–9) : " You must know diseases, not as the zoologist knows his species and his genera and his orders, by descriptions of comparative characters, but as the hunter knows his tigers and panthers and wild boars. . . . ' Familiarity ' is the word, not mere knowledge." In *Guy's Hospital Reports*, vol. xv, Moxon writes : " When we are dealing with the public or social function of names, we must keep in view the distinction between a science nomenclature and an art nomenclature. The aim of a science is the increasing and unlimited knowledge of the things it concerns itself with ; a science seeks out and names with no other object than to know. The scope of any art is, on the contrary, limited and prescribed ; it has its proper sphere of work, and it must borrow from the nomenclature of the sciences which it rests upon such names only as are useful for its practical purposes."

The following is the first division in our empirical or clinical arrangement of cases of epilepsy. There are two types :

1. *Epilepsy Proper.*
2. *Epileptiform Seizures.*

Partly in order to show that I do not advocate the absolute separation of clinical from scientific investigation, but only the temporary separation, I will consider several broad differences and resemblances betwixt the two divisions of cases from a scientific as well as empirical standpoint.

(*a*) *As to Affection of Consciousness.*—The distinction is not that consciousness is lost in one and not lost in the other, but that consciousness is lost first thing, or very soon, in the paroxysm of epilepsy proper, and late or not at all in the epileptiform seizures.

To say that an epileptic paroxysm begins with loss of consciousness is equivalent to saying that the epileptic discharge begins in some part of the highest of the cerebral centres. This is an irresistible inference, be those highest centres where they may.[1]

(*b*) *As to Spasm or Convulsion.*—Convulsion begins more nearly bilaterally in the former ; is more nearly universal at once, is more rapid, and is sooner over. In the latter, it begins very locally on one side—hand, side of face, or foot—and *becomes* universal more gradually, the spasm being comparatively slow, especially at the outset.

(*c*) *As to Seat of Changes.*—The latter depends on disease in some part of Hitzig and Ferrier's region ; the former (this is hypothetical) on disease in some part in front of that region, or *behind Ferrier's sensory region*—that is, on disease in some part of what I suggest are the highest cerebral centres : the so-called motor and sensory regions are only, I think, middle motor and middle sensory cerebral centres ; the parts in front of the middle motor centres being the highest motor centres ; *those behind the middle sensory centres the highest sensory centres.*

The vague term " disease " or " changes " has to be analysed ; the term " disease " is frequently used without regard to the distinction betwixt the two things, physiological abnormality (*d*) and abnormality of nutrition (pathology) (*e*).

(*d*) *As to Abnormal Physiological Condition of Centres.*—In each of necessity there is increased instability of cells, since there occasionally occur excessive liberations of energy ; in each there is a " discharging lesion " ; there is, then, no essential difference in the abnormal physiological condition in cases of the two divisions ; yet the paroxysms of epilepsy proper are more " intense " (more spasm in a short time) than those of epileptiform seizures, and this possibly depends in part on the fact that the highest centres have most small cells (compare *b*).

(*e*) *As to Pathology.*—In each there is increased nutrition ; the excessive liberation of energy in the paroxysm of necessity implies increased taking in of nutrient substances having potential energy ; increased nutrition is the other side of high instability. We have as yet little more than this very general, but inevitable, inference as to pathology in either. How the increased nutrition is

[1] By highest centres we do not mean geographically highest : a better term would be " latest centres "—anatomically speaking, " latest developed centres " (individually and in race of organisms) ; physiologically speaking, centres which are the seat of the activities during which our latest mentation, or present highest consciousness, arises.

brought about we do not know in most cases; in some cases (see *f*) it is determined by tumour.[1]

(*f*) *As to Morbid Anatomy*, we can say that the former are rarely caused by gross organic disease such as tumour; the latter are often so caused, syphilitic gross disease in particular. Sometimes, however, in cerebral tumour there are attacks difficult to distinguish from the epileptic vertigo of epilepsy proper.

Of course, the gross organic disease only "causes" the seizures in the sense that it leads to high instability of cells in its neighbourhood; it acts like a foreign body. The probability is that it leads to the hyper-physiological condition of instability (see *d*) by producing a subinflammatory change, and thus increased nutrition (see *e*).[2] This difference as to morbid anatomy in the two seizures can only mean, of course, either that gross organic disease most often occurs in some particular places or that in some particular places it more easily leads to instability of nerve cells.

Several of the foregoing are to a great extent but detached statements from different standpoints of what Bright and Wilks long ago asserted, *viz.* that epileptic or epileptiform attacks without loss of consciousness point to gross organic disease, such as tumour of the brain.

As implied, however (*a* and *c*), the essential difference betwixt the two kinds of seizures is chiefly as to the degree of evolution of the centre, part of which has become unstable. This leads me on to say that several of the above statements (*a*, *c*, *d*) as to differences in the two seizures are implied in the following highly interesting generalisation by Herpin: "En résumé: plus le début est long, moins la crise est violente; plus il est instantané, plus l'accès est intense."

I shall pass over the second division of seizures, and consider only epilepsy proper—what most nosologists call genuine, or idiopathic, epilepsy. I exclude the epileptiform seizures, partly to shorten my subject, but chiefly because I could do little more than repeat what I have elsewhere said about them. I learn from Charcot's writings that they were fully described by Bravais in 1824.

[1] I have suggested that increased afflux of blood to the cells unstable may result in some of those cases where there is no local gross organic disease from embolism or thrombosis. I do not mean that there is a new blocking in each fit, but that the blocking determines increased afflux of blood to a certain cortical region, and that, in consequence of increased nutrition, the cells therein have a highly raised instability. In other words, the hypothesis is that in some cases the "cortical regions" unstable in epileptics are "arterial cortical regions." Other things equal, the smallest cells will soonest become unstable. A mass of nervous matter in many small cells will "present a very much larger surface to the contact" of the nutrient fluid than the same mass in a few large cells. It is to be observed that in most cases of epileptiform seizures the attacks are for some time limited to small muscles; epileptic seizures generally begin by spasm of small muscles or in muscles the chief movements of which require little energy for the displacements they have to effect.

[2] MM. Pitres and Franck have made an important communication of facts bearing on the production of changes of instability, as the following quotation from *Le Progrès Médical*, January 5, 1878, shows. The quotation refers, first, to the results of destroying one of the centres in Hitzig and Ferrier's region: "Whilst the underlying white substance of the destroyed centre progressively loses its excitability, the grey substance of the neighbouring centres becomes turgid and inflamed, and if the inflammation be not sufficiently intense to alter the structure profoundly, a considerable augmentation of its excitability can be proved [a discharging lesion]. Epilepsy is then produced with the greatest facility. To make the animal walk, to exercise pressure upon the skin which has covered the cerebral wound, to pass a sponge over that portion of the brain which is uncovered, etc., often suffices to produce convulsive attacks. It is even very curious to see the grey substance react by convulsive phenomena under the influence of mechanical excitations which, in the physiological state, give place to no appreciable motor reaction. Under these conditions, partial epilepsy may remain limited to those parts of the body the centres of which have become abnormally excited, and respect the limb corresponding to the destroyed centre."

Their study has been placed on a scientific basis by the researches of Hitzig and Ferrier. These researches show that epileptiform seizures are developments, although excessive and brutal developments, of the movements normally represented in some particular parts of the cerebral cortex ; and thus the notion that epilepsy is a sort of entity attacking the patient is finally got rid of. An epileptic is a person certain of whose own cortical nerve cells have become highly unstable ; and in their discharge, the movements or impressions they represent are excessively developed.

More recently, eminent French physicians (Charcot, Lepine, Landouzy, Carville, Duret, Pitres, Franck, etc.) have given more definite clinical and scientific form to this most important—because least complex—group of epileptic seizures. Gowers, Dreschfeld, Byrom Bramwell, Ringrose Atkins, Bevan Lewis, and others in this country, have made most important additions to our knowledge of these. Charcot and others have added very greatly to our knowledge of the anatomy and physiology of the brain by their discoveries of the cortical origin of monoplegias corresponding to monospasms. Their researches merit the highest of all praise, that of introducing method, by a kind of work which can be rated highly as clinical, or physiological, or anatomical, or pathological.

I am strongly of opinion that the epileptiform group should be studied first, and although I pass over it in these lectures for the reasons given, I shall now and then illustrate complex phenomena of epilepsy proper by corresponding simpler phenomena of epileptiform seizures.

Taking, then, epilepsy proper, we say that it is a paroxysmal loss of consciousness. That is only a statement from the psychical side ; it is the first statement as to type. We have, speaking of the physical side, to add that there is with the loss of consciousness more or less spasm of muscles (including in that expression spasm of muscular coats of arteries and the like), or equivalent effects of cortical discharges. This is the second statement on the type. The third statement is, that the loss of consciousness is the first, or nearly the first, thing in the paroxysm.

There are degrees of involvement of consciousness, from slight confusion of mind to complete insensibility, or, after the attack, to coma. There are also degrees of the accompanying spasm,from,for example, such as slight twitchings of the hands, or that signified by facial pallor, to universal severe convulsion. Presumably there is an exact correspondence betwixt the psychical loss and the discharge, but it would be difficult to show it from cases. But we must not suppose that the correspondence is betwixt degree of affection of consciousness and degree of the physical condition of spasm ; inferentially the correspondence is betwixt the degree of affection of consciousness and the degree of the physcial condition of gravity of the discharge.

It would be very remarkable if there were not very many degrees of seizures, from those with most transitory and trifling manifestations, to severe universal convulsion, followed by universal paralysis and coma. It would be contrary to all analogy if there were not. In epileptiform seizures it is common for the patient to have very partial convulsions before widespread or universal ones. Thus, a patient of mine had, first, attacks of spasm beginning in her right index-finger, and " working " up to the elbow ; months later she had severe convulsions, with loss of consciousness, attended by much spasm. A patient may have spasm limited to the big toe, that is, to him apparently so limited, and at other times widespread convulsion. One of my patients used to show his twitching hand to his fellow-workmen " as a curiosity," before he had severe seizures which appeared to him of moment.

To return from this illustration to epilepsy proper ; we see that there are numerous degrees. At the one end of the scale is the case of a patient whose seizures are so slight and transient that a stranger to him might think he only bungled for a moment in conversation ; and at the other end is the case of a patient who has loss of consciousness with severe and violent convulsion, followed by deep coma (apoplexy), quite undistinguishable at the first from coma (apoplexy) produced by fatal cerebral hæmorrhage.

The slight seizures are often at the beginning of a case of epilepsy so slight and transient, that the patient takes no notice of them ; only when a convulsive seizure comes on does he find out what his slight transitory mental confusion, etc., meant.

Upon this basis of degrees we now divide epilepsy proper. At first glance, we should expect the division to be founded on both the width and degree of spasm and the degree of affection of consciousness. This, however, cannot be done ; there is not a discoverable exact correspondence (*vide supra*). We cannot make a clear division on this double basis. For this reason, and because there are degrees of affection of consciousness and degrees of spasm, the division must be not only arbitrary, but rough. We make one which seems very rough indeed. It is into slight and severe, or, using French names, into *le petit-mal* and *le grand-mal*—freely translatable as " little fit " and " big fit."

I do not think the division is quite so arbitrary as it appears to be at first glance ; the discharge beginning in the highest cerebral centres has, it is suggested, to overcome the resistance of the middle cerebral centres, *i.e.* the so-called " motor region," before it can produce peripheral effects (spasm, etc.). If there be such a thing as epileptic loss of consciousness without any peripheral manifestations, I suppose the explanation is that the effects of the discharge are limited to the highest centres ; the currents developed by the primary discharge of some part of the highest centres pass by lateral lines to other collateral parts of the highest centres and discharge them. This is equivalent to saying that the currents developed, whilst strong enough to overcome the resistance of collateral parts of the highest centres, are not strong enough to overcome the resistance of, that is, to discharge, the middle cerebral centres. And when not strong enough to discharge some of the middle cerebral centres, the currents may be strong enough to discharge others. The peripheral effects in slight seizures are manifested on small muscles ; the discharge is then strong enough to overcome partially the resistance of the centres in Hitzig and Ferrier's region (middle centres), those representing small muscles and containing fewest large cells (Bevan Lewis). If this be so, we see that the correspondence is not betwixt the affection of consciousness and the peripheral effects of the discharge ; there may be a discharge strong enough to abolish consciousness, and yet not strong enough to produce any, or very slight, peripheral effects.

By the expression " severe," we mean those cases in which there is very much spasm and often universal convulsion with tongue-biting. I exclude these cases.

To recapitulate briefly : We have excluded one large division of cases (epileptiform), leaving epilepsy proper, and then from this remaining division we have excluded the severe seizures. We have only to consider slight cases of epilepsy proper. I must, then, give a type of a slight case, and this will be some indirect account of the severe ones excluded from consideration. To prevent a possible misunderstanding, let me remark that the terms " slight " and "severe" used empirically refer to quantity of manifestation, especially to range of spasm, not to gravity of the case. The slight seizures are said to be the worst for mind : this accords with the hypothesis that the currents develop by discharges of some part of the highest centres, or are chiefly limited to the highest centres.

The type of the slight cases is sudden and transient loss of consciousness, closely followed or accompanied by but little spasm, and that of small muscles, such as is signified by pallor of face (spasm of facial arteries), slight spasm of the eyes, hands, etc.

Two things are said about the spasm in these type cases (*les petits-maux*) : it is slight in degree ; it is limited (may affect parts in many different regions, however, and in this sense be widespread, or, more figuratively speaking, widely scattered). In contrast, the spasm in the severe seizures (*les grands-maux*) is very great ; it is not simply widespread, but universal ; at any rate, in severe seizures, all the " visible " muscles, small and large, are affected. In some of the cases we call slight there is apparently universal slight stiffness ; there is a miniature universal convulsion, and possibly the " tremor," " shivering," " shocks," " starts," etc., described by some patients are miniature universal clonic convulsions ; still, the most striking effects are manifested in small muscles. Instead of saying " small muscles " *we should in strictness* say " parts, the movements of which require little force for the displacements they have to effect."

There is a kind of spasm which is not obvious. A " vacant " look may depend on slight rigidity of the facial muscles. A patient is sometimes said " to look vacant " ; a patient is said to " look fixedly." A loss of expression is essentially an unvarying expression, and very likely it is a matter of opinion whether a given facial aspect in a slight seizure is to be described as a " vacant look " or as a " fixed look." In the stiffened face of paralysis agitans, there is either " loss of expression " or a " puritanical expression," according as we take it. In double facial paralysis, we may take the physiognomy to be either " loss of expression " or a " sulky look." I only say that the so-called " vacant look " in a slight seizure may signify slight even-spread facial spasm, admitting that it may also signify relaxation of the facial muscles. In some seizures, there is at the onset a real expression, which cannot be put down either to a wave of facial spasm, or to a relaxation of facial muscles. There is a very definite emotional expression ; one of fear is common. We not uncommonly hear a mother assert of her epileptic child's slight attacks, " She looks frightened, and runs to me." There is also the antithetical expression of indignation in other cases. There are minor degrees of each emotional expression, as astonishment, " looking startled," etc. It is important to notice these expressions ; for possibly they will help us to account for the " form " of the actions which in some cases follow seizures ; whether the actions when excessive are those of " attack " or of " escape."

Again, there may be more spasm in slight seizures than we see. If we look at the face and limbs only, we may see very little, although the respiration is altogether suspended, as is shown by dark lips ; we infer that there is either spasm of the glottis or of other parts of the respiratory apparatus.

The slightness of spasm in some slight seizures is occasionally shown by the persistence of movements which widespread spasm would render impossible. In slight seizures the patient may go on walking apparently well ; he may sway about, but so far as he does work, so far is spasm absent from the parts concerned in locomotion.

Then, on the other hand, there are conditions which are, or simulate, loss of power : if the attack be sudden, the patient falls down ; in some cases he drops what is in his hands ; the head drops when the patient is sitting, is not pulled down by spasm ; he may look like a person going off to sleep in a chair. These conditions are not easy of explanation ; *to say that a man falls or drops things because he loses consciousness is an explanation which explains nothing, and may pair off with such an " explanation " as that chorea is due to "disorder of volition."* He may fall, either because some muscles over-contract and destroy his equilibrium, or because he loses power in some.

There are certain movements occurring in slight epileptic seizure which, I submit, should be distinguished from spasm, either tonic or clonic. A common one is a movement of mastication ; another is a swallowing movement ; there is such a one as rubbing the hands ; and there is sometimes writhing of the arms during suspended respiration. To call them *movements* is to tacitly deny them to be *spasm.*

Of course, all movements, as well as all spasms, imply nervous discharges ; but the former imply slight discharges at particular intervals. I submit that the movements of mastication, swallowing, etc., occurring in a slight fit cannot depend on an excessive discharge—that is, on an epileptic discharge.

It is well to mention some of the names patients or their friends give to slight seizures : " sensations," " turns," " spells," " thinkings," " stupidities," " reveries," " forgetfulness," " faints," " giddiness," " becoming absent," " quiet faints." I was consulted by one epileptic for " dropping off to sleep in the most extraordinary way."

Now, the slightest of these so-called sensations are very often the sole seizures for weeks, or months, or years, before the severe fits come on.

When slight seizures have preceded the severe fits, the patient may, until questioned, tell us nothing about the slight ones ; he dates his illness from the first severe fit ; or, if the slight seizures occur mixed up with severer ones, he mentions the severer ones only. He does not call his slight seizures fits, but " sensations," " symptoms," etc. He may say, " I've not had a single fit since I saw you, but I have had many sensations." These " sensations " are really slight fits, or, when considered in relation to the severe ones, incipient or abortive fits.

We speak first of the mental side of the slight cases—of the affection of consciousness. As the definition or type of the slight seizure is vague, it may be well to give an example.

A boy, 10 years of age, had been subject to fits for two years. At the first, they were so slight that his mother said they thought he was " in a deep study " ; he used to sit " as if he were thinking." The attack was only of a few seconds' duration, and no alteration of complexion was noticed. Later on, in his fits he would turn up his eyes—slight spasm of very small muscles. Later still, there was, besides this, occasional shaking of the body (imitated before me by tremor). I saw one. Whilst sitting, the boy blinked his eyes ; he did not alter in colour ; he then drew in a deep breath, and rapidly all was over. The paroxysm was so sudden and short that I could not make any special investigations.

Now for cases which do not fully resemble the type, for cases which are subtypical. This boy lost consciousness, but it is to be insisted upon that there may be epilepsy proper without *loss* of consciousness. There may be defect of consciousness only. For example, a patient may say that he is not unconscious in his attacks, but add that he does not know where he is, that he hears people talking, but does not know what they say ; this shows that he has not *lost* consciousness, but it shows also that he is defectively conscious ; in popular language, he is " confused," becoming so suddenly, and remaining so for a few seconds only. " To be confused " and " to be defectively conscious " are synonymous expressions.

Then we have evidence from what we observe that a patient in an epileptic paroxysm is not absolutely unconscious. The patient may not only utter incoherent words, but may reply to questions vaguely, as, " What do you say ? " or, more definitely, he may reply quite correctly. There is the difficulty here that the talking, vague or definite, may be just after a very slight and transient fit ; but in an empirical or clinical inquiry for diagnosis the distinction is of little moment.

So our first exception or subtype is that the patient may be only defectively conscious, or, popularly speaking, simply confused.

More than this, there may be, according to the patient's report, no defect of consciousness at all. It is well known that a common precursor of affection of consciousness in a paroxysm of epilepsy proper (slight or severe fits) is a strange sensation at or near to the epigastrium, " in the chest," or " at the heart," some patients may say. Children call it " pain " or " stomach-ache." The sensation is variously described by adults as " sinking," " nausea," and it is frequently said to be accompanied by fear. Now, patients will tell us that, for months before they had any affection of consciousness preceded by an " epigastric sensation," they occasionally had that sensation alone, and thought little or nothing of it ; some thinking it to be owing to " disorder of the liver," although it was sudden and transient (paroxysmal). This, then, would be a second subtype of epilepsy ; it would be for a time all the paroxysm.

It may be said, your " definition " by type here breaks down utterly for practical purposes, for in this subtype consciousness is not affected at all. If literally taken it does break down ; we ought and must take such cases as subtypes. It is certain that these sensations may occur paroxysmally for months without anything further. The fact that such a paroxysmal sensation is often epileptic in nature is shown by the future of the cases : undoubted epileptic affections, attacks with convulsion and tongue-biting, come on, and each of these severe paroxysms is preceded by the sensation. What was once all is now the so-called warning of the severe fit. Strictly speaking, it was when it occurred alone a rudimentary or incipient fit of epilepsy ; and when it becomes what we call a warning, since a severe fit follows, it is the inception of the severe fit. Besides, I should doubt whether consciousness was not affected to some trifling extent. However, I state what patients say, and at any rate the affection of consciousness is insignificant or most transient, or both.

Then there are cases of slight epileptic vertigo. By epileptic vertigo I do not mean any sort of " confusion in the head," I mean real vertigo : a sensation of movement of external objects, or a sensation of turning of the body itself; at the beginning of some severe attacks of epilepsy proper, the patient does actually turn to one side, " turns right round," as the friends say. Vertigo, with apparent displacement of external objects, is, I think, a sensation accompanying turning of eyes (to right side only?) Hence I do not use the term "epileptic vertigo" as the name for a slight *degree* of seizure, but specially for a slight seizure of a particular *kind*, or for a seizure beginning in a particular way. I will not say there is no defect of consciousness in cases of epileptic vertigo, but it may be very slight and transient, and, according to the patient and his friends, none. I do not believe that consciousness is entirely unaffected in any sort of giddiness, however caused. Let a man try to think, when giddy, of something complex and difficult to him, to tackle some problem he could just manage to solve when well ; he would fail when giddy.

So, then, whilst we take paroxysmal *loss* of consciousness as our type, there are subtypes. There is not only loss of consciousness, there is defect of consciousness, and there is also no affection of consciousness. The paroxysmalness of the seizure and the sequel show that each is truly epileptic ; they occur at different periods of the same case. Indeed, we may have each of the three degrees at different times in one case.

## Lecture II

So far we have spoken of the type case and of the subtypical cases as if there were paroxysmal affections of consciousness only, or the crude sensations, vertigo and the epigastric warning. Indeed, we may hear of nothing else than affection of consciousness ; but often there are decided physical accompaniments, if not always some. Necessarily there is always a physical condition—*viz.* a discharge of some part of the nervous centres, even if there be cases of epilepsy with loss of consciousness only. I now come to speak of visible or inferable *peripheral* effects of the central discharge.

Visible effects of the discharge are spasms ; such effects of it as that the salivary glands hypersecrete are inferred from witnessing flow of saliva, and perhaps from hearing swallowing movements. We infer that the bladder contracts from finding that the patient has passed urine. There is a large and important class of inferable effects, from, or rather accompaniments of, the discharges ; these are " crude sensations." With regard to all " crude sensations," we can—since, although abnormal, they are psychical states—only translate what the patient tells us into physical conditions. Thus, if a patient say that at the onset of his fits he has " balls of fire " before his eyes, we infer the physical condition of excessive discharge of sensory elements of centres especially representing the retinæ. Of course, any sensation, healthy or morbid, is only to be called peripheral in the sense that it is referred to the periphery (epi- or ento-periphery), or that it is, as in vision, considered as in the environment in relation to some part of the periphery.

Here we must pause to remark on several matters. First, we speak of the nature of the epileptic discharge, partly restating in a different way the substance of what was said in the last lecture, when speaking of movements of mastication, etc.

Whenever we speak of discharges in epilepsy it is to be inferred that nervous discharges in a degree far above normal are meant. There are, of course, nervous discharges in the operations of health. But in epilepsy the spasm is plainly the result of an *excessive* discharge ; there is a strong development of a great number of movements of parts at once. The crude sensations at the onset of severe fits, " balls of fire," etc., *imply* correlative strong discharges. During excessive discharges of parts of the very highest centres, nothing like normal mental states arise ; time is required for consciousness ; consciousness ceases during the rapid and excessive discharges of vast numbers of the nervous arrangements which are the substrata of consciousness. The psychical states arising during an epileptic discharge of the highest centres are only crude sensations, such as vertigo and the epigastric sensation.

There are certain peripheral effects equivalent to spasm. The flow of saliva is equivalent to spasm, being the result, it is supposed, of strong currents along efferent, if we may not say motor, nerves. The stopping or slowing of the heart is supposed to be owing to effects produced through the inhibitory fibres of the pneumogastric nerve, efferent although not motor fibres. The effects of epileptic discharge on the circulatory apparatus have not been minutely studied. At the onset of some slight attacks the pulse stops. A patient not unfrequently tells us that his heart palpitates at the onset ; but whether it then goes slower, whether the palpitation means intermittence, is hard to determine. Increased frequency of cardiac action, *after a slight fit*, might be ascribed to partial exhaustion of the inhibitory fibres or their centres—a condition analogous to that of centres in epileptic hemiplegia (post-epileptic paralysis significant of exhaustion of centres from the excessive discharge in the prior paroxysms).

It is to be understood that the term " sensation " is used as a name for a psychical state, and not as convertible with an active state, or discharge, of sensory nerves or centres.

There are sensations occurring during excitations or discharges of motor centres, as well as during excitations or discharges of sensory centres : thus epileptic vertigo is an abnormal sensation as much as coloured vision is ; the former is a crude psychical state occurring during (not from) excessive discharges of central sensory elements representing retinal elements, the latter a crude sensation occurring during (not from) excessive discharges of central motor elements representing ocular and perhaps other movements. It will be convenient occasionally to use the terms " motor sensation " and " sensory sensation." It is not meant that muscular movement, nascent or actual, is any part of a sensation, nor is it meant that a sensation is a mode of motion of either motor or sensory nervous elements. The expressions are to be taken simply as abbreviations of the expressions " sensation *occurring during* activity of a motor centre," and " sensation *occurring during* activity of a sensory centre."

We must not limit the term " sensation " to the so-called special sensations —sight, touch, etc. In the expression " sensation " are included all sensations whose corresponding physical organs are on the periphery. Using mixed anatomical and psychological terms, on the same understanding as the expression " motor sensation " is used, these may be called epi-peripheral sensations. But there is also the large class of sensations—ento-peripheral sensations— called by Lewes " systemic," and by Bain " organic." This division into two classes of normal sensation corresponds to the division to be made later on into two classes of " crude sensations."

We divide the peripheral effects of epileptic discharges into three rough groups. It must be borne in mind that we are speaking solely of epilepsy proper, and only of slight fits, under this division. (1) Affection of animal parts; (2) affection of organic parts. Then under each we consider (*a*) what we see, *viz.* spasms or equivalent effects of central discharge; (*b*) what we infer from the patient's statement about his crude sensations before he loses consciousness.

1. *Affection of Parts serving in Animal Functions.*—(*a*) Visible movements. The most pronounced of these are stiff or gliding movements of the hands, of the eyes, or of the face, or perhaps of all these parts—that is to say, spasms of those regions of the animal parts having small muscles;[1] or, in other words, of those parts directly concerned in the most intellectual operations and most voluntary actions. (*b*) Crude sensations (special senses). The patient may have preluding stench in the nose, or "balls of fire" before the eyes, or noises in the ear, or numbness of the hands. These we interpret to be owing to central discharge of different sensory elements of the highest centres of the cerebral hemispheres, representing the regions of the body concerned in the several senses named. There is also the motor sensation vertigo.

2. *Affections of Parts serving in Organic Functions.*—(*a*) Visible changes from spasm or effects equivalent to spasm. The face and the lips may turn pale, or become red and then pale. There may be a flow of saliva; the pulse may stop; there may be eructation. (*b*) Crude sensations (systemic) of suffocation, of dying, of "sinking into the ground," nausea, the epigastric sensation already mentioned, chilliness, warmth, etc.

3. *Common to both Animal and Organic.*—Then, as a third division, we must consider affections of respiration. Respiration belongs, or at any rate respiratory movements belong, both to the animal and to the organic group; for we not only breathe to aerate the blood (organic function), but we fix the chest-walls after a full inspiration, possibly by closure of the glottis in "effort," as, for example, in lifting a weight (animal function).

It is a common thing for there to be entire suspension of respiration with but little true spasm of the face and limbs. The feeling of suffocation in an early stage of epileptic fits is probably owing to the beginning of this suspension.

Now let us state some facts of scientific bearing, and in such a way as to bring us to a clearer consideration of the empirical value of certain symptoms in the diagnosis of slight seizures. We gave as one of the things distinguishing the paroxysm of epilepsy proper from the epileptiform seizure that the former began by loss of consciousness, or that loss of consciousness was nearly the first thing. In other words, these (the epileptic) are the cases in which there is no warning, or in which it is short. Now, such a mode of beginning implies that the correlative physical condition, the excessive discharge, begins in the highest cerebral centres; for these, of course, are the centres engaged during our highest and latest mental states; only another way of saying engaged during

[1] It is significant that the rule is that all sorts of epileptic and epileptiform convulsions begin in small muscles, or in muscles whose ordinary movements require little energy for the displacements they have to effect. I have advanced the hypothesis that small *muscles* are represented in the cerebrum by small cells, or rather that *movements* of parts which require little energy for the displacements they have to effect are represented by small cells. As the researches of Bevan Lewis show, this is not altogether an hypothesis, in so far as "centres" in Ferrier's region are concerned. "Centres" chiefly representing "small movements" are those which have fewest large cells. This matter has wide bearings.

our consciousness. For we have not got a consciousness *and* latest and highest mental states ; we have only two names for one thing. Moreover, if analytically we speak of ourhighest mental states under thenames of will, memory,emotion, and reason, we are only giving names to different aspects of consciousness. Thus there are not separate centres for the will, nor for memory, nor for reason, nor for emotion ; all four arise simultaneously during activity of the highest cerebral centres—that is, they necessarily all arise when consciousness arises, being only names for different aspects of consciousness itself. The term " substrata of consciousness " (in detail, substrata of the simultaneously arising states, will, memory, etc.) is only another name for highest and latest developed centres (racially and individually).

The following are equivalent expressions :

*As to the Paroxysms.*—1. The fit begins with loss of consciousness ; 2. The fit begins without a warning.

*As to the Centres.*—3. The discharge begins in the highest cerebral centres ; 4. The discharge begins in the substrata of consciousness ; 5. The discharge begins in the centres engaged during the fourfold state—will, memory, reason, and emotion ; 6. The discharge begins in centres which especially contain substrata of numerous tactual and visual images, words, emotions, etc. ; 7. The discharge begins in parts which especially represent movements in which small muscles are concerned.

With obvious modifications, the statements apply to cases in which the loss of consciousness quickly follows the onset—quickly follows a warning.

Thus we see that not only the animal parts, but that the organic parts also, are the fields of symptoms from epileptic discharges ; and, as the paroxysms are such as begin with loss of consciousness, we declare them to result from discharges of the highest centres. This is only another way of saying that the highest centres represent the parts concerned, both organic and animal ; not the face and limbs only, but the heart, salivary glands, stomach, etc. The epileptic discharge is an " experiment " showing that the highest centres contain nervous arrangements representing these parts. When we bear in mind that emotional manifestations are activities of deeply organic parts as well as of animal parts, we see that psychology is in absolute harmony with the facts of epilepsy proper ; for emotion—like memory, reason, and will, the remaining other sides of conscious states—begins to arise during activity of our highest cerebral centres. So now we add to the above seven statements the following equivalent statement :

8. The discharge begins in a part representing both organic and animal parts.

Let us for a moment consider the facts of severe fits. In these cases, both animal and organic parts are affected by the severe discharge ; but not only the small muscles, but all the visible muscles of the body, are affected. Moreover, some organic parts are affected ; we cannot say all. The following statement is hypothetical ; it is only supposed to be equivalent to the others :

9. The discharge begins in centres representing the whole organism.

In these lectures we deal with slight cases in which there is little more than loss of consciousness, in which the peripheral effects are slight. Now, it is a singular thing, at first glance, that it is in these very cases that the slight symptoms we have are not only those referable to animal parts, but also symptoms referable to organic parts, as pallor of the face, flow of saliva, slowing and stoppage of the pulse. With either set of symptoms there may be stoppage of respiration, with little spasm of the limbs. Do not these facts show that organic as well as animal parts of the body are represented in the cerebrum? Do not they show that they are both represented in the very highest of the cerebral centres? For the seizures begin by discharge of these highest centres. Besides, how would anyone set about explaining what occurs physically during the emotional manifestations of fear, joy, etc., unless he assumed that the organic parts are represented in the highest centres? And everybody does tacitly assume it in ordinary discourse. To say that "he is frightened" implies it; for what represents the "he" or the "ego" of every passing moment but the then highest consciousness, and what should be the substrata of highest consciousness except the highest nervous centres? When we say anyone is frightened, we imply that there are occurring physical manifestations from discharges of the highest correlative centres. The facts of emotional manifestations are indeed very striking. To take the case of fear, and to speak only of what can be seen or inferred from involvement of the organic parts, we find that the heart is quickened, the respiration is hurried, the mouth is dry, there is increased perspiration, the face is pale, there may be intestinal evacuations, and in anxiety (fear spread out thin) there is increased renal secretion or increased flow of the watery elements. The criticism that these are only "caused by emotion" is invalid. A psychical state cannot cause anything physical; an emotion is not the cause, but the psychical accompaniment, of what are physically nervous changes, and the central changes are those causing, directly or indirectly, disturbances of the organs named as well as of animal parts omitted from our catalogue. And if it be possible for a person to feel afraid only, in the sense of no external manifestations appearing, then the only difference is that the central changes are slight, or are antagonised by others; that is to say, they are limited to the highest nervous centres.

A slight digression to facts of other kinds of brain disease is justifiable. Epilepsy cannot be understood if it be not regarded in relation to all other cerebral diseases. This digression will lead round about to a practical consideration of certain important matters connected with the diagnosis of epilepsy. Although a digression from our principal topic—epilepsy—it is a continuation of that part of our subject which is to show that the cerebral centres represent organic as well as animal parts.

The above-mentioned facts, showing implication of organic parts in epilepsy, find their parallel in the occurrence during meningitis, and some other acute primary brain diseases, of vomiting, constipation (occasionally volvulus), irregularity of pulse and respiration. These cases show, exactly as slight cases of epilepsy do, that organic parts are represented in the organ of mind. It is exceedingly important to note for practical purposes that from disease of "the organ of mind" we have such peripheral physical symptoms; the more so that, whilst they are of great value in the diagnosis of acute *primary* disease of the brain, positive mental symptoms (delirium, etc.) are of little value—none, I think—in diagnosis of such acute *primary* disease.

If it were admitted that the "organ of mind" was, like lower centres, representative of nothing else than impressions and movements, it would save us from many blunders. Surely there is nothing strange, *a priori*, in supposing that the higher and highest cerebral centres have the same fundamental kind of constitution as the lowest centres in the pons, medulla oblongata, and spinal cord. And, *a posteriori*, we find that very frequently disease of the cerebrum does cause motor or sensory symptoms, or some of both ; we find that with tumours in the middle cerebral centres there are definite partial convulsions, or convulsions becoming universal ; we find that faradaic or galvanic stimulation of those centres produces definite movements. But some of those who admit that Hitzig and Ferrier's regions contain movement centres still think the rest of the cerebrum is " for mind." But there is no incongruity whatever in holding this opinion, and in holding also that the rest of the cerebrum is made up of nervous arrangements representing impressions and movements. To hold that " the organ of mind " is made up of nervous arrangements representing impressions and movements seems strange when the two little words " organ of " are read over so that one is misunderstood to mean that the " *mind* is made up of nervous arrangements representing impressions and movements." All that is said is that the *substrata* of mind have this sort of constitution. So that I think, as others do, that the parts beyond Hitzig and Ferrier's centres are " for mind " ; in the sense that they contain the substrata of highest mental states. But this belief leaves me perfectly free to hold the opinion that these substrata are nervous arrangements for impressions and movements.

These remarks are not of mere theoretical interest ; from not admitting this kind of constitution of the cerebrum, acute brain disease in its earliest stages is nearly always put down to fault in some non-cerebral organ, whose activity is particularly disturbed, directly or indirectly, by disease in that part of the brain which represents that organ. Effects are taken as causes. Is not migraine frequently put down to digestive derangement ? Are not cases of tubercular meningitis and cerebral tumour in their earliest stages constantly ascribed to stomach and liver derangements ? Would these mistakes be so common if it were recognised that the liver and stomach, as well as the hand and foot, were represented in the organ of mind ?

Now, to come back to epilepsy. Because a patient's pulse is irregular during or just after an epileptic fit, the fit, supposing it be slight, is put down to cardiac affection, even when the patient is suddenly seized when sitting reading or at dinner, turns deadly pale, and yet does not fall. Again, because a patient's fits begin with an epigastric sensation, described as nausea, or if there be eructation, it is not at all uncommon for the attacks to be ascribed to indigestion, notwithstanding that these stomach symptoms occur paroxysmally, and in face of the facts that ordinarily the patient may eat a big dinner and forget it, have after it no pain, no flatulence, no feeling of distension, no nausea, but go on digesting it unconsciously. So that if such a case is to be looked on as dyspepsia, it is paroxysmal dyspepsia causing loss of consciousness. Supposing the patient had dyspepsia, and supposing that he was invariably much more dyspeptic just before each fit occurred, we ought to wonder why dyspepsia " caused " loss of consciousness, and caused it suddenly, and caused it transitorily, when there are scores of cases of aggravated dyspepsia without such complication. Trousseau mentions a case in which attacks of violent giddiness, with deadly pallor, occurred, after a sensation of pressure at the pit of the stomach, soon followed by vomiting. These attacks were put down to dyspepsia. The boy's father and his medical attendant refused to believe in Trousseau's diagnosis of epilepsy ; the sequel of the case showed Trousseau to be right. Trousseau says, of what he calls a " visceral aura," that it escapes the observation of the physician all the more easily from its simulating other affections in a numerous class of cases. The " visceral aura," or " warning " of an epileptic fit, is nothing more than the first effect of the central discharge; it is some change produced in the viscus, or it is some sensation referred to the viscus, the sensation arising with the central discharge. In this way of regarding the term, Trousseau's meaning is, that the disturbance is supposed to originate in the viscus, whereas it is produced there by the central discharge; the discharge being of a part which especially represents that viscus. Herpin asks: " Is there anything more strange in the tonic convulsion beginning in the muscles of the digestive canal than in its beginning in those of the hand and foot ? " Herpin's question is very pertinent, since, as facial pallor shows, spasm in epilepsy frequently does begin, or occurs very early, in the muscles (muscular coats) of equally organic parts (facial arteries). Here an inconsistency may be pointed out. Some organic symptoms are admitted by everybody to result from the central discharges, as pallor of the face, flow of saliva; some, as eructation, are looked upon as not resulting from it, but (*i.e.* the dyspepsia it implies) as causing the other symptoms with which they occur.

To resume: cases of meningitis, cerebral tumour, undoubted cases of epilepsy, show that the organic or visceral parts are disturbed by cerebral disease in many cases, in which visceral disease is supposed to disturb the brain. Two things are plain to the laity: that digestion influences the brain, and that the brain influences the digestion; a heavy meal produces in some people sluggishness of mind and depression of spirits; joy or grief takes away the appetite.

There is still another way of regarding the relation of visceral states to the organ of mind. It is well known that visceral diseases, or slightly abnormal visceral conditions, influence the mind (the brain). We have the so-called *spes phthisica*, and there is the melancholy of abdominal disease. Milner Fothergill has stated with great clearness the relations of affections of different thoracic and abdominal organs to different mental conditions. From such considerations we pass on to a clearer view of the relations of mental (properly cerebral) to organic states.

We may fairly assume that the viscera and all other parts of the organism are doubly connected with the cerebral centres, even with the highest of them. There are nerve fibres efferent downwards from centres to part of body; nerve fibres afferent upwards from part of body to centres. Thus there is harmonious action, consent, betwixt the part and the centre; and when one gets out of order the other suffers. If, to speak figuratively, the brain (as in an epileptic fit) fixes the chest, the chest crams, or tries to cram, the brain with blood. If the brain stop or slow the heart, as in some cases of *le petit-mal*, the heart would supply the brain with blood. It is, " You bother me, I'll bother you." There is a multiplication of effects. Hence, a study of the several " visceral auras " is of great practical moment. I doubt not that when there is a discharging lesion in a cerebral centre representing especially the stomach (when the patient at the outset of his seizure has a sensation of nausea), that centre, being in an unstable condition, is easily worried into discharging when the digestion is overworked. Indeed, for more reasons than this, attention to the diet of epileptics is one of the most important things in their treatment, as Dr. Paget, of Cambridge, long ago insisted.

There are two other things referable to internal organs, which occur in slight cases, and more frequently in slight cases than in severe ones, *viz.* passing urine and fæces. It may be doubted whether these are owing to epileptic spasm ; they may occur after the fit, and be due to " loss of control." They occur after death. However, be these two things direct or indirect results of the paroxysms, they occur at any rate practically with the other symptoms. They are exceedingly valuable helps to the diagnosis of epilepsy, especially in its slighter forms. I say in the slighter forms, for it is said that the urinary and fæcal discharges occur most often, as Herpin long ago asserted, in the slight attacks. Passage of urine is most common, and is a valuable help to diagnosis. If a child, but especially if an adult, pass urine in bed, epilepsy is one of the things to be carefully investigated for. If passage of urine occur in a so-called " faint," or in a " giddy attack " in the daytime, there is probably epilepsy—almost certainly.

I will now make some general remarks on the diagnosis of epilepsy, and remark briefly on the question of pathology.

Perhaps one reason why, on the occurrence of a few slight attacks, there is a hesitation in carrying the evidence to its logical conclusion is, that the patient may, to all appearance, be in first-rate health. Unfortunately, this goes, so far as we can yet tell, for nothing at all against the diagnosis of epilepsy. I submit that, before the first attack, however slight, something must have been going wrong in the nervous centres. I take it for granted that everyone admits every sort of epilepsy to depend on discharge of highly unstable nerve cells. The nervous elements must have become unstable before the first sudden " explosion " ; a gun must be charged before it can be discharged. Suppose a person, feeling well and in no way discoverably out of health, has suddenly one morning, when reading a book, a violent convulsion with loss of consciousness. Surely we must admit that some part of his nervous system had been changed before that unlucky morning ; the nerve cells do not become suddenly unstable, and then suddenly discharge. Such a case is a startling one ; but we must, I submit, make the like supposition in the case of a first slight fit, however slight it may be.

Possibly another reason for hesitation in diagnosing epilepsy is the absence of anything likely to be a cause of so serious a thing. The patient is well, and has had a healthy, ordinary life. But we are not always content to say of a case of epilepsy that we do not know the cause. Thus there is a tendency to fall back on the nearest most striking event, and to explain away the symptoms by fright, by temporary dyspepsia, by overwork, and so forth. We have not yet discovered the cause of epilepsy proper in any sense of the word " cause." Nor is there any morbid anatomy of it. We note carefully the facts of the above and other so-called causes, but until we find some morbid anatomy we are not justified in anything more than stating, as an hypothesis, that epileptic fits occurred during this or that condition or circumstance. And when we have found the morbid anatomy, we shall then have to discover how fright, dyspepsia, etc., produce the unstable condition of nerve cells, on the discharge of which the first and every subsequent fit depend. The hypothesis is stated that such causes as fright are simply " exciting causes " of the first discharge of nerve cells which have, by prior pathological processes, reached a high degree of instability.

As regarding pathology, I would repeat that there is a negative pathology ; epilepsy proper, slight or severe, is rarely owing to gross organic disease such as tumour, whilst epileptiform seizures frequently are. The changes in epilepsy proper are minute, as is evident enough by their having never been found. When opportunity serves we ought to look into the state of each tissue of the part. For here comes the great question, Is the change primarily arterial and secondarily nervous ; or is it a change beginning first of all in the nerve cell ? There are many nervous diseases which are not nervous at all in the sense that the nervous elements are first to go wrong. In most cases of nervous diseases of which there is an anatomy, the nervous elements are quite innocent ; they suffer because their arteries get blocked up or break, because tumours grow in their connective tissue, etc. This leads to the question of hereditariness, and thus once more to the question of diagnosis of epilepsy.

It is not denied that epilepsy is a disease of some nervous organ ; whatever view anyone takes of the seat of epilepsy, he believes some nervous centre or centres to be affected. But now comes the critical question—There being several ingredients in any nervous organ, which one is *primarily* affected ? That the nerve cells are changed no one denies ; but, repeating the above question in two questions, we ask, Does the change begin in the nerve cells of the centre ; or do these suffer secondarily from a change beginning in some non-nervous element of the centres ? The answer can only be hypothetical in cases of epilepsy proper, for the simple reason that as yet there is no morbid anatomy of epilepsy proper. Let us see how the two questions stand with regard to current notions of inheritance of nervous diseases.

Supposing there were nervous diseases in many of the patient's near blood-relatives, we must be careful how we interpret this evidence as showing that his epilepsy is a nervous affection. We must consider what sort of pathology these " nervous diseases " have ; are they nervous in the sense that the morbid process begins in the true nervous elements of the centres diseased, or only in the sense that it begins in the non-nervous element, and leads to damage of the true nervous elements ? The fact that his relatives had hemiplegia or apoplexy from cerebral hæmorrhage is simply no evidence that he inherits a disease of the nervous system in the sense that the changes begin in the nervous elements of nervous organs, for the very plain reason that the pathological processes causing paralysis and apoplexy are of a non-nervous kind ; if they have a bearing, as I think they have, they point unmistakably to arterial or cardiac changes. But then the nervous affections in the epileptic's family may be such as chorea, neuralgia, migraine, or epilepsy proper. Since nothing is decided as to the pathology of any one of these affections, we cannot possibly say that they point to an inheritance of epilepsy, or tendency thereto, in the sense that they point to changes *beginning* in nervous elements. I should not make these remarks were they not to lead to a practical inquiry. The hypothesis in possession is that epilepsy is owing to changes beginning in the nervous elements of nervous organs, and it is supposed to be supported by the fact that there are often in the patient's family persons who have that or some other neurosis ; that is, some other nervous affection of which there is no morbid anatomy. Why is it that we speak with most confidence of the inheritance and interchangeability of those very diseases of which there is no morbid anatomy ? The occurrence of these neuroses cannot be adduced as evidence that epilepsy is a disease primarily nervous. I wish to put forward, again, another hypothesis, *viz.* that the cells suffer secondarily, as a consequence of arterial disease ; that there is thrombosis or embolism of small arteries in most cases of epilepsy proper. I have held this opinion since 1864 as regards those epileptiform seizures in which there were no signs of gross organic disease. It first occurred to me on finding epileptiform seizures in patients who had valvular disease of the heart. I have since applied it to epilepsy proper. It may be said, " Your statement is only an hypothesis." So is any other view which can be taken of a disease of which there is no morbid anatomy.

## Lecture III

So far we have spoken of negative mental states in slight epileptic seizures. We said the patient had in, and also after, his attacks defect of consciousness, or loss of consciousness. But occasionally there is *also* an exactly opposite mental state, a positive one. There is then a double mental state—a negative and a positive element together. A patient seized with a slight fit suddenly becomes vague as to his present surroundings, and at the very same time, or in instant sequence, he has a " dreamy " feeling, often of some apparently former surroundings. This double mental state helps the diagnosis of slight seizures greatly.

Let me give an example. One of my patients stated, as the onset of his fits, two diametrically opposite conditions of mind. He said: (1) " The ordinary operations of the mind seemed to stop; (2) " I seem to think of a thousand different things all in a moment." He put it again thus, still making a double statement: (1) " If writing a letter, it becomes a blank; and (2) the thoughts before-mentioned come." Here there were very clearly (1) a negative state, defect of consciousness as to his then surroundings; and (2) a positive state of increased consciousness, a " rising up " of formerly organised mental states. The patient next lost consciousness; then the negative state became deeper, and his dreamy state vanished.

But sometimes there is no " dreamy state," but there are actions; there is an " epileptic somnambulism " as well as an " epileptic dream." An epileptic, after a slight fit, took his boots off in church; one of my patients began to undress at a wharf—his fellow-servants stopped him when he had got one leg of his trousers off. Such cases are very common.

We have, then, two divisions of positive conditions in or after slight fits of epilepsy proper:

(1) " Dreamy " states without actions.

(2) Actions more or less elaborate.

There is a distinction betwixt the two classes [1]—one akin to the distinction, made by many authorities, betwixt ordinary dreaming and ordinary somnambulism. The rule is that the patient, in the cases under the first division, remembers his positive mental state—remembers his dream—or, of course, we should know nothing about it, there being nothing for us from which to infer it, as he does not act. But when a patient does anything in or after his fits, he remembers no mental state during his actions, nor does he remember

[1] In no case do I believe it possible that *elaborate* states (" dreamy " states, " actions," or " movements ") can occur from an *epileptic* discharge. I believe all *elaborate* positive states occur from, or arise during, an increased energising of centres permitted by removal of control of higher centres (Anstie, Dickson Thompson). In the case mentioned in the text, we note that there was a double mental state: the patient had defect of object consciousness (negative) and (positively) increase of subject consciousness; in another way of stating it, he had loss of function of the now-organising nervous arrangements and increased function of the earlier organised.

what he has done. As will be seen by the examples, the memory of the so-called "dream" is often very slight, sometimes only that there has been some vague mental state; it is then rather a belief that he had dreamt than a remembrance of a dream.

There are cases which in one of their stages come under the first, and in another stage under the second, division. The patient has a "dreamy state"; then becomes unconscious and acts. He remembers his dream, but knows nothing of his actions.

I confess that I believe there is some sort of mental state attending the actions in the patient who is said to be unconscious, and who, on recovery, knows nothing of them; I believe that he has lost *highest* consciousness, and that his automatism has an accompaniment of some degree of consciousness or subconsciousness.

But, not to raise a difficult question, we will simply say that, in the cases under the first division, there are dreamy states and no actions; and that, in the second, there are actions and either no dreams or no remembered dreams attending *them*.

1. *Dreamy States without Actions*.—There is in cases of this division some defect of consciousness, and, at the very same time, some mental activity of a sort—what is commonly called an Intellectual Aura, but which is here called "a dream."[1] Besides other objections to the term "intellectual aura," it does not bring into prominence the fact that the condition it should name is duplex.

Now let me mention more cases. It is not uncommon to find that a patient gives as the warning of his fits such an account as this. "It begins," said one of my patients, "by a sort of referring to old things, things that have happened," which he could not further describe; he added, too, that he lost himself. That is to say, he used two expressions which seem, but are not, contradictory; he had defect of highest, that is, latest, consciousness; to some extent he lost himself to his then surroundings, and yet at the same time had the mental state which was the psychical accompaniment of a revival of some organised processes, if not exactly, as he averred, of some particular former events. Next he lost consciousness altogether, was convulsed, and bit his tongue.

I am not leaving the subject of slight seizures and straying into the consideration of severe ones in mentioning the above case, in which convulsion with tongue-biting occurred. The interest of this illustration lies in the fact that, for several months, the patient had occasionally a slight fit, exactly like what was ultimately the so-called warning (really first stage) of his severe ones; he said that, during some months, he occasionally had "*this* reference to old things," and "lost himself" for a moment, before anything he thought to be serious occurred.

A patient subject to very slight attacks said that he occasionally passed into a "dreamy state," and would fancy he saw the same things under the same

[1] The expression covers states which are doubtless dissimilar; Voluminous Mental State would be a better name to include them all. Another term I use for some of them is "Reminiscence." I use it "without prejudice," as the lawyers say. I do not adopt the patients' statements in their literal meaning, either when they say that they have again had an old dream, or when they say their state is a reversion of "things that have happened," or anything else; I simply tell what they have told me. Of necessity, the positive mental state—as also that of ordinary dreaming and the positive mental state in ordinary insanity—must be a revival of *formerly acquired* states of some sort, although in new and grotesque combinations.

combination of circumstances as he had once before seen them. To illustrate this, he said, pointing to it: " If I were to see that fender, I should say: ' Dear me! I saw that fender before.' " *The sensation is to him pleasing*; if " he thinks of something else," he can shake it off. All this patient's fits were slight; the greatest abnormality towards severity was that in one he slipped off his chair suddenly unconscious, but many of his fits were slighter; he would turn pale and " livid " in some. It was certain that they were epileptic; he had been subject to them eight years. In the first he passed urine, and so he did in one six years later. In his earliest attacks *he had a metallic taste in his mouth.*

Such reminiscences as this patient had occur in healthy people, or in trivial and transitory disorders of health. I speak of cases in which the mental state occurs frequently, and with some decided affection of consciousness, in such slight paroxysmal conditions as we know do merge into severe undoubted epileptic seizures. The fact that they are like normal or nearly normal states is a matter of great interest.

It may be said that such mental states are mere curiosities. Not so, if they are, as they are, the precursors of epileptic convulsion, with tongue-biting. I dwell on these cases because they are somewhat unusual, and because I think they have not attracted due attention in this country.[1]

In the following there was an account given of a mental state, which reminds one of the hyperbolical accounts given by persons rescued from drowning, of their mental states during submersion.

A female patient, 34 years of age, gave as her warning of her epileptic seizure: " It seems as if I went back to all that occurred in my childhood, as if I see everything, but so quick and soon gone that I cannot describe it." She next, as a rule, became unconscious, but occasionally she has this feeling of " reminiscence " only. Unfortunately, except that she always passed urine in her fits, no account of the severe paroxysm was obtainable, except the so-called intellectual aura of it. The account of this warning was given in reply to the simple question, " How does the fit begin? "

This patient was only a domestic servant, and thus being little educated it may be said that her account, besides being vague, was untrustworthy. Yet she gave it spontaneously; one does not ask leading questions in such things. Of course, I do not mean that the poor woman remembered all the events of her life, but simply that she had some sort of voluminous mental state. That her attacks were epileptic is practically certain, as at other times she lost consciousness altogether and passed her urine in the paroxysm.

A boy, 14 years of age, stated his dreamy state in boyish language. About every day he had two or three fits in succession. He said, " I come over queer." " I feel as if I was lost—as if I were in some strange country." That his slight seizures were epileptic is proven by his having had also undoubted epileptic seizures.

Let me now mention other expressions of other patients as to the dreamy state. Most vaguely it is described as a " dreamy state "; often it is said to

[1] Besides, they are of great scientific interest. These cases stand at the top of a series of different degrees of dissolution, of which the lowest degrees are coma; midway come cases of actions more or less elaborate. It is understood that the condition in each degree is duplex, and that the negative and positive elements vary inversely, and that the comparisons and contrasts to be instituted are betwixt the negative elements and betwixt the positive elements of the several degrees.

be a feeling or thought which is indescribable. One patient used the expression, " Old scenes revert for hours before the fit." Another said, " If I were walking along and had a fit, I should think, Oh ! I saw that before." This patient had also an epigastric sensation, which he described as " a sudden fear," " a pang," " as if passing through an ordeal." A patient, whose case will be alluded to later on, said, " A feeling of being somewhere else." His fits began by a sensation of smell. A highly educated man described his mental state as one of double consciousness. In detail he said it was " the past as if present, a blending of past ideas with present." (Again, " a peculiar train of ideas as of reminiscence of a former life, or rather, perhaps, of a former psychologic state." He then lost consciousness ; returning consciousness was like awakening from a dream or trance ; the vision vanishing in spite of every effort to retain recollection of it. He said, " Sometimes I think I have it, and then it is gone." It may seem that this patient was reading philosophy into his symptoms, but a poor boy described the feeling " in his head " at the beginning of the seizure as if he had " two minds "—an exactly equivalent expression. I believe that the expression " double consciousness " is literally correct.[1] Another patient said, a feeling " as if dreams were mixed up with present thoughts." Another said, he had " a trace of last night's dream," and also " a thought accompanies it " ; " can't usually remember it,—in the last it was about gipsies." The attacks were also attended by an unreal smell—so-called subjective sensation of smell. Another patient saw " various visions when not quite unconscious." It was once " a wood and some people " ; another time, " pillars of an old Gothic church, and people standing in it." This patient also had a sensation of smell.

Such mental states in the early stages of epileptic paroxysm have attracted little attention in this country. Dr. Joseph Coats of Glasgow has recorded such a case (*British Medical Journal*, November 18, 1876). They have long been described by the French—Falret and others. Voisin, in his admirable article on Epilepsy, speaks of them.

It has been said that the intellectual aura (or what I call " dreamy state ") in slight attacks, or when ushering in severe ones, is usually the same in the same patient. So far as I can judge, it is not often so. Always, apparently, some voluminous mental state, the dreamy state is not always the same. Falret and Trousseau say that the " remembrance " is often what, on a former occasion, caused, or at least accompanied, the fit. Falret says that many become epileptic after some strong emotion or profound terror, and, at each fresh attack, see in their mind or under their eyes the painful circumstances or the frightful scenes which produced the disease in them the first time.

2. *Post-Epileptic Actions.*—We redivide, and still only empirically for clinical purposes, the second division into five groups ; in other words, we make five types.

(*a*) The patient acts nearly normally ; often the actions are a continuance, although in an imperfect and perhaps grotesque way, of what he was doing, or was about to do, before the fit. For example, a patient seized with a slight fit when about to wash himself, twirls his hands about the basin ; or going

[1] Of course I am not, in saying this, referring to the duplex negative and positive condition ; that is, no consciousness and subconsciousness, not double-consciousness. The " double-consciousness " is made up of the remains of object consciousness and of increased subject consciousness—a revelation, by " experiment of disease," of the normal rhythm in all mentation.

upstairs to make slight alterations in dress for dinner, he has a slight fit and undresses altogether.

(*b*) The patient walks quietly the wrong road, and finds himself in some strange place ; or he runs away from the place where he was seized with the fit as if terrified ; or he appears to be acting as if he wanted to go home, when really he is at home.

(*c*) We have the so-called co-ordinated convulsion. The patient, directly after his fit—or in it, as his friends will say—lies on the floor, sprawling about, kicking with his heels, etc.

(*d*) She rolls about, struggling and kicking, shouting, laughing, and often tries to bite. This condition in a woman is often taken for hysteria, and the mistake is easy, as the prior fit may be slight and transient. It is only for this reason that I state the condition separately from (*c*).

(*e*) The patient is up and about, and violently maniacal.

It is not pretended that the above is a good arrangement of cases ; it is the best *empirical grouping* I can at present make. Above all, it must not be taken as a scientific classification. Scientifically, all cases of insanity should, I submit, be classified, as each is an example of Dissolution. This term is used, not in its popular meaning, but as the opposite of Evolution ; it is so used by Herbert Spencer. Time will not suffice to do more than give one illustration of post-epileptic actions, from a case which comes more nearly under (*a*) than any other which I have not yet published.

A patient, aged 43, had been subject for three or four years to occasional attacks of loss of consciousness. I could get no account of any warning, and the patient denied having any actions after a seizure ; yet he really had. In a letter, after this visit, the patient wrote : " I have also had an attack to-day out-of-doors before dinner. I was walking home from the City, and had got as far as the London Hospital, but ultimately found myself walking the contrary way, under some impression that I was going to the City." Of course, if " under the impression " means that he remembered some " dreamy reason " for going to the City, the case is exceptional ; but I imagine, considering what follows, that it was his hypothesis to explain his conduct. Later on, he came with his assistant. He told me that the patient used to turn blue in the attack, but lately pale. There is movement of the hands and one leg is lifted : whether these movements were really spasms or only vague movements, whether parts of the paroxysm or post-paroxysmal, I could not ascertain. The assistant gave clear evidence of actions in or, as I believe, after the attacks. Thus, in the last attack but one, or rather, as I believe, just *after* it, he became violent, caught hold of various parts of his assistant's body and tried to drag him upstairs. The patient did get upstairs, and tried to take his clothes off ; looked at his watch, and then looked out of the window. He was well in about fifteen minutes. The last attack I heard of was in a place of worship, whilst sitting in his pew ; when his assistant spoke to him, the patient said : " Do you want to see me on business ? " (This reminds me of an illustration in *Punch*. A suburban resident, disturbed by the collector at church, woke up and cried " Season," apparently supposing that he was in the train, and that the guard was asking him for his ticket.) The last-mentioned attack in my patient was so slight that it attracted the attention of no one but his assistant. In, or, as I suppose, just after, an epileptic fit, and when yet " unconscious," this patient might read a page correctly and yet know nothing of it afterwards ; for example, he once read a parish notice.

Having now illustrated the first division, and also the first set of cases under the second division, I will relate a case showing both " dreamy states " and actions ; it is to be observed that " loss of consciousness " comes betwixt. There are in each case three stages.

1. The double state of (1) defect of consciousness along with (2) the positive, the dreamy state.

2. A further stage, one of loss of consciousness.

3. A stage of actions.

In these cases, we find that the patient remembers something of the first stage—his dream—but knows nothing of his actions.

The following case is that of a poor girl, a labourer's daughter, and herself on the parish. She is 29 years of age ; she has had severe fits for about eight years.

Her severe fits occur at night ; she bites her tongue in them, and, possibly because they occur in sleep, she has no warning of them. But, besides these severe fits, she has slight ones, which she calls " sensations." The feeling arises in her mind that she is miles away, but where she knows not. This is the only mental state. After the dreamy state, this patient becomes unconscious, and then actions follow ; she runs about the house. Of this running about she knows nothing. She remembers her " dream " without actions, but not the actions. Once she had a slight fit—a " sensation "—in bed, got up and ran about, and knocked her head against the bedpost. The woman who brought her remarked that the door was closed, adding that once, after a sensation, the patient had fallen downstairs in her hurry. The patient passes urine in these " sensations " ; so that, were there no severe fits, with tongue-biting, we should declare the " sensations " to be epileptic. If shaken in her runnings about, she stops, and in about twenty minutes comes to herself.

Colour, sound, taste, and smell are psychical states *attending* nervous discharges ; these sensations must not be spoken of as if they *were* nervous discharges. What we have called " crude sensations "—*e.g.* " balls of fire," " noises in the ear," etc.—are also psychical states as much as normal sensations are ; they *attend* excessive (epileptic) nervous discharges. These crude sensations, although as certainly psychical states as the " dreamy states " previously spoken of, are infinitely less elaborate ; they are also far less elaborate than certain other psychical states now to be mentioned.

Let us give an example to show broadly the difference betwixt a crude sensation and an elaborate psychical state. Coloured vision—a crude sensation warning at the onset of some epileptic paroxysms—is sometimes quickly followed by " seeing faces." The mere statement declares the immense difference in elaborateness ; the numerous different relations of sensations of colours, of extensions and distances, which make up the spectral image of a face, constitute a vastly more complex phenomenon than any development of colours and outlines attending an epileptic discharge. The most elaborate visual phenomena of some migrainous paroxysms—fortification outline, differently arranged colours, appearance of vibration, etc.—are far less elaborate than a spectral face. There is as much difference betwixt " balls of fire " and a spectral face as there is betwixt a house and heaps of materials of that house when pulled down ; or betwixt a series of elaborate musical chords and the noise made by playing the notes of those chords in a few seconds. But such elaborate phenomena as spectral faces are, it is supposed, *less* elaborate than those psychical states we have called "dreamy states," and sometimes spoken of as being voluminous. Thus, a spectral face is a much less complex psychical state than the feeling of "being somewhere else," or of imagining that a thing now seen was formerly seen under the very same circumstances.

The inference from the foregoing is, that whilst the several crude sensations are due to (attend) the onset of the epileptic discharge, such a highly compound phenomenon as that of slightly developed sensations constituting by intricate relations a spectral face does not occur from (attend) an epileptic—that is, an excessive nervous—discharge; it is supposed that the elaborate psychical states occur during slightly raised activity, slightly increased discharges, of those nervous arrangements most definitely connected with the one in which the epileptic discharge begins. Let us now state crude sensation warnings in relation to corresponding elaborate psychical states.

It must not be forgotten that we are speaking of cases of epilepsy proper—that is to say, of cases in which loss of consciousness is an early event in the paroxysm. The crude sensation of coloured vision not unfrequently attends the onset of epileptiform seizures; it occurs often in migrainous paroxysms, which in a scientific classification are (sensory) epilepsies.

1. *Paroxysms beginning by an Epigastric Sensation.*—This is often accompanied or quickly followed by an emotion of fear; the patient may *look* frightened ("startled," "guilty," etc.). Patients have used the following expressions: "I feel frightened," "dread," "horror," "perfect anguish and despair." There is not always an epigastric sensation with the feeling of fear. One epileptic patient used the several expressions "come over very melancholy," "intense fear," "frightful feeling, worse than any pain"; this patient had no epigastric sensation. One patient, who referred his warning to the mid-sternal region, said he "felt bowed down with trouble," and then said it was not trouble, but as if he "had some difficulty to overcome"; it is possible that the crude systemic sensation in this case was respiratory. I suppose there will be two sorts of respiratory sensations, or two sensations referable to the active part of the respiratory apparatus; for the chest not only moves rhythmically in breathing (organic function), but is fixed for short intervals in "effort" (animal function); if so, there will be the two crude sensations, suffocation and sense of impediment to exertion.[1] Possibly the feeling of fear at the onset of an epileptic paroxysm determines the epileptic cry (Herpin).

It may of course be suggested that the fear is a normal fear, that the patient is naturally frightened because experience tells him that a fit is coming on. Patients usually repudiate this interpretation. Such an interpretation is not supported by analogy of some other morbid conditions. It is common enough for hypochondriacs to have intense fear or misery, and yet to declare that they have no outward cause for anxiety. It is notorious that suicides are not often

[1] Some patients suffering from nervous exhaustion "come over frightened," and associate this emotional state with a disagreeable feeling at the epigastrium. Curiously, some patients so complaining add that they feel "as if they had done something wrong." These are slight cases of melancholia, although practically they differ vastly in degree from cases of melancholia commonly so-called. A girl, aged 11, had slight epileptic seizures, which began, she said, by a feeling as if she had "done something very wrong," "as if she were going to be beaten." I have no note about epigastric sensations in her case; she had a feeling as if something were going to choke her. Some healthy but nervous people, when actually frightened, feel "something turn over," etc., at the epigastrium. I have heard this feeling called "blue pain."

those who have any real and, so to speak, external calamity, but often those who, as their friends, or even themselves, may put it, " have every worldly blessing." People *are* according to the state of their nervous systems ; they may have the nervous conditions for fear or misery when there is no cause for either, just as a man in ague has the nervous condition for cold, and feels cold when he is hot. In some hypochondriacs, when a cause for their fear is alleged (*e.g.* the belief that they will be eternally lost), it is plain that nervous exhaustion came first, and " appropriated " some commonly thought of cause for alarm. In many people remorse is a sign, not of true repentance, but of nervous exhaustion. Then in some few epileptics the stage of warning is declared to be pleasing. The epigastric sensation is sometimes accompanied by the " dreamy " state.

2. *Paroxysms beginning by Noises in the Ear.*—Not unfrequently the noise is followed by " hearing voices." In many cases, at least, the term " voices " is inappropriate, for the patient may hear words or sentences ; he may " hear speeches," not vocal tones only.[1] I have heard a patient say that he heard the words " in his head," another that he " heard words without any sound." What these expressions mean I do not know.[2] This " hearing voices " would, I think, in a slight seizure, be strong evidence against auditory vertigo, supposing the other facts of the case were difficult of interpretation. For it should be remarked that the noise in the ear, and the sequent " voices," may sometimes be the sole seizure, although in all the cases in which I have yet observed this sequence, the patients have had also at other times severe epileptic paroxysms.

3. *If a fit begins by Coloured Vision* (" balls of fire," " flashes of light," etc.), there may follow " spectral faces," etc. This sequence would be valuable in diagnosis, because now and then the coloured vision and spectral faces might constitute the sole seizures. The sequence would be strong evidence against migraine, and in favour of epilepsy.

4. *Taste.*—I know nothing of any elaborate psychical state which corresponds to a crude sensation of taste, in the same definite way as spectral faces do to coloured vision, or the so-called " voices " to noise in the ear. In one case there was " the dreamy state " in a patient whose earliest fits began by a " metallic taste." [3]

[1] In an ordinary case of complete aphasia (loss of all speech except for some recurring utterance and rare occasional utterances) we note not only that the patient cannot use words in speech, having lost nervous arrangements for words by disease of one side of his brain, but also, what is not one whit less important, that he retains a service of words by which he understands what we say to him, and words which serve him in that part of his mentation which needs words (or symbols of some sort) ; he is speechless, but it is easily demonstrable that he is not wordless. The hearing " voices," or rather speeches or words, I presume, depends on increased excitation of the sensori-motor substrata of words which serve in receiving speech of others.

[2] It calls to one's mind the assertion of some persons that when under laughing-gas they felt the extraction of a tooth but had no pain. I have notes of the case of an epileptic who said his fits were preceded by a " tasteless taste." In some dreams developed by a noise, whilst the noise of necessity acts first, the corresponding noise in the dream comes last.

[3] I would suggest that such movements as those of mastication, of spitting out, and " smacking the lips," imply an excitation of some centres for taste analogous to that excitation of other centres during which " balls of fire," " noises in the ear," etc., arise ; similarly that rubbing the hands implies an excitation of some part of the tactual centres. (These statements will call to the reader's mind the case of a headless frog rubbing an irritated part of its body with a hind leg.) In the cases of epilepsy the supposed physical condition leading to the adapted movement is central ; but the reference is to the periphery. An ataxic patient of mine had only one hand, but had numbness not only in that hand, but in the spectral hand. Neither the masticatory nor the hand-rubbing movement can be put down to an *epileptic* discharge ; that would produce spasm of the masticatory and hand muscles, " running them up " into a contention in which all movement properly so-called would be absent.

I have notes of one case in which the patient has a taste at the beginning of his seizure, and then, on going into unconsciousness, masticates and spits out. But this patient has no sort of elaborate psychical state along with or just after the taste, and before loss of consciousness ; he acts elaborately after his paroxysm, remembering nothing of his actions. I have notes of a case of slight seizures in a boy, who spoke of them as " sensations of grease " ; but I could never get to know what " grease " meant. This boy, in attacks, put different substances into his mouth : at the seaside, sand ; at school he drank ink ; in the country he bit pieces of butterflies ; he smacked his lips in the attacks, and his brother said he had a look of disgust. I infer that there was here a sensation of taste, or at least an excitation of centres for taste. He passes urine in his attacks ; after them he sometimes acts " foolishly " and irrelevantly. He has no " dreamy state," nor any other sort of elaborate psychical state, attending the onset of his seizures.

5. *A Crude Sensation of Smell* is sometimes a precursor of epileptic attacks ; it is very much commoner than a taste—a rare thing,—and commoner, too, than a noise, but very much less common than colours. In one case so beginning, the patient had the delusion that the smell was external. In another case a patient held his nose when the attack began, from which the inference is that the smell was supposed to be external. Here, again, I know of no mental state which corresponds to smell *as directly* as spectral faces correspond to coloured vision, unless the " externalisation " of the smell is the analogue of the spectral faces. It must be added that the rule is that the patient feels the smell " in his nose " ; probably this is at a stage when he is fully conscious. The sense of smell, rudimentary though it be, is at once one of the most " commonplace " and the most intellectual. A scent or stink makes us sick, and, on the other hand, some scents develop in us very voluminous reminiscences.

A crude sensation of smell in some cases of epilepsy is followed by the voluminous psychical state called " dreamy state," although such voluminous psychical states occur without the crude sensation of smell, and, so far as I know, such states may not follow it.

The relation of the crude sensation to its corresponding elaborate mental state is, I presume, analogous to that of epi- or ento-peripheral sensations to ordinary dreams.

I think it will be found that in many, I dare not say in most, cases the voluminous mental state occurs in patients who have at the onset of their seizures some " digestive " sensation—smell, epigastric sensations, taste, or, in cases where there are movements implying excitation of centres for some such sensations, such movements as those of mastication.

We ought, I think, to say with sensations " subjectively serving." Taste serves subjectively in estimation of the agreeable or disagreeable, objectively in recognition of a quality in an external object. It seems strange at first glance that the *most* elaborate psychical states—the dreamy states—should attend or follow those warnings which refer to the less " intellectual " of the special senses, and to the epigastric sensation. It may be that there are errors of observation on my part : I have, however, no notes of cases in which the dreamy state attended a warning of vertigo. I have not heard of the dreamy state in association with coloured vision or noises in the ear. (I have never heard of it attending the onset of any epileptiform convulsion.) Yet it occurs in some cases wherein there is no crude sensation warning at all, and these may, for aught I know, be cases in which the part of the cerebrum discharged serves during some objective sensation. It may be well to say that I have not arrived at the provisional conclusion that the most elaborate psychical—the dreamy—states attend the more subjective of the sensations by theorising; it is a mere matter of observation, and possibly of very inadequate observation. It is possible that whilst the crude subjective sensation occurs during epileptic discharge of the sensory region of the left cerebral hemisphere, the dreamy sensations arise during raised activity of the right cerebral hemisphere.

There cannot be any doubt but that the crude warning sensations, sight and hearing, are sometimes followed by intelligibly related elaborate mental states.

The still more elaborate psychical states, the so-called "dreamy states," have not been carefully analysed. Judging from the statements of patients, they are diverse. Some are spoken of as being very elaborate, and yet the particulars are not remembered. There is the feeling of being somewhere else; there is the feeling of having seen things then present as they were seen some former time; occasionally there is a definite vision, one more elaborate than a spectral face. We should consider each kind of dreamy state in relation to its crude sensation warning when there is one; but sometimes there is no such warning, and for the rest I am at present unable to trace any definite relation betwixt particular warning sensations and particular "dreamy states." I have as yet only notes of fourteen cases.

To discriminate betwixt the dreamy states is important for another reason. It is possible that when they are followed by loss of consciousness (or of highest consciousness), and then by actions, some kinship may be discovered betwixt the particular "dreamy state" and what is done after the paroxysm. For example (see p. 300), there may be some relation betwixt the woman's dreamy state at the onset of her paroxysm of being "miles away," and her "running about" when the paroxysm is over. A patient of mine had the "dreamy state" of "being somewhere else," and after his paroxysm he, as his friends put it, "made for the door." Similarly, there may be a relation betwixt the several less elaborate psychical states, the spectral "faces" and "voices" (which in some cases follow corresponding crude sensations and precede the loss of consciousness, or of highest consciousness) and the post-epileptic conduct.

With regard to post-epileptic actions we should carefully note whether the "form" of the conduct is that of fear, the great subjective emotion, or anger, the great objective emotion, or of both; the states are often, if not always, mixed, even in health. Does conduct with fear (trying to escape, etc.) follow those seizures heralded in by an epigastric sensation? What sort of warning, if any, ushers in those seizures which are followed by conduct seemingly guided by anger, by fury, and attack? The warning most antithetical to the epigastric sensation, which is often attended by the emotion fear, is, I suppose, the sensation of vertigo. I suppose the crude "motor sensation" vertigo (see p. 287) is a brutal development of that sensation which is most representative in object consciousness, and that the crude "sensory sensation," the epigastric sensation, is of one most representative in subject consciousness. Let me state the double hypothesis in greater detail.

The most representative of objective sensations is that "motor sensation" which stands for relations established betwixt the organism and the environment—as *reacting on* the environment; in other words, that which estimates relations of external objects one to another. The physical basis of this sensation is ocular movement with central nervous arrangements representing ocular movements. Epileptic vertigo is a crude sensation corresponding to what is normally sense of orientation (vertigo is practically desorientation, as coloured vision is practically blindness, although not darkness), and the physical side of it is an excessive discharge of cerebral nervous arrangements representing ocular movements.

The most representative of subjective sensations will be that "sensory sensation" standing for the relations of tissues as to their state of nutrition. The state of nutrition is the physical basis on which the parts of the organisms are related one to another, as they are *affected by* the environment. Perfect nutrition or health has a correlative sensation, for which there is no name, except perhaps the name of "satisfaction." A quasi-healthy, imperfect, or incomplete nutrition is attended by hunger. I submit the further hypothesis that the epigastric sensation (sensation referred to solar plexus ?) is the crude sensation corresponding to the systemic sensation of hunger, or to the state of widespread need of repair of tissues ; that it is a feeling occurring during excessive central discharge, equivalent to that given by real widespread ill nutrition : if so there is nothing remarkable in its being attended by fear, for fear is the emotion of pain—using the term "pain" in the wide psychological sense as the reverse of pleasure, and as implying conditions injurious to the organism. Its manifestations show this clearly. Anger is the emotion of combat, as its manifestations show (Spencer, *Psychology*). What kind of warning, if any, mostly precedes loss of consciousness in those paroxysms after which the patient's conduct is seemingly as if guided by anger, I do not know.

It is certainly singular that vertigo and a sensation referred to the epigastrium are the two common warnings of epilepsy proper. I would urge that when studying post-epileptic actions, as they are of different kinds and have different degrees of elaborateness, and as they seem to be related to "dreamy" or to any other less elaborate psychical state, ushering in the paroxysm, we should note whether the form of the conduct is that of fear, or anger, or both.

In some cases the actions seem to be, popularly speaking, an unemotional carrying out of a simple dream. (Strictly speaking, no intellectual state can be quite free from emotion.)

Sometimes the post-epileptic actions are plainly determined by what was done or doing just before the paroxysm set in ; sometimes they are a going through some performances highly habitual in the patient. In the first case the very *recent* organisation of the ideas rivals in effect the stronger organisation of the habit, so far as revivability during unconsciousness or subconsciousness goes.[1] So then the post-epileptic actions are certainly not always in relation to the mode of onset of the paroxysm. Thus the methodical study of post-epileptic actions in relation to the early stages of the paroxysm is difficult. We should, I think, see whether or not there may be in some cases intelligible

[1] We usually say that in failing memory old events (or strictly the most organised) are remembered, and recent (the least organised) are forgotten. This is not without a very obvious qualification : it would be better to say that recent events are *soon* forgotten. In some cases of partial loss of speech, the inferior speech which is left consists in the substitution of a word more organised in, or more automatic to, the patient. But it is not always so ; the substitution may, I think, be explained in some cases by the fact that the patient has recently uttered the substituted word. There is indeed barrel-organism, to use a modification of Gairdner's expression for a temporary condition of some aphasics who get out a word in reply to a question and then must utter it in reply to further different questions.

relations betwixt the stages—(1) warning; (2) "dreamy" or less elaborate mental state; (3) actions after loss of consciousness and the emotional form of the conduct.

No doubt there are, strictly speaking, as many varieties of epilepsy proper as there are different warnings of paroxysms. It is to be hoped that, by the kind of investigation above mentioned, we may break up epilepsy proper into natural groups. If one patient's fits always begin by vertigo, and another's always by the epigastric sensation, it follows of necessity that different parts of the nervous system are diseased in the two patients. This is more striking, but not really more certain, when we adduce such different special-sense warnings as noise in the ear and coloured vision. What is especially desirable is a careful notation of the next events after the warning, and above all as to the affection of organic parts, particularly in those cases where the warning is either vertigo or the epigastric sensation.

The investigation of the different kinds of paroxysm of epilepsy proper is a matter of extreme difficulty. We shall, I think, be much helped by a careful preliminary study of the two great emotions—fear and anger. Certainly, those who believe that fright "causes epilepsy" ought to try to be well up in the physical phenomena occurring during this great emotion. So should those also who think fear—or, rather, the physical changes during it—to be an exciting cause of the first fit; for it may be that severe fright has something to do with determining which shall be the lines of least resistance to the first and subsequent discharges of the part of the highest centres which has become unstable.

I hope a clear knowledge of the mode of onset, and of the sequence of affection of parts, especially of the organic parts, will facilitate a rational therapeutics. For now we have, as Fraser, Brunton, Ringer, Fothergill, and others have shown, remedies which have, what for brevity I may call "an elective affinity" for certain parts, and remedies like atropin and muscarin, which are largely antagonistic in their action. Is there a variety of epilepsy proper in which belladonna is especially useful? Is there one in which its "antagonists" muscarin and pilocarpin are useful? To this question I can give no answer yet; enough is not yet known of the sequence of affection of parts in different varieties of epilepsy proper to enable one to give even an hypothetical answer. Both belladonna and the fungus from which muscarin is taken have been long used in epilepsy.

*Note.*—In these lectures, some modifications I have recently made in my opinion as to the relations to one another of the several cerebral centres are omitted. I have called the centres of the corpus striatum the lowest cerebral motor centres; Hitzig and Ferrier's centres, the middle; and the parts in front of these, the highest motor centres. But since many fibres from the spinal and higher homologous nuclei gain centres in Hitzig and Ferrier's region direct, passing through without joining the centres in the corpus striatum, the so-called middle centres stand, at least in part, in the same relation to the spinal motor centres as do the centres in the corpus striatum. I may here indicate in outline an hypothesis as to the relations of the several cerebral motor centres: (1) That the centres in the corpora striata represent more especially the movements concerned in tactual and visual images (ideas). (2) That the highest of the centres in Ferrier's region represent especially those locomotor movements, such as putting forth the hand, etc., which do not require displacement of the organism as a whole. (3) That the lower centres in this region represent especially manipulatory movements, such as writing, buttoning, manipulations of trade, etc. (4) There are movements, organic and animal, concerned during emotional states which will have an exceedingly wide representation in the cerebrum, and probably more directly in the highest centres than any other class of movements. Stating no suppositions on the relations betwixt these several cerebral centres, it is supposed that the highest motor centres represent or re-represent all four classes of movements in intricate combinations.

[Opposite the above note there is, in Dr. Jackson's writing, " I have greatly modified my opinion on this matter.—J. H. J."]

# ON RIGHT- OR LEFT-SIDED SPASM AT THE ONSET OF EPILEPTIC PAROXYSMS, AND ON CRUDE SENSATION WARNINGS AND ELABORATE MENTAL STATES[1]

In this paper I speak of the epilepsy of nosologists, sometimes called " genuine " epilepsy, or epilepsy proper. In this epilepsy consciousness is either lost first of all or very early in the paroxysm. Loss of consciousness, as the first, or nearly the first, thing in a paroxysm, is, I presume, a sign that the central discharge begins in some part of the highest cerebral centres. In epileptiform seizures consciousness is lost late, and is not affected at all when the convulsion is very limited in range ; in these seizures the discharge begins in some part of the lower cerebral centres (in some part of Hitzig and Ferrier's region). I think it is important to note, not only in epileptiform seizures but in epileptic seizures, on which side the first spasm or other abnormal condition is. Hence we ought to inquire whether the patient be left- or right-handed. In many cases of epilepsy proper the spasm is for the most part bilateral, but rarely is it quite equal and contemporaneous on the two sides at its onset. In many cases the head or eyes or both turn to one side at the onset. We ought to try to get to know to which side the first turning is. Unfortunately, the accounts given by the patient or his friends are often little trustworthy. Besides, sometimes the head first turns to one side and then to the other ; I mean that sometimes turning to each side occurs before spasm spreads to the limbs or trunk, or, at any rate, before it involves either of these regions in any marked degree. I had recently under care a case of convulsion in which, in one seizure, the head turned to one side at the onset, and in the very next seizure to the other. If we find, however, that the first spasm is always on the same side in every seizure, we may reasonably infer that the " discharging lesion " is of some part of the opposite cerebral hemisphere. In some cases there is no turning to one side ; the eyes may go up and the head back. I suppose this is owing to great rapidity of the discharge.

I think the time has come for recognising that many different epilepsies are grouped under the one term " epilepsy " ; we have come to recognise that at least several different epileptiform seizures are grouped under the term " epileptiform." The paroxysm of epilepsy which begins by vertigo is a different epilepsy from that beginning by a sensation referred to or near to the epigastrium (solar plexus ? ). The seats of the " discharging lesion " must differ when there are these two different paroxysms. There are, at any rate, as many different epilepsies as there are different warnings ; the so-called warning is simply the first result from, or during, the central discharge ; it is the thing of most localising value. Besides, it would appear to be very evident that the " discharging lesion " may be in either the right or in the left cerebral hemisphere. I wish to urge, firstly, that we should study, not the epilepsy of nosologists, but each different epilepsy as distinguished by its particular warning. I

[1] *Brain*, vol. iii, 1880–1, p. 192.

fully believe that it is a good thing to take epilepsy to be a sort of clinical entity, and, for an example, to work up the " warnings of epilepsy." In this way we can say that of sensation " warnings of epilepsy," coloured vision is common, noise in the ear rare, and taste very rare. Such are empirical generalisations of value. Like other physicians I have long worked in this way. But to make rational generalisations we should also work in another way. Instead of speaking only of different warnings " of epilepsy," I think we should say, too, that there are different epilepsies each with its own warning, and some with no warning. Secondly, we should observe each epilepsy throughout, from the warning, if there be one, through the paroxysm, to the after-condition of actions, when there are any. To begin with, we must study groups of cases according to the warnings. This kind of study is extremely difficult. It is to be understood that some of the statements I put forward as results of such study are made with great diffidence as to their exactness. He who undertakes a task of this kind is sure to make mistakes, however careful he may be. This short paper, I may say, represents great labour.

I dare not state it as a fact, but my impression is that when an attack of epilepsy starts by vertigo, *in the sense of there being apparent movement of objects to one side*, the first part of the convulsion is usually right-sided, and that external objects appear to be displaced to the right. Such vertigo would signify discharge of some part of the left cerebral hemisphere. I have put this doubtfully, partly on account of the difficulty there is in getting trustworthy information from the patients and their friends, and partly because some observations made at my request do not support impressions from what I have personally gathered from patients. It may here be remarked that the term " vertigo " is often used somewhat loosely. I do not take the expression " giddiness " from a patient's mouth to always mean true giddiness. We have to put down not his name for, but the description he gives of, the sensation he calls giddiness. Unless we take pains to be accurate in our examinations as to the question propounded, our observations will be of little value. The investigator who simply asks leading questions on this and some other matters to be mentioned shortly is not accumulating " facts," but is " organising confusion." He will make errors enough without adopting a clumsy plan of investigating which renders blundering certain. I would expressly remark that by the expression " epileptic vertigo," a slight fit of epilepsy is not meant, but vertigo in a slight fit of epilepsy, or at the onset of a severe one—that the patient has the sensation of external things moving or of himself turning. I submit that it is inconvenient to use the term " epileptic vertigo " for slight epileptic paroxysm in which there is no vertigo.

Some patients have a " warning " of smell ; others a sensation referred to, or to the neighbourhood of, the epigastrium ; others have, sometimes in addition to one of the above-mentioned crude sensations, movements of mastication, or movements like those of tasting. With these warnings the first spasm, if there be any, is usually on the left side. I suppose the movements mentioned indicate discharge of centres for taste, although the patient has no sensation of taste. It is very rare to find any sensation of taste as a " warning " of any kind of seizure.

I must stay to remark on the movements above-mentioned. It is submitted that they cannot result directly from an epileptic discharge. An epileptic (that is a sudden and an excessive) discharge of the nervous arrangements for these movements would produce that contention of movements which is spasm, not movements properly so-called. I suppose they are indirect (reflex) consequences of discharge of nervous arrangements serving during taste. *Mutatis mutandis* for rubbing the hands (discharge of tactual centres ?), and writhing of arms during suspended respiration, in other seizures. The hypothesis put forward is quite in accord with one of Ferrier's deductions from an experiment, is indeed a restatement of it with application to disease. Ferrier (*Functions of the Brain*, p. 189) writes : " As regards taste, I think that the phenomena occasionally observed in monkeys on irritation of the lower part of the middle temporo-sphenoidal convolution, *viz.* movements of the lips, tongue, and cheek-pouches, may be taken as reflex movements consequent on the excitation of gustatory sensations." In some slight cases of epilepsy the patient spits. I suppose no one would imagine such a highly compound movement to result (directly) from an epileptic discharge. It might, I submit, be plausibly put down as an indirect consequence of discharge of gustatory central nervous arrangements. So then in some slight fits of epilepsy we have not only that " clotted mass " of movements we call spasm, but also movements properly so-called. (I think too that there is in some cases, besides spasm, inhibition of lower motor centres and consequent paralysis.)

There is another way in which the warnings mentioned may be considered, as they are excessive and crude developments of objective or of subjective sensations. Unfortunately the terms " objective " and " subjective," so frequently used by medical men, are used in different senses. Thus, sometimes the term " subjective " is used for psychical states in contrast to the accompanying nervous states, which latter are then called objective. Sometimes the term " subjective," or the subject, is used for mind, or even without distinction between mind and organism, in contrast to the environment, which latter is then considered objective, or the object. Sometimes the term " subjective " is used for a sensation internally initiated, and the term " objective " for a sensation peripherally initiated ; thus, a patient who can smell nothing, and yet has stenches in his nose (at the onset of epileptic seizures, for example), is said to have no objective sense of smell, but to have subjective smell. Sometimes the term " subjective " is used for the patient's abnormal states of mind, pain, for an example, as when it is said " all his symptoms are subjective," in contrast to the symptoms the medical man can himself testify to, spasm, paralysis, cardiac murmurs, etc. These different contrasted applications of the two terms lead to great confusion in medical writings, and particularly when the same writer uses them sometimes one way and sometimes another. I imagine even that some philosophical writings are difficult to understand because the term " subjective " is used sometimes for mind and sometimes for organism ; and the term " objective " sometimes for nervous states and sometimes for environment (both the organism and the environment are " outside " mind). Hence, without venturing to say how the two terms ought to be used, I may properly say how I use them in this article. I use them both as psychical terms ; the term " subjective " answers to what is physically the effect of the environment on the organism ; the term " objective " to what is physically the reacting of the organism on the environment. The reader will note that it is not said that " subjective " stands for what is on the physical side of the organism, and " objective " for what is environment, but that they are used for what are on the physical side the two conditions of the organism in its correspondence with the environment. The correspondence is duplex, and all mental action is a rhythm of subjective and objective states.

Whether vertigo of the kind defined can be shown to occur most often during discharge of the *left* cerebral hemisphere or not, it is, at any rate, a crude development of the most representative of all objective sensations. Ocular movements represent the most special adjustments of the organism to—of all its reactions upon—the environment. They are the movements especially concerned during orientation. The vertigo mentioned is a crude sensation occurring during strong discharge of the nervous arrangements for these movements, and is desorientation, as coloured vision is blindness. In fact the so-called warning (vertigo) is itself consciousness ceasing in a particular way. What is physically a losing of the most special adjustments of the organism to the environment (desorientation) corresponds to what is psychically (object) consciousness ceasing.

Since most people are right-handed, the left cerebral hemisphere in most people represents the most objective movements, those movements for most specially operating on the environment. Moreover, speech is a process by which are symbolised relations of things in, or as if in, the environment[1] or things considered objectively ; nearly all evidence goes to show that the left cerebral hemisphere is in most people the one concerned during speech. I make these remarks on speech in order to ask if temporary aphasia does not more often occur after those epileptic seizures which start by vertigo ? I am not speaking of the well-marked and very definite temporary aphasia which is found after some right-sided epileptiform seizures. After some epileptic seizures there is temporary " abnormal talking," and this is sometimes aphasic.

Smell and taste are the two of the five special senses which, even popularly speaking, are the most subjective. Besides the five special senses there are sensations which Bain calls " organic " and Lewes " systemic." The common epigastric sensation preluding epileptic attacks is, I suppose, a crude development of the sensation of hunger—the most representative of systemic sensations. If so, the epigastric warning sensation is (subject) consciousness ceasing. Hunger is, on the one hand, a desire for food, on the other hand it represents the whole of our tissues as to their state of nutrition. At any rate the epigastric sensation is a systemic and subjective sensation.

I do not make the statements as to the side first in spasm in relation with " subjective " sensation warnings for any theoretical reason. On the contrary, they are antagonistic to certain conclusions I have come to from a different kind of evidence. It was a matter of surprise to me to find evidence of left-sided spasm at the onset of convulsions with these " warnings." I used to think the more " subjective " of sensations were chiefly represented in the posterior part of the left cerebral hemisphere. The inference that they occur most often in cases when the first spasm is left-sided is from observations, and I say again, observations all of which cannot be certainly trusted, the reports of patients and their friends not being always to be relied on.

We have always to note the side first in spasm in cases of " warnings," by crude development of the " objective " sensations, sight and hearing. I think it is usually, but certainly not always, the left. Here, again, we must

[1] Of course one does not use the term " environment " in its narrow dictionary meaning. If a man says his leg is longer than his arm, he is as much making a statement of things objective as when he says this stick is longer than that.

inquire about right- and left-handedness. It is certain that in some *epileptiform* seizures with coloured vision, the first or sole spasm is right-sided. Alexander Robertson (*British Medical Journal*, April 18, 1874) narrates a case of right-sided (epileptiform) convulsion with red vision. I have recorded the case (*Medical Times and Gazette*, June 6, 1863) of a woman who had right-side-beginning seizures, and at other times "attacks" of coloured vision. A left-handed man under my care in the Hospital for the Epileptic and Paralysed had fits beginning by a noise in the *left* ear. There was in that case tumour of the right cerebral hemisphere within the upper temporo-sphenoidal convolution—Ferrier's auditory centre. Gowers examined the specimen for me, and mentions the case in his second Gulstonian Lecture.

All the crude sensations above mentioned are psychical states, as indeed the term "sensation" implies. It is a grievous error to consider sensations as being active states of sensory nerves or sensory centres; doing so leads to taking such warnings as coloured vision to be of the same order as spasm of ocular muscles, or discharge of centres for them; the coloured vision is of the same order as vertigo. When we say that a patient has numbness and spasm of his hand at the onset of an epileptiform seizure, we are speaking of things different in two ways: the numbness is a crude sensation, a crude psychical state; the spasm is a physical symptom: the former occurs *during* discharge of sensory, the latter *from* discharge of motor elements of the centre. Confusing sensations with states of sensory nerves or centres leads also to ignoring that sensations occur during energising of motor centres. Nor should we use the term "bodily sensation," unless it is understood to mean a sensation referred to some part of the body. All sensations are in our minds, neither in the body nor in the environment; the correlative physical states are in the body. The peasant supposes redness, sweetness, heat, etc., to be in external objects, although, inconsistently, he does not suppose pain to be in the pin which pricks him. The physical changes during sensations are always in our own bodies. The best classification of sensations is into those which are objective—sensations referred to, or as if standing for, things in the environment—and subjective sensations—sensations referred to the body. But this classification, for obvious reasons, is largely arbitrary. For an example, taste serves chiefly subjectively, if it is a question of the agreeable or disagreeable, how the thing affects me; it serves chiefly objectively when it is a question whether this thing is bitterer than that, when it is chiefly a question of relations of things outside me one to another.

We can now consider certain psychical states during the onset of epileptic seizures which are much more elaborate than crude sensations. Once more there are reasons for noting in cases of epilepsy the side first in spasm, and whether the patient be right- or left-handed. I speak first of certain highly elaborate mental states, sometimes called "intellectual auræ." I submit that the term "intellectual aura" is not a good one. The state is often like that occasionally experienced by healthy people as a feeling of "reminiscence," that on which Coleridge, Tennyson, Dickens,[1] and many others have written. It is sometimes called "dreamy feelings," or is described as "dreams mixing up with present thoughts," "double consciousness," "feeling of being somewhere else," "as if I went back to all that occurred in my childhood." Some-

[1] Quotations are given from these authors by Quaerens, a medical man, who reports his own case—epileptic attacks beginning by "reminiscence"—in *The Practitioner*, May 1870.

times there is a definite elaborate vision. Very often the patient is sure of some thought, but cannot describe it in the least. Dr. Coats, of Glasgow, has reported such a case. The patient may describe the state vaguely as "silly thoughts." . . . These are all voluminous mental states and yet of different kinds; no doubt they ought to be classified, but for my present purpose they may be considered together.

These "dreamy states" mostly occur with the "subjective" warning—sensations, smell, and epigastric sensation, and with the supposed gustatory movements and sometimes with spitting. They cannot be owing to an epileptic discharge. It would be a remarkably well-directed and distributed epileptic discharge which would give rise to the exceedingly compound mental state of being somewhere else. Besides, it must not be forgotten that there very often is along with the dreamy state one of the crude subjective sensations mentioned. It is scarcely likely that one thing, an epileptic discharge, should be the physical condition for a sudden stench in the nose—a crude sensation—and also the physical condition for an infinitely more elaborate psychical state. I submit that the former occurs during the epileptic discharge, and that the latter is owing to but slightly raised activity of healthy nervous arrangements consequent on "loss of control"—possibly of some in the cerebral hemisphere opposite the one, which I believe to be nearly always the right, in which the discharge begins.

The elaborate mental state alluded to occurs sometimes without any crude sensation warning, but in some at least of these cases the first spasm or one-sided affection is left. In one case, with the dreamy state, the patient's head at the onset of every convulsion turned to the right. I was interested in finding that he was a left-handed man. This was the exception proving the rule. In one case, that of Quaerens (see footnote, p. 312), in which the patient had a "reminiscence," the only local symptom was in the right hand, and the patient was not a left-handed person; this case is a clear exception.

In some cases with the dreamy state, the patient spits. In one case beginning by sensation of smell the patient spat out, and had no dreamy state. I suppose the spitting had similar significance to the chewing, etc., movements.

It is, so far as I know, rare for the dreamy state to attend warnings of coloured vision and noises in the ear. I do not know of a clear case of such association. This is the more remarkable, as each of these crude objective sensations is sometimes followed by a less elaborate mental state, "seeing faces" and "hearing voices" (words), respectively. "Seeing faces" is a vastly less elaborate state than the dreamy feelings spoken of, such a one as "being somewhere else," although much more elaborate than crude sensations. Coloured vision and "seeing faces" are not likely to be both owing to an epileptic discharge. Both are psychical states, but the latter is far more elaborate.

I have notes of but one case in which the dreamy state occurred with the objective warning of definite vertigo.[1]

In but one of all his fits had this patient any sort of warning. The dreamy state attending vertigo in that fit was a feeling of being in some other place,

[1] Dr. Joseph Coats has recorded a case, already alluded to (*British Medical Journal*, November 18, 1876), of an epileptic, each of whose fits, with few exceptions, was preceded by giddiness and a peculiar "thought." "Sometimes the fit only consists of the aura, followed by a peculiar feeling in the abdomen, which passes up to the head and back to the abdomen, when vomiting results."

" several places," not any particular place. I use the expression " definite vertigo," for I have known two cases in which with sensation of external objects moving in front of the patients, not to one side, there was the dreamy state ; in one (the carpenter's case, *vide infra*) described as " silly thoughts." This patient has the feeling as if objects were coming upon him. I think this sensation, and that of objects appearing to move away, ought to be distinguished from the feeling of objects moving to one side. I have seen a patient in whom, according to his account, a " dreamy " feeling did not occur with his " giddy attacks," but with other attacks beginning by some thoracic or epigastric sensation. So far the case is very striking, and is particularly so as to the occurrence of mouth movements with the seizures in which there was the dreamy state. I admit, however, that there are apparently some discrepancies, to which I shall try to give prominence. The patient recorded his own case, which was published with additions, some years ago, by Dr. Weir Mitchell, who kindly advised him to see me. He had attacks of several kinds. Weir Mitchell writes : " The spells of pure giddiness have been frequent of late. They come on suddenly, and there are none of the strange mental conditions which attend other spells." The giddiness was clearly paroxysmal, and was attended by a feeling of turning to one side. When I saw him, I had no idea of the importance of noting the particular side to which the tendency to turn was, and had paid no particular attention to " dreamy states." The " other spells " began by, what I gathered when I saw the patient to be, an epigastric sensation, but which he, in his printed account, speaks of as " severe oppression across the chest," making it difficult for him to breathe. He states in his account, " I unconsciously move my mouth as if chewing, and sometimes will also grit my teeth." He describes his mental condition as comparable to that of one suddenly awakened out of a sound sleep. " He cannot catch hold of the dream, which seems to be quickly passing from him, and at the same time he cannot yet appreciate the state of unconsciousness into which he has so suddenly awakened." He writes also : " The things around me seem to be moving ; and if I am reading, the book will appear to be going from me, when at once I feel as if all must be a dream, though well knowing at the same time it must be reality . . . through it all the fear of some impending catastrophe seems to be hanging over me."

Here we have together epigastric sensation, chewing movements, fear, and dreamy state. But we have to note that there is in these seizures apparent movement of objects ; so then it may be taken that this is exceptional. The apparent movement of objects of course implies changes in himself, some ocular movements or discharge of centres for them. It may be said that he had vertigo ; yet in what he himself called his giddy fits he had no dreamy state. I did not ascertain whether the movement was of *all* objects from him as it was of the book. When there is apparent alteration of the distance of objects at the onset of epileptic seizures they usually appear to come nearer or to be larger, but may seem to go farther off. It may be mentioned that on awaking from sleep objects appear to be nearer, and as we get fully awake they recede. Such apparent displacements of objects at the onset of epileptic seizures no doubt depend on abnormal states of the accommodative apparatus or their centres (under atropine objects appear smaller or farther off ; the reverse for calabar bean). This is very different from displacement of objects to one side attended by a feeling of giddiness. Lateral movements of the eyes will have to do with estimation of the figure (superficial extension) of objects, and symbolise tactual movements; accommodation has to do with distance: it symbolises locomotor movements (of arms as well as locomotor movements ordinarily so-called).

I heard of no one-sided affection in the attacks with the dreamy state. It is to be mentioned that he could talk in them. In other attacks, which he calls "paralysing attacks," there was movement of the mouth; but he is then aphasic, and probably the movement is one of spasm. In these attacks his *right* hand becomes fixed across his chest, and he loses "all control over his words." There is no mention of giddiness in these seizures. He adds: "The same feeling of uncertainty usually surrounds me as in the other." If this refers to the dreamy feeling, the case is so far exceptional. He has, however, attacks of severe giddiness without any dreamy sensation.

The day I had written the above I was consulted by a right-handed patient, who had left-hemiplegia since 1875, and afterwards, since 1876, occasional seizures, like those of genuine epilepsy. All his attacks began by the same "dreamy" feeling, as if he were falling down a coalmine.[1] In this case there was no other premonitory sensation except something referable to the ear. There was not, at the onset, a sensation of smell, nor any epigastric sensation, nor any fear. I positively could not get to know whether or not he had a noise in the ear, or in the head, nor even with certainty that it was a noise at all; for the patient, after describing his sensation as a singing, said it was not a real singing, but rather a "dullness." But the interest of the case is that upon a damaged *right* cerebral hemisphere there should ensue seizures beginning with the voluminous mental state mentioned. This patient had slight seizures, and also occasionally severe ones; in the severer ones the spasm preponderated on the left side. I have (*Lancet*, March 11, 1876) recorded cases in which noise in the ear occurred at the onset of epileptic seizures; in the second case this was followed by hearing "voices," a fact, however, which was not mentioned in that report. I have seen many such cases, but the case of the left-hemiplegic patient above referred to is the only one I have seen in which there was a voluminous mental state with a "warning" of noise; if, indeed, there was in that case such warning.

There are other kinds of psychical states in connection with some epileptic paroxysms. It is not uncommon for a patient to have the emotion of terror and to look terrified at the onset of his seizures. When so, there is usually the epigastric sensation with it. It is to be observed that sometimes there is fear without any epigastric sensation,[2] and that sometimes, although very rarely, there is with the epigastric sensation a pleasurable feeling.

I never remember hearing a patient mention the antithetical (objective) emotion of anger; but friends of patients sometimes describe a look of indignation. Yet some patients say that at the onset of their seizure they feel they must attack someone, or have a hatred against some person present. As anger is the emotion of combat, this is equivalent to confession of feeling of anger. I do not know anything definite as to crude warning sensation with look of anger, at the onset of epileptic paroxysm. Theoretically, one would expect it to be an

[1] He had had nothing to do with coalmines at any time, and could discover no reason for this particular recurring "dream."

[2] After some slight paroxysms, beginning either by the epigastric sensation or by fear without it, the patient's bowels are moved; a fact, I submit, of some significance.

objective sensation. I believe that when the emotion of fear occurs at the onset of a paroxysm, with or without the epigastric sensation, the first spasm is on the left. I have, however, one patient whose fits always begin by fear—as if, to use his words, " something had given me a sudden fright "—and whose first spasm is always right-sided. He, however, is a left-handed man (his father was also left-handed). This patient has a sensation, not at his epigastrium, but at the middle of his chest. (The case has been referred to, p. 314, as the case of the carpenter.)

It is not uncommon for a patient to have the epigastric sensation, to look frightened, to feel frightened, and to have also the dreamy state. In this regard another thing is to be considered. Some patients act elaborately after their paroxysms. I would ask, " Are the actions after the fit apparently coloured by fear, actions of escape, when the seizures start by a feeling of fear ? Is the same emotion carried out in each stage ? "

When there is a dreamy feeling, the " dream " also may influence the post-epileptic actions. In one case actions of " running away " occurred after a fit beginning by sensation of smell, and with a " feeling of being somewhere else." Another patient always used to run away after fits, at the onset of which she had the feeling of " being miles away." (Correspondingly for spectral faces, voices, etc., after coloured vision and noises in the ear ? ) As with the epigastric sensation and fear there is often also a " dreamy state," we may have actions in accord with the " dream," and also coloured by fear. I imagine the actions in some cases, wherein there is the dreamy feeling, except, perhaps, that of reminiscence (which is, I presume, nothing other than a revelation of the earlier subconscious part of the normal process of recognition), are more likely to be adjustments to some " ideal " environment ; the dream being made up chiefly of long-past experiences ; the actions may be very elaborate and yet not purposive-looking as to the present environment.

I would suggest a corresponding series of inquiries as to seizures beginning by objective sensations, and especially by vertigo. " Are the actions after these seizures more seemingly purposive to the patient's present surroundings, and often those of anger ? " " Are they the result of an ' unremembered ' or vaguely remembered ' dream,' made up chiefly of recent experiences ? " The expression " unremembered dream " may seem absurd at first glance ; but we must bear in mind that Descartes, Leibnitz, Kant, Jouffroy, and Hamilton believed there to be no dreamless sleep. It may, however, be held that there is nervous activity without any attendant mental state in deep sleep, that it is really dreamless, and that any " mental modifications " come during waking. Similarly it may be held that when actions after a fit are very purposive-looking there is no " dream," but yet such kind of activity of nervous arrangements as would in imperfect sleep give rise to a dream, made up chiefly of recent experiences.

When actions are always the same in a patient after every fit, it may be that that they are in accord with what occurred about the time of his first seizure.

To repeat. I ask, on which side is the first spasm, or other abnormal condition, in cases beginning by crude sensation of smell, by movements of chewing, etc., by the epigastric sensation with or without fear, and in cases where there is fear without any epigastric sensation ? I think it is usually the left side. Again I ask, on which side is the first spasm, or other abnormal condition, when there is a " dreamy state " with or without any of the above-mentioned phenomena? I think it is usually the left. We ought to inquire also whether the patient be right- or left-handed. Correspondingly for cases in which there is a crude objective sensation as a warning.

I would also ask that the nature of the actions, when they occur after a fit, should be considered (*a*) as being complex or simple; (*b*) as purposive-looking, or seemingly purposeless; (*c*) as unemotional, or as coloured by anger or fear.

I doubt not that there is some order throughout, from the warning to the end of the post-paroxysmal stage. The above imperfect sketch, the best I can do, is the result of much labour, as a contribution towards discovering this order. I am far from asserting that I have done anything of value towards this end, and trust I have fairly acknowledged the difficulties and uncertainties necessary to investigations in which we have to trust so much to our patients.

# ON TEMPORARY PARALYSIS AFTER EPILEPTIFORM AND EPILEPTIC SEIZURES: A CONTRIBUTION TO THE STUDY OF DISSOLUTION OF THE NERVOUS SYSTEM[1]

In the Mirror of the *Lancet*, December 13, 1873, and October 26, 1878, are reported, with remarks, cases of temporary local paralysis after epileptiform convulsions; after those convulsions, that is to say, in which spasm begins in the terminal part of a limb or in the side of the face: these convulsions were first described by Bravais in 1824. As I there stated, the paralysis is supposed to depend on exhaustion of nerve fibres consequent on the excessive discharge in the paroxysm. I do not now, however, speak so confidently as to the geographical position of the fibres exhausted; physiologically speaking, they are, I suppose, those connected with the discharging cells, and presumably some fibres of the internal capsule. Since the remarks in the first report appeared, I have found that the hypothesis advanced is in all essential respects the hypothesis of Todd and Alexander Robertson. It is briefly that the temporary post-epileptiform paralysis depends on temporary central exhaustion consequent on the excessive discharge during the paroxysm. During the paroxysm there is a severe nervous discharge (liberation of energy) beginning from highly unstable cells ("discharging lesion"[2]) of some portion of the cerebral cortex; the currents developed of course "flow" in the order of lines from those of least to those of most resistance; in other words, the movements of the external parts represented are developed in the order of their speciality of representation by the nervous arrangements (cells and fibres) of the portion of the cortex in question. Spasm in convulsion is nothing more than a contention, or sequence of contentions, of many of the movements represented by unstable cells of some part of the cerebral cortex; numerous movements being developed in a short time.

The convulsion is the external positive event answering to the internal positive event of excessive nervous discharge (great liberation of energy). The local paralysis remaining when the convulsion is over, when the discharge has ceased, is of the parts first and most convulsed, and is supposed to be the external negative condition answering to the internal negative condition of exhaus-

[1] *Brain*, vol. iii, 1880–1, p. 433.

The term "dissolution" has long been used by Herbert Spencer as the opposite of "evolution." I use it in that sense in this, as I have done in former papers. Great objections are made to this application of the term, but I submit that it is inexpedient to coin a new word for the opposite of evolution of the nervous system, when "dissolution" has been used for at least fifteen years for the opposite of evolution in general. The term is none of my choosing; it was used as I am now using it, long before I thought of the process it names.

[2] The very simple expression "discharging lesion" has, I find, led to difficulties. It has been taken to mean that some morbid product discharges, just as the expression "the kettle boils" might be taken to mean that the copper vessel and not the water boils. A "discharging lesion" consists in some alteration (excess of function) of some part of the patient; certain of his nerve cells, representing some movements of some parts of his body, have by some pathological process become highly unstable; on their discharge, the movements they represent are suddenly developed in great numbers in a very short time. The contention of these movements is spasm.

tion of some fibres overworked from the excessive discharge of cells connected with those fibres. The nerve fibres being only exhausted, and not destroyed, as in some other kinds of paralysis, post-epileptiform paralysis is temporary, unless, of course, the fit recurs soon.

The condition following an excessive cerebral discharge is supposed to be analogous to exhaustion, by strong faradisation, of a nerve going to the cut-off leg of a frog. A closer analogy is the temporary paralysis of a frog after a tetaniform attack induced by a large dose of strychnia ; the functional power of the motor nerves is temporarily destroyed. Since after an enormous dose of strychnia there is paralysis without prior convulsion, it is believed that strychnia may act directly on the motor nerves. However, Vulpian concludes [1] : " Les nerfs d'un membre privé de circulation chez une grenouille strychnisée perdent donc *une partie* de leur motricité sous l'influence des excitations prolongées, répétées et violentes, qu'ils subissent dans ces conditions."

A still closer analogy is that, on strong faradisation of a frog from mouth to anus there is a tetanic condition, and after it a *temporary* " résolution flasque et générale de toutes les parties du corps." [2]

The above is not the accepted explanation. Some physicians believe the temporary post-epileptiform paralysis to result from the cerebral congestion of asphyxia induced by arrested respiration in the paroxysm. In reply, it may be said that such congestion being universal in the brain cannot account for *local* paralysis. Again, the paralysis has been attributed to small extravasations of blood caused by congestion from arrested respiration. But the paralysis is of the parts first and most convulsed in the prior paroxysm, and it would be very remarkable if the extravasations in each succeeding fit always occurred in the same centre—in that representing parts first and most convulsed. I do not adduce against this opinion the fact that the paralysis is temporary, for I admit that small clots may produce only temporary paralysis. There are other strong arguments against the accepted explanation. We find local paralysis after some epileptiform seizures in which there has been no interference with respiration whatever ; paralysis so occurring cannot be caused by cerebral congestion, nor by extravasations in the nervous centres. On the other hand, local paralysis does not occur after severe seizures of epilepsy proper, in which there often is extreme asphyxia from spasm of respiratory muscles. To repeat : absolute, although temporary, local paralysis may be found where there has been no asphyxia in the prior paroxysm, and is not found after paroxysms of epilepsy proper when the asphyxia has been suddenly induced and extreme in degree.

It is asserted by some authorities that the local paralysis after epileptiform seizures is *not* always of the parts first and most convulsed. In my experience, it has always been so. This being no answer, I can only ask that further observation may be made on the matter.

It is understood, of course, that we are speaking of paralysis following seizures which we may call chronic ; we are not speaking of cases of meningeal or cerebral hæmorrhage ; in some cases of cerebral hæmorrhage the clot which destroys some part of the brain, and which in this way produces hemiplegia, also causes convulsion. We speak of cases such as those in which a small tumour or other " foreign body " in the mid-cortical region of the brain leads to instability of cells near it—leads to what I have called a " discharging lesion " ;

[1] *Arch. de Phys.*, vol. iii, 1870, p. 128. [2] Vulpian.

the cells rendered unstable occasionally " explode " or liberate much energy, or, in other words, discharge excessively, and all of them much more nearly simultaneously than the comparatively stable cells do in health. After their excessive discharge has ceased, as signified by cessation of spasm, there *is* often paralysis, and that paralysis is temporary.[1]

It is supposed that the following is the sequence from a growth in the cortex to the temporary post-epileptiform paralysis : (1) A growth, often a syphilitic one, in the cortex cerebri ; so far apparently there are no convulsive or paralytic symptoms. But the growth, in its character as a foreign body, (2) induces (presumably slowly) changes of instability in nerve cells near it. Still there may be no outward signs of it, or rather of these changes it induces. Next (3) some day the unstable cells discharge and produce a convulsive paroxysm. (4) After the paroxysm there is paralysis of the parts which were first and most convulsed. (5) The patient is apparently well again in a few hours or days, and keeps so until the next fit comes. (Of course the " foreign body " may produce the general symptoms of tumour, optic neuritis, headache, etc., which do not here specially concern us.)

It is recognised nowadays, thanks especially to Hitzig, Ferrier, and Charcot, that tumours in the mid-region of the brain, when very large and when much softening is induced, may be the cause of some permanent paralysis ; here the paralysis is owing to permanent destruction. In this paper temporary paralysis after convulsion is alone considered, and so far only local temporary paralysis after epileptiform seizures.

It is not denied, of course, that convulsion may occur in a part which is already paralysed, partially or completely. For example, a patient may become hemiplegic without convulsion, and then on partial, or, indeed, on apparently complete, recovery, he may become subject to convulsions beginning in the hand, side of face, or foot. This I believe happens most often when the hemiplegia has resulted from embolism or thrombosis.

Cases of transient paralysis not preceded by convulsion, however often repeated, and however much like one another the recurring palsies may be, do not come here under our notice. Transient paralysis may be owing to a small clot, or to softening from blocking of a small vessel. Repetitions of similar local paralyses, each transitory, are hard to explain ; but, as above said, we are not here concerned with them. Again, a patient subject to localised convulsion may have a batch of them, and in the intervals of the convulsions the parts occasionally severely convulsed may remain absolutely paralysed. It is very singular to witness spasm beginning in and spreading over a

[1] I have suggested that the size and shape of cells, as well as their nearness to the tumour, or other source of irritation, will have to do with their becoming unstable ; other things equal, the same quantity of matter in many small cells will present a vastly greater surface to the contact of nutrient material than the same quantity in one large cell. I have also suggested that small muscles, or, more properly, movements which require little energy for the displacements they have to effect (those of face and of the hands in touch, for example), are represented by small cells. Such movements are rapidly changing during many of the operations they serve in—writing, for example—and require repetitions of short liberations of energy, and necessitate quick recuperation of the cells concerned. Movements of the upper arm are, in comparison, little changing, and require persistent steady liberation of energy. That small muscles are represented by small cells is not altogether a mere hypothesis. The masterly researches of Bevan Lewis seem to me to show that those parts of Hitzig and Ferrier's region which especially represent small muscles have most small cells. It is to be noted that parts like the hand will be represented in a great number of different movements, and therefore by numerous ganglion cells. It may be mentioned too that epileptic and epileptiform seizures usually begin in small muscles, and it often happens that for a time a patient's seizures are limited to small muscles.

limb which the patient can at no time move in the slightest degree.[1] In this paper, I repeat, temporary paralysis after convulsion is alone considered.

Let us note the sequence of phenomena in a very simple case, recorded in the *Lancet*, October 26, 1878, intercalating hypothetical explanations in brackets, and thus keeping them separate from the facts. A patient subject to epileptiform attacks (having permanently a local " discharging lesion ") has no obvious paralysis (since if the nervous arrangements, their cells being highly unstable, are useless for normal function, there is large compensation by neighbouring parts). One afternoon she has a fit (an excessive discharge, beginning from the part of the cortex the cells of which are unstable), the spasm affecting chiefly the right arm (brutal, that is excessive, development and more nearly simultaneous development of the movements which the unstable cells discharging represent than would occur in healthy operations) : after the fit the arm is *absolutely* paralysed (exhaustion of central nerve fibres has been effected by the discharge) ; all paralysis is gone in five hours (there being only exhaustion, recuperation is soon complete).

Of course there are cases in which the post-epileptiform paralysis is trifling, and more transitory than in the case above instanced ; the patient may say his hand is a " little numb," and we may find that he grasps firmly, but cannot pick up a pin or button his shirt. It is convenient to take for illustration a simple case ; the reasoning is essentially the same. In the case instanced we have not merely to account for (1) local paralysis after a localised convulsion, but for two other things also ; (2) for the absoluteness of the paralysis ; (3) for the paralysis being very transient.

We have so far, except in passing illustration, spoken only of epileptiform seizures. Logically, if Todd and Robertson's hypothesis is to be sustained, there ought to be paralysis after seizures of epilepsy proper. It would usually be said that there is none. So that whilst after the comparatively slight seizures called epileptiform there is often decided paralysis, there is, according to current opinions, none after the much severer paroxysms of epilepsy proper. At first glance this seems decisive against Todd and Robertson's hypothesis, as well as against the hypothesis of congestion and extravasation already combated. But local paralysis (of the face, or of a limb, or of one side of the body) is not the sole paralysis met with ; there is such a thing as paralysis spread all over the body. The patient, after a severe paroxysm of epilepsy proper, has not, it is true, any paralysis of but one limb ; he is not hemiplegic. He is, however, I submit, biplegic, if such a word may be coined. I mean that there is some, however slight, paralysis of both sides of the body ; the paralysis is nearly evenly, I do not say absolutely equally, spread on both sides of his body. How does it happen that such paralysis is ignored ? One reason I submit is, that being slight, evenly spread, and transient—there being no difference, or no obvious difference, betwixt the two sides of the body—it is not easily recognisable as paralysis. Another reason is, that here, as in other cases, abnormal physical conditions are erroneously " explained " as being owing to abnormal psychical states. After a very severe fit of epilepsy proper, the patient does not

[1] Perhaps it may seem that such cases are counter to the hypothesis. But that the comparatively slight discharges during " volition " should fail to move a part, and that an excessive discharge should move it, is not extraordinary. Yet if the fibres be exhausted, how is it that by them the excessive discharge can effect convulsion of the part they pass towards ? We must suppose that they are either not absolutely exhausted, or that they soon recuperate enough to be affected by the excessive discharge.

move his limbs ; all admit that. He seems a mere breathing, circulatory, etc., mechanism, lying otherwise inert on the floor. As he is then comatose, it would generally be said that he does not move *because he is unconscious*. A moment's consideration, however, will show that this is an explanation which verbally explains everything, and yet in reality explains nothing. It may pair off with such a pseudo-explanation as that a patient does not move a limb because there is loss of volition, or with that which accounts for an aphasic's inability to speak, or for his speaking badly, by saying that it is " *because* he has lost the memory of words." It belongs to a whole family of psychologico-materialistic confusions ; it is akin to that which has it that ideas or sensations (psychical states) produce movements (physical states) ; to that also which declares that the mind affects the body. Nothing is said against the popular or clinical use of these expressions. No one objects in a clinical conference to the expressions that ideas or emotions affect, or, more inclusively, that the mind affects, the body, when it is understood that what is meant is that centres, *during activity of which mental states arise*, can affect other centres, and thus the body. But much is to be said against the use, or rather abuse, of such expressions in what purport to be scientific explanations. It is, to say the very least, inexpedient in a scientific exposition to attempt to explain physical conditions by invoking crude popular psychological doctrines.

To return to the case. I submit that the post-epileptic comatose patient does not move, for the very simple reason that there is some negative *physical condition* of his nervous centres. It is an intelligible, if it be an erroneous, explanation to say that his highest nervous arrangements, and no doubt many lower ones too, are exhausted by the excessive discharge in the prior paroxysm. Surely the patient's not moving, if it be not owing to exhaustion of nervous arrangements, is at any rate owing to *some* negative *physical* condition ; this negative physical condition is not loss of consciousness, but is only correlative with that negative *psychical* condition, if one may be allowed to speak of two negative conditions being correlative. I submit that it is not an intelligible explanation to say that the patient does not move because he is unconscious. Why should he not move if unconsciousness were all, his nervous system being sound ? The fact is, he cannot be unconscious without having some negative physical condition of his nervous system answering to that negative psychical condition, and it is the central negative physical condition alone which we have to take count of in our explanations of his other physical condition of immobility.

The paralysis after a paroxysm of epilepsy proper, although widespread, is not necessarily, I suppose never is, total everywhere ; it varies in different cases from slight to severe. In some cases of post-epileptic coma, there is considerable movement on disturbing the patient. This is not in the least counter to the hypothesis, for besides the possibility that but few of the patient's highest nervous arrangements are exhausted, many others, and also some of lower centres, are capable of functioning. There is no *a priori* reason why there should not be slight quasi-trifling paralysis spread all over the body—in other words, loss of some movements of every part of the body, with retention of many other movements of every part of the body—than that there should be slight quasi-trifling paralysis throughout an arm as there often is—in which case there is loss of some movements of the limb as a whole, with retention of many other movements of it. To speak of a part as being both paralysed and also as being movable by the patient, is not even unusual in ordinary clinical language. For to say that an arm is partially paralysed means that there is both some paralysis and also some movement remaining. We should not speak of paralysis of *muscles* from central lesions. Nervous centres do not represent muscles, but, or except as, movements. Hemiplegia appears as loss of power in certain muscles, but really is a loss of a number of movements of the parts paralysed. Similarly a convulsion appears as spasm of muscles, but is really a development of numerous movements of the parts, or rather an attempt at such development; spasm being a contention of many movements. From a small destructive lesion of a centre a few movements of muscles may be lost, and many other movements of the same muscles be retained; the hemiplegic man, who cannot easily button his waistcoat, and yet can lift a chair, has only lost some power in the muscles of the arm, in the sense that he has lost some of the most special or " delicate " movements of this limb. Similarly there may be loss of some of the most special or " delicate " movements all over the body, with retention of very many more general or " coarser " movements all over the body.

I do not shirk the logical consequences of the doctrine that the highest centres are, like all lower centres, sensori-motor—that from loss of function of more or fewer of them there is paralysis. Let me go into detail. I believe that in every case of insanity, however slight it may be, there is, so long as it lasts, defect [1] of consciousness. I believe, too, that there is necessarily correlative with this negative psychical condition a negative physical condition of the highest nervous arrangements. Putting this otherwise, consciousness in health attends but is not activity of these highest nervous arrangements; and when the function of them or some of them is lost by any pathological process there is correspondingly loss or defect of consciousness. The highest centres are not consciousness, they are only the anatomical substrata of consciousness. Since the anatomical substrata of consciousness are like all other centres made up of sensori-motor arrangements, there should be widespread, however slight, paralysis in every case of insanity. I believe there is. Of course in many cases it would be difficult or impossible to demonstrate any. Some of those who might deny there to be any in a case of insanity might nevertheless admit it by saying that there was loss of expression, shambling gait, and slowness of movement. To take an extreme case, one of temporary acute mania after an epileptic paroxysm. The furious post-epileptic maniac is unconscious as well as maniacal. His symptomatic condition is double: there is a negative and there is also a positive element. I believe there is during his mania widespread paralysis consequent on temporary exhaustion of many of his highest nervous arrangements, which exhaustion is the negative physical condition answering to his negative psychical condition. I do not mean that his maniacal actions are the outcome of the exhaustion; that is an impossible explanation; there is supposed to be paralysis answering to that exhaustion. How, then, do we account for the co-existing over-movements of mania? The case is an example of dissolution, using this term as the opposite of evolution.

[1] I dare say it may be denied that in some slight cases of insanity there is any defect of consciousness, partly because it is erroneously inferred that what is clinically called insensibility is meant. Yet probably some of those who would deny defect of consciousness in a slight case of insanity would tacitly admit it by saying that the patient's judgment, power of attention, emotional control, or will was defective. A person has not got a consciousness in addition to will, memory, and emotion; these are only names applied to artificially distinguished aspects of consciousness; defective judgment, etc., is defect of consciousness.

Evolution does not simply imply a progressing increase of complexity and speciality only, but also that the higher (more complex and special) nervous arrangements control or inhibit the lower. There are two things : " the adding on " of the higher is at the same time " a keeping down " of the lower. Now as to the reverse process of dissolution. It also is a double process. " The taking off " of the higher is a " letting go " of the lower. On removal of the influence of some of the highest nervous arrangements (on loss of their function in case of post-epileptic mania by exhaustion), the next lower nervous arrangements, no longer controlled (Anstie, Dickson), spring into activity, and it is from *their* activity that the maniacal movements result. On the physical side there is loss of function of some of the highest nervous arrangements, and increased activity of the next lower. Correspondingly on the psychical side is loss of consciousness and mania. In all other cases of insanity there is a negative and a positive condition ; in some, as in post-epileptic mania, the positive condition is hyperpositive.[1]

There is no inconsistency in supposing that there is paralysis in the sense of there being loss of some of the most special movements all over the body, and that there is also retention of very many others, and over-increased activity of them, any more than there is in supposing there to be loss of some movements of the arm in cases of chorea, where other movements of that limb are over-developed. I submit that what has been called defect of voluntary co-ordination of the arm in chorea, is simply loss of so many movements of the limb, that it is so much paralysis ; and what has been called morbid involuntary co-ordination, is simply over-development of some others. Besides, we daily see co-existing the diametrically opposite conditions of paralysis and spasm, as in the rigidity of hemiplegia. So we do more rarely in the tremor of disseminated sclerosis, in which there is loss of some movements and retention of others.

As aforesaid, the immobility of the post-epileptic comatose patient, which is here called paralysis, is commonly " explained " as being owing to a psychical loss. It would be denied that there is any paralysis. Yet after all, what is denied in technical terms is admitted in simple ones. On return of consciousness after the paroxysm, or of some consciousness, whilst it would be said that the patient is not paralysed, paralysis is really admitted in the statements that he is " prostrated " or " weak " after his fits. Even after slight epileptic attacks (*le petit-mal*) there is veritable paralysis ; the patient is weak (" unfit for anything," " thoroughly done up," are the kind of expressions

[1] I consider that there are many degrees of dissolution consequent on exhaustion of different amounts effected by epileptic discharges of different degrees of severity. To make, perhaps with some arbitrariness, three degrees, there is (1) post-epileptic " ideation " ; (2) post-epileptic action (mania for example) ; and (3) post-epileptic coma. This is using ordinary nomenclature, which is misleading. There is a negative and a positive element in each degree. Along with post-epileptic ideation there is (*a*) defect of consciousness ; with the post-epileptic actions there is (*b*) loss of consciousness and in the third degree there is (*c*) coma. We compare these three negative conditions, saying they signify respectively shallow, deep, and deepest dissolution, the central condition being " shallow," " deep," and " deepest " exhaustion of nervous arrangements of the highest and perhaps also of lowest centres. The positive elements comparable are (*a*) the " ideation," (*b*) the actions, and (*c*) not the coma, but the vital operations, circulatory, respiratory, etc., going on in the comatose state. These are owing to activity of nervous arrangements which are healthy except for being uncontrolled by their now exhausted higher nervous arrangements. Unless the duplex conditions in each be recognised, the three degrees cannot be shown to be analogous, nor can the cases be shown to come under the principle of dissolution of the nervous system. It is understood, too, that what we really compare and contrast are the physical conditions in the several degrees.

patients use). Let me say explicitly that if the paralysis is to mean only local paralysis, the patient after a slight or severe epileptic paroxysm is *not* paralysed. I admit that most willingly, indeed I assert it. But it is not fair to make such a limit to the meaning of the term. I submit that the patient is paralysed. His " weakness " is veritable paralysis, even if it be owing especially to exhaustion of nervous arrangements for vital organs (cardiac, respiratory, etc.).

I venture, then, to submit (1) that the psychological " explanation " is really no explanation of the comatose patient's immobility; the explanation of a materialistic condition should be in materialistic terms. Our concern, as physicians, with negative or positive psychical conditions is simply to get to know what is going wrong in the *nervous system*. The absolute distinction betwixt mind and body is insisted on, not, as some seem to suppose, because a psychological view is taken of any nervous diseases, but for the diametrically opposite reason. *The distinction is made in order that we may be thoroughly materialistic in our dealings with disease*, and that we may methodically consider the nervous system from top to bottom as a mere sensori-motor mechanism.[1]

Next I submit (2) that there is paralysis after epileptic seizures and that (3) this paralysis is universally spread, and (4) is owing to exhaustion of some nervous arrangements of the highest centres and perhaps of lower ones too.

That loss of function of nervous arrangements of the highest centres (which centres, although neither they nor their activities are consciousness, are yet the anatomical substrata of consciousness) should entail paralysis in the sense of universal weakness, is in accord with the doctrine of evolution of the nervous system. And that it should not entail local paralysis is equally in accord with that doctrine. I have long held that the very highest centres are, like all other centres, sensori-motor. In other words, parts of the brain other than Hitzig and Ferrier's centres (lower cerebral centres) are, I think, made up of sensori-motor arrangements. I do not say this in consequence of their experiments; I urged it before their experiments were begun, and urge it still. For various reasons I think that the nervous arrangements of the highest centres are the most special and complex of all sensori-motor arrangements. Each unit of the highest centres represents, I believe, the organism as a whole (complexity) and each unit represents the whole organism differently (speciality). There is, to speak figuratively, " an experiment made by disease," which seems to me to demonstrate that the highest nervous arrangements represent the whole organism. In a severe paroxysm of epilepsy proper, one setting in with loss of consciousness (when of necessity, therefore, the corresponding physical process of discharge begins in some part of the highest centres) the whole

[1] Scientific materialism is quite a different thing from crude popular materialism. Scientific materialism distinguishes betwixt mind and nervous system in order to study each thoroughly. Popular materialism does not separate the two, and mixes up in its " explanations " psychical factors and physical states. Scientific materialism is only materialistic as to what is material, the nervous system. Popular crude materialism, making no distinctions, confuses two utterly different things, psychical states and physical states. It is said that in an early stage of paralysis agitans the patient can keep his hand still by an act of volition. No one objects to this phrase used clinically if the physical process corresponding to what is psychically volition be meant; if it be meant, for example, that a cerebral discharge can inhibit the movements, or inhibit spinal or other centres for them. But if it be really meant that the will can arrest a physical process, the statement is most unwarrantable. It amounts to saying that the will influences matter. Let anyone try to conceive how the will can stop a movement; it is on the other hand conceivable, if not believable, that a nervous discharge *during* " volition " may stop a movement, for both are material things. Clifford writes: " . . . . If anybody says that the will influences matter, the statement is not untrue, but it is nonsense. The will is not a material thing, it is not a mode of material motion. Such an assertion belongs to the crude materialism of the savage."

organism is involved ; there is universal convulsion. The convulsion in epilepsy proper is, I take it, a brutal development of movements represented in the highest centres primarily discharged, and doubtless too in lower centres secondarily discharged. The discharge " by disease " beginning in some part of the highest centres of either side of the brain shows that they represent movements of all parts of both sides of the organism ; they show this as certainly as artificially induced discharge (by galvanism or faradism) of any centre in Hitzig and Ferrier's region shows it to especially represent movements of some external part. This conclusion from an " experiment by disease " is strictly in accord with the doctrine of evolution. As consciousness, or most vivid consciousness, represents the whole subject (subject-object), so the anatomical substrata of consciousness, or in other words the highest nervous centres, represent the whole organism. There is still another way of looking at this aspect of the question.

In many cases of epileptiform seizures beginning by discharge of some part of the mid-region of one side of the brain, and developing first local one-sided spasm, the convulsion *becomes* universal. The difference betwixt such a convulsion from discharge of part of lower cerebral centres and one of epilepsy proper from discharge of a part of the highest centre, is only a difference in compound degree ; it is such a difference as great difference in evolution of the two centres would lead us to expect. The doctrine of evolution implies that the highest centres of one side are evolved out of the lower cerebral centres of the same side ; that they represent all the parts which the lower centres have represented but in more numerous, more complex and more special combinations.[1]

The two convulsions, (1) epileptic, from discharge of part of the highest centres and (2) epileptiform, from discharge of part of lower cerebral centres, are in accord with these statements. The severe convulsion of epilepsy proper is more quickly universal, the parts on the two sides of the body are convulsed more nearly simultaneously, and the different movements of every part are developed more nearly contemporaneously, than in the severe epileptiform seizure. That it is a difference of degree is shown, in part at least, by the fact that in most cases of epilepsy proper the convulsion affects one side a little earlier and a little more than the other.

Frequently, however, the epileptiform convulsion is limited ; the spasm is local. Just as after localised convulsion (epileptiform seizure) there is local paralysis, so after universal or widespread convulsion there is, I submit, universal or widespread paralysis. The explanation given of post-epileptic immobility is, it seems to me, at any rate as good as the psychological explanation ; if indeed the latter deserves the name of explanation.

To return now to cases of patients locally paralysed after localised epileptiform seizures. It may be alleged against the hypothesis put forward, that there is no proportion betwixt the severity of the seizure (the severity of the discharge) and the subsequent paralysis (amount of exhaustion). But once more it is pointed out, that decided local paralysis is usually what is solely called paralysis. Widespread slight temporary paralysis is not easily recognised as

[1] That both sides of the body are represented in each half of the brain is quite certain, as " descending " wasting in certain cases of one-sided cerebral disease proves. And since the fibres wasted in the spinal cord are some of those of the opposite lateral column and some of those of the anterior column of the same side as the cerebral lesion, there is warrant for the inference that the two sides of the body are differently represented in each half of the brain.

paralysis. If a man has total weakness of one arm, or even slight weakness of it after an epileptiform convulsion affecting that limb, that weakness is called paralysis. But if there be universal transitory slight weakness after a seizure, it is not called, but really is, paralysis.

On the hypothesis, there ought logically to be an exact relation of proportionality betwixt the discharge and the subsequent central exhaustion ; betwixt the convulsion and the subsequent paralysis. I submit that there is. The relation is, however, not easy to see at first glance. I ask the reader to remember that I expressly admit, that after the severest epileptiform seizures, there is less paralysis than after the slight ones, *if by paralysis local paralysis be meant*, and that I expressly deny that there is less, if paralysis be used, as I submit it ought to be, for widespread or universal weakness as well as for local weakness after a fit.

We must in the remainder of this paper discard the vague word " severe " as applied to nervous discharges in disease, and speak of quantities of energy liberable and rates of liberation. Different quantities of grey matter will be unstable in different cases, and there will be differences of degree of instability of cells in different cases. Thus, in different cases there will be different quantities of energy liberable and liberated in the paroxysms. It is quite a certain thing that there are all degrees of spasm in unilaterally beginning convulsions from slight paroxysmal twitching of a few fingers, or " starting " of the big toe, to the severest universally-becoming convulsion ; hence there are different quantities of energy liberable. But we must consider not only the quantity of energy liberated by discharging cells, but the rapidity of its liberation. Of course the conditions are complex, different quantities of energy will in different cases be liberated in different times. We estimate the two things respectively, but of course very roughly indeed, by the amount of spasm, and by the suddenness of onset and rapidity of spreading of spasm.

I think as a matter of observation that, other things equal, the more deliberately spasm sets in, and the more slowly it spreads, the more local it is, and also the longer it continues ; and further, that the paralysis after such spasm is correspondingly more local, is greater in degree, and more persistent. If so, we may, on Todd and Robertson's hypothesis, say of the central process, that the more deliberately the discharge begins, and the slower it is, the less widespread are the nerve currents developed, and the longer they continue ; and that consequently the post-epileptiform exhaustion of centres is more local, more complete, and more persisting. On the other hand, the more suddenly spasm sets in, and the faster it begins to spread, the greater, I think, is the range it attains ; and further, that the paralysis after it is more widespread, less in degree, and more transient. If so, we may, on Todd and Robertson's hypothesis, say, that the more suddenly the discharge begins, and the more rapid it is, the more widespread are the currents developed, and the less time do they continue ; and that the post-epileptiform exhaustion of centres is more widespread, less extreme and more transient. The paralysis in the latter cases is *apparently* less, because it is not so localised, because it is slighter in degree, and because it soon passes off—in a word, it is not easily recognisable as paralysis, and may yet be admitted to be so, being called weakness.

Suppose two patients, in each of whom the same cortical area is affected, and so affected in one that a certain quantity of energy is occasionally liberated slowly, say in ten minutes, and so affected in the other that an equal quantity is occasionally liberated rapidly, say in two minutes. Let us suppose that the part of the cortex represents especially movements of the arm. I suggest that the currents developed in the first case might " flow " almost exclusively to the arm, to the parts most specially represented in the part of the cortex discharged, and that in the second case they would " flow " less exclusively to the arm, but also to parts more generally represented, and finally to lower and collateral centres.

The rapid and sudden spreading of spasm implies a sudden rapid liberation of energy, and thus a shorter liberation of what is liberable ; the currents developed will have greater force than those from a slow liberation of an equal quantity of energy. It is not asserted that nerve impulses travel faster in cases of rapid liberation than in cases of slow liberation ; but that there is in the former a greater " quantity of motion " in a short time against an equal quantity in a long time in the latter. The more rapid short liberation (since currents of greater force, although over a shorter time, are developed) will overcome greater resistances than currents of less force over a larger time from slow, lengthy liberation. As will be seen, I do not use the term " force " as synonymous either with momentum or energy ; it is, however, difficult for me to use the term " force " without misgivings, since, among other reasons, it is a term used differently by different people. Supposing every molecule of a nerve to be of the same mass, and to always travel or vibrate with the same velocity, the momentum (quantity of motion) of each impulse is equal. Suppose the quantity of energy liberated to be equal in two cases, the more rapid liberation will lead to a current in which a greater number of such momenta occur in a short time, against an equal number in a long time during the slower liberation.

The movements of external parts which any centre *most* specially represents are, physiologically speaking, those united to it by lines of *least* resistance. We must bear in mind that any centre represents external parts by lines of different degrees of resistance, and no doubt often represents parts indirectly by intermediation of other centres, lower or collateral. The more force resulting from liberation of energy upon nerve fibres, the greater are the resistances which can be overcome. When greater resistances are overcome of course the wider range has the spasm, and thus the more widespread will be the subsequent paralysis.

But why is there not, after rapid discharge, as much local paralysis in the parts which were first convulsed as after the slower discharges, as well as paralysis in those parts which are next convulsed ? Let me put this again. Supposing there is such a discharging lesion that there occurs a slow discharge upon an arm leaving it completely paralysed. Let us imagine, simply in order to state the question more clearly, the cells of the discharging lesion to become so much more unstable, or many more to become unstable, that in the next paroxysm the discharge is much more rapid, and that the whole body is convulsed. Why in the latter case is not the arm as much paralysed as in the former case, although there is also some slighter paralysis of the rest of the body ? As a matter of fact, I submit that the paralysis is really less in degree in the part first convulsed when the spreading of spasm is rapid, and goes beyond the part, than when it is slow and is confined to that part. There is less spasm of the part first convulsed, that is, of the part most specially represented by the cells discharging. When by more rapid discharges the next more resisting lines (of lower or collateral centres) *are* overcome they are *then* paths of less resistance than before. The energy when more rapidly liberated by the discharging cells may be said to escape in more ways ; the currents developed are less concentrated on the external part which the discharging cells more specially represent ; the currents developed overcome lines of next and next greater resistance ; hence parts most specially represented in the centre are less convulsed than in slow discharges and those less specially represented more than in slow discharges.

On the other hand, in slow discharges the currents developed will keep more to lines of least of all resistance, will " flow " to parts most specially represented ; being unable to overcome lines of greater resistance, they will *continue* to flow only on the lines which can be most easily overcome ; thus the spasm is local and lengthy.

If the above reasoning be valid we should expect, after sudden rapid short discharges, no decided local persisting paralysis, but slight widespread temporary paralysis, often so slight, so widespread and so temporary that it is ignored as paralysis and called prostration. If, to speak roughly, as much paralysis as makes one arm useless for four hours could be spread out thin all over the body for perhaps a quarter of an hour, it would not be recognised as paralysis at all, but as weakness, etc.

No doubt, after the more rapid discharges there is really more paralysis. The discharging lesion is like a fulminate ; by the rapidity of the discharge it overcomes the resistance of the normally unstable (comparatively stable) cells of physiologically connected centres, and the more rapidly it discharges, the more of healthy and collateral centres is it likely to overcome ; it will produce effects in more ways more nearly at once. The currents developed by a rapid local discharge having overcome healthy collateral or lower centres, the energy of these centres will be added on to that of the primal liberation ; there will be a compound effect from a more rapid discharge.

# EPILEPTIFORM CONVULSIONS FROM CEREBRAL DISEASE[1]

For some years before the brilliant researches of Hitzig and Ferrier, I held, as I do still, that the *whole* nervous system is a sensori-motor mechanism. The cerebrum differs from the rest, I consider, only in being the most complicated part of the nervous system. No one denies nowadays that all mental phenomena have for their physical side or basis active conditions (discharges) of cells and fibres ; this, however, is only a morphological statement as to the composition of the highest nervous centres. I submit that the facts of disease warrant the inference, which is strictly in accord with the doctrine of evolution, that the cells and fibres of all centres are grouped in sensori-motor arrangements—the very highest centres, those most concerned with mental phenomena, being only the most special and complex of these arrangements.

We should endeavour to study diseases of the nervous system, including so-called " diseases of the mind," in a brutally materialistic manner. The attention we, as physicians, give to mental phenomena, is given in order that we may study the nature of their physical basis definitely.

I do not see how it is possible to study diseases of the nervous system materialistically, unless we clearly distinguish betwixt psychical states and physical states. Moreover, it seems to me that the occurrence of such symptoms as convulsions from disease of the " organ of mind " (cerebral hemispheres) is incomprehensible unless that organ is made up of sensori-motor nervous arrangements. The view I take is, briefly : (1) that psychical states and nervous states are utterly different ; and yet that (2) nervous states are always concomitant with psychical states ; (3) that the nervous states are active conditions of cells and fibres, making up sensori-motor arrangements.

As regards some parts of the brain, it may be said that they are " for mind." The proper expression is that they represent or re-represent parts of the body, and are only the anatomical substrata of mind. Popular psychology ignores the fact that movement enters into the anatomical substrata of ideas, volitions and emotions, or perhaps consciously repudiates that notion altogether, erroneously supposing the averment to be that movements enter into ideas, emotions, etc. The physical basis of a visual idea (or image) is constituted by central nervous arrangements representing certain retinal impressions and certain ocular movements, but the idea (or image) is not an active state of those nervous arrangements ; the idea or image arises during, that is to say, in concomitance with, an active state of such nervous arrangements.

No one is fitted to begin the materialistic study of diseases of the brain unless he has a good knowledge of psychology. It is ignorance of psychology which tends to giving metaphysical explanations of certain symptoms, such as that " a patient does not move his arm, because he has lost volition over it " ; " a patient does not move after a severe fit of epilepsy proper, because he is unconscious " ; " a patient does not speak, because he has lost the memory of words." These are explanations which explain nothing.

[1] *Transactions International Medical Congress*, vol. ii, 1881, p. 6.

To say that ideas or sensations produce movements is to use neither psychological nor materialistic language, but a mixture of both. Such expressions have the appearance of clearness, but are really incoherent.

From a physiological point of view, nervous symptoms are divisible into two groups : (1) negative—those owing to a destructive lesion, or a temporary loss of function of nervous tissues ; and (2) positive—those owing to excess of function of nervous tissues—to over-liberations of energy, or, in other words, to hypernormal nervous discharges.

I look on a convulsion from disease of some part of the brain as a sudden, simultaneous, or very rapid development of many movements represented in that part, and in associated parts ; or rather, a convulsion is a contention in which many movements are " run up " into spasms. There is a sudden and excessive discharge of many nervous arrangements representing movements, at once or nearly together, because the cells of those arrangements have by some pathological process become highly unstable. The discharges are of nervous arrangements which are not ideas, voluntary actions and emotions, but are the anatomical substrata for these mental states.

The simplest cases for the study of positive symptoms are the convulsions first described by Bravais (1824). The pathology of this class of seizure has been greatly cleared up by Bright, Todd, Wilks, and other physicians. They have recently been specially elucidated by the physiological researches of Hitzig and Ferrier, and by the clinical researches of Charcot, Lepine, Landouzy, and many other physicians. I speak as much as possible of the clinical side, acknowledging, however, that recent important advances in our knowledge of cerebral localisation are due mainly to the physiological researches of Hitzig and Ferrier.

In the class of seizure I speak of in this paper, the spasm begins comparatively deliberately in (1) the hand, or (2) in the face or tongue, or in both these parts, or (3) in the foot. This is the order of frequency of place of onset, the onset being usually always the same in the same patient. The evidence from morbid anatomy, agreeing with that of the physiological experiments alluded to, is that there is in these cases cortical disease, and that the part of the cortex affected is within the mid-region of the brain—of convolutions bordering the fissure of Rolando. We call these seizures epileptiform, reserving the term " epileptic " for cases of the epilepsy of nosologists—epilepsy proper, as it is sometimes called.

Of necessity, whatever special view may be taken as to localisation, each of the three kinds of epileptiform seizures depends on disease of some particular part. We make, then, from the three places of onset, three kinds (varieties) of epileptiform seizures, owing to disease of different parts of the cortex in the mid-region of the brain.

The term " disease " is vague. Whatever pathological condition is discovered post-mortem in such case, the proximate cause of the paroxysm is an abnormally high unstable condition of some cells, resulting in occasional discharge. The first outward spasm, although sometimes called a " warning," is, really, the evidence of the starting of the internal hypernormal discharge. Probably, few cells are abnormally highly unstable ; in severe seizures the sudden and excessive discharge of those highly unstable cells overcomes, it is supposed, the resistance of healthy cells in physiological connection with those highly unstable.

The ascertainment of the starting-point of the spasm is the basis for methodical localisation: or, speaking more simply, we learn from this what it is which it is most important to localise in any case under observation. If one patient's fits always begin in his thumb, and another patient's always begin in his little finger, the elements of the cortex highly unstable (over-dischargeable) in the two cannot be quite the same, however closely they may lie together in the cortex cerebri.

In the study of these cases we have to consider: (1) the starting-point of the spasm; (2) the range of the spasm, how far it spreads; (3) the march of the spasm, the order of spreading; (4) the suddenness of onset, rapidity of spreading, and duration of the paroxysm; (5) the post-paroxysmal condition (temporary paralysis); (6) post-epileptic aphasia; (7) affection of consciousness; (8) we have to ascertain the particular part of the cortex diseased; (9) the physiology of the lesion; (10) the pathology of the lesion; (11) treatment.

1. *Starting-points.*—We have already spoken of three starting-points. Those seizures starting in the hand are clinically analogous to cases of hemiplegia, in which the arm suffers more than the leg; those starting in the side of the face are probably clinically analogous to cases of partial aphasia, with slight and transient hemiplegia. Those starting in the foot are clinically analogous to cases of hemiplegia, in which the leg suffers more than the arm.

The important matter, with a view to localisation, being the starting-point of the spasm, our clinical study of it must be minute and precise. When the spasm starts in the hand, it is most frequently in the index-finger, or thumb, or both; when in the face, it begins near the mouth, or in the tongue, or in both these parts; when in the leg, in the foot, and the starting is nearly always referred by the patient to the great toe.

In some cases, if not in most, there is premonitory numbness, tingling, or some other abnormal sensation in the parts first seized by spasm; evidence, I think, that the centres engaged are not solely motor. In some cases, almost contemporaneous with the onset of the spasm, there are colours before the eyes; occasionally, but very rarely, there is a stench in the nose. In one case, where the spasm started in one leg, there was a noise in the ear of the same side. For brevity, these important facts are omitted from consideration.

2. *Range.*—It is certain that there are many ranges of the spasm, from, for example, slight spasm, apparently limited to the thumb and index-finger, to universal convulsion. It frequently happens that a patient has very limited convulsion, of which he may take no notice, before he has widespread ones. The same patient may have, on different occasions, convulsions of widely different ranges.

A seizure, in which the spasm is seemingly limited to the thumb and index-finger, is not a different kind [variety] of fit from one so beginning and becoming universal; they are but two vastly differing degrees of one kind of seizure. This, obviously, bears on localisation. It means that a discharge, starting in some cells of a small part of the cortex, may be very limited, or, no doubt, by overcoming the resistance of physiologically associated healthy nervous arrangements, may spread widely. Of necessity, the spasm depends on liberation of energy, and it is supposed that the degree and range of convulsion varies as the quantity liberated by unstable cells, and the rapidity of its liberation. We may, although the division is of necessity largely arbitrary, speak of ranges thus: (1) monospasm (of arm, or of face, or of leg). These are clinically analogous to

Charcot's monoplegias from cortical destructive lesions. (2) Hemispasm, in two degrees. There is (*a*) convulsion of the face, arm, and leg, analogous clinically to chronic cases of hemiplegia ; (*b*) such convulsion with, in addition, turning of the eyes and head to the side convulsed and some spasm of respiratory muscles of both sides, the analogue of cases of hemiplegia described by Vulpian and Prévost, in which the eyes and head turn from the side paralysed. (3) There is a still further range ; part or the whole of the other side of the body is sometimes gained, the convulsion becomes universal. This range, I suppose, is clinically analogous to cases in which, upon a vast one-sided cerebral lesion, such as a large hæmorrhage, the patient moves none of his limbs on either side. It is, however, asserted by some physicians (the patient in these cases of large cerebral hæmorrhage being unconscious or comatose) that he does not move " because he is unconscious." This is only a verbal explanation. It is certain, from the facts of " descending wasting," that both sides of the body are to some extent represented in each side of the brain, and it is a legitimate hypothesis that discharge beginning in part of one half of the brain, and not reaching the other half, can produce some convulsion of the same as well as of the opposite side of the body. This hypothesis does not say that the opposite half of the brain may be reached ; but is, that discharge limited to one half can convulse both sides of the body. In this connection Broadbent's well-known views as to representation of unilateral and bilateral movements in the brain should be considered. These views will be referred to again later.

3. *March of Spasm.*—Clinically we have for localisation, not only to note the range attained, but to observe the method of spreading over that range. For in localisation we have not simply to ascertain the movements chiefly represented in any part of the cortex (presumably those of the part in which the spasm starts), but all the movements represented in it or in other parts in physiological connection with it, those united with the part primarily discharged by lines of least resistance. It is not enough to say of a seizure, for an example, that " the arm was convulsed " ; we have to note whereabouts in the limb the spasm starts and how it spreads in it. In one case of convulsion of the arm the spasm spread down the limb from shoulder to finger in every fit I saw (and I saw many). In other cases of spasm limited, or nearly limited, to the arm, it spreads up. We must not use the unqualified expression, of two cases, " in each the right arm was convulsed," when the spasm in one " went up," in the other " went down." Manifestly two different parts of the cortex must have been diseased in these different spreadings of spasm, although in each it was over the same limb ; the movements in each must at least have been represented as differently grouped. Whilst the starting-point of the spasm is the clue to the seat of the lesion, and whilst the range of it is a clue to the movements the diseased centre represents, and to movements represented in nervous arrangements physiologically connected by lines of least resistance with it, the order of spreading is our clue to representation of movements in relations of subordination or sequence one to another—their time relations. Suppose, for the sake of argument, all the parts of one side were equally convulsed in two cases of hemispasm ; yet, if the spasm started in the hand in one and in the foot in the other, the parts of the cortex primarily discharged must be different. If in cases of hemispasm the seizure begins in the arm, the rule is that the spasm goes up the arm and down the leg ; if in the foot, up the leg and down the arm ; to the latter there appear to be numerous exceptions.

As stated, the spasm, in some cases, after affecting what we shall call the "first side," gains the other side of the body, which we shall call the "second side." I presume that the spasm of the first side is caused in part by intermediation of the decussating cerebro-spinal fibres, which in the cord lie in the lateral column; the second side I have suggested, is convulsed by the intermediation of the direct fibres in the anterior column. Pitres and Franck have shown that (in dogs) bilateral convulsions may occur from excessive irritation of one cerebral hemisphere, even when the "motor centres" of the other have been extirpated. On Broadbent's hypothesis it may be said that at least part of the convulsion of the second side is owing to active conditions of the decussating fibres putting in action the associated nuclei of both sides of the cord, and thence the bilaterally acting muscles of both sides of the body. On either hypothesis one would infer that the convulsion of the second side would not be a facsimile of that of the first side. However, Ferrier says that the artificially induced bilateral convulsion in a monkey from irritation of a part of the cortex cerebri of one hemisphere is the same on both sides of the animal's body. Apart from any hypothesis, we have, with a view to localisation in man, to note how the second side is affected. In some cases only a part of the second side is affected, and usually, I think, the leg when the earliest part of the seizure on the first side was of the arm. I would ask the following questions, with a view to further observation. Of course we note the particular part of the first side which is first in spasm. In regard to the following questions, it is supposed to begin in the right hand; the right is the first side, and the left the second side.

(1) Does the spasm of the left side begin in the leg? (2) Does it go *down* or *up* these limbs? (3) Does it affect the extensors more than the flexors? (4) Is the spasm more tonic than that on the first side?

The spreading of spasm in these convulsions has to be considered from another point of view. It is not in simple order; the spasm does not leave one part when the next is attacked. It is in compound order. In cases of slowly spreading spasm, we easily see that the part the seizure begins in is at first a little in spasm, next it is more in spasm, and other parts are in spasm also. There is the double difference: (1) more spasm, and (2) greater range of spasm. This is best seen in convulsions starting in one side of the face. Speaking roughly, there is, first, spasm of the muscles of the side, so far as their movements are chiefly unilateral; and then, before this is over, there is the compound spasm of the unilaterally acting muscles of one side, and the bilaterally acting of both sides. We may see in this complex struggle that the mouth becomes ovoid; the wider part being to the side first in spasm. Such cases are strictly in accord with Broadbent's hypothesis. The order of spreading in these convulsions may be rudely symbolised as $x$, then $x^2$, $y$, then $x^3$, $y^2$, $z$, and so on.

In some cases, after rapidly recurring convulsions, the part which in the earliest attacks was first seized is not affected; the fit begins at what would be a later stage of the earliest seizures. So far for a series of rapidly recurring attacks. But in some cases, where the fit occurs at long intervals (perhaps from destruction of part of the cortex corresponding to the parts which in early seizures were first in spasm), the parts first convulsed in the patient's earlier fits cease to be convulsed in his later ones.

4. *Suddenness of Onset, Rapidity, and Duration of Spasm.*—It is important

to note the suddenness with which spasm sets in, the rate of its spreading, and the duration of the paroxysm.

I think the more suddenly the spasm sets in, and the more rapidly it begins to spread, the greater range does the convulsion ultimately attain, and the sooner over is the paroxysm. On the contrary, when the spasm starts deliberately, and spreads slowly, it is more likely to be limited in range, say nearly limited to one arm, and to be lengthy. The bearing of this will be best seen when we come to speak of post-epileptiform paralysis. The duration of seizures varies exceedingly—from a minute or two, to more than two hours. I am not here speaking of repetition of fits at short intervals. General remarks on duration, however, are necessarily indefinite, for we should consider duration of seizure and range of seizure together.

5. *Post-paroxysmal State* (*Temporary Paralysis*).—With a view to more precise localisation, or rather for clearer interpretation of the particular effect any lesion discovered has, we must consider very carefully some relations of convulsions and paralysis.

The fact that after an epileptiform seizure the patient may be temporarily and locally paralysed is one of extreme importance. There may be complete paralysis, which paralysis is temporary unless the fits recur. Some preliminary remarks are needed before we consider this relation or sequence. Let us put the question we are thus concerned with in a particular way.

When in a case where a cortical lesion is found post-mortem there had been any paralysis, it is a matter of great moment to note whether or not that paralysis was after convulsion and temporary ; or, if it had been permanent, whether the convulsions were rapidly repeated. For not denying (on the contrary, after Ferrier's and Charcot's researches, affirming) that cortical destructive lesions produce paralysis, and admitting, too, that such paralysis might be temporary, it still remains that a few hours' complete paralysis after a convulsion belongs to a different category ; it cannot be ascribed to the destructive effects of the gross lesion discovered post-mortem. A man may be seemingly well ; he has monospasm, then he is monoplegic, and in a few hours, unless the fit recurs, he is seemingly well again.

In this inquiry we are not concerned with paralysis occurring after convulsion in cases of meningeal or cerebral hæmorrhage, ordinary, or from vascular tumour, nor with cases of so-called uræmic convulsion ; we deal with chronic cases only. (*a*) Spasm may begin in parts already partially paralysed (hemiplegic), or which have seemingly recovered from hemiplegia, the paralysis having set in without convulsion. (There is often a condition for embolism in these cases.) (*b*) It may begin in, and affect severely, a part which, after recent prior convulsion, is partially or even absolutely paralysed. (*c*) Some cases are complicated. We have carefully to distinguish betwixt slowly creeping paralysis from destructive changes and the temporary paralysis after a convulsion. (*d*) There may be the complication of slow paralysis and occasional temporary paralysis after seizures. (*e*) In intra-cranial syphilis we may first have convulsion, followed by temporary paralysis (cortical gumma), and then the very different thing, hemiplegia from blocking of a syphilitically diseased artery. (*f*) There may be indirect evidence of paralysis, as well as direct ; an arm may, when the patient tries to use it, move in a way closely like that in disseminated sclerosis. Such erratic movements are to be distinguished from quasi-spontaneous little spasms, jerks, "jumpings," etc., and from increased reflexes (?)

on disturbing the parts. (*g*) A patient may cease to be subject to sharp-cut paroxysms beginning in the hand, and become liable to over-movements of the arm and hand for hours or days, movements like, but more gliding than, those of chorea.

Admitting these complications and difficulties, only ordinary temporary paralysis after convulsion, beginning in a patient who, before the seizure, had no obvious paralysis, will be spoken of in this paper. I now make three remarks on such cases : (*a*) The paralysis is, in my experience, always of the parts first and most convulsed. (*b*) It varies in degree, from such as mere inability to pick up a pin, to absolute powerlessness of the hand and arm. (*c*) It varies greatly in range, from paralysis of the hand to hemiplegia, with (Julius Mickle) lateral deviation of the eyes, and probably to greater ranges still.

We have such a sequence as the following to consider : (*a*) A man is seemingly well. (*b*) His leg is convulsed strongly, and the arm slightly, for about ten minutes. (*c*) The leg is much paralysed for a few hours. (*d*) He is seemingly well again. When a cortical lesion is found, we have to note whether any paralysis there had been was after a convulsion or not.

*Various Hypotheses as to the Nature of the Paralysis.*—(*a*) Post-epileptiform local paralysis has been ascribed to congestion of the brain during asphyxia produced in the prior paroxysms. Besides the difficulty of understanding how uniform brain congestion can produce localised paralysis, there is the fatal objection that absolute local paralysis may remain after a seizure in which there has been no asphyxia. (It may be mentioned, too, that the occurrence of clonic spasm in such cases shows that cerebral congestion is not essential for the production of that kind of spasm.) Thus, during spasm of an arm, leaving the limb paralysed, the patient may stand all the while and talk to bystanders, have no affection of consciousness, and no trouble of respiration. (*b*) Another hypothesis ascribes the temporary paralysis to extravasation of blood. Not denying here that temporary paralysis might, in other kinds of cases, be owing to small clots, there is the objection that in temporary monoplegias after monospasms there is nothing to cause such extravasation. Further, it may be urged that it would be very remarkable were the extravasation in each succeeding paralysis always to affect that part of the nervous system which specially empowers the part seized in the prior convulsion. Besides, if cerebral congestion or extravasation were producible by these paroxysms in such a degree as to cause local paralysis, we ought to find local paralysis after the very much severer paroxysms of epilepsy proper, and we do not find it. (*c*) It seems to me that Todd and Alexander Robertson's hypothesis accounts best for the facts. This hypothesis is that temporary paralysis, after a convulsion, indicates not simply that discharged cells have " run down," but exhaustion in nerve tracts between the cortical lesion and the muscles convulsed. It is manifest that during the convulsion there is an excessive activity from the cortex through some nerve tracts to the muscles convulsed—cortex in so-called motor region, internal capsule, nerve fibres in cord, anterior horns, nerve fibres of nerve trunks. It is reasonable to infer *a priori* that any subsequent and yet temporary local paralysis is owing to exhaustion of nerve fibres produced by that hypernormal process, especially when the paralysis is found where the spasm had been and is temporary. At any rate, there is some negative condition of the nervous system which, being temporary, cannot be put down to any local disease discovered post-mortem.

It has been asserted that there is no proportion betwixt the degree of the seizure and the degree of the post-epileptiform paralysis. I admit that after the severest fits there may be less paralysis than after the slighter ones, if we are to take note only of decided local paralysis, of which so far alone I have spoken. But I think there may be more paralysis after the severest seizures, if we take count of what goes by the name of " weakness." There are many ranges of post-epileptiform paralyses. We have spoken of monoplegias. Long ago Todd described what he called " epileptic hemiplegia."

If spasm begins deliberately, and spreads slowly, it is more limited in range and continues for a longer time. After such paroxysms, the paralysis also is limited in range—there is obvious local paralysis. If spasm begins suddenly, and spreads rapidly, it may become universal ; and then there may be, after the paroxysm, no, or but little, obvious local paralysis, but yet widespread slight paralysis—a condition spoken of as one of " weakness." Let us for one moment consider a patient's condition after a severe seizure of epilepsy proper.

I submit that there is often paralysis after even severe seizures of this kind, although there is no decided local paralysis. Since the patient is, after such fits, unconscious, it may be asserted that he does not move, " because he is unconscious." This is a verbal explanation, identical in kind with the explanation that a man monoplegic, after monospasm, does not move the part affected, " because he has lost volition over it " ; these explanations explain nothing. Our explanation of materialistic conditions must be brutally materialistic. Whenever a man is unconscious, there is some abnormal physical condition of some part of his nervous system, and it seems to me more reasonable to put his immobility down to this. Besides, I think paralysis is admitted to exist after paroxysms of epilepsy proper, by the statement that the patient on recovery from loss of consciousness is " prostrated," etc. If, so to speak, as much paralysis as constitutes immobility of one arm for four hours could be " spread out thin " all over the body, it would not then be called paralysis, but " prostration," etc.

*On Reflexes after Epileptiform Seizure.*—There is a further field of investigation as to the nature of post-epileptiform paralysis. Observations on the conditions of reflexes after epileptic seizures have been made by Westphal. After one convulsion I saw, which began in the foot and affected the left leg chiefly, and the left arm slightly, there was very great paralysis of the leg and slight paralysis of the arm. There was greatly exaggerated knee-jerk and there was foot clonus on the paralysed side during the paralytic stage. These conditions were not found on recovery. In some other cases of post-epileptiform paralysis observed for me by Mr. Neatby, the conditions were too complicated for brief analysis. For the most part they were in harmony with the observation just cited. We should consider the condition of reflexes after epileptic paroxysms. In some cases, immediately after epileptic attacks, there is, Dr. Beevor has ascertained for me, exaggerated knee-phenomenon, and also foot clonus. But Westphal has found the knee-jerk sometimes absent after epileptic seizures, and so has Gowers in one case he has briefly reported ; in that case it was absent for a minute or less. Hence there are discrepancies.

The cases of post-epileptiform paralysis, besides differing in being temporary, differ from paralysis in ordinary cases of hemiplegia from clot and local softening, in that in the former there has been some active process through the cord during the paroxysm, whereas in the latter the cord becomes affected after a time, and slowly. On Todd and Robertson's hypothesis, we might say that a temporary negative condition in the cord was established when the paralysis appeared, and explain the absence or presence of the deep reflexes on the degree or range of that negative condition. Gowers has suggested that, in the case he mentions, there may have been temporary exhaustion of the lumbar nuclei ; in my patient it may be that the knee-jerk would have been found absent had I tested for it instantly when the spasm ceased. The subject is a complicated one ; in my patient's case, as in others, little spasms came on now and then "spontaneously," and in some cases touching a limb after a fit will make it jerk. There are other complications. We have particularly to bear in mind that there may be some persisting paralysis from permanent destructive lesion of the cortex, as well as, in addition, some temporary paralysis after a seizure ; and thus there might be increase of the reflex mentioned at all times, although perhaps they would be more marked after a paroxysm. I have found foot clonus in one case several weeks after a patient's last seizure, and at a time when there was no obvious paralysis ; the patient walked well and felt well. I would suggest that we should most carefully note, not only the region and range of post-epileptiform paralysis, but also the condition of reflexes instantly on the cessation, and at various times up to and after recovery.

6. *Post-epileptiform Aphasia.*—In some cases (all right-sided, so far as I have yet personally observed) there is, after the seizure, temporary partial aphasia. I have but once known this so-called complication to occur after fits beginning in the foot. Perhaps that case was exceptional, as there were found post-mortem, months later, large blood cysts, which had compressed each hemisphere from front to back. Aphasia is certainly most frequently found after fits beginning in the hand, or in the side of the face, or in the tongue. It may occur when the spasm is limited to the cheek and is trifling in degree. These cases must not be confounded with cases of so-called emotional aphasia. There may be temporary, partial, or even complete aphasia without any spasm, for example, in patients with valvular disease of the heart ; these are probably cases of very limited softening from embolism. I, however, limit myself to cases in which there was clear evidence of precursory local (right-sided) spasm. In some cases the aphasia is discovered after recovery from loss of consciousness following severe epileptiform seizures ; in others there is no loss of consciousness in the prior seizure.[1] My belief is, that when the fit begins in the face or tongue, or both, the defect after it is rather ataxy of articulation, a jumbling of syllables ; and that when it follows a seizure starting in the hand, it is more often one in which words are well uttered, but either mistakenly or only in short, well-organised sentences, such as "very well." It must be borne in mind that in some cases of post-epileptiform aphasia, as in some cases of aphasia otherwise caused, there is inability to put out the tongue when told, although the patient moves it well in eating, swallowing, and puts it out "by accident."

Temporary aphasia, after epileptiform seizures, may exist with temporary paralysis of the arm, or of one side of the body. The presumption is, that the internal negative local condition is the same both for the aphasia and the paralysis.

[1] It is worth noting, that in many such cases, when the spasm affects the face, the patient will say that his arm on the same side "falls dead." Gowers suggests that epileptic discharges sometimes inhibit.

In considering the explanation of post-epileptiform paralysis we ought to consider it along with post-epileptiform aphasia, with which, as has been said, it sometimes occurs, and also with post-epileptic conditions. It seems to me that Todd and Robertson's hypothesis gives the simplest explanation of post-epileptiform paralysis, of the physical condition of the negative element of post-epileptiform aphasia, and of the physical condition in post-epileptic loss of consciousness. Of course the erroneous and limited utterances of the aphasic are not supposed to be owing to local nervous exhaustion, that is supposed to account for his inability to say anything else or better. And in a case of post-epileptic mania, local exhaustion is only supposed to be the physical condition for the loss of consciousness accompanying the maniacal action. It is impossible that a negative condition can cause the positive manifestations in a case of aphasia, or those of mania after an epileptic seizure.

7. *On Affection of Consciousness.*—So far we have said nothing, excepting incidentally, about cessation of consciousness. In some epileptiform seizures it is lost and in some not. It is lost in severe cases ; it is not possible for me to use a more precise expression. There may be spasm limited to the arm or to the leg, or affecting one arm and leg, and even the face also, without any evidence of even defect of consciousness ; the patient converses with us about his condition. Roughly speaking, consciousness usually ceases when the head and eyes begin to turn after the limbs of one side have been affected. I suppose that the more rapidly the spasm sets in and spreads, the less is the range attained before consciousness is lost.

It is worth while to speak of the difference betwixt epileptiform seizures and epileptic seizures, with regard to negative affection of consciousness.

The difference is not that in the epileptiform paroxysm consciousness is not lost, and that in the epileptic it is lost ; but that in the former it is lost late in the paroxysm, whilst in the epileptic it is lost, or is defective, first thing, or nearly first thing.

8. *Localisation of Lesion.*—The observations made, recording local lesions found after death in different cases of epileptiform seizures, are now very numerous. The cases I have recorded have for the most part been cases of tumour, and the disease has been too often so wide that most of them are not of much beyond clinical value. These cases have been many times quoted, and I need not refer to them. Nor need I give an account of their observations ; they are very numerous, and many of them have been already collated by Ferrier and others.

9. *The Physiology of the Lesion.*—It is a truism to say that a healthy movement implies a liberation of energy or nervous discharge—initially by cerebral cells, at any rate if the movement be a voluntary one. A convulsion—that is to say, a sudden, excessive, rapid, and temporary development of movements—many movements " run up " into spasm—implies of necessity a corresponding sudden, etc., discharge. A local convulsion, if only local at the onset, implies that the excessive discharge begins locally. I say begins locally, for I suppose the discharging lesion to be, so to speak, a " fulminate," which, by the rapidity of its " decomposition," discharges healthy associated (collateral and lower) nervous arrangements. When fits (always of the same style) recur, although often in different degrees and ranges, the inference is that there is persistent change in some cells in one locality, such that they occasionally attain high instability and occasionally discharge excessively.

10. *The Pathology of the Lesion.*—The question in pathology is, What is the process by which cells become highly unstable? Without pretending to determine the steps of it, we may say that the primary change is frequently tumour, and very often a syphilitic tumour. In some cases I have failed to discover, have no doubt overlooked, a local lesion. It is not necessary to go into the evidence as to the pathology of these cases here. The diagnosis of the nature of the lesion is a general question in diagnosis, not one about these seizures in particular. I refer to but two things. From my earliest studies[1] I have been struck by the occurrence of epileptiform seizures in some cases of complete or partial recovery from hemiplegia, presumably due to embolism (sometimes occurring in young patients who have valvular disease of the heart), and in some patients with valvular disease without previous hemiplegia. But in no such case have I had a post-mortem examination. It is, then, but an hypothesis that plugging of vessels may lead to instability of cells. The empirical association is, I think, too frequent to be a mere coincidence. So far as the process produces softening, so far, of course, it produces a condition from which spasm, or any other positive symptom, is impossible.

Sometimes a patient who had had an injury to the head, followed by general brain symptoms (loss of consciousness, etc.), recovers, except that he remains liable to convulsive seizures. And sometimes the seizures are of the class we are considering.

I am convinced that in some syphilised patients a blow on the head is followed by cortical syphilitic disease. Dr. Clifford Allbutt long since asserted this. It ought to be borne in mind when we consider the propriety of trephining in cases of epilepsy or of epileptiform seizures after injury to the head.

In one case already referred to of seizures beginning in the right foot there were found post-mortem two very large blood cysts, one over the left, the other over the right cerebral hemisphere.

11. *Treatment.*—It is not necessary to go into the question of treatment with regard to these cases, for the obvious reason that the question of their treatment is but part of the question of treatment of various morbid conditions of brain. There are certain valuable empirical methods of treatment by drugs too well known to need pointing out. Everyone knows that a ligature and certain other procedures allied in effect will sometimes stop epileptiform seizures. No one fails to conceive the possibility of syphilis in such cases, and to treat the patient anti-syphilitically when necessary. The question of trephining in some cases of epileptiform seizures is very important, but is too large a one for me to consider here; besides, I have had no personal experience of it. In some cases of epileptiform seizures, after injuries to the head, there is depression of bone; there is now in the London hospital a patient who has such a depression consequent on an old injury in the left postero-frontal region; he is subject to seizures beginning in the right arm.

[1] *London Hospital Reports,* vol. i, 1864.

## LOCALISED CONVULSIONS FROM TUMOUR OF THE BRAIN [1]

THIS is the case of a patient who for twelve years was subject to occasional convulsive seizures, beginning in his right foot. Post-mortem, there was a tumour in the cortex of the left side of the brain, as shown in the two drawings. For these drawings, and much more, I have to thank Dr. James Anderson. The case belongs to a class which was described by Bravais in 1824. Their pathology has been greatly cleared up by Bright, Todd, Wilks, Ferrier, and others in this country; and by Hitzig, Charcot, Lepine, Landouzy, and others abroad. A valuable case is reported by Dr. Franz Müller of Graz.[2]

On October 15, 1872, the patient, then 30 years of age, was admitted under my care in the London Hospital. He had had fits about two or three times a week over a period of two years; their duration, he said, varied, lasting five or ten minutes, but sometimes an hour. Perhaps when, as he said, he had a fit for an hour, there was a succession of convulsions, but it is quite certain that one fit may last many hours—may affect the whole of one side for hours, the patient remaining conscious all the time. The patient gave the following account of his attacks. After some dizziness his right big toe begins to "cramp," and gets drawn towards the sole of the foot, then he feels a twitching of the leg, chiefly of the calf; the leg and knee are drawn up. Most of his fits stop here. He called these "weak fits," others he called "strong fits." In the latter the arm is affected, but always after the leg; the spasm begins in the fingers and passes up the arm; his arm and hand may be drawn above his head; his mouth works about. During this further range of convulsion the leg continues working. After a severe fit he loses consciousness: he knows nothing about affection of the left side, possibly because he is unconscious.

He remembers his first attack; he was astonished and amused, so he said, by the lifting of his right leg when standing talking. Soon he fell to the ground, both right limbs "working"; in this attack he lost consciousness. Some patients suffering from seizure of this class are subject to quasi-trifling limited seizures before they have one which they think severe enough to make them consult a doctor.

He had many attacks of the two degrees when in the hospital in 1872, but none were witnessed; he lost consciousness in the stronger seizures. Occasionally also he had attacks of dizziness, with apparent movement of objects and dimness of sight, but with these there was no limb affection.

I saw him several times in 1872 when he was an out-patient; he always gave the same account of the starting-point of his seizures, and so he did on a second admission, September 1875, and on his third, January 28, 1882.

*Second admission.*—In 1875 my then house physician, Mr. Richard Atkinson, saw several seizures, and noted some important facts as to the condition of the limbs when the seizures were over. On his admission he was examined carefully and in great detail for paralysis. None was discovered. The man said he was weak on the right side after his fits. One was seen, September 1,

[1] *Brain*, vol. v, p. 364, 1882. [2] *Transactions International Medical Congress*, vol. ii, p. 15.

by Mr. Atkinson just after an examination, revealing no paralysis. There was first hurried respiration, and then tonic movements of the right hand and arm and right side of face, then clonic spasm. Paralysis of the arm was very marked after the fits; the convulsion began in the leg, but nothing is said of its movements in the notes, as the fit so described occurred, as I suppose, when the patient's legs were covered in bed. Mr. Atkinson saw an attack on September 2; it set in during a conversation. The patient began to answer vaguely and ceased speaking; his legs were seized with tonic spasm; their muscles felt hard and rigid; the right leg was the one more affected, the left in a much slighter degree. In about half a minute the clonic spasm began, the contractions became fewer and fewer, and in about a minute from the onset ceased. In this fit the legs only were engaged. The patient denied that his left leg was affected, and said it appeared to be so from movements of his body. But affection of the left leg along with greater spasm of the right was observed four times. On another occasion the man said the stiffness of the left leg was voluntary. Probably Mr. Atkinson was right. In another patient [1] I saw such a fit; the spasm, starting in the left foot, affected the whole leg and slightly the left arm; the right leg vibrated rhythmically.

To return to the present case. Observations as to the leg in which the spasm does not begin are important. It is quite certain, from the facts of "descending Wallerian wasting," that each side of the brain sends fibres to both sides of the cord. It is not very rare for both legs to be affected in convulsions of this class starting from one arm. Gowers has recorded such a case. But since the fibres sent from one side of the brain into the cord lie in different columns of the cord, one would *a priori* expect some difference in the seizure on the two sides. On one occasion the spasm, Mr. Atkinson observed, was such that the right leg was flexed at the knee and the left at the ankle. On September 3 Mr. Atkinson saw another fit just the same as the one detailed, and after this he found more loss of power in the right leg, as he did after others; the patient was not unconscious in this seizure. He had many fits of this kind. He had twelve in one night, of the exact range of which we know nothing, and one night so many that he did not count them; the morning after these numerous fits the only movement of the leg remaining was slight flexion of the knee; he could not lift it from the bed; sensation was unimpaired. Often his fits began by inability to talk, probably aphasia. On one occasion he was unable to speak for three minutes and a half, but no spasm was then observed; the patient, however, felt "twittering" in his right great toe. He had at other times fits in which, as in the one on September 1, the arm became affected after the leg; but on their cessation Mr. Atkinson found only paralysis of the leg, not of the arm, as on September 1. It is not, however, stated whether the man's hand was tested in delicate operations.

I remember nearly making a mistake in saying there was no paralysis of the left hand, after a seizure beginning in the left leg, because the patient seemed to grasp as strongly with the left as with the right hand. But I found, a little later, that he had great difficulty in using the left hand in delicate operations.

To return to the case, the subject of the paper. Facial paralysis was never noticed. He had fits daily, sometimes twenty or thirty. On September 11, having had but two fits the day before, and none since, he could move the leg better, but could not walk unaided.

[1] *Medical Times and Gazette*, February 12, 1881.

On September 17 he ceased to have fits ; his paralysis passed off, but unfortunately there is no note about the date of its disappearance. On October 15 there is the statement that there was no paralysis at all. On the 20th he went out. On December 21 he came to see a surgeon for fistula ; he had had no fit for ten weeks ; there was no trace of paralysis.

*Third admission.*—He came in again Saturday, January 28, 1882, hemiplegic of the right side. Mr. Coates, my present house physician, got just the same account of the starting of the fits as we did in 1872 and in 1875. The patient said that he rarely become unconscious ; but when conscious in them, could not speak ; he could at the same time recognise people, and understand what they said. He was not paralysed on Thursday, the 26th, having on that day helped his father, an undertaker, in a funeral. He was found paralysed on Friday morning, the 27th. Whether he had a fit or a series of fits in the night or not was not ascertainable. His face and tongue were normal ; his speech good ; the right arm was quite paralysed, and the only movement of the right leg was that he could, when lying in bed, draw it up slightly. Superficial reflexes (in front) were not obtained on either side. There was ankle clonus on the right side only ; the knee, wrist, triceps and biceps' jerks were greater on the right side. So much for his nervous condition. His temperature was 104·5°, respirations 40 ; and there were physical signs of right-sided pneumonia. He died on Monday, January 30.

At the autopsy the right lung was found to be consolidated. A tumour was seen on the surface of the right cerebral hemisphere.

The following is Dr. James Anderson's report of his examination of the brain : The brain has been preserved in spirit. Part of the dura mater has been left in the middle line opposite the fissure of Rolando. Both this and the rest of the meninges present a normal appearance, except in front of the upper half of the fissure of Rolando, where the pia mater is dark brown in colour from extravasated blood. Opposite the posterior extremity of each superior frontal convolution in the longitudinal fissure is a marked depression corresponding to a Pacchionian body. The pia mater detaches readily from the surface of both hemispheres, including the area of extravasation mentioned above.

After removal of the pia mater the surface of both hemispheres presents a perfectly normal appearance, except an area on the upper surface of the *left hemisphere*, *including the posterior half of the superior frontal convolution* and *that portion of the ascending frontal convolution from which it arises*, *viz.* here *the upper half*. About half an inch of the upper extremity of the ascending frontal convolution is normal in appearance. In the centre of the above area is a hæmorrhage about the size of a sixpence (Fig. 1, E), and round this to the area of a crown-piece are numerous miliary haemorrhages. The whole area has a wrinkled (from numerous blood vessels grooving it) nodular aspect, while the fissures are almost obliterated (by adhesion of their walls) and the convolutions are depressed. The area is sharply limited by *the fissure of Rolando* posteriorly, the *superior frontal fissure* externally, and by the *longitudinal fissure* internally ; while anteriorly the above appearances shade off gradually and as stated, the anterior half (in length) of the superior frontal convolution is to all appearance normal. The fissure of Rolando and the superior frontal fissure are both deep, the latter being prolonged back into the former. The portion of the cerebrum thus defined is harder to the touch and more resistant, especially at and internal to the central hæmorrhage, than the rest of the brain. *In the longitudinal fissure* the same wrinkling nodulation and flattening of the convolutions exist opposite the above area *down to the level of the calloso-marginal fissure*, not, however, so marked as on the superior surface. The area included by the tumour (Fig. 1, A, B, C, D) is manifestly larger than that corresponding to it on the right side. The length of A, B (Fig. 1) is $2\frac{1}{8}$ inches, while that of $A^1$, $B^1$ is $1\frac{1}{2}$ inch.

A transverse vertical section throughout the central hæmorrhage (E), that is, through the posterior extremity of the superior frontal convolution, shows the

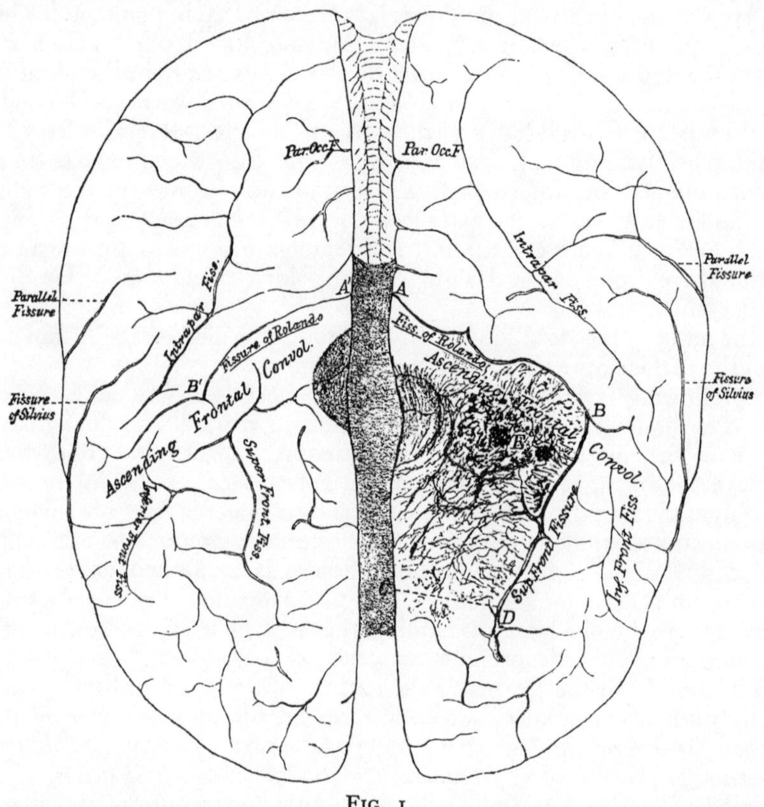


FIG. 1.

tumour to be limited in the deeper parts also to the area defined. The tumour cuts stiffly, and about an inch below the central hæmorrhage is a calcareous mass about the size of a pea (Fig. 2, F). The great bulk of the hard part of the tumour lies above and internal to this calcareous nodule, and is of a dull grey colour. Throughout the cortex are numerous miliary hæmorrhages; the central hæmorrhage (Fig. 2, E) extends to the depth of $\frac{1}{2}$ inch; a second smaller hæmorrhage (Fig. 2, G) lies about 1 inch external to it, and below this is a patch of gelatinous softening (Fig. 2, H) in the inner wall of the superior frontal fissure. The outer wall of that fissure, and the neighbouring brain tissue outside the area defined on the surface, present in successive parallel transverse vertical sections a perfectly normal colour and consistency. On laying open the interior of the brain in the usual way, the ventricles were found of normal size, the choroid plexuses and velum interpositum were gorged with blood. The ganglia at the base of the brain, as also the pons, medulla oblongata, and cerebellum, were to all appearance perfectly normal.

Microscopic examination shows the tumour to be a glioma composed of round and spindle cells, but varying much in the amount and arrangement of these at different parts. At certain points, especially externally, there is extensive fatty change, and in that part beginning external to the central hæmorrhage the tumour contains numerous calcareous particles (" brain sand "). The tumour shows numerous recent hæmorrhages. Microscopic examination of the tissue of the ascending parietal convolution shows that the tumour does not extend behind the fissure of Rolando.

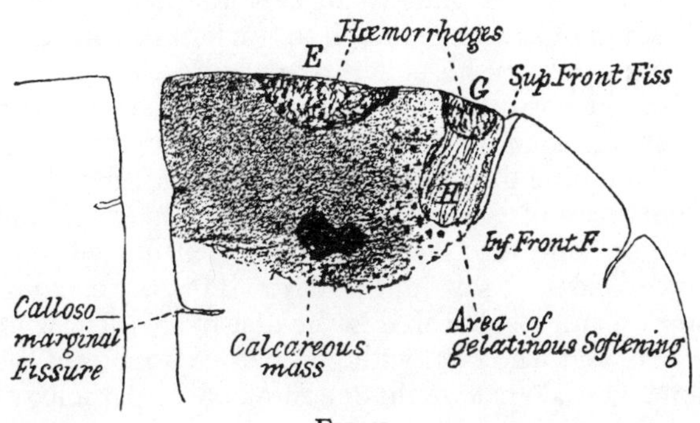


Fig. 2.

*Remarks.*—This man's fits always began, so far as I was told, in the foot, and affected the leg first and most. But he was several times under the care of Dr. Stephen Mackenzie, who tells me that the man declared in 1877 that the fits usually began in the right hand. Dr. Mackenzie feels confident that for the last two years of the man's life the fits began as frequently in the right hand as in the right foot. That the disease was in the mid-region of the brain (the so-called motor region) is in accord with many observations. The difference in the starting-points of the spasm, sometimes foot, sometimes hand, renders the case of comparatively little value for precise localisation. Even supposing that the fits had begun either always in the hand or always in the foot, the locality of the tumour is neither in accord with other observations I have made, nor with the recent experiments of Hitzig and Ferrier. It is of little use saying anything on localisation in such a case, and therefore I omit what I said when reading the case before the Medical Society of London before I was acquainted with the facts Dr. Stephen Mackenzie supplied me with. Besides, the damage by tumours is mostly widespread, coarse, and indefinite. The experiments of Hitzig and Ferrier, and the researches of Charcot on cases of monoplegia from limited cortical softening, are more definite for purposes of localisation than anything we can conclude from the doings of most cases of cerebral tumours.

Now for clinical facts.

The duration of the case, considering that we found a gliomatous tumour post-mortem, is noteworthy—about twelve years from the first attack. That there was tumour all that time I cannot know. One of the cases of fits beginning in the right leg I have recorded was that of a man who was under my observation three years, and he had had fits of just the same kind seven years before. Ten years from the first fit we found cerebral tumour post-mortem. Moreover in that case there were none of the common symptoms of tumour until about a month before he died (when he had double optic neuritis), not even severe headache. Dr. Young, of Aldershot, diagnosed tumour of the cerebellum in a boy whom he sent to me in 1870. This patient died from meningeal hæmorrhage, the result of a fall seven years later ; there was a tumour of the cerebellum.[1]

Now I speak of the ordinary symptoms of local gross brain disease.

On the first admission (1872), the patient said that since the fits, that is, for two years, he had been subject to severe headache ; for some time the pain was over the left temple, but mostly all over the head. But I do not think it was very severe, not of severity enough to warrant the diagnosis of local gross organic disease as the cause of his convulsive seizures, and on his next admission (1875) he said he did not often suffer from headache. At none of the three admissions was anything found wrong ophthalmoscopically. Nevertheless, it is possible that some time during the six years or so I did not see him he had double optic neuritis, and got rid of it. I have known a man who had fits beginning in his left hand who got rid of optic neuritis entirely, and of his fits too, for ten years at least. I saw him to-day. This was a syphilitic case. But neuritis has come on and disappeared in the case of a patient who had fits affecting mostly one arm, and who died with gliomatous tumour of the brain.

The question comes, What would one think of the pathology of the case of a patient who had only fits of this kind and no headache, or no severe headache and no affection of his optic nerves ? Perhaps we may say that, as a matter of fact, most seizures of this kind are owing to syphilitic brain disease ; but supposing there to be no evidence of syphilis, as in the case I relate ? What should we conclude ? There was no history of a blow—which Virchow believes to be one cause or starting of gliomatous brain tumour—and no ear disease. There was nothing definite except the fits, which are only localising—do not point to the nature of the disease.[2]

I do not think we could conclude with certainty as to the pathology of such a case. I suppose I thought, in 1872 and 1875, it most likely that there was no tumour ; that there was some cortical lesion, I felt sure. I have had two autopsies on patients who had epileptiform seizures beginning very locally, and yet I found no local central disease ; there was universally spread atrophy of both sides of the brain. Such widely spread disease would not account for localised fits, and besides, atrophied brain tissue is for function nothing at all, and could not cause anything. No doubt in each of these two cases a minute local lesion existed, which I failed to discover.

In some cases of cortical syphilis I believe the gumma is absorbed or disappears, leaving a sort of scar, as syphilitic liver disease does. I have published[3] the case of a man who had fits beginning in the right hand ; we

[1] *British Medical Journal*, May 17, 1873, and March 24, 1877.

[2] The abnormal physiology of such cases is quite certain ; there is highly raised instability of some nerve cells. The question in pathology is, " By what process does this great local instability result ? " And part of this question is, " Is the instability the indirect result of gross organic disease ? " If local gross organic disease be decided for, then arises the further question, " Is it syphilitic or not ? "

[3] *Medical Times and Gazette*, December 28, 1872.

found adhesions of the dura mater over convolutions of the left cerebral hemisphere, where the grey matter had disappeared, leaving an œdematous tough scar. There was a large ordinary gumma in the opposite cerebral hemisphere. But I do not believe that I overlooked any such changes in the two cases of cerebral atrophy I have just mentioned.

Now that we have had the autopsy, we feel sure that the patient was always, so long as a large tumour existed, on the brink of death ; for at any time a large hæmorrhage might have occurred from the tumour and killed him. It is well known that patients, seemingly well, or not very ill, die suddenly in this way by hæmorrhage from cerebral tumour.[1]

Hæmorrhage from such tumour is one cause of hemiplegia. It is hard to believe, however, that the small hæmorrhages found post-mortem in the case I have narrated had anything to do with the patient's hemiplegia on his last admission. The nature of this hemiplegia is a very difficult clinical problem. It could not be due to the destruction effected by the tumour. I think it possible that it was a sequence of some seizures in the night, and that the patient would have recovered from it had he not died of pneumonia. Of course I cannot know that he had fits in the night. Before (in 1875) he had had almost perfect paralysis of the leg ; he told us (in 1882) that he had been hemiplegic several times. I think this is likely, but I must add that the patient was mistaken as to another matter, the date of his last hemiplegia ; he was too ill to be thoroughly trusted ; his father said his son had never been hemiplegic. I will allude only to the paralysis in 1875. This was clearly a sequence of his seizures. The most reasonable explanation of paralysis after such convulsions seems to me that given by Todd (who first described what he called epileptic hemiplegia, and what I call post-epileptiform hemiplegia) and Alexander Robertson—exhaustion of nerve fibres by the excessive discharge in the paroxysm. I have seen perfect hemiplegia come on after convulsive seizures, and pass off again several times in the same patient ; a cortical lesion was found post-mortem in that case.

It is very important to note the condition of the reflexes in cases of paralysis after local convulsive seizures, but I say nothing about them in this case ; they were only tested for when the patient was hemiplegic on his last admission.

For many reasons it is important to note the condition of the deep reflexes in cases of local paralysis after epileptiform seizures. The matter is somewhat complicated. I have known foot clonus of the side affected by fits, when there was no paralysis, and several weeks after the last fit. But we sometimes find temporary foot clonus and temporarily exaggerated knee-jerk on the side temporarily paralysed after a convulsive seizure affecting that side, in a patient who before his seizure had normal reflexes.

[1] Hence a young person with double optic neuritis is to be considered in danger of sudden or rapid death, not on account of the neuritis of course, but because in young people it often results somehow from vascular glioma.

# A CONTRIBUTION TO THE COMPARATIVE STUDY OF CONVULSIONS [1]

## 1. *Introductory*

WHEN I first began the investigation of nervous diseases I supposed, as most other physicians then did, and as perhaps most still do, the seat of epilepsy to be the medulla oblongata. But I soon came to the conclusion that the cerebrum is the seat of epileptiform seizures (convulsion beginning unilaterally). I supposed the particular parts diseased to lie within the region of the middle cerebral artery; that rough localisation was before I had the advantage of the experimental researches of Hitzig and Ferrier. Later on, I supposed that, as I crudely put it, epilepsy (the epilepsy proper of authorities) depended on discharges of convolutions " at a greater distance from the motor tract " than epileptiform seizures did.[2] I believed then, that no variety of convulsion in man arose from any sort of change below the cerebrum proper. But very lately I have come back to the belief, that *some* convulsions (I do not call them epileptic) in children (and, I suspect some in adults which are *called* epileptic) depend on lesions of the pons or medulla oblongata. The fits in children to which I especially allude are " inward fits," otherwise called laryngismus stridulus; they are " respiratory convulsions."

Of course I knew long ago that Brown-Séquard had demonstrated that in guinea-pigs a *liability to* convulsions could be experimentally produced (in ways everybody knows), and that the fits could be artificially brought on when the brain proper had been taken away. And I knew that Kussmaul and Tenner had produced convulsion by rapidly bleeding rabbits when the brain proper had been removed. It is plain that the convulsions in these animals do not depend on the cerebrum. Moreover there are the most valuable experiments of Westphal, another way of producing a liability to convulsions in guinea-pigs. But I supposed, erroneously I now think, that no sort of convulsion occurred *in man* from any kind of disease lower than the cerebrum proper. I thought the reason why convulsion occurred in certain lower animals deprived of the cerebrum, and not in man from disease of parts lower than the cerebrum, was explainable by the manifest great differences in the degree of evolution of the nervous systems of those animals from that of the nervous system of man. Seeing that the convulsions in the animals just mentioned were demonstrably owing to changes in the medulla oblongata, or pons, or both, I tried to show why such convulsions occurred in these lower animals and not in man.[3] Having now modified my belief on this matter, I come to attach even a greater value than I once did to the researches of Marshall Hall, Brown-Séquard, Kussmaul and Tenner, and Westphal. This by way of mere preliminary. I now think, as above stated, that there are three classes of fits in man. I go on to speak more particularly of the three.

[1] *Brain*, vol. ix, 1886, p. 1.

[2] " Study of Convulsions," *St. Andrews Medical Graduates' Transactions*, vol. iii, 1870. (See p. 8.)

[3] *West Riding Asylum Reports*, vol. iii, p. 342, " On Evolution of Nervous Centres." (See p. 106.)

## 2. *The Scale of Fits*

I believe (1) epileptic fits (epilepsy proper) to depend on discharging lesions of parts of the highest level of evolution, and (2) epileptiform seizures to depend on discharging lesions of parts of the middle level of evolution. Both (1 and 2) are cerebral convulsions. Both, to my thinking, are " cortical." (3) Inward fits (respiratory convulsions) and some other fits depend, I submit, on discharges beginning in parts of the lowest level of evolution.

## 3. *The Three Levels of Evolution of the Central Nervous System*

I now give a brief outline of the hierarchy of the nervous centres. It is admittedly imperfect ; it is incomplete, too, by omission of the sympathetic chain, peripheral ganglia, and ganglia of the posterior roots of the spinal nerves. (Strictly, we ought to speak of four levels, the periphery being the real lowest.) It will be seen that the scheme is not after the morphological divisions, spinal cord, pons Varolii, etc., but is, especially, according to degree of indirectness with which centres represent parts of the body, and is thus an anatomico-physiological scheme. The motor nuclei of the pons Varolii and medulla oblongata are some lowest motor centres as much as the anterior spinal horns are some others.

(1) The lowest level of evolution, or series of lowest centres, is pretty much what Marshall Hall called " the True Spinal System," which, according to him, especially consisted of spinal cord, medulla oblongata, and pons Varolii. The nuclei for ocular muscles in the floor of the aqueduct of Sylvius are, no doubt, the topographically highest known lowest motor centres.[1]

The lowest sensori-motor centres represent all parts of the body, animal and organic, " from nose to feet," in simplest, etc., combinations.

Besides the centres we have spoken of, anterior and posterior spinal horns and their homologues higher up, and besides Clarke's visceral column and its lower and higher representatives, there are what are called " regulating centres," —micturition centre, vaso-motor centre, respiratory centre, etc. It may be that these are simply recombinations of elements of the nuclei mentioned. I think that these centres are products of internal evolution.

(2) The middle level of evolution consists of Hitzig and Ferrier's motor centres, and of Schäfer and Victor Horsley's trunk centres, and also of Ferrier's sensory region.[2]

The middle sensori-motor centres re-represent all parts of the body, organic and animal, from nose to feet, in more complex, etc., combinations.

(3) The highest level of evolution consists of parts of the brain in front of the middle motor centres (frontal or prefrontal, lobes), highest motor centres, and of parts behind the middle sensory centres (occipital lobes), highest sensory centres.

The highest centres re-re-represent all parts of the body, organic and animal, from nose to feet, in most complex, etc., combinations.

The lowest level of central evolution being evolved out of the periphery (epi- and ento-) represents all parts indirectly, but yet most nearly directly

[1] There is no impropriety in this expression, nor in such a one as " two lowest centres," since " lowest centre " is a proper name.

[2] Since Hitzig and Ferrier are not agreed on details of motor representation by the cortex, it will be seen that by using the expression " Hitzig and Ferrier's motor centres " I do not pretend to demarcate exactly the middle and highest motor centres.

of all the levels ; the middle, evolved out of the lowest, represents (re-represents) all parts doubly indirectly ; the highest evolved out of the middle, represents (re-re-represents) all parts triply indirectly.

The highest centres, the climax of the evolution, are in popular language the " organ of the mind." I again insist, as I have done for many years, that this " organ " is as certainly of sensori-motor constitution as is the lumbar enlargement (some lowest centres). But the constitution of the highest centres differs vastly in degree from that of the lowest centres. They (*a*) represent most indirectly (re-re-represent) (*b*) literally all parts of the body having nerves (as the lower levels do), but they (*c*) represent all parts in most numerous and most complex, etc., combinations. Just as any state of consciousness is a state of a whole person psychical, so the correlative activity is of nervous arrangements representing a whole person physical (the whole organism). When a person is having a particular mental state, there are occurring physically, of course, activities of his highest centres. But what I urge is that the nervous arrangements then engaged represent his body, and some parts of it most especially.

I believe that the cerebellum also represents all parts of the body, but in ways different from the cerebrum. It will be seen that the lowest level of evolution is at once lowest cerebral and lowest cerebellar.

### 4. *The Comparative Study of Convulsions ; Varieties of Lowest Level Fits*

One object is to make a comparative study of the three classes of convulsions or fits depending on discharges on the three different levels of evolution—lowest, middle and highest levels of evolution. Speaking roughly, there are supposed to be lowest, middle, and highest " level fits." [1] Several things qualifying a direct comparison and contrast of the three classes of fits will be spoken of later.

An " inward fit," or respiratory convulsion, is but one variety of fits on the lowest level, just as convulsion beginning in one hand is but one variety of epileptiform seizures (middle level fits), and just as convulsion ushered in by an " epigastric sensation " is but one variety of epilepsy proper (highest level fits). Moreover, what we call respiratory convulsion should in many cases, since the convulsion becomes universal, be called respiratorily beginning convulsion. In each class of fits the convulsion is universal if the discharge be severe enough. Ordinary spasmodic asthma in the child or adult is a respiratory convulsion, and is also a lowest level fit. Both it and inward fits are, I submit, owing to sudden, etc., discharges beginning in some part of the respiratory centres. Rigor is another lowest level fit, dependent on discharge beginning in some part of the vasomotor centre. I suppose, as implied in some foregoing remarks, that the fits induced by Brown-Séquard and Westphal in guinea-pigs, and by Kussmaul and Tenner in rabbits, are lowest level fits in those animals. I shall consider later whether, as I have said I suspect, some fits in the adult called epileptic are really epileptic (epilepsy proper), or are lowest level fits—fits analogous to those occurring in Brown-

[1] In still other words, which must not be taken literally, there are " least evolved," " higher evolved," and " most evolved " fits. Thus a severe epileptic seizure is a " more evolved fit " than a severe epileptiform seizure is, even when in each the convulsion is universal. I shall no longer use such expressions, for strictly the three classes of fits are three different dissolutions *being effected*.

Séquard's guinea-pigs. But I ought to say now, that I fear I shall not be able to make out anything like a demonstration on this matter. In any case we should have to consider the vast differences in the degree of evolution of the nervous centres in man and in the guinea-pig.[1]

It may be well to say very explicitly, what is, however, repeating part of the foregoing, that I do not believe epilepsy, the epilepsy proper of nosologists, and epileptiform seizures to be owing to any sort of lesion on the lowest level of evolution, although of course the motor centres on this lowest level are secondarily engaged in epileptiform seizures, and tertiarily in epileptic seizures.

" Inward fits," or respiratory convulsions, some lowest level fits, are the main subject of this paper ; epileptic seizures, highest level fits, have been spoken of at the outset for the sake of order, and will be considered again in comparison and contrast with " inward fits," and other lowest level fits.

### 5. *Inward Fits*

" Inward fits," or laryngismus stridulus (respiratory convulsions), occur mostly in children under 1 year of age, not often after 2. Laryngismus stridulus occurs especially, Niemeyer says, during the first year of life ; Charles West found that out of thirty-seven cases, thirty-one occurred between the age of 6 months and 2 years. Meigs and Pepper write [2] : " Of thirty cases selected indifferently from our practice, and from authors in which the age is given, thirteen were 6 months or less of age, eleven between 6 months and 1 year, four between 1 and 2 years of age, one of 2 and one of 4 years of age ; so that of the thirty, twenty-four were under 1 year." " Laryngismus seldom attacks children more than a year old." [3] Henoch writes that it is " confined almost exclusively to the period between the sixth and twenty-fourth months. I have hardly ever observed it at a later age, but have seen cases as early as the fifth or sixth week." [4] What is the significance of this limitation by age ?

### 6. *The Infant's Nervous System*

The lowest level of evolution is probably nearly the whole of the new-born infant's developed nervous system ; the higher levels, in so far as they are not yet organised, are masses of " nervous stuff " and not centres proper ; they are almost a fœtal part of the new-born infant. No doubt development goes on with increased activity in the higher two levels after birth ; the nervous masses, as we called them, will be rapidly becoming middle and highest centres. But their development will be far behind that of the lowest (" earliest ") level. " Inward fits " are rare under 6 months of age, when the lowest level itself will be very imperfectly developed ; but probably the main reason why these fits do not often occur until the age of 6 months is that rickets is rare before that age.

[1] Since writing this sentence, I have seen fits in a boy whose case is, I think, very like the cases of Brown-Séquard's guinea-pigs. A boy of 7 falls suddenly to the ground when his head or face, either side, is touched ; his face flushes, his eyes turn up and to the right, his respiration stops, and there is a sudden jerk of his limbs. Since his fits began a few months before the age of 2½ years (when he had " an ordinary epileptic fit "), as he has imperfect left hemiplegia, and for other reasons to be given when the case is reported, the supposition of pretence is about as reasonable as that Brown-Séquard's guinea-pigs should pretend to have fits when the epileptogenous zone is touched. (See p. 362).

[2] *Diseases of Children*, 7th ed.

[3] Ringer, *Therapeutics*, 10th ed, p. 67.

[4] *Lectures on Diseases of Children*, p. 70.

According to Soltmann, the convolutions in the " motor region " (I call this region the middle motor centres) in new-born dogs, cats, and rabbits is unexcitable at birth, and epileptiform seizures cannot be provoked in them by excitation of that region. Albertoni has confirmed these observations. Franck and Pitres write of Albertoni's researches : " Il résulte de cette série d'expériences que l'épilepsie par la faradisation de l'écorce du cerveau n'a pu être provoqué chez un chien de treize jours, tandis qu'elle s'est produite chez les animaux âgés de dix-neuf jours et plus." Soltmann's conclusions have, however, been recently disputed by Dr. Joseph Pareth, who says the dog's cortex *is* excitable in the first days after birth. Still we cannot but suppose that the higher centres must, in new-born animals, be a long way behind the lowest in their degree of development.

The infancy of a dog in comparison with that of man is of slight duration. The higher the animal, the longer its infancy. Man's infancy is the longest of all. The following quotation from Fiske is of profound importance to the medical evolutionist in many ways.

" The gulf by which the lowest known man is separated from the highest known ape consists in the great increase of his cerebral surface, with the accompanying intelligence, and in the very long duration of his infancy. These two things have gone hand-in-hand. The increase of cerebral surface due to the working of natural selection in that direction alone has entailed a vast increase in the amount of cerebral organisation that must be left to be completed after birth, and thus has prolonged the period of infancy." [1]

Much is said of the " great excitability " of the nervous system of infants. I should not speak so generally, but would say that the lowest level of evolution is in the new-born infant almost the whole of its then developed nervous system, and thus almost the sole part there is to be excitable. Putting this otherwise, the lowest level is, the younger the infant, the more nearly *its* highest level ; it is indeed more nearly its highest and lowest at once, although, later in life, on full development of its middle and highest nervous masses into centres proper, that level will be the real lowest. It itself in the infant will be at once imperfectly developed and actively developing, and thus *naturally very excitable.* The parts most actively developing on the infant's lowest, his then nearly highest, level will be the centres for organic parts ; the centres for animal parts will be far behind them in degree of development. No doubt the order of degree of development of the centres for the three great organic functions, although nearly contemporaneous, will be, both before and after birth, digestive, circulatory, and respiratory ; the respiratory will be, of the three, the most actively developing in infancy. The lowest centres for the three systems are seated in that part of the lowest level which is, morphologically, the medulla oblongata, and as Lauder Brunton, in some very important remarks, says : " the medulla oblongata in the vertebrata may be looked on as a lower and more fundamental centre than the brain or spinal cord." [2]

Another side of some of the foregoing statements is that the higher levels being in the infant little organised (being there morphologically, but not being there functionally to any great extent) the lowest level will be less " controlled " or less " kept down " than in older persons. *Pari passu* with the later develop-

[1] *Destiny of Man*, p. 54. For a full account of Fiske's opinions on the importance of prolongation of infancy, see his *Cosmic Philosophy*, vol. ii.

[2] *Pharmacology*, etc., p. 197.

ment, or evolution, of the higher levels, the lowest will be more and more " kept down." Putting this otherwise: the process of evolution is not only an " adding on," but is thereby, at the same time, a " keeping down "; the newly added (properly the higher and newer *evolved out of* the lower and older) controls its lower. Using popular language, we gradually get above our mechanical selves as evolution of our middle and highest centres (and especially their internal evolution) proceeds.

Here I refer to Soltmann's important researches on imperfect development of inhibitory arrangements in very young dogs, cerebral, he thinks, as well as spinal. If Soltmann's observations are correct, they are a very important contribution to the doctrine of evolution of the nervous system. The younger the infant, the more of a mere ordinary reflex mechanism will be what there then is of its nervous system; the less check there will be of one part by another. The accelerating cardiac centres will develop ahead of the cardio-inhibitory centres; the respiratory ahead of its checking nervous arrangements, the vaso-motor ahead of the vaso-dilator nervous arrangements.

### 7. *Recapitulation*

So now we find that " inward fits " occur in the very young, in those persons, that is, whose lowest level of evolution is the most developed and yet most actively developing level, and which, from the comparatively little development of higher centres, is little controlled. This is saying that what we call the infant's lowest centres are its *then* nearly highest centres or highest and lowest at once. " Inward fits " occur in those persons whose *then* nearly highest centres are *naturally very excitable*. Bearing in mind Soltmann's observations, we add that these nearly highest centres (which later in life will be the lowest centres) are more nearly ordinary reflex centres, are less checked in their actions and interactions by inhibitory nervous arrangements. But why have some and not other infants " inward fits "? In other words, what is the determining cause of such discharges of the infant's " naturally very excitable " respiratory centres as produce, not respiratory movements, but respiratory convulsions? That inward fits nearly always occur in the rickety is now (Elsasser, Jenner, Gee) accepted doctrine. But what is the relation? Henoch writes: " All attempts fail to explain the connection between rachitis and spasm of the glottis." It is, then, somewhat rash in me to submit an explanation. The question is, " By what steps does rachitis bring about sudden and excessive discharges of the respiratory centres in infants? What is the intermediary between rickets and inward fits?" As a preliminary, some general remarks on nervous discharges must be made.

### 8. *Digression on Nervous Discharge*

All movements are the results of nervous discharges (or liberations of energy by nerve cells), but in the case of convulsion there are sudden excessive and rapid discharges; such discharges of any motor centre do not produce movements proper.[1] Besides developing movements strongly, they develop many

[1] Many years ago Moxon remarked, " muscle is only in degree less nervous than nerve." There is, in severe epileptic fits, a sequence of discharges of four levels of motor evolution—highest, middle, and lowest nervous centres and of " muscle centres "—muscles being in one aspect, in accord with Moxon's remark, nervous centres; in another aspect they are glands. I continue, however, to speak of three levels of evolution.

together—produce that contention of many movements which we call convulsion. Any motor centre suddenly, excessively and rapidly discharging is, for the time being, a " convulsive centre." What I call " discharging lesions " in epileptic and epileptiform seizures are small persistent " convulsive centres." A " discharging lesion " (or part of a motor centre become a " convulsive centre ") is a local persisting hyperphysiological state of nerve cells induced by some pathological changes, which changes lead to increased, but yet, I think, inferior nutrition.[1]

It is to be insisted on that convulsion, in any case, is nothing whatever else than a sudden excessive and rapid development of the *normal* movements which the centre, suddenly and excessively discharging, represents. The great thing to bear in mind is, that such discharges lead not only to excessive, but also to contemporaneous development of many movements, so that the name " movements " is no longer properly applicable to the motor affection produced, and we call it convulsion. Let any motor centre be discharged strongly enough, and rapidly enough, and we have convulsion of the parts the centre represents.

There is, of course, something more. Since a " discharging lesion " is a physiological fulminate (normal cells of a centre having become a quasi-parasitical hyperfunctioning part of it), the sudden excessive and rapid discharge of its *highly* unstable elements upsets the equilibrium of (discharges) anatomically connected nervous arrangements of normal instability ; normal elements which, in the case of a " destructive lesion," serve towards compensating a loss, are in the case of a " discharging lesion " compelled to co-operate in an excess (co-operation in excess is compensation inverted). So it is always to be understood, when not stated, that not only are the movements of the parts most especially represented by cells constituting a " discharging lesion " developed, but that the movements of other parts also, represented by normal cells which are (by collateral and downward currents) compelled to discharge, are developed. (The discharges in both cases being sudden, etc., what we just called the development of movements is really the " running them up " into convulsion.) Hence from sudden and rapid discharges of a small part of the highest centres (in epilepsy proper) we may have from wide collateral and downward discharges universal severe convulsion (co-operation in excess).

Convulsion, although very different from a series of normal movements, is not something altogether *sui generis*. I do not now believe, as I once said, that all metaphysic has died out of the expression " attacked by convulsion " ; it is not always thoroughly realised that a convulsion is simply a brutish development of many of the patient's ordinary movements. A severe epileptic convulsion, to take that case for illustration, is nothing whatever else than a sudden, excessive, rapid, and consequently a nearly contemporaneous, development of many of the patient's commonplace daily movements—of movements of the eyes in looking ; of the face in its various expressions ; of articulatory movements ; of manipulatory and of other movements of the arms ; of movements of the trunk and legs in walking ; of digestive, respiratory, and circulatory movements, etc. But from such developments there is no looking, smiling, talking, etc., because all the movements which are developed, being nearly contemporaneously developed, are " run up " into a muscular fight. Speaking figuratively,

[1] I have been said to have put forward the " theory of discharges " as the *pathology* of epilepsies. I have really tried hard to show that certain pathological processes only *induce* " discharging lesions " which are *hyperphysiological* states.

we may say that the epileptic discharge is trying to develop all the functions of the body excessively, and all at once ; a severe fit is a fairly successful attempt. Let me give a very simple illustration. If there be a centre for locomotion, then during slight sequent discharges of its elements in health, there is walking or running ; but if very many of those elements were to discharge, suddenly, rapidly, and excessively, the man walking or running would not go faster ; on the contrary, he would be stopped, would be stiffened up into a tetanus-like attitude by the *contemporaneous* development of many locomotor movements.[1]

We must not speak of " disorderly discharges," but simply of degrees of discharges above the normal—of degrees of suddenness, excessiveness, and of rapidity of discharges. Coming close to our particular topic, we say that whilst normal discharges of the respiratory centres produce a sequence of respiratory movements, sudden excessive and rapid discharges of those centres produce a respiratory convulsion, which is a sudden excessive and contemporaneous development of, and therefore a strong contention of, normal respiratory movements.

### 9. *The Determining Cause of Sudden, etc., Discharges of Respiratory Centres in Inward Fits*

It is agreed upon that the normal stimulus to the respiratory centres is venous blood. It has long been recognised that rapidly induced asphyxia in animals produces a certain kind of convulsion, a respiratory one. I believe the determining cause of the sudden excessive and rapid (convulsion-producing) discharge of the respiratory centres in cases of " inward fits " to be an excess of their " natural stimulant," venosity of blood. There is no persistent " discharging lesion," as I believe there to be in epileptic and epileptiform seizures. The normally " very excitable " respiratory centres are occasionally goaded into excessive activity. It is not necessary for me to deny, and I do not deny, that besides being naturally very excitable, the centres developed in the infant, and especially those most actively developing, are *morbidly* over-excitable in rickets and in some other diseases. But I make no use of that hypothesis. But how comes about this excess of the " natural stimulant "—excess of venosity of the blood in rickets ?

Mentioning the circular shape of the young child's chest (its respiration being chiefly diaphragmatic), I remark next that " inward fits " occur, not only in persons with such an imperfectly developed respiratory apparatus, but, as is well known, most often in those of them who, from rickets, have abnormally soft ribs. The ribs being abnormally soft in the rickety, and thus not " holding out " during the descent of the diaphragm, the efforts of that muscle are more or less neutralised. Thus there is in young rickety children a condition for venosity (which may in part account for the great sweating in these subjects). Further, the attacks of laryngismus occur chiefly at night when, from sleep, there is still less perfect respiratory action and thus a condition for still greater venosity. A crying fit many bring on a paroxysm (as, anticipating, laughing may bring on an attack of spasmodic asthma in an adult). Henoch [2] writes in his article " Spasm of the Glottis," " In fact, many characteristics of the affec-

[1] It will be seen that I do not believe that an attack of mania ever replaces an epileptic convulsion ; if cells of the nervous arrangements discharging so as to produce movements in mania were to begin to discharge so suddenly, etc., as nerve cells do in an epileptic fit, the maniacal movements would be " run up " into convulsion.

[2] Op. cit., p. 70.

tion can be seen in a *healthy* child who, in the midst of a severe crying spell, suddenly "holds the breath"; *i.e.* lies with the head thrown back, face dark red, somewhat cyanotic, respiration interrupted, and rigid limbs. The excessive crying and the excitement appear to cause spasm of certain respiratory muscles, which disappears, as a rule, after a few seconds." I submit that the thing first caused by the crying in such cases is super-venosity, and that this, over-stimulating the respiratory centres, causes respiratory spasm. Henoch then goes on to speak of *abnormal* conditions: "attacks [of laryngismus] may occur during complete quiet, and *even on awakening from sleep*; but even then it is favoured *by every respiratory exertion*, *viz.* crying, drinking, eating, as well as by psychical influences, anger and fright." The parts I have italicised in the second half of the quotation seem to me in favour of my hypothesis.

Great venosity of the blood will much over-stimulate the "naturally very excitable" respiratory centres in infants, and thus produce respiratory convulsion.[1]

No doubt the respiratory centres are also acted on indirectly through the vagi, the venous blood stimulating the endings of these nerves in the lungs. For when the vagi are cut across, respiration is slower, but yet deeper. Stimulating the central end of one of the vagi quickens respiratory movements; indeed great stimulation so accelerates the rhythm, that it ceases to be rhythm, ordinarily so-called; there is tetanus of the diaphragm, and standstill of respiration in an extreme inspiratory phase. Here we see that, increasing the rapidity of the discharges of the respiratory centres fuses the respiratory movements into convulsion.

Of course no one can ignore that there is very great venosity of blood in the paroxysm of laryngismus, but my contention is that too great venosity is the first thing, that it precedes any part of the paroxysm. Whilst healthy breathing depends on slight venosity—the respiratory centres acting in healthy states from some slight deficiency of oxygen, or possibly, as some think, from stimulation by carbonic acid, too great venosity will stimulate the respiratory centres so overmuch as to produce, not a sequence of normal respiratory movements, but that excessive development and contention of them which is convulsion—will produce arrest of respiration by fixation of the respiratory apparatus. In healthy respiration the inspiratory part is chief; expiration being to a great extent recoil from inspiration. But even if we could conceive that the inspiratory movements were alone suddenly, etc., developed, the chest would be more or less fixed, fixed in a high inspiratory attitude. In dyspnœa, the expiratory movements come into greater prominence.

When there has been first set up any degree of spasm of any part of the respiratory apparatus, the venosity will become greater still, and thus there will be a rapid multiplication of effects. There are degrees of "inward fits," from that local convulsion signified by "crowing inspiration" (perhaps after temporary complete closure of the glottis), to universal convulsion probably consequent on prolonged closure of the glottis, or on partial closure of it with also fixation of other parts of the respiratory apparatus. The supposition is, that the more rapid the initial discharges (that is, the more elements of the respiratory

[1] Possibly, in so far as the higher levels are developed in infants, sleep, which in all persons is, among other things, the going out of function of the highest nervous arrangements (a normal dissolution), leaves the respiratory and other lowest level centres less controlled, and thus more excitable than during waking.

centres suddenly discharging at once, and thus the greater the rate of transfer of energy), the more is it likely for the convulsion to become universal.

That the convulsion, even when universal, is not owing to discharge of higher levels (not of the so-called motor region, middle level, at least) is proved by the fact that asphyxia renders the "motor area" of the cortex inexcitable.[1]

## 10. *Universalisation of Convulsion beginning Respiratorily*

Supposing, then, the first sudden, etc., discharge in inward fits to be of the respiratory centres in seizures becoming universal, the universalisation of the convulsion may be owing to secondarily induced discharge of other centres on the lowest level. Nearly all the muscles of the body must on demand, so to speak, serve in respiration. This implies that the respiratory centres, whilst representing some movements of the nose, larynx, and chest nearly directly, represent also movements of nearly all other parts of the body with various degrees of greater indirectness ; means that they can "call on" other motor centres to act with them in a certain order ; means that their discharges, when strong enough, "find their own" in other centres—flow in lines which are of least resistance *to them*. It is not then necessary to suppose that there are big permanent respiratory centres for all parts of the body, but to hold that there are centres representing most especially the respiratory apparatus, from great over-action of which centres other centres, not ordinarily respiratory, can be called out as reserves, called upon to suspend their own individual duties to serve respiratorily, to join in the fight for breath. The term "centre," in any case, is an arbitrary expression.[2]

I refer to remarks made in the section *Digression on Nervous Discharge* on secondary discharges of normal elements consequent on a primary sudden, etc., discharge of highly unstable elements.

It may perhaps be that the same cause, super-venosity, acts directly on other lowest centres, discharging them after discharging more or less of the respiratory centres. Indeed there certainly is action on some other lowest centres ; for in artificially produced asphyxia there are discharges of the vaso-motor and sweat centres, as well as of the respiratory centres.

The presumption is that there are the two effects ; that universalisation of the convulsion depends partly on discharges spreading from the primarily discharging respiratory centres to other centres on the lowest level, and partly on elements of these other centres being also discharged by the direct action of over-venous blood upon them.

[1] It may be said that some clinical facts show that great venosity of the blood, in adults, "excites the brain." In some cases of emphysema with bronchitis, the patient may be delirious at night. To take a stronger case A man was recently admitted into the London Hospital under Mr. McCarthy's care for injury of the spine, which reduced the patient to diaphragmatic respiration. He became delirious, when he was evidently undergoing asphyxia. For my part I cannot see how these facts show that venosity *excites* the brain. I should say that the venosity accounted for the negative half only of the patient's condition when delirious—for the physical condition answering to his defect of consciousness—that it put out of use some of the highest nervous arrangements of the highest centres. I submit that the positive part of the condition, the delirium proper, was the outcome of raised activity of lower nervous arrangements of his highest centres, consequent on loss of control. We remarked before that evolution is not only an "adding on," but a "keeping down" also ; so in the case of dissolution from venosity just mentioned, the "taking off" of the highest nervous arrangement is a "letting go" of the lower.

[2] For admirable remarks on the term "centre," see Lauder Brunton, *Pharmacology*, etc., 1st ed., p. 199.

In the foregoing is a detailed acknowledgment of what was stated generally in saying that the convulsions in the respiratory fits of children sometimes become universal. There are effects produced by asphyxia in many centres, if not in centres " all along the line " of the lowest level. In children we see turning up of the eyes ; asphyxia produces sweating, raised arterial tension ; there are carpo-pedal contractions as well as the severer universal convulsion. Hence severe respiratory seizures, there being universal effects, are more thoroughly comparable and contrastable with severe epileptiform and epileptic seizures, in each of which also there are universal effects, than the too limited name " respiratory " I give to them implies.

If venosity in the rickety causes the respiratory fits we call laryngismus in infants, other causes of venosity in very young children should do the same.

11. *Respiratory Convulsions in Laryngitis of Young Children*

I refer to convulsions in young children, subjects of laryngitis (" spasmodic laryngitis ") ; they are respiratory convulsions, but may become universal. I suggest that the age of the patients, the fact that there is a manifest impediment to respiration at the gateway of the respiratory apparatus, and the occurrence of the attacks mostly at night (in sleep), point to an over-stimulation of the respiratory centres by too great venosity. If so, the hypothesis that attacks of laryngismus are similarly caused is favoured. " Spasmodic " laryngitis usually occurs in children under 2 or 3 years of age ; the attacks usually occur suddenly during sleep, and next day the child may be seemingly well except for a little hoarseness and cough ; the attacks are sometimes mistaken for laryngismus.

12. *Treatment of Inward Fits*

Let us now see if the results of treatment favour the hypothesis put forward. It is good practice not to let the child who is the subject of laryngitis sleep too long at a time—not to let it remain too long in a condition favouring venosity ; I suppose the same applies to laryngismus stridulus, to which morbid affection I confine further remarks on treatment.

It is understood, of course, that attention is given to diet, digestion, and state of the bowels. No one fails to treat the rickets, the most approved medicine being cod-liver oil. The good effect of the highly valued remedy, cold sponging, favours my hypothesis ; manifestly it will stimulate the respiratory centres. So do the good results of carrying the child out even in cold weather, and change from town to country air. The several remedies will tend to reduce venosity. Now for drugs, more especially in the treatment of what we may call laryngismus itself. The best remedies should, on the hypothesis, be those which stimulate the respiratory centres. Eustace Smith writes[1] : " Of special drugs, musk and belladonna are most useful [in laryngismus stridulus]. The former can be given to a child of twelve months old in doses of one-third of a grain every six hours, and will be found to have a powerful influence in checking the tendency to spasm. Belladonna, to be of service, must be given in sufficient doses. A baby twelve months old will take well fifteen drops [of the tincture] three times in the day." Musk[2] is a stimulant to the respiratory centre, as is also belladonna. It is well known that children tolerate large doses of belladonna ; bearing in mind Soltmann's researches, this may be

[1] *Diseases of Children*, p. 273. [2] Brunton's *Pharmacology*, etc., p. 988.

because in them it acts more as a stimulant, or rather that the parts it can render negative (inhibitory and secretory nervous arrangements) are not as yet largely enough present in the infant to be paralysed.

What is said of the beneficial effect of the stimulating action of belladonna on the respiratory centres is not inconsistent with the hypothesis, that great excess of the " natural stimulus " (venosity) produces the fits ; for to keep respiration going on actively will prevent great venosity. But anything which makes the respiratory centres act excessively causes so rapid a succession of impulses from them to respiratory muscles as to fix the chest in one persistent inspiratory condition, and brings about next similar impulses to expiratory muscles. Thus there results a fight in which the chest is still in infinite effort, as two well-matched wrestlers are at a certain stage of their contest, the full power of each being developed.

Chloral is a remedy for fits of laryngismus lauded by high authorities. It is the best remedy for a rapid succession of fits of any kind—for putting an end to the seizures, that is. It is not, I presume, actually curative of the morbid condition inducing them. It may be given when fits of laryngismus are frequent.

Now for treatment after the paroxysm. When the fit is over, the child usually comes round spontaneously. But supposing that after a severe attack respiration no longer goes on. The respiratory centres are exhausted, or what remains of them unexhausted is not enough to produce respiratory movements ; the child is seemingly dead. There is paralysis of the respiratory apparatus after respiratory convulsions, just as there may be of a limb after an epileptiform convulsion which had affected that limb first and most.[1] Here we must bear in mind that, after asphyxia fits produced in lower animals, the heart, as a rule, continues to beat for a short time after respiration has stopped. Hence if luckily present when a child is seemingly dead after a fit, we should give him a chance of recovery by artificial respiration. We should not waste time to see whether the heart has or has not stopped. The following quotation [2] justifies the above remark, and is of value in several other ways. Brunton is speaking of asphyxia fits artificially produced in lower animals. The first paragraph in the quotation refers to the paroxysm, the second to the after-paralytic stage, the third is directly relevant to what was just said on attempts to restore infants apparently dead after their respiratory convulsion.

" As the blood becomes venous, the activity of the respiratory centre increases, the respirations becoming quicker and deeper, and the accessory respiratory muscles are thrown into action. This condition is called *dyspnœa*. Finally, the excitement extends to all the muscles of the body, and we get general *convulsions*, which have generally an opisthotonic character. The eyeballs very often protrude during these convulsions, and the blood pressure rises greatly from stimulation of sympathetic and vaso-motor centres in the medulla.

" After the convulsions cease, the animal usually lies motionless, and the heart, as a rule, continues to beat for a short time after the respirations have ceased.

" The excessive venosity of the blood in this condition has paralysed the nerve centres ; but if artificial respiration be now commenced, and the blood

[1] I believe there to be paralysis after epileptic fits also ; but, so far as I know, no one agrees with me in this supposition.

[2] Brunton, op. cit., p. 202.

becomes gradually aerated, the conditions just described are again passed through in the reverse order; convulsions first reappearing, then dyspnœa, next normal breathing, and if the respiration be pushed far enough, apnœa."

I say nothing further here of carpo-pedal contractions which so often complicate laryngismus; their interpretation is difficult. If we take a mere general view of them, as "spasms," there is no difficulty; but the question is, "Why are the most terminal parts of the limbs so specially subject to spasm in this disease?"

### 13. *On Convulsions in some other Morbid Affections of Young Children*

Besides convulsion in rickety infants, and in those infants whose blood aeration is more acutely in arrears from catarrhal laryngitis, I suppose that in some other diseases in which there is great venosity in very young children there are respiratory convulsions. Probably convulsions in young children who have congenital heart disease are of that nature.

Eustace Smith writes,[1] dealing with congenital heart disease; "Convulsions are very common, especially in infants; and startings and twitchings during sleep are seldom absent whatever be the age of the patients.

"Nearly one-half of the cases die before they have completed the first year, and two-thirds before they are two years old. Death often occurs in a convulsive fit; and infants usually die in or directly after such a seizure."

We have convulsions in some cases of whooping-cough, if indeed the ordinary attacks are not allied to convulsion. Judging from what Henoch says,[2] I should say that some convulsions in patients who have pertussis are very closely like the severe convulsions of laryngismus. The parts I have italicised in the following quotation are particularly interesting in this regard—the first as to age; the second as to contractions, resembling, if not identical with, carpo-pedal and other contractions. Henoch calls attention to "the unfavourable significance of those paroxysms [of whooping-cough], which are characterised by protracted apnœa [?], in which cough, with very few or no inspirations, is alone observed, and therefore no whooping tone is heard. *Such attacks are chiefly observed in little children during the first year of life.* The cyanosis rapidly reaches its highest grade; the suffocation is threatening, and may indeed prove fatal, especially when the disease is complicated with diffuse catarrh or broncho-pneumonia. *Under these circumstances partial spasm* (*deviations of the eyes, contracture of the fingers, toes, arms, etc.*), or even *general and fatal convulsions*, may occur during the attack, or immediately afterward, either in consequence of the protracted venous stasis in the brain, or the accumulation of carbonic acid in the blood, which must ensue in the absence of sufficient inspirations."

### 14. *On So-called Excentric Irritations; Excess of "Natural Stimulants"; Epileptogenous Zones*

I have said nothing so far of excentric irritations in cases of laryngismus, not being convinced that they have any share in the production of the seizures.[3] I except, of course, that "excess of the natural stimulus" of the respiratory

[1] *Diseases of Children*, p. 540.

[2] Op. cit., p. 173.

[3] Of course, excitation of very many parts of the body (nose in sneezing, ear in producing cough, sudden application of cold) act on the respiratory centres. I speak of more definite or particular stimuli, and of excessive stimuli.

centres which may consist in strong excitation of the vagal ends in the lungs. Dyspepsia may act, if causing flatulence, by interfering with the play of the infant's diaphragm, and thus indirectly help towards increasing the venosity of its blood. In cases of catarrhal laryngitis there may be excentric irritations from the larynx as part causes of the respiratory convulsions ; but if so, here again there is an excess of a natural stimulus, although of a different kind from venosity. I should doubt whether dyspepsia (*vide supra*) would by " stomach irritation " cause any kind of fits. What I find hard to believe is, that excentric irritations of any sort, of any part, can act on " the nervous centres " when they are healthy, so as to produce convulsion. I can understand that convulsion may result if the peripheral part irritated is particularly related to (specially represented in) the centre which is compelled to discharge—is its " natural stimulus "—but not then unless the centre is from some other cause already morbidly over-excitable. The part of the periphery (ento- or epi-) especially united by afferent nerve fibres to any motor centre, by the intermediation of sensory centres, is, when that centre has become by disease a " convulsive centre," its epileptogenous zone. I can easily understand, to illustrate by epileptiform seizures, that if a man have already a discharging lesion of part of the so-called " arm centre," a tap on some of the tendons of his hand may *start* a fit. And I do not deny that if a man has epileptic fits (epilepsy proper) with a " stomach warning," indigestion may provoke a fit by producing stomach irritation—the stomach being the epileptogenous zone in that patient. On this topic more later. We next consider cases of respiratory fits, experimentally produced in healthy lower animals, when such excentric irritations need not be invoked, even as part causes. This will be the subject of a future paper.

# ON A CASE OF FITS RESEMBLING THOSE ARTIFICIALLY PRODUCED IN GUINEA-PIGS[1]

THIS is the case of a boy who has fits when his head is touched. The case is in many respects very like that of a guinea-pig rendered " epileptic " by some operation on its spinal cord or sciatic nerve (Brown-Séquard). The patient has an epileptogenous zone, as the guinea-pig comes to have some time after the operation.[2]

Before going further, I would remark that, using the term " epilepsy " generically, there are, I think, three classes of epileptic fits: (1) epilepsy proper; (2) epileptiform seizures ; (3) fits depending on discharges beginning in parts of the pons Varolii and medulla oblongata.[3] The fits my patient have belong, I think, to the third class. In there being persistent local disease (as evidenced particularly by the hemiplegia), the case very much resembles the cases of Brown-Séquard's guinea-pig, and closely in that there is an epileptogenous zone. I say little of Brown-Séquard's researches on epilepsy, because Mr. Victor Horsley has recently repeated this distinguished physician's experiments, and can speak more definitely of them than I can. That the fits in the case of the guinea-pigs depend on discharges beginning in some part of the pons Varolii or medulla oblongata, or both these divisions of the nervous system, is clear, if they are producible when the higher parts have been taken away (Brown-Séquard). Convulsions are producible in rabbits by rapid bleeding them when the higher parts are removed. These are similar to asphyxia fits, and depend, like them, on discharges beginning in the respiratory centre. I submit that laryngismus stridulus and spasmodic asthma are owing to discharges beginning in the same centres started by super-venosity.

I do not wish to make too much of one case, the only one of the kind I have seen. I particularly draw attention to the fact that the attacks are not opisthotonic, as malingering boys' fits commonly are. In this patient's case pretence is out of the question. The fits date from the tender age of 2½ years ; they occur during sleep.[4] When awake the fit is not producible if the boy knows he is going to be touched. There is in the hemiplegia clear evidence of local disease of some part of the nervous system. The fits have been witnessed by Sir James Paget, Dr. Bristowe, Mr. Hutchinson, Mr. Savory, Dr. Hughes Bennett, Dr. James Anderson, and Mr. Victor Horsley.

A boy, first seen in consultation with Mr. R. W. Dunn, of Surrey Street, on January 19, 1886. The patient's age was 7 on February 2 of that year. When about 3 years old, the patient had a convulsion, about which I obtained no information, except that he " turned up his eyes." His mother

[1] *Medical Society's Proceedings*, vol. x, 1886.

[2] I think it very likely that every patient subject to fits of any class has an epileptogenous zone—that disturbance of the part of the periphery (ento- or epi-periphery) most especially represented in the " discharging lesion " may provoke a fit.

[3] I refer to a paper in *Brain*, April 1886, for details of this classification—" A Contribution to the Comparative Study of Convulsions." (See p. 348.)

[4] I have known epileptiform seizures, beginning in one thumb and affecting one arm, and turning the head to the same side, to occur during sleep.

attributed this fit to exposure to cold, by the carelessness of his nurse. After this he was " delicate " ; he walked at the age of 2 years and 3 months, and did not talk till between 5 and 6.

At the age of 2½ years he had a fit, called by his medical man " an ordinary epileptic fit " ; it is said to have lasted an hour, but there may have been a succession of fits. There was foaming of the mouth and heavy breathing, and he was convulsed. He has since had four attacks of this kind, or perhaps, we should say of this degree ; the last of them was three months ago. Ever since the first " ordinary epileptic fit," he has had imperfect use of the left arm and leg (*vide infra*).

The most noteworthy thing in this case is that he " began to fall down " occasionally about a month or six weeks before the first fit, that is, before the first so-called " ordinary epileptic fit," which occurred at the age of 2½ years. Ever since he has been subject to these " fallings," which are really fits also. But so far as his father knows the boy never has these seizures unless his head or face be touched ; it is to be particularly mentioned that a fit would not occur if he knew he was going to be touched. His mother, to show me what happened, flicked his face with her handkerchief ; the boy suddenly collapsed, and would have gone down to the ground had he not at the time been held by his father. He turned red, looked vacant, his respiration stopped and his eyes were turned to one side. The affair was rapid and soon over—perhaps fifteen seconds or less—so that I did not then accurately note details. Stoppage of respiration was very evident ; it had been noticed by other (non-medical) people besides his father and mother. Later, when percussing his head to see if there was a tender spot, he fell down suddenly, having the same symptoms as before. His father said that the boy would have some days fifty " falls " of this sort, and did not believe that ever a day passed without a fit—for fits, no doubt, these " falls " are. Accidentally brushing his head against a curtain would send him down. Touching any part of either side of his head or face would bring on the attacks ; according to his father's account it made no difference what part of his head or face was touched. The boy could tell me nothing whatever about the attacks. I think he was unconscious in them, but cannot be certain.[1] The fits would occur in sleep, as his father supposes, from the boy's head being inadvertently touched by movements of his hands. He carried about with him clear evidences of sudden inopportune falls occurring during his play. When I saw him first there was a sore on one side of his head, the left frontal eminence was much hypertrophied (his father not inaptly, for a layman, said of this swelling that from repeated falls it had become " a permanent ossification "), the right frontal eminence was not so large, and yet it was abnormally large. Continuing this part of the subject, I pass on to the next visit, when I had the advantage of the help of Dr. James Anderson and Mr. Victor Horsley in investigating the case more fully.

January 25, 1886. There is a bruise on the right cheek. His mother told him to shut his mouth before she touched his head ; she explained that he had bitten his tongue in a recent " fall." He had a habit of running with his tongue protruded ; shutting his mouth and bringing his teeth together prevented

[1] In the case of the patient who had some of his fits during sleep (see a previous footnote), there was no negative affection of consciousness at the climax of those fits, which began when he was awake. He spoke when his head was much turned to the left. Until on one occasion he made at that stage of the fit a remark relevant to what I was saying, I had supposed him to be then unconscious.

tongue-biting when he " fell." However, he had only once bitten his tongue ; he never bit it in the " severe epileptic attacks."

In the fits we saw he fell down, and seemed to be unconscious ; the two eyes turned to the right and upwards in parallelism ; his respiration stopped for a few seconds. His father had noticed that in every attack observed since the last visit the eyes turned to the right. When lying down the fits, on touching his head, seemed to be slighter. When his head was touched whilst he was recumbent his limbs moved ; there was but one movement—a sudden jerk—which was soon over. In some the left leg moved alone, or it moved more than the other ; possibly the right arm moved more than the left.

*Permanent condition of the left limbs.*—The face and tongue were moved normally, and so it is believed were the right limbs. The left arm was slightly less than the right in circumference ; his father reported that he moved it clumsily, but his grasps were about equal. His father said that when the boy was using the right hand in such an operation as drawing, the left hand was always " going," showing us in imitation movements of his own hand somewhat like those of athetosis. The boy limped slightly with the left leg ; it was decidedly less in circumference than the right. There was no foot clonus on either side, and his knee-jerks were supposed to be normal. The patient's chest was well shaped. There was no evidence of rickets.

At my request his father made particular observations on the fits in sleep. He had frequently seen attacks brought on in sleep, when the boy was accidentally touched either by himself or by others. On purposely touching him in sleep, his father observed that (letter, January 27, 1886) " the movements of the body were exactly the same as when awake ; the duration of the apparent unconsciousness the same, and, unless my observations deceived me, the eyes were turned upwards and to the right." It will be seen that his father, in the part of the letter quoted, does not speak confidently as to the position of the eyes in the fits during sleep. In a further letter, dated February 2, he writes : " I have touched him twenty or thirty times during sleep the past two nights, with the result simply of waking him. Three or four times, however, the touch has given him a momentary shock, and his eyes turned up, but I believe not to the right side. The shocks are of such short duration it is difficult to open the lid in time and watch result. If I open the eye preparatory to giving the touch, he awakes." " His aunt, who generally bathes and dresses him, maintains that he is more sensitive on the left side of the head than the right." (" Sensitive " here refers to degree of excitability, of what we may call the epileptogenous zone.) " I have often tried to discover a place on his head more sensitive than another, but have failed to do so ; he may be more sensitive on the left side an inch to 2 inches above the ear, but I must not, for fear of misleading you, say that he is ; his aunt thinks so, and she has opportunities of observation.

" The last four days he has stated that sometimes he feels his left arm heavy, as though a weight were pulling it down. This may be fatigue from using it. He has been very sensitive the past four days, and has had some severe falls, one on his forehead, and to-day on his chin, which is cut, bruised, and swelled."

February 6. I saw the patient again. He bore marks of sudden " falls " ; there was a cut near the right angle of the mouth ; in this " fall " his teeth made a mark on the floor. There was a bruise on his forehead ; this was owing to his head coming in contact with the window-sill; this "fall" was consequent on the curtain being blown by the wind against his head. He had had many attacks, and looked dull and apathetic; his father attributed the increased frequency of the attacks to dyspepsia.

The following extract from a letter written by his father (dated March 4) is important: "At the last interview with you, one of the gentlemen present made the remark that when the boy fell he appeared to be violently drawn by a muscular contraction. This, I think, is a true remark, for the boy says that he feels pulled down. I had rather a forcible illustration of this recently. He was sitting on my knee whilst I adjusted the band over his eye; in untying the knot, my finger slipped, the vibration caused him a shock, and his eyebrow struck me on the upper lip. Though the fall was only a few inches—say 3 or 4—the blow was so heavy that my lip was cut, and, at first, I thought my tooth was broken; the blow of his head, by simple gravitation, could not, at the distance of 3 or 4 inches, have struck so heavy a blow. There evidently was a power imparted by muscular contraction. He tells me that he sometimes feels a weight in the left arm. After a shock this morning, he had convulsive movements for a minute in his left arm; the middle finger especially was moved."

I saw the boy again March 10. He had cut his upper lip and bruised his nose; one of his recent falls was consequent on his head being brushed by the window curtain. I saw him once more on April 18. His father said there was a change in the fits. Thus, in one the night before (his brother had put his arm round the patient's neck) he raised his arms above his head, and shrieked and fell; he continued to shriek during less than a minute, and was much exhausted after the fit. The boy could tell nothing about the attack. He had twenty attacks one day; they still never occur unless he be touched. The eyes turn to the right, but sometimes go straight up.

# ON POST-EPILEPTIC STATES

## A Contribution to the Comparative Study of Insanities [1]

### *Section I. Difficulties of the Subject.*

I find that I have not made my opinions as to the nature of post-epileptic states clear to many of my medical brethren. I may plead in extenuation that, as the subject involves consideration of psychology, the anatomy and physiology of the nervous system, and clinical medicine, it is not easily presented in a simple way. It would be an absurdity to attempt to simplify it by ignoring its difficulties, and, before such an audience as this, it would be impertinent to deal with it in a popular way.[2] In the investigation of so large a subject, having the several very different aspects mentioned, we ought to take into very particular account many things which are, I think, commonly little regarded in connection with it, or which are passed over as being irrelevant to it. As I deal with post-epileptic states as they form part of the subject, Comparative Study of Insanities, I must consider the three topics recently mentioned ; and, as one of my aims is to show that the same general principles apply to diseases of all parts of the nervous system, I shall frequently take cases of non-mental diseases for illustration.

### *Section II. Need of Psychological Knowledge.*

It would be vain to attempt the scientific elucidation of mental diseases, some of which are post-epileptic states, if we ignored their psychological aspect. This aspect is practically ignored when psychical states and any nervous states are spoken of as being the same thing, or, as it is sometimes said, " different sides of one thing." The confusion of the anatomy and physiology of the nervous system, or of some parts of that system, with psychology is the bane both of neurology and psychology. It leads to superficial simplifications, and to crude popular " explanations," most of which are merely verbal. No one is any the wiser for the " information " that a man comatose after an epileptic fit does not move because he has lost consciousness, that an emotion makes the heart beat, or that ideas or sensations produce movements. Such expressions are permissible in ordinary talk, and, perhaps, at a clinical conference, but they ought to be turned out of scientific expositions of diseases of the nervous system. We must be particularly careful not to speak of sensations (psychical states) as if they were activities of sensory elements (physical states). An expression I shall frequently use, " sensori-motor," must never be taken to mean " sensa-

[1] *Journal of Mental Science*, October 1888 and January 1889.

[2] This paper is an expansion of an address read before the Medical Psychological Association during the presidency of Dr. Needham. I have not always kept to the style of speaking before an audience. I have divided the matter into Sections. Anyone who has read Herbert Spencer's works will find that I have borrowed largely from them. There is nothing in this article which I can imagine to be of any value which has not been inspired by him. I should, however, be sorry if any crudities of mine were imputed to Mr. Spencer. I strongly urge all neurologists to study his works, and also Fiske's very valuable book, *Cosmic Philosophy*.

tion-motor." Movements always arise from liberations of energy, and never from sensations or any other kind of states of consciousness.

A medical man's aim should be to deal with what are called diseases of the mind (really diseases of the highest cerebral centres) as materialistically as possible. But to be thoroughly materialistic as to the nervous system we must not be materialistic at all as to mind. The popular evolutionist, when he appears in our medical ranks, will very likely try to show how, by stages of increasing evolution, mind is at length " got out " of the body. But no evolutionist as yet, so far as I know, has attempted that marvellous feat.[1] We should be content with " getting " the " organ of mind " (highest centres) out of the rest of the body. States of consciousness are assumed, in this address, to be merely concomitant with certain nervous states, those of the highest cerebral centres. I have nothing whatever to say of the nature of the relation of the two utterly different and yet concomitant things, cerebration and mentation, to one another. As an evolutionist I am not concerned with this question, and for medical purposes I do not care about it. Even if consciousness was known to be a " function of the brain," it would be necessary, in order to simplify our studies of the most difficult of all diseases—insanity—to artificially separate this function for a time from that other " function of the brain," which is to co-ordinate all parts of the body in most complex, etc., ways.

The nervous states concomitant (correlative) with psychical states are, according to the doctrine of evolution, sensori-motor. The highest centres (popularly the " organ of mind," " mental centres," etc.), are, according to this doctrine, only the most complex, etc., and latest developed of a series of centres, every one of which represents impressions or movements, or both. I must remark on the term " impression." It is sometimes used for a kind of mental state, as in the couple " impressions and ideas." I always use it as a name for something purely physical, for a state of sensory nerve " endings " (properly beginnings); for activities of peripheral structures from which afferent nerves pass to the central nervous system. It is not a good term, but I must have some word, which does not imply anything psychical, for what occurs at the sensory periphery. I can think of no better term than " impression," which, when any psychical implications it ordinarily has are eliminated by definition, will serve to go with the term " movement." Nervous centres are called sensori-motor because they represent impressions and movements.

It being quite certain that the lower centres are sensori-motor, it is surely a legitimate hypothesis that the highest are so too. Negative lesions of the lower centres produce paralysis, sensory or motor, or both, and it is a legitimate hypothesis that such lesions of the highest centres do too. If the highest centres are not sensori-motor, the comparative study of insanities, some diseases of those highest centres, with diseases of lower centres, is an impossible study. I will at once deal with this dictum.

Manifestly, it is frivolous to compare, or even to contrast, any mental

[1] Herbert Spencer says : " The doctrine of evolution under its purely scientific form does not involve materialism, though its opponents persistently represent it as doing so." He speaks of the materialistic hypothesis as being " utterly futile." He frequently insists on the absolute difference between states of consciousness and nervous states. Here is a most explicit declaration. After a consideration of increasing complication of mental states and nervous states, he writes (*Psychology*, vol. i, p. 403) : " Of course, I do not mean that material actions thus become mental actions. As was said in Sections 41–51, 62, 63 : ' No effort enables us to assimilate ' mind and motion. I am merely showing a *parallelism* " (italics in original) " between a certain physical evolution and the correlative psychical evolution."

symptoms in cases of disease of the highest centres with any physical symptoms from disease of any lower centres. For example, to compare or even to contrast the negative psychical state, loss of consciousness, with the negative physical lesion producing hemiplegia is absurd. Ignoring such pseudo-comparative studies, I urge that unless the comparison and contrast attempted be between *paralysis* resulting from the negative lesion of the highest centres, *signified by the loss of consciousness*, and the paralysis resulting from the negative lesion in the case of hemiplegia, we do not really enter upon the proper comparative study of the two dissolutions. Paralysis from negative lesions of motor central nervous elements is always loss of *movements*. (See Section V.)

It is one of the chief aims of this address to show that a negative lesion of the highest centres (implied by the negative affection of consciousness which exists in every case of insanity) causes some paralysis, sensory or motor, or both. I have never held the hypothesis that any part of the cerebral cortex is either purely sensory or purely motor, but that some parts are preponderatingly sensory, and others preponderatingly motor. I suppose that in the fore part of the prefrontal lobes sensory representation is a vanishing point, and that motor representation in the occipital lobes is a vanishing point. Hence I consider that from a negative lesion of any part of the cortex there is both sensory and motor paralysis, although the proportions of the two may be enormously different in differently seated lesions.

On the basis that all centres are sensori-motor the comparative study of insanities with diseases of lower centres can be instituted. Thus I shall try to show that in the insanity of post-epileptic coma (acute temporary dementia) there is some universal, I do not say total, paralysis. I wrote (Bowman Lecture, *Transactions Ophth. Society*, vol. vi, p. 12, 1886) : " Deep post-epileptic coma is psychically dementia, but is, on the physical side, nothing else than some universal, almost total, paralysis—paralysis not only of animal, but of organic parts also, proportionate to the degree of the prior epileptic process.[1] This contention of mine is, however, denied ; let us say, what cannot be denied, that the patient is nearly dead. I dare say my calling the psychical side of the condition insanity (dementia) will be objected to. Let us say that the patient is, or is nearly, mentally dead ; this cannot be denied." I here refer those interested in the Comparative Study of Insanities to Dr. Mercier's article " On Coma," *Brain*, January 1887. I gave from that very important article a quotation regarding the psychical and physical nature of Coma, in this Journal, April 1887 (*Remarks on Evolution and Dissolution of the Nervous System*, in a footnote to Section I).

### *Section III. Remarks on the Anatomy, Physiology, and Pathology of Diseases of the Nervous System—the Three Elements of a Clinical Problem.*

That a knowledge of the anatomy and physiology of the nervous system is necessary in such an inquiry as this is plain enough. Yet some remarks may not be out of place here. And first as to the use of terms.

The anatomy of the nervous system must be very carefully distinguished from its morphology. Nervous morphology deals with the sizes, shapes, and topographical relations of nervous masses, of convolutions for example.

[1] Of course we cannot say that such super-positive phenomena as foot clonus, passage of fæces, etc., after epileptic fits, are paralytic ; but they signify exhaustion of " controlling " nervous elements and are indirect evidences of paralysis (or of exhaustion of efferent nerves).

Minute nervous morphology deals with the sizes and shapes of nerve cells and with thicknesses and lengths of nerve fibres. Nervous anatomy deals with centres, that is, with regions of the nervous system *as they represent parts of the body*. Minute nervous anatomy deals with cells and fibres, as they make up nervous arrangements representing impressions or movements, or both. The morphology of parts of the Rolandic area was well known before the researches of Hitzig and Ferrier ; but until their experiments nothing, at least in the opinion of nearly all medical men, was known of the anatomy of these parts. By his discovery of the trunk-centres Horsley has added greatly to our knowledge of the anatomy, in the proper sense of the term, of the cortex cerebri. Moreover, Horlsey and Beevor have done inestimable work in the same direction by their minute and precise investigation of the "motor area."[1] As an evolutionist I pay little respect to morphological divisions ; for example, I ignore the division of the lower part of the central nervous system into the morphological masses, spinal cord, medulla oblongata; and pons Varolii, and speak of a lowest level of evolution, an anatomico-physiological unity, made up of some elements of all these masses.

A great part of our clinical knowledge is nothing else than anatomical and physiological ; pathology is only the third element of a clinical problem. In other words, we have in every case of disease to deal with an abnormality of structure (anatomy), function (physiology), and nutrition (pathology). I have illustrated this dogma at length (*British Medical Journal*, July 21, 1888). To locate a lesion in any centre is an anatomical proceeding. All about nervous discharges (liberations of energy), the amounts and rates of those discharges (the quantity of energy liberated and the rates of its liberation), and the degrees of resistance encountered by nerve impulses in cases of diseases of the nervous system is as much abnormal physiology as consideration of these things in healthy people is normal physiology. Pathology, an abnormality of the nutritive process, ought to be most carefully distinguished from abnormal physiology. (Nutrition is the taking in of materials having potential energy ; physiology is concerned with the liberation of energy thus acquired.) The pathological process (abnormal nutrition) is that which, directly or indirectly, *leads to* abnormal functional (that is, abnormal physiological) states.

There are two diametrically opposite kinds of abnormal functional states of nervous elements, negative and positive. That pathological processes produce negative functional states, negative lesions, I need not stay to illustrate. There are two very different degrees of positive or super-positive functional states which should be very carefully distinguished.

The condition of nerve cells in what I call a " discharging lesion " is an example of the first degree. It is not a pathological condition ; it is a crude physiological state *resulting from* a pathological process, resulting *directly* from it. In the case of epileptiform seizures the " discharging lesion " is most often the result of a tumour or, more correctly, of a secondary abnormal nutritive process, probably a local encephalitis produced by the tumour. In cases of this degree of positive functional change there are occasional sudden and excessive discharges. The second degree of positive functional change is not the *direct* result of any pathological process whatever. There *is* in these cases a pathological process, but it produces a negative functional state of the elements, normally inhibiting (controlling) those other elements in which the second

[1] *Philosophical Transactions*, vol. clxxviii, 1887, B, pp. 153–67, and vol. clxxix, 1888.

degree of positive functional change exists. Thus foot clonus in a recent case of hemiplegia results directly from co-operating agency of certain over-active anterior horns. But no pathological process has touched these lowest motor centres ; that process is morphological miles above them ; it has produced a negative state of fibres of the internal capsule ; the motor centres immediately concerned with the foot clonus are only in physiological over-activity from loss of control. This degree of functional change does not issue in occasional, sudden, and excessive discharges, not, at any rate, without afferent excitation.

It may seem strange to speak of *symptoms* resulting from nervous activities abnormal in degree, which are not of pathological origin, that is, not of direct pathological causation. But a little thought will show that this is so, especially if we consider simple cases. Thus such symptoms as foot clonus after epileptiform seizures, and erection of the penis in cases of transverse lesion of the lower part of the cervical cord,[1] evidently signify hyper-physiological activities from " loss of control " only. No sort of pathological process has touched the nervous elements immediately concerned in the production of these symptoms. Experiments on lower animals, equivalent to the effects of pathological processes in man, are even more strikingly proving. After section of the vagus (equivalent to a pathological process) the heart goes faster ; the heart itself is simply " let go," is only in hyper-physiological activity. " Paralytic secretion " is a more obtrusive example of over-physiological activity merely ; the over-active gland has not been touched, only nerves going to it have been cut.

*Section IV. On the Duplex Condition of Nervous Symptomatologies—Positive and Negative Elements in Symptomatologies.*

To distinguish between symptoms owing to the direct action of disease in the sense of pathological process and those which are its indirect consequences—which are owing directly to activities of quite healthy nervous arrangements, and which are normal, too, except often for hyper-physiological exaltation—is of supreme importance in the study of diseases of the nervous system. I shall again illustrate the distinction regarding insanities in a later section. I now give other kinds of illustrations of it from simpler morbid affections of the nervous system.

It is not an exaggeration to say that more than " half " the symptomatology of a case of paralysis of an external rectus from lesion of the trunk of a sixth nerve is owing to over-activity of nervous arrangements which are beyond all question perfectly healthy. Disease, in the sense of pathological change, is responsible only for the very local paralysis, that of one small muscle. The double vision is impossible without activity of *intact* nervous arrangements of centres for moving both eyes ; the " erroneous projection " (with consequent vertigo and reeling) is owing to over-activity of certain nervous arrangements of all orders of centres, highest included, which are perfectly healthy. In a paper in this Journal (April 1887, Section X, " Disorders of Co-ordination with

[1] This is a complex illustration, but one worth giving as part of the evidence towards showing a series of inhibitions in the central nervous system. The nervi erigentes inhibit the arteries of the penis. But the part of the visceral column (Stilling's sacral nucleus) from which these nerves come is itself inhibited so that the penis is ordinarily flaccid. In cases of complete transverse lesion of the lower cervical cord or upper dorsal cord inhibition is subtracted from Stilling's inhibitory nucleus, whereupon it, being " let go," inhibits the arteries of the penis, they become dilated, and then the organ is turgid.

Negative Lesions") I have illustrated the same principles. " Half " of the symptomatology of " disorders of co-ordination " with negative central lesions is paralysis owing to that negative lesion—is loss of some *movements*. But the other " half " is from forcing of other movements by over-activity of perfectly healthy nervous arrangements.

The getting along, however imperfectly, of patients ataxic in tabes, or of patients who, having disease of the cerebellum, reel from one place to another, is by agency of quite healthy nervous arrangements made to do more than normal owing to lack of others which have been destroyed by pathological changes. Taking the second case, the smallest degree of thought will show that the movements made in the reeling about, the movements by which the patient does in some way go along, cannot possibly result from the pathological change which has *destroyed* some elements of the cerebellum, which has made a hole in that organ. To say that they do, is asserting that they are caused by a void, caused by nothing at all. It is only by entertaining vague notions about " a co-ordinating centre " (the lineal descendant of " faculty of co-ordination ") that we can speak of a destructive lesion of the cerebellum as " causing inco-ordination of locomotion." A negative lesion of this organ causes only that " half " of the symptomatic condition which is paralysis (loss of movements) ; the patient gets along by agency of other movements, the nervous arrangements for which are intact ; he gets along by them badly from lack of those lost. I suppose that in an early stage of tumour of the middle lobe of the cerebellum the paralysis is loss of some of the movements of the spinal muscles ; the erratic gait is owing to over-development (" forcing ") of other movements of the same muscles, and also of some of those of the muscles of the legs. The " forced " movements of the legs serve to some extent to compensate for the movements lost. The essential state of things, the state produced by disease, pathological process, is paralysis. If we cannot say that in the ataxy of tabes there is loss of central *motor* elements effected by pathological changes, it is evident enough that in an early stage of this inco-ordination there is underdoing of some movements, those in which the peroneus longus is chiefly concerned (equivalent to paralysis), and overdoing (forcing) of others, those in which the tibialis anticus is chiefly concerned. I will illustrate the duplex symptomatology of nervous diseases by another series of cases.

I submit, it must be taken quite hypothetically, that the tremor in paralysis agitans, the rigidity, exaggerated knee jerk, and foot clonus in some cases of hemiplegia, the movements in athetosis and those in spasmodic wry-neck are owing to over-activity, or to non-antagonised activity, of nervous elements which are perfectly healthy ; these over-movements are, I believe, very indirect consequences of negative lesions which directly produce paralysis, loss of some movements. The supposition is that there is loss of some movements of muscles from a negative lesion and over-development of other movements *of the very same muscles*. In other words, I do not believe that continuous and persistent liberations of energy (discharges) by nerve cells in these cases are the direct results of pathological processes inducing exaltation of function of those cells. Pathological processes do induce those excessive exaltations of function which I call " discharging lesions " (first degree of functional change), but they issue in occasional, in " explosive," discharges.

The hypothesis is that the principle of duality of symptomatology applies, with a very obvious exception, to all nervous diseases with negative lesions, insanity included; that negative lesion alone is the result of pathological change and produces negative symptoms; the other symptoms, completing the symptomatology, are owing to activity, often over-activity, of healthy nervous arrangements, and are abnormal physiological states.

*Section V. The Three Levels of Evolution of the Central Nervous System. Evolutionary Differences between the Lowest and Highest Levels. Movements v. Muscles. Positive and Negative Movements.*

I urge that to limit attention to the anatomy and physiology of the brain proper in the scientific study of "disease of the mind" is misleading. I submit that there are three levels of evolution (roughly stated in this Journal, April 1887, Section 5) of the central nervous system. The highest centres (popularly "mental centres") of the cerebral system make up the highest level. This level is only a most complex evolution out of the middle level, as the middle is a less complex one out of the lowest, and as the lowest is a least complex one out of parts of the body,[1] which parts that lowest level represents most nearly directly.[2] Speaking very roughly indeed, we may say that from the separate, detailed representation of parts of the body by the lowest centres up to the highest cerebral centres there is a gradual "mixing up" by stages of increasingly complex representation, so that at the acme of representation each unit of the highest centres represents (re-represents) the whole organism in most complex ways, no two units of those centres representing all parts of the body in exactly the same degree and order. In this way the "*organ* of mind," not the *mind*, is "got" out of the rest of the body.

If anyone is interested in the nervous system so far only as its anatomy and physiology correspond to psychology, he should begin his studies of it with the lowest level and the parts of the body this level directly represents. It consists of the centres of the cord, medulla and pons, or, more carefully, of all centres from and to which spinal and cranial nerves come and go. We certainly should begin with this level for the comparative study of what are called diseases of the mind, for they are really some diseases of the highest level, which has inevitable relations with the middle and lowest levels. It is an impossibility to take a realistic view of an ordinary epileptic fit (epilepsy being a disease of the highest cerebral centres) unless we consider the lowest level. The epileptic process begins in some part of the highest level (in some part of the "mental centres") and when the fit is a severe one all the levels are greatly involved; the peripheral effects (convulsion and its equivalents) are directly dependent on discharges (tertiary) of the lowest level. The post-epileptic condition, supposing the fit to have been a severe one, is the sum of the after-effects of discharges of all the levels; this condition is, I urge again, some universal paralysis. Moreover, in post-epileptic mania, the lower levels are engaged in producing the movements, engaged subordinately to all that is left intact of the highest; another reason why we must take them into account in this inquiry. Before I go further, I must remark on movements.

It is necessary to bear in mind that motor nervous centres represent move-

[1] By the expression "parts of the body" is here meant all parts other than the nervous system; they make up the lowest level of the whole organism.

[2] The lowest level is cerebro-cerebellar; it is the lowest level of both the cerebral and the cerebellar systems. I ignore the cerebellar system for the most part in this address, so that by highest centres highest centres of the cerebral system are meant.

ments of muscles, not, so to put it, muscles in their individual character. The simplest movement is not the arithmetical sum of the contractions of all the muscles engaged in effecting it ; it is the algebraical sum of the co-operating and antagonising contractions of those muscles. (The same, *mutatis mutandis*, for sensory centres and impressions.) Paralysis from negative lesions of motor nervous centres is always loss of movements.

There are differences of evolutionary rank of movements of the same muscles. We can illustrate this by losses of movements. In progressive muscular atrophy there is loss of simplest movements of the hands (cerebral and cerebellar) from negative lesion of certain motor centres (anterior horns) of the lowest level ; in paralysis agitans there is loss of more complex (cerebral) movements of the hands from negative lesion of certain motor centres of the middle level ; in general paralysis there is loss of some of the most complex movements of the hands, from negative lesion of motor centres of the highest level, from destruction of motor elements of the sensori-motor bases of tactual ideas. These illustrations may be considered to be hypothetical, but they will serve my present purpose ; they are intentionally artificialised. Referring back to a previous statement on the compound paralysis of the post-epileptic condition, I now say that when the fit has been a severe one there is loss of very many most complex, or many less complex, and of a few simplest movements.

One thing to be insisted on is that from destruction of a part of a motor centre there may be loss of some movements of all the muscles of a muscular region with retention of other movements of all those same muscles. This is the state of things in imperfect paralysis of limbs in hemiplegia, and is an illustration of duplex symptomatology. Referring to the statements, Section IV, as to tremor, rigidity, and athetosis, but taking only the case of rigidity in perfect hemiplegia for illustration and limiting illustration to the hand, we see that there is loss of some movements of muscles of the hand and over-development of other movements of those muscles ; there is, or is in effect, loss of all the complex cerebral movements of it and over-development of all the simple spinal (lowest level) movements of it (possibly the cerebellum is also concerned in this over-development).

When we speak of representation of movements we tacitly take into account motor elements of centres empowering inhibitory nerves ; they effect what may be called negative movements. Similarly, with proper changes, for sensory elements : the depressor nerve may be called a negative sensory, or afferent, nerve. So, then, centres represent positive and negative movements, and positive and negative impressions ; this qualification is always to be understood when the expressions " loss of movements " and " loss of impressions " are used.

Negative lesions of the nervous system, or any part of it, " organ of mind " not excluded, never produce anything else than loss of impressions or of movements, or of both. There *is* something more in the symptomatology of cases, as I have recently (Section IV) illustrated by very different symptomatologies.

Although it involves great recapitulation from the paper (this Journal, April 1887) several times referred to, I must speak here in detail of the evolutionary differences of the lowest and highest levels of the central nervous system. I neglect the middle level in the following remarks, one reason being that, so far as I know, no one agrees with me in dividing the brain proper into middle and highest centres. But I take it for granted that at least two levels of the central nervous system will be admitted by all.

The lowest level, in comparison with the highest level, represents impressions and movements of all parts of the body most nearly directly ; it is a series of centres (properly segments), representing parts of the body in (1) few and simplest combinations (little differentiation), (2) in most general ways (little specialisation), (3) in greatest detail (smallest districts of the body, least integration, " for local affairs ") ; (4) the centres on this level have fewest interconnections (little co-operation). If we take note only of the organic centres on the lowest level I think it is plain that this formula applies closely. The cardiac and respiratory centres obviously are : (1) most simple ; they have few, if any, *different* movements ; there is, indeed, practically a succession of similar movements at equal intervals. (2) These centres have little speciality; obviously they are for most general ends, they serve the body as a whole, in essentially the same way at all times from birth to death. (3) That most [1] of the lowest centres represent limited regions of the body is plain (pupillary, respiratory, cardiac, bladder, etc., centres). (4) The interconnections the organic centres have are certainly few ; obviously pupillary activities, respiration with circulation, digestion, micturition, etc., go on with a great degree of distinctness from one another and with much independence of one another.

The highest level differs from the lowest only in grade of evolution. The centres of this level represent impressions and movements of all parts of the body triply indirectly and in comparision with the lowest level, in : (1) most complex combinations ; in (2) most special ways ; (3) each represents very extensive areas of the body, if not the whole body (greatest integration) ; (4) these centres have the most numerous interconnections. That this formula applies to the highest centres is essentially in accord with current doctrines. It is certain that the " organ of mind " is (1) concerned with most numerous different things ; (2) of high degrees of speciality ; (3) that every psychical process is an act of a person, and, therefore, the inference is irresistible that there are, correlatively, activities of most highly integrated centres, of centres each representing all parts of the body as a whole ; (4) and that by it most elaborate relations of—(1) very complex, (2) special and (3) highly integrated combinations of—impressions and movements in co-existence and sequence are effected.

That the centres or units of the highest level have, during their activities, attendant psychical states, and that the centres of the lowest level have not, if they have not, makes no difference whatever as to what has been said of the evolutionary differences of the two levels ; we have been dealing in this section with things physical, with a sensori-motor mechanism. I cannot too often repudiate the notion that any account of the *organ* of mind is an attempted explanation of *mind*.

[1] It may be said that the vaso-motor centre does not represent a limited region of the body, but the whole arterial system, and therefore that the formula does not apply. It may, however, be that this great centre is a sort of mosaic of minor centres; there seems to be one part of it which especially represents the arterial system of the liver. Moreover, there are minor vaso-motor centres in the spinal cord. In the text I am only considering the lowest level passingly. In another article I shall try to show that in the fore part of the lowest level there is a rudimentary highest centre ; I mean a centre co-ordinating all parts of this lowly evolved level in a simple way. This hypothetical highest centre will be very rudimentary in man. One would suppose that the amphioxus must have such a centre to give some degree of unity to its simple self. Evolution is not, as we state it in the text, an even process, not one to be symbolised by what is called involution in algebra.

*Section VI. On Degrees of Detachment and Degrees of Independence of Levels of Evolution.*

Another way of regarding the evolutionary process is to say that the several levels, in spite of their dependence on one another, attain, as evolution progresses, a degree of independence of one another.

As evolution progresses the highest centres not only gradually develop (become increasingly complex, etc.), but also become more and more detached from, and more independent of, the lower centres out of which they have been evolved. Their detachment and independence are never complete, except hypothetically, in the case of those elements of them which are the physical bases of constants (" forms of thought "). There are degrees of detachment and of independence. By the double process of increasing complexity and increasing detachment we gradually " get above " our lower mere animal selves ; in popular language, we become less and less at the mercy of our lower instincts. Our highest sensory and highest motor centres (together the " organ of mind ") can energise, to a large degree, independently of the lower centres out of which they have been evolved, and by aid of which they have been developed ; consequently they can act independently of the environment. Spencer writes (*Principles of Psychology*, vol. i, p. 546) : " . . . Manifestly, the more extensive and more intricate the central plexus [highest centres] grows, the more *detached* may these [what under their subjective aspects we call feelings and ideas] become from the actions—the more may the impressions produced by things and relations reverberate through the nervous system—the more may there arise trains of thought." Fiske writes (*Destiny of Man*, pp. 46–7) : " . . . There is no consciousness except when molecular disturbance is generated in the cerebrum and cerebellum faster than it can be drafted off to the lower centres. It is the surplus of molecular disturbance remaining in the cerebrum and cerebellum *and reflected back and forth among the cells and fibres of which these highest centres are composed, that affords the physical condition for the manifestation of consciousness.* Memory, emotion, reason, and volition begin with this retention of a surplus of molecular motion in the highest centres." The part I have italicised is very important.

Not committing Mr. Spencer or Mr. Fiske to any crudities of my own, I would thus illustrate. Thanks to the protection of the highest sensory centres by the lower sensory centres (which are " resisting positions," as well as " reservoirs of energy "), the highest sensory centres can energise uninterfered with by the environment. Again, the sister highest motor centres, thanks to the resistance of the lower motor centres, can act without producing peripheral reactions upon the environment ; the muscular periphery is " protected " from the highest motor centres. There can be activities limited to the highest links of the great sensori-motor chain. Here we have the physical conditions answering to faint states of (object) consciousness. When the highest centres are acted on from the sensory periphery, and are thus put in strong activity, they do react on the muscular periphery ; the whole of the sensori-motor chain is then engaged, and there are correlatively vivid states of (object) consciousness.

Thanks to the " protections " spoken of, there occurs internal evolution in our highest centres ; we can have combinations never actually experienced (" ideal combinations "), as, indeed, we obviously must have when dreaming, and certainly have, too, during much of our waking lives. I here give a quotation from my Croonian Lectures (*British Medical Journal*, April 12, 1884): "There is something more: there is what I will call Internal Evolution, a process which goes on most actively in the highest centres. On account of its great preponderance in the highest centres of man, he differs so greatly from lower animals. We acquire numerous different ideas: that is to say, there is, on the physical side, an organisation of many different nervous arrangements of our highest centres during actual converse with the environment. When, as in sleep, and in 'reflection,' this actual converse ceases, the quasi-spontaneous slight activity of the highest sensory centres is uninterfered with by the environment, they being protected from it by the lowest and middle sensory centres; and, consequently, there are no reactions on the environment, the highest motor centres being resisted by the middle and lowest centres. In such case (sleep, reverie, reflection, etc.) the very highest nervous arrangements of the highest centres, those in which entirely new organisations can be made, will be in least activity and the next lower [nervous arrangements] of those centres in greater activity. The nervous arrangements of the highest centres, or some elements of them, are 'left to fight it out among themselves'; new combinations arise, the survival of the fittest [and 'the effecting of the possible']. Manifestly new, although evanescent, combinations are made during dreaming, but I contend that permanent rearrangements (internal evolutions) are made during so-called dreamless sleep (I believe that the late Dr. Symonds, of Bristol, stated this in effect)."

*Section VII. Evolution of the Physical Basis of Consciousness.*

I will state a particular case to illustrate relations of the two levels (still neglecting the middle level) to one another and their degrees of detachment and independence. I will speak arbitrarily of one element of a state of (object) consciousness, artificialising greatly for ease of illustration. I will use the term "emotional centre" (of course, there is no such separate centre), making it mean a part of the highest centres concomitant with the activities of which emotions arise. (One part of the artificialisation is by neglect of the representation of animal parts in this centre; the so-called emotional centre represents all parts of the body, although doubtless the heart and other viscera first and most.)

Certain parts of the body are represented directly by centres on the lowest level in simple and in general ways, in detail, and with comparatively few interconnections, as they serve in doing the menial work of digestion, circulation, respiration, etc. But all these same parts are represented indirectly, in most complex and special ways, in intricate combinations and with many interconnections in the highest centres, being represented again (re-represented) in those centres through the intermediation of the centres of the lowest level, which, as we said, represent them directly as serving in menial work. The indirect and very complex, etc., re-representation of these parts of the body by some of the nervous arrangements of the highest centres is the "emotional centre." The anatomical substratum of an emotion (let it not be forgotten that I am artificialising), the "emotional centre," is not the sum of those centres on the lowest level serving in menial work which I mentioned above; it is part of their evolutionary sum. The "emotional centre" so constituted has become detached from, largely independent of, the very centres of the lowest level out of which it has itself been evolved. For we can have faint emotions (without manifestations) during slight activity of the " emotional centre " whilst the lowest centres out of which that so-called centre has been evolved are at the same time steadily engaged in mere menial work. But during vivid emotions the " emotional centre " is in strong activity, and there are then manifestations. Now the centres on the lowest level are, subordinately, engaged, too ; and, so far as they are engaged in this way, their service in menial work is much interfered with ; it is suspended when sudden fright causes fainting, and is put an end to when it kills.

In a paper in this Journal, April 1887 (last paragraph but one), I gave an outline of the evolution of the anatomical substrata of the four artificially separated elements of states of (object) consciousness ; that is, of the evolution of the physical bases (together, the highest centres) of will, memory, reason, and emotion (together states of consciousness) out of the lowest centres, which centres represent limbs, viscera, etc., directly, in simple ways, and, so to say, for commonplace duties and as serving in menial work. I did this in more detail in the Croonian Lectures, *British Medical Journal*, April 12, 1884.[1]

The foregoing remarks on the evolution of the physical basis of consciousness bear very closely indeed on our subject. For the epileptic fit is nothing whatever else than the result of a sudden, excessive, and rapid discharge beginning in the sensori-motor nervous arrangements which are the physical bases of will, memory, reason, and emotion (together states of consciousness). There is after it paralysis owing to negative functional state (exhaustion) of these nervous arrangements, and also, in the less degree, of those of the lower centres out of which the physical bases of the four elements of states of consciousness have been evolved.

### *Section VIII. Need of Wide Clinical Knowledge.*

If anyone thinks that the study of diseases of the nervous system as they are dissolutions will take his attention from their clinical or practical consideration he is mistaken. I urge two methods of study, one scientific and one clinical. Without a considerable clinical knowledge of cases no one is fitted to begin the scientific, comparative, study of nervous diseases. For the scientific study of insanities a very wide clinical knowledge is necessary. It would never do to confine attention to cases described in textbooks by alienist physicians, to what I may call " orthodox " cases of insanity. Not being an alienist physician I say this, and what follows in the present section, under correction by the Members of this Society, who of necessity know very much more of " diseases of the mind " than I do. I should not presume to address alienist physicians on their special subject had I not the hope that from a long study of simpler diseases of the nervous system, I might contribute something of at least indirect value for the elucidation of the most complex problems they have to deal with. In a later section I shall urge a study of cases of abnormal mental affections, many of which are not, in a clinical regard, cases of insanity at all, and, so far as I know, are not dwelt upon in books on insanity.

Further, we must, in such an inquiry as this, study diseases of the nervous

[1] There is an unfortunate misprint in the latter account. For " volition of the movement " (an expression mixing up the psychical and the physical) read " volition of the moment."

system which are in no reasonable sense cases of insanity regarded from any standpoint. It is a legitimate hypothesis that the same fundamental principles apply to all nervous diseases whatsoever, from such as paralysis of an external rectus up to insanity. I have illustrated this (Section IV). The alienist physician, above all other physicians, should have a large general knowledge of the simpler nervous diseases before he tries to explain the most difficult of all diseases whatsoever. On the principle of studying simple things as a basis for the elucidation of the more complex we should deal with foot clonus after an epileptic fit as well as with elaborate and universal movements, as in epileptic mania, after one; both symptoms exemplify the same principle, "loss of control." Before anyone studies epileptic paroxysms, surely he ought to study epileptiform paroxysms, which are vastly simpler. If we do not know well what is found after these comparatively simple seizures we ought to be diffident in concluding as to the nature of post-epileptic states. Finding unmistakable paralysis after the simple fits, we are justified in stating the hypothesis that there is paralysis after epileptic fits; we can then seek evidence of very different kinds towards proving and disproving the existence of that paralysis. Towards this end we should study cases of aphasia; especially should we study temporary aphasia after certain epileptiform seizures; all the more because this aphasia is often associated with paralysis of the face or arm, or both. That the physical condition correlative with loss of words is loss of nervous arrangements, representing complex, etc., movements of the tongue, palate, lips, etc., is, I think, as certain as that the paralysis of the arm and leg that so often goes with the aphasia is loss of movements of those limbs.

In the preceding remarks is the excuse, if any be needed, for going so much further afield than is the custom when dealing with one subject. But the "one" subject, post-epileptic states, refuses methodical consideration apart from other nervous diseases. Every nervous disease, being a flaw in one great evolutionary system, demands consideration as wide as we can make it with precision.

That certain general principles, implicitly stated in the formula of evolution, apply to all diseases of the nervous system is an hypothesis verified only in some cases. It is quite certain that both hemiplegia and aphasia display reduction from the complex, special, etc., towards the simple, general, etc., and that the principle exemplified in these two cases applies to some simple cases of insanity is equally certain. It is quite fair to apply the hypothesis in all cases of nervous disease; this remark will sound strangely, of course, to those who erroneously suppose that an hypothesis, a supposition, is a conclusion, which it is not.

Since, according to the doctrine of evolution, the highest centres (Section V) represent all parts of the body, a case of insanity, being a disease of these centres, is physically the evolutionary sum of something out of disease of every part of the body; speaking very crudely, it is the representative of diseases of all parts of the body. Hence we should study the simple diseases of the spinal cord, medulla oblongata, and pons Varolii (which are, so to say, "detailed nervous diseases," being of small regions of the body), as a preparation for the study of insanities, exceedingly complex diseases of the highest centres (which are diseases of centres representing all parts of the body in wholes). Moreover, just as in the study of insanity we do not limit attention to cases described in textbooks on that disease, so we should not limit attention to cases of disease of the cord, medulla, and pons described in ordinary neurological textbooks.

*Section IX. Limitation of the Inquiry into Mental Disorders of Epileptics.*

It is frequently said that temporary elaborate abnormal actions sometimes occur periodically in epileptics, whilst they are " unconscious," unpreceded by an epileptic fit of even a slight degree. Dr. Clouston, in his very valuable work, *Mental Diseases*, says that mental symptoms essentially periodic and paroxysmal most often occur after the fits. But he mentions five other ways in which " epileptic insanity " occurs in relation with them. Dr. Savage, in a most important article, entitled " Some of the Relationships between Epilepsy and Insanity," *Brain*, January 1887, when speaking of what is called masked epilepsy, expresses the opinion that in most of these cases a fit of some sort, great or small, does occur before the strange acts. Again, to give a quotation from that article : " I have met with but few cases of true masked epilepsy, and in none have I been convinced that no fit had occurred." In his work *Insanity and Allied Neuroses*, p. 384, Dr. Savage writes : " It is common to meet with cases in which, immediately before or after the fit, an outburst of uncontrollable fury of the most destructive kind takes place." But he speaks, too, of such outbursts as most commonly occurring after the fits, and on sudden return to consciousness.

I believe I may assume that the majority of alienist physicians admit that *suddenly* occurring *temporary* abnormal elaborate actions during unconsciousness in epileptics (and it is with such cases only that I deal) are in most instances preceded by a fit, although not, as my hypothesis is, in all instances. I do not undertake to show the converse—that there are actions after every epileptic fit. In the process of slow re-evolution, during return to complete consciousness after slight fits, there are really often actions which are little heeded as post-epileptic states ; the patient may take out his watch, look at his papers, ask what day it is, what o'clock it is, etc. (re-orientation).

I may here express my surprise that I have not succeeded in making evident that my belief is that elaborate actions during unconsciousness in epileptics occur *after* paroxysms. The title of an article I published, *Medical Times and Gazette*, July 19, 1873, is " Remarks on the Double Condition of Loss of Consciousness and Mental Automatism *following* certain Epileptic Seizures." I now give a quotation from that article : " . . . Dr. Hughlings Jackson does not believe, as he used to do (see this Journal [*Medical Times and Gazette*], December 14, 1867, p. 642), that the Mental Automatism of Epileptics—epileptic mania, for example—is the result of the discharge [epileptic] of any part of the brain, that is to say, *not the direct result*. The duplex condition is found, he considers, when the discharge is *over*. The mental automatism is one of the indirect results of the [epileptic] discharge. It is true that in some cases of sudden mania [in epileptics] a prior seizure is not witnessed. Hence, some say that mania occasionally ' replaces ' a fit. (This is the very opposite of the view now being stated.)" (Italics in original. The words in square brackets alone are new.) The title of another paper (" On Temporary Mental Disorders *after* Epileptic Paroxysms," *West Riding Asylum Reports*, vol. v, 1875, see p. 119) shows that I have continued to hold the doctrine that suddenly occuring elaborate abnormal states in epileptics occur *after* their fits. I argued to the same effect (Croonian Lectures, *British Medical Journal*, April 5, 1884).

*Section X. Degrees of Post-Epileptic States.*

There are three degrees. (1) What may roughly be called " Confusion of thought " ; there is here a mental condition of two opposite elements, (*a*) slight defect of consciousness, and (*b*) persistence of the rest of consciousness.[1] (2) (*a*) So-called " loss " of consciousness with (*b*) actions. (3) (*a*) Coma with (*b*) persistence, seemingly, of " vital " operations only.

That the three degrees do occur after epileptic fits of different severities is certain ; therefore, each of them ought to be considered in this inquiry. Yet I think the custom is to deal only with the second degree, as if the first and third required no explanation as post-epileptic states. But surely coma after an epileptic fit ought to be considered in the same inquiry as that in which unconsciousness with mania after such a fit is considered. Is it not unmethodical to cut off the first and third degrees and to deal only with the second degree of one series of states found after epileptic paroxysms ?

*Section XI. Three Depths of Dissolution : Shallows of Evolution Corresponding.*

It is convenient here, although somewhat out of order, to remark in mere outline on the physical conditions of the three degrees as they are three different depths of dissolution of the highest centres with correspondingly three different shallows of evolution remaining.[2] I shall, for convenience' sake, speak of the highest centres as if they were made up of " layers," which of course they are not: I say particularly that I am not thinking of layers of cells of the cerebral cortex ; I am speaking quite artificially, and, so to say, diagrammatically. I shall assume that there are four layers.[3]

(1) In the first degree there is loss of function (effected by the prior epileptic discharge) of the first, highest layer (first depth of dissolution). To this answers the negative affection of consciousness. The lower level of evolution (we should say sublevel ) is the second layer during activities of which the consciousness remaining arises.

(2) In the second degree, the first and second layers are functionless (second depth of dissolution). To this answers the " loss " of consciousness. The level of evolution, being the third layer, is shallower, and during its activities (or, as some would say, from them) the actions[4] arise.

(3) In the third degree the dissolution is still deeper. It is of the first, second, and third layers, and, correspondingly, there is still greater negative affection of consciousness, coma. The lower level of evolution is the fourth layer, and possibly no consciousness attends its activities. Of course, it may

[1] In former papers (see this Journal, April 1887, Section XVIII), I have spoken of what is known as the Intellectual Aura (I call it " dreamy state ") as being the positive element in some cases of the first degree of post-epileptic states. In this paper a more inclusive expression is used. I now feel uncertain as to the exact symptomatological nature of the " dreamy state."

[2] I never use the expressions " evolution " and " dissolution of the mind." It would be convenient perhaps to use them sometimes if one could be sure that they would be taken to imply mere parallelism with evolution and dissolution of the highest cerebral centres of the nervous system.

[3] I speak at present of dissolution after epileptic fits as being uniform, as if, that is, all the divisions of the highest centres were evenly lowered in function. Yet, I believe that the dissolution in these cases preponderates in one lateral half of the brain ; that there is local dissolution of the highest centres. I shall rectify the statement made in the text later on.

[4] I use the term " action " in a psychical sense ; actions are psychical states corresponding to certain movements of the limbs, etc., in the same way as in the psychical states words (also actions) correspond to certain complex, etc., movements of the tongue, palate, lips, etc.

be held that in this degree all four layers of the highest centres are quite out of function, a view I do not take.

In all cases, whether in health or in disease, the activities of the highest layer are determined from below. The lower level of evolution in the second degree, although we spoke of it as being the third layer, is the whole of the nervous system except the highest two layers of the highest centres. If there be any psychical states in this degree they attend activities of the third layer, which is the highest there is then.

It is not held that in any of the three degrees the dissolution is confined to the highest centres, although the illustration by the artifice of layers literally taken declares that it is. But the illustrations are purely artificial. And even supposing that the highest centres were in layers the dissolution would not really be abruptly limited to this or those layers, as I have, for convenience, stated it to be. Unquestionably, plainly after severe fits, the lowest of all centres undergo some dissolution. Loss of the knee jerks after some epileptic fits (Westphal, Gowers, Beevor) shows that some spinal centres have lost function. The dissolution in deep post-epileptic coma is highly compound ; it may be rudely symbolised (using the initial letters of highest, middle, and lowest centres with indices, but with no pretence of exact quantification) as $h^3 + m^2 + 1$. This is only a way of saying over again that there is (Section V) loss of some of three orders of movements, most complex, less complex, and most simple. We are at present neglecting the important fact that post-epileptic dissolution is in this way compound.[1]

*Section XII. The Comparative Study of Insanities.*

The Comparative Study of Insanities is by regarding all " mental diseases," of which post-epileptic states are some, as dissolutions beginning in the highest (cerebral) centres of a great sensori-motor mechanism. Such a study is of three kinds.

(1) We may consider different kinds of insanity in comparison and contrast with one another ; that is, as they are physically owing to dissolutions beginning, or preponderating, in different divisions of the highest centres (local dissolutions of these centres). For example, we might compare and contrast cases of melancholia with cases of general paralysis ; hypothetically in the former there is dissolution beginning in the posterior, in the latter beginning in the anterior lobes of the cerebrum.

(2) We may compare and contrast different degrees of the same kind of

[1] There is nothing more important regarding evolution and dissolution than that they are processes, respectively, of increase and decrease in compound order. I have long been possessed by this notion. I gave an example of it (*Medical Times and Gazette,* December 19, 1868) when stating details of the sequence of spasm in a case of epileptiform fits. It may be that in the sensory sphere compound order is analogous to Weber's law. But speaking of the sensory sphere I would put it as follows, without any attempt at exact quantification : A certain degree of stimulus at the sensory periphery produces no effect (I mean that no sensation ultimately arises), as the stimulus does not overcome the resistance of elements of any lowest sensory centre. A stimulus somewhat stronger produces a very great effect ; for being, the supposition is, just sufficiently stronger to overcome the resistance of elements of some lowest sensory centre, there is liberation of a large quantity of energy of those elements, and ultimately a great effect is produced on the highest sensory centres. An increase of the strength of a nervous discharge produces a compound effect. This applies to normal and abnormal discharges of sensory and of motor elements. The principle is exceedingly important with regard to differences in the physical processes during faint and vivid states of object consciousness, ideation, and perception for example.

insanity ; that is, as each is a different depth of dissolution of the same division of the highest centres, the three degrees of the post-epileptic condition for example.

(3) We may consider insanities (as they are diseases of the highest centres) in comparison and contrast with diseases of lower centres, with aphasia and hemiplegia for example.

The comparisons and contrasts we mean are (1) of the *physical* conditions of different insanities with one another ; (2) of degrees of the *physical* conditions in the same kind of insanity, and (3) of the *physical* conditions in insanities with those which are lesions of lower centres. I do not mean, of course, that we may not profitably compare and contrast mental symptoms of one kind of insanity with those of another kind ; for example, the mental symptoms of melancholia with those of general paralysis. With such comparisons and contrasts I do not here occupy myself. I deal with mental symptoms as signs only of what is not going on or of what is going on wrongly in the nervous system.

*Section XIII. On the Significance of Positive Mental Symptoms.*

We must be careful not to compare and contrast the wrong things, as we may easily err in doing if we confound the physical with the psychical. Further, we shall get wrong if we think of " mental symptoms " without analysing them into negative and positive (often super-positive). Whilst it is absurd to compare and contrast negative mental symptoms with negative physical symptoms, it is, if possible, more absurd still to compare and contrast a *mélange* of negative and positive mental symptoms with any physical symptoms. Dissolution alone is owing to disease in the sense of pathological process. It is a negative functional state caused by a pathological process ; the negative symptoms of a patient's insanity alone answer to it. Positive mental symptoms in all cases of insanity answer to activities of healthy nervous arrangements on the level of evolution remaining. These two statements on the symptomatology of insanities are so important in the comparative study of these diseases that I will illustrate them at length, although in doing so I shall have to repeat particularly still more of what was said generally in Section IV.

Repeating statements of the preceding paragraph otherwise, the assertion is that the physical condition for positive mental symptoms [1] is never caused by *pathological* processes ; on the contrary, these symptoms occur during activities of parts which are healthy and which are normal too, except often for *physiological* over-activity ; they attend activities of all which is left intact in a nervous system maimed by dissolution, activities of that which dissolution has spared. We ought to avoid such expressions as that disease " causes mental symptoms," or that it " disorders the functions of the brain." These expressions hide the fact that we have to deal with a symptomatology made up of two diametrical opposites.

What to medical men are positive mental *symptoms* are, or are parts of, mentation which is perfectly normal in the patient, as certainly normal in him as the mentation of the sane is normal in them. The mentation of the sane attends activities of the proper highest layer of evolution, the mentation of the insane of *their* highest layer. Thus in the first degree of post-epileptic states the patient's *then* highest layer is the second layer of his normal highest centres

[1] I exclude " crude sensations " such as occur at the onset of epileptic fits.

and his mentation is correlative with activities of that layer. What we call the insane man's extravagant conduct displays his will; what we call his illusions are his perceptions (memory); what we call his delusions are his beliefs (his reasoning); and what we call his caprice is evidence of his emotional change.

The insane man is a different person from his sane self, and we should take him up for investigation as that new person. For although we speak, as is the custom, of defect of consciousness as if it were a something, it is a nothing; it is so much consciousness eliminated, got rid of. The correlative functionlessness of nervous arrangements, dissolution, is a physical nothing; it is so much of the highest centres eliminated, temporarily or permanently, as the case may be. The insane man, the new person, has, in this way, a lower consciousness and a shallower nervous system than the former person, his sane self. But this shallowed nervous system, with the parts of the body it represents, is all there then is of him physically, and thus no wonder that correlatively *he* (all the " he " there is) believes in what *we* call his delusions. Indeed, if, as I assert, the delusions are the patient's beliefs, it is tautological to say he " believes in his delusions," that being equivalent to saying " he believes in his beliefs."

As just said, the insane man is a different person from his former sane self. In a case of post-epileptic unconsciousness with mania, the second person, as we shall call him, differs from the first, the normal, person by a minus and by a plus. Physically there is less of him by lack of the highest two layers of his highest centres, and there is too much of what is left of him in the sense that there is greatly increased activity of the layer reduced down to.

By taking a simpler case, I can show how we are misled if we do not distinguish the two persons when we use the same pronoun for each of them. I take the normal dissolution of sleep, the first depth of it. No one denies that the " positive mental symptoms " in this case of " normal insanity " are correlative with activities of perfectly healthy nervous arrangements.[1] " I am awake now, but in my sleep *I* was dreaming. I wonder that in my dream *I* could have believed that the Emperor of China was a steam engine." The I's and the *I*'s, the same for the grammarian, symbolise two different persons for the student of mental diseases. *I*, we may call him B, is I, we may call him A, *minus* the use of the higher nervous arrangements of the highest centres (dissolution), and *plus* increased activity of the next lower evolution remaining. The dreamer does not wonder because his mentation is correlative with all there then is of him. For A to wonder that B did not wonder implies a confused notion that he (A) was present with, and was being tricked by, the temporarily existing B. But when B existed there was no such person as A. It is rather the other way. B is present with A on re-evolution; or, to speak more carefully, B's dream, his mentation, remains quasi-parasitical in A for a short time, as much as and so long as A remembers it, or, more simply, *has it* after awaking, after ceasing to be B.

Whilst popularly it is permissible to say that the sane man " lives in the real world," and that the insane man, say the dreamer, " lives in a world of his own," the statements are, when regarded scientifically, very misleading. Everybody, sane or insane, " lives in a world of his own "; everybody's real world, what seems real to him, is made up of " projections " of his own images. The only

[1] The images in dreams and in insanity are as certainly objective as the images of the sane man's ordinary, waking, perception are.

thing outside which we can suppose to be " common to all " is that which makes each have images peculiar to himself. I will now illustrate this.

A cabman is standing dressed by his bed in one of my wards. On my coming up to him he asks me to get into his cab, and to tell him where he shall drive me. I ask, " Where is your cab ? " With a sneer and a manner which amounts to saying, " What a fool you must be," he exclaims, pointing to his bed, " Why, there ! " This patient saw a cab, had that image strongly " projected," his objective state, at a time when I saw a bed, when I had that image strongly projected, my objective state. It is of no avail for trustworthy witnesses to assert that the patient *could not have seen* a cab, because there was no cab present, and, therefore, that the patient " only fancied," etc., that he saw one. Something, not himself, " got out of " himself the image cab, " out of " the bystanders the image bed.[1] It might be said that this doctrine confuses reality and unreality. But what reality and whose reality ? The image cab was the patient's reality ; the image bed was the healthy bystanders' reality.

[1] I do not say " image *of* a cab " and " image *of* a bed." I am not endorsing a crude popular psychological hypothesis that " real " outer objects, in themselves coloured, shaped, etc., photograph their colour, shape, etc., on us. What I call the image is a state of the mind (each person's), a " ghost," standing as a symbol of something not us, of the nature of which something we know nothing.

*Editorial Note.*—This was marked, " To be continued." No continuation has been found in subsequent numbers of the Journal.

# ON A PARTICULAR VARIETY OF EPILEPSY ("INTELLECTUAL AURA"), ONE CASE WITH SYMPTOMS OF ORGANIC BRAIN DISEASE [1]

I HAVE notes of about fifty cases of the variety of epilepsy I am about to speak of. I have seen very many patients with symptoms of local gross organic brain disease (optic neuritis, etc.); in many of the latter, as subsequent necropsies showed, there was intracranial tumour. But one of the cases (Case 1, p. 392) I am about to relate and remark on (I have referred to it briefly, Bowman Lecture, "On Ophthalmology and Diseases of the Nervous System," *Transactions Ophth. Society*, vol. vi) is the only one I have seen in my own practice in which this variety of epilepsy was found associated with marked symptoms of local gross organic brain disease.[2] Although necropsy was forbidden, the case is of great clinical importance. The variety of epilepsy alluded to is one in which (1) the so-called "intellectual aura" (I call it "dreamy state") is a striking symptom. This is a very elaborate or "voluminous" mental state. One kind of it is "reminiscence"; a feeling many people have had when apparently in good health (see p. 388 the case of Quærens and that of Dr. Ferrier's patient, Case 3, p. 398). Along with this voluminous mental state, there is frequently a "crude sensation" ("warning") of (*a*) smell or (*b*) taste; (or, when there is no taste, there may be movements, chewing, tasting, spitting, *implying* (?) an epileptic discharge beginning in some part of the gustatory centres), or (*c*), the "epigastric" or some other "systemic" sensation. The wording of this statement implies, at any rate it is meant to imply, that the "dreamy state" sometimes occurs without any of the crude sensations mentioned, or movements supposed to imply discharges of gustatory elements, and that sometimes those crude sensations and movements occur without the "dreamy state"; this will be exemplified in cases shortly to be given for incidental illustration.

I have been struck by certain non-associations. In my experience vertigo in the sense of external objects seeming to move to one side, rarely occurs with the "dreamy state." In this paper I have to state exceptions (see Case 2) to this. The other variety of vertigo, that is, the feeling of the patient himself turning, does not so rarely occur with the "dreamy state." Again, I have no account of crude sensations of sight (colour projections) associated with the "dreamy state," but I have notes of one case in which the patient, *at other times*, had migrainous paroxysms with visual projections. In cases of epilepsy beginning by colour projections, the much less elaborate mental state "seeing faces" is not uncommon. I have thought that crude sensations of hearing are not associated with the "dreamy state." Until recently I have known

[1] *Brain*, vol. xi, 1888, p. 179.

[2] Since this was written I have had a necropsy of a woman who had had paroxysms with the "dreamy state," and crude sensation "warnings" of smell. She had left hemiplegia and double optic neuritis. I can now only say that there was a tumour in the right temporo-sphenoidal lobe. My colleague, Dr. Beevor, who sent the patient to me, has kindly undertaken the examination of the specimen; on receiving his report I shall publish the case. (See p. 406.)

of no exception, but I shall have to relate one in a case, the notes of which are supplied to me by Dr. James Anderson. Auditory sensation warnings are not rarely followed by " hearing voices " (really words as if spoken to the patient), a less elaborate state than the " dreamy state." I now return to the variety epilepsy with the " dreamy state."

There is not always *loss*, but there is, I believe, always, at least *defect*, of consciousness co-existing with the over-consciousness (" dreamy state "). *After* some paroxysms in which consciousness has been lost there are exceedingly complex and very purposive-seeming actions during continuing unconsciousness ; in a few cases the actions appear to be in accord with the " dreamy state."

It will have been seen that I do not consider the " dreamy state " to be a " warning " (" aura "), that is to say, not a phenomenon of the same order as the crude sensations of smell, etc. Hence my objection to the term " intellectual aura," and adoption of the less question-begging adjective " dreamy," one which is sometimes used by the patients. It is very important in this inquiry to distinguish mental states according to their degree of elaborateness—from crude, such as the crude sensation warnings of smell, etc., to the vastly more elaborate, such as the " dreamy state "—in order that we may infer the physical condition proper to each. The crude sensations are properly called warnings ; they occur during *epileptic* (sudden, excessive and rapid) discharges ; the elaborate state I call " dreamy state " arises during but slightly raised activities (slightly increased discharges) of healthy nervous arrangements.

I have previously considered this variety of epilepsy, *Medical Times and Gazette*, December 2, 1876, and February 1 and March 1, 1879 ; *Brain*, July 1880. These papers have attracted very little attention ; they have, however, been referred to by Dr. Mercier ; by Dr. Beevor, in his important article " On the Relation of the ' Aura ' Giddiness to Epileptic Seizures," *Brain*, January 1884, p. 488 ; and by Dr. James Anderson (*vide infra*, p. 386). The following quotation is from a lecture I published, *Medical Times and Gazette*, March 1, 1879, p. 224 : " I think it will be found that in many, I dare not say in most, cases the voluminous mental [' dreamy '] state occurs in patients who have at the onset of their seizures some ' digestive ' sensation—smell, epigastric sensation, taste, or, in cases where there are movements implying excitations of centres for some such sensations, such movements as those of mastication."

Under the name " intellectual aura," the " dreamy state " has long been known to occur in epileptics. The case of Quærens (*vide infra*, p. 388) is, so far as I know, the first definite case of epilepsy with that phenomenon published in this country. Dr. Joseph Coats, *British Medical Journal*, November 18, 1876, has recorded a very important case of an epileptic whose fits, with few exceptions, were preceded by giddiness and a " peculiar thought." " Sometimes the fit only consists of the aura [the thought], followed by a peculiar feeling in the abdomen which passes up to the head and back to the abdomen, when vomiting results."

Dr. James Anderson has recorded a case of this variety [1] of epilepsy in which, from symptoms, ocular and cerebral, detailed in his report, he correctly predicated tumour, and its position. This case has several important bearings, but for my present purpose it will suffice to say that the patient's " dreamy

[1] " On Sensory Epilepsy. Case of Basal Cerebral Tumour, affecting the left Temporo-Sphenoidal Lobe, and giving rise to a Paroxysmal Taste-sensation and Dreamy State," *Brain*, October 1886.

state " was associated with a rough " bitter sensation " in his mouth. It is the only case published which I know of in which a necropsy has been had revealing any local morbid changes in a case of the variety of epilepsy mentioned. Dr. Anderson refers to a case, closely like that of his own patient, recorded by Mr. Nettleship, *Transactions Ophth. Society*, vol. iv (necropsy by Dr. Sharkey). In the report of that case, however, the " dreamy state " is not mentioned ; there was a crude sensation warning in the patient's fits, " a sudden feeling of suffocation in the nose and mouth." I think it not impossible that the " dreamy state " was present in the slight seizures (the patient did not always lose consciousness). I doubt not that I have in former years disregarded this important symptom. I have suggested (" Bowman Lecture," op. cit.) that ophthalmic surgeons who see very many cases of optic neuritis (that is, cases in most of which there is local gross organic intracranial disease, such as tumour) should minutely investigate any paroxysms, however slight and transient, their patients may have, especially when there is any kind of defect of smell or taste. Just as the most exact knowledge we have of the seats of " discharging lesions " in different epilepti-*form* seizures is from cases of gross local organic brain disease, so no doubt our most exact knowledge of the seats of " discharging lesions " in epilep*tic* seizures will be obtained from cases of such kind of disease. Some preliminary remarks on *slight* epileptic fits are necessary. I mean fits commonly called attacks of epilepsy proper.[1]

The slighter paroxysms are, the more deserving are they of minute and precise investigation, both for the patient's sake and for scientific purposes ; for the patient's sake since, unless we give most careful attention to the details of them, we shall sometimes altogether overlook epilepsy ; for scientific purposes, because the analysis of slight seizures is more easy and fruitful than that of severe ones. It often happens that a patient has sometimes severe seizures of the variety of epilepsy under remark, and at other times severe seizures ; and not rarely he has no " warning," in any sense of the term, of the latter. Obviously the clue to the seat of the " discharging lesion " is only given definitely by the " warning " (such as the crude sensations mentioned) ; so that of the patient's slight seizures we may learn much, of the severe ones without warning very little that is definite.

I urge strongly that the great thing as to the diagnosis of epilepsy is not the " quantity " of the symptoms, nor the severity of the fits, but paroxysmalness. Again, *loss* of consciousness is not essential for the diagnosis of epilepsy ; there may be *defect* of consciousness only ; and, as we have been saying, there may be " over-consciousness " (" dreamy state ") co-existing with the defect of con-

[1] Using the colourless word " fits " generically, I make three classes of fits (see *Brain*, April 1886) : (1) ponto-bulbar ; (2) epileptiform ; (3) epileptic (epilepsy proper of nosologists). As the name implies, (1) depends on discharges beginning in bulbar and pontal centres (laryngismus stridulus, certain uræmic fits (?) and asthma (?) and I imagine some fits *called* epileptic). I have published (*British Medical Journal*, November 20, 1886) the case of a boy who had fits started by touching his head, a case analogous to fits artificially produced in guinea-pigs (Brown-Séquard), and due, I presume, to abnormal changes in the ponto-bulbar region. (See p. 362.) Class (2) is of fits depending on discharge beginning in some part of convolutions of the so-called " motor region." I imagine that (3) is owing to discharge beginning in some part of convolutions of the cerebrum other than those of the " motor region." Both (2) and (3) are to my mind " cortical," although that term is commonly given to (2) only. I think it most likely that migrainous paroxysms are " fits " which are the (chiefly) sensory analogues of (2) epileptiform seizures. I feel confident that (3), epilepsy proper, will have to be subdivided very considerably, and possibly some seizures we call epileptic will have to be classified apart. I hope the above classification will be useful provisionally.

sciousness ; with defect of consciousness as to present surroundings there may be a rise of consciousness as to some other and often quasi-former surroundings (" dreamy state ") ; the latter may attract exclusive attention, the co-existing defect of consciousness being ignored. The most seemingly trifling symptoms, when occurring paroxysmally, deserve careful analysis in proportion to their paroxysmalness ; suddenly " coming over queer " for a moment or two may be a slight epileptic attack and the forerunner of severe attacks. Of course it is a very old story that veritable epileptic fits may be very slight indeed, and, often enough, so slight and transitory that bystanders do not notice them ; but there are particular reasons for insisting on this point with regard to cases of the variety of epilepsy the subject of this paper. I particularly wish to remark that, in many of them, the slight seizures are so very slight, that the patient unfortunately disregards or underrates them until a severe fit comes and declares their evil significance. As bearing closely on this neglect, I here say that such slight seizures are not always disagreeable, but sometimes positively agreeable. I have heard patients say that they used to " encourage " the feeling, before they knew what it meant. The day I write this, a patient told me that he used to try to bring the feelings on when he first had the attacks ; they are now disagreeable. The symptoms often seem to be so fanciful to the patients that they may reckon them for a time as mere oddities. Even when they have found out the bad meaning of their slight attacks, they are often seemingly unwilling to give any details of the " dreamy state." Dr. James Anderson's patient " showed some reluctance to talk about the scene." They and their friends do not seem to care for questions as to movements of chewing, smacking the lips, etc., thinking, probably, that such little things have no real bearing on a serious condition. I would go further and say, that some medical men seem to think questionings on the " dreamy state," inquiries about spitting, champing movements, etc., are unpractical. I now stay to illustrate some of the preceding remarks.

One of my patients (*vide infra*, Case 5), a medical man, had seizures of this variety of epilepsy in so slight degree at first, that he took no more notice of them than to make them a subject of joking (to use the words from the report he made of his own case, he " regarded the matter playfully, as of no practical importance "). He now has severe as well as slight fits. I refer also to the case of a medical man who reported it himself under the pseudonym Quærens (*Practitioner*, May 1874, p. 284). The title is, " A Prognostic and Therapeutical Indication in Epilepsy." When he consulted me, February 1880, he had had eighteen severe fits (loss of consciousness, convulsion, tongue-biting), and had had " many hundreds " of slight attacks. The *slight* attacks which he still had when I first saw him were so slight that strangers noticed nothing wrong with him ; he is never quite unconscious in them ; the severest of these slight fits only " bemaze " him for a minute or two ; he can go on talking. Here are epileptic attacks with defect (" bemazement "), but not with loss of consciousness. A medical friend who sees much of Quærens observes a little flushing of the patient's face, that he is " as if considering something," but only to his intimate friends is it known that he has any kind of seizure. The only local symptom I heard of is a peculiar feeling in the right hand. In each slight fit he has that variety of the " dreamy state " which I call Reminiscence ; this peculiar feeling occasionally occurs in many people who are supposed to be healthy. Quærens quotes Tennyson, Coleridge, and Dickens about it. I reproduce the quotation from Dickens, and after it the whole of the patient's report of his own case (op. cit.):

" We have all some experience of a feeling which comes over us occasionally, of what we are saying and doing having been said or done before, in a remote time—of our having been surrounded, dim ages ago, by the same faces, objects, and circumstances—of our knowing perfectly what will be said next, as if we suddenly remembered it."—*David Copperfield.*

" Last year I had the misfortune to become, for the first time in my life, subject to occasional epilepsy. I well remember that the sensation above described, with which I had been familiar from boyhood, had, shortly before my first seizures at a time of over-work, become more intense and more frequent than usual. Since my first attack, I have had only few recurrences of the feeling in question. On two occasions, however, it was followed next day by an epileptic seizure, and I have since treated its occurrence as an indication for immediate rest and treatment.

" There seems to me a twofold therapeutic interest in this experience. First that, whatever pretty suggestions Coleridge and Tennyson may make to account for it, and however universal its occurrence may be regarded by Dickens, it probably ought to be regarded as showing disturbance of brain function; and that, perhaps, its recognition and removal might sometimes prevent the development of a more important disorder. Secondly, that inquiry in cases of epilepsy may detect a something of this sort, put aside as not being of sufficient consequence to speak of; and yet in truth being a minimised form of *petit-mal*, warning to precautions against a larger seizure."

The following is also a striking illustration of slight epileptic seizures with the " dreamy state," before severe fits. A man, H., aged 29, who consulted me, March 1882, began to be ill in 1873 or 1874 (he could not be more precise). He had " curious sensations," " a sort of transplantation to another world, lasting a second or so." He otherwise described them by saying that whatever he was doing at the time he (now I use his words) " imagined I have done this before, imagined I was in exactly the same position years ago." He said, too, that it was as if waking from sleep. At first he had these " sensations " at long intervals (he could make statements no more definite), but they became more frequent, two or three a day. He was not quite unconscious in them; he had defect of consciousness only. He thought nothing of them; took no notice of them. Now, suppose he had at this stage consulted a medical man, what would have been said of such seizures? The patient had no crude sensation warning. I got no more than the facts stated. There might be a natural hesitation to diagnose epilepsy from the " dreamy state " alone, as in this case it was very like, if not quite like, ordinary " reminiscence." I should never, in spite of Quærens' case, diagnose epilepsy from the paroxysmal occurrence of " reminiscence " without other symptoms, although I should suspect epilepsy, if that super-positive mental state began to occur very frequently, and should treat the patient according to these suspicions were I consulted for it. I never have been consulted for " reminiscence " only; there have always been in the cases I have seen, at the time I have seen them, with this and other forms of " dreamy state," ordinary, although often very slight, symptoms of epilepsy. Some of the patients who have " reminiscence " with other symptoms in epileptic paroxysms know quite well that its occurrence in healthy people is part of popular knowledge. This case of H. was then, however, most certainly one of epilepsy ; the sequel showed it. To go on with the report of his case. One morning (March 1875) he found his tongue bitten ; of anything occurring in the night he knew nothing. He did not consult a medical man until he found his tongue bitten another morning. In February 1882 he had a severe fit in the day ; twice he fell in a fit in public places. His friends told him of other attacks in the day, of which he knew nothing. In them he became unconscious, and after some of them, whilst continuing unconscious, he acted elaborately and strangely.

Another way of showing how slight paroxysms of epilepsy may be is by the fact that the patient does not mention them when he has severe attacks. This remark applies to slight fits of other kinds. A man (W.) who consulted me for severe fits (and who then had quasi-trifling seizure with the " dreamy state "), came to me a year later, saying that he had had no fits. He had had, however, many slight seizures, but so slight were they that he said no one else knew he had them ; he goes on walking in them. His crude sensation is the " epigastric " sensation. I give his own words as to the " dreamy state " ; a " double self " and a " thought."—" I get an idea in my head different from what I am thinking of." He might have twelve of these slight fits, for fits they certainly are, a day.

Before leaving this part of my subject I remark, by way of recapitulation, that he who neglects the " dreamy state," because it is indefinite and " merely curious," and such symptoms as chewing, etc., movements, and apparent alteration in the size and distance of external objects, because they seem trifling things, may not even surmise that his patient has the serious disease epilepsy in a rudimentary form, until a severe fit comes to tell him so. Even then it may be said that the slight paroxysms " developed into " epilepsy ; but I insist that such slight paroxysms are themselves epileptic. Such slight seizures may be erroneously put down as hysterical, or may be fancifully ascribed to indigestion, malaria, etc.

I have confessed that in former years I have underrated, and even, I find, neglected, the " dreamy state." Both to acknowledge a great clinical fault and for the importance of illustrating elaborate actions *after* epileptic fits with the " dreamy state," I give the following extract. In an article, *West Riding Asylum Reports*, vol. v, 1875, pp. 116–17 (" On Temporary Mental Disorders after[1] Epileptic Paroxysms " (see p. 126)), I mention the case of an epileptic patient who after some of his slight seizures (he had severe ones, too) would act very elaborately. After one he was found " standing by the table mixing cocoa in a dirty gallipot, half filled with bread and milk intended for the cat, and stirring the mixture with a mustard spoon which I must have gone to the cupboard to obtain." But I omitted to state what I find in my notes of this case, that at the onset of his fits the patient had " a sort of dreamy state coming on suddenly." I fear I then thought this symptom too indefinite to be worth inquiring into and recording, or possibly, to adopt Quærens' words, I put it " aside as not being of sufficient consequence to speak of," though I hope the

[1] I draw attention to the word " after," as I have been said to adopt the explanation that " epileptic mania " is the outcome of the same degree of discharge as that which produces convulsion. But I hold almost the very contrary doctrine. I have contended strenuously that *elaborate* mental states *never* occur during, and that *elaborate* series of movements *never* occur from (directly from) *such* a discharge. Only such mental symptoms as crude sensations occur during that degree of discharge ; such elaborate mental states as the " dreamy state," in my opinion, *never* do.

omission was only a blunder. In this patient's case I have no note of any crude sensation warning.

No better neurological work can be done than the precise investigation of epileptic paroxysms. Whilst epilepti*form* convulsions have been minutely studied, comparatively little attention has been given to the analysis of epilep*tic* fits. Speaking only of epileptic fits and solely of slight seizures of this kind, the endeavour should be not merely to ascertain whether a case is one of "genuine epilepsy" or not, but to describe all that happens in the paroxysm. For although I use the expression "variety of epilepsy" as if there were a clinical entity "epilepsy," with complications, peculiarities, etc., warranting subdivisions of it, there can be no question that there are at least as many epilep*sies* as there are paroxysms beginning with different "warnings." What we call the warning,[1] this being the first event from, or during, the onset of the local, sudden, rapid and excessive (or briefly the "epileptic") discharge, is the clue to the seat of the "discharging lesion." There are at least as many differently seated "discharging lesions"[2] as there are different warnings of the paroxysms. So that I admit that the grouping together of cases of epilepsy which present, in the paroxysms, the "dreamy state" is an entirely arbitrary proceeding, as much so as taking any other striking symptom to mark a group would be; all the more that not only, as I have said and illustrated, does the "dreamy state" sometimes occur without a crude sensation of smell, etc., but that these crude sensations may occur in slight fits without the "dreamy state." And in the group itself, as arbitrarily indicated, there are at least several different epilepsies; certainly a paroxysm beginning with a crude sensation of smell is a subvariety, and one beginning with the "epigastric" sensation is another, although in both cases there may be the "dreamy state." The "discharging lesion" must be differently seated in the two cases; most likely the former is a "discharging lesion" in some part of Ferrier's centre for smell. (See also Dr. James Anderson's patient's case, in which there was a "warning" by a taste.) But artificial separations, studies of cases as they approach certain types, are absolutely necessary for clinical purposes. Hence I shall continue to use the expression "variety of epilepsy" for a group of different epilepsies, each of these agreeing in presenting the "dreamy state;" this will not be harmful if we investigate each case on its own merits. But I hope that this empirical method, one much less empirical than the current method, will aid

[1] As before said, the "dreamy state" is not a warning in the sense of the word used in the text; crude sensations are warnings in the proper sense.

[2] The expression "discharging lesion" is objected to by some of my medical friends. I have been told that we can understand an ulcer discharging, but not nerve cells. Apart from this kind of criticism, the term may be objected to for better reasons, especially when the word "seated" is used with it. I only mean by "discharging lesion" a vast exaltation of the function (hyper-physiological alteration) of cells of small parts of the cortex caused by an abnormal nutritive (pathological) process involving an increased but an inferior kind of nutrition. By "seated" here or there I simply mean that the cells so altered are of this or that part of the cortex. A "discharging lesion," or "physiological fulminate," is an alteration of cells of nervous arrangements of the cortex, representing some impressions or movements, or both, of parts of the body. That the "discharging lesion" (or whatever it is to be called) is often small and local in epilepti*form* seizures (of a few cells of the middle motor centres ("motor region") of one half of the brain) is not, I think, doubtful. I have suggested that the radical cure of fits in such cases is for the surgeon to cut out that "discharging lesion," as well as the tumour, if there be one, producing it. I think too that in epilep*tic* fits the discharging lesion is similarly "doubly local," but of the highest centres. A most excellent name for what I call "discharging lesion" is Horsley's term "epileptogenous focus." My reason for continuing to use the term "discharging lesion" is that it keeps us well in mind that the epileptic process is but an exaggeration, although a vast one, of normal nervous discharges—of a normal *physiological* process.

us towards a scientific classification; that we shall ultimately be able not only to speak of certain symptoms as constituting genuine epilepsy or some variety of it, but of these or those particular symptoms as pointing to a "discharging lesion" of this or that particular part of the cortex. This will be trying to do for epilepsy what has been done to a great extent for epileptiform seizures. We may speak of "varieties of epileptiform seizures," but we speak of each case as showing that there is a "discharging lesion" of this or that part of the cortex in the Rolandic region.

Before we can make good generalisations we must carefully analyse. To group together as "visual warnings" colour projections, apparent alteration in the distance of external objects and "dreamy states" with definite scenes, is generalising without previous analysis, and is an attempt to organise confusion; they are exceedingly different things. He who is faithfully analysing many different cases of epilepsy is doing far more than studying epilepsy. The highest centres ("organ of mind"), those concerned in such fits, represent all, literally all, parts of the body sensorily and motorily, in most complex ways, in most intricate combinations, etc. A careful study of many varieties of epileptic fits is one way of analysing this kind of representation by the "organ of mind." Again, it is not, I think, an extravagant supposition that there are, after slight epileptic fits of different kinds, many temporary morbid affections resembling those persistent ones produced by destructive lesions of different parts of the cortex. To illustrate for a moment by epileptiform seizures; there is temporary aphasia after some fits beginning in the face or hand (more "elaborate" utterances, I think, when the exact starting-point is in the ulnar fingers); this is the analogue of aphasia from a destructive lesion (softening, etc.) To return to epilepsy. There is, I am convinced, in, or after, certain paroxysms of epilepsy temporary "word-blindness"; certainly in one patient of mine who had a "warning" by noise. I could not make out that this patient was at the same time "word-deaf," but thought his temporary deafness was ordinary deafness. Still there may have been word-deafness. In another patient, who called his attacks "losses of understanding," there was clearly both "word-deafness" and "word-blindness," with retention of ordinary sight and hearing; this patient's attack used to begin with a warning of noise, but he has recently had his "losses of understanding" without that warning.

I have given brief details of some cases of the variety of epilepsy with the "dreamy state" in the preceding introductory remarks. I now narrate other cases at more length.

*Case* 1.—*Epileptic attacks with crude sensation warnings, by smells in the nose and by the "epigastric" sensation; "intellectual aura" or "dreamy state"; double optic neuritis. Attacks of left-sided tremor—apoplexy and left hemiplegia. No necropsy.*

It is well to say at once, that there was no evidence of disease of the digestive, renal, circulatory, or respiratory systems. There was no history of syphilis. For most of the notes of the case I am indebted to Mr. Wholey.

A. B., a man 37 years of age, was sent from the out-patient room to George Ward, London Hospital, to see me, November 7, 1884. He was subject to attacks of *le petit-mal*. The first attack was in 1882; it only lasted about five minutes. He had no more until May 1884; since which date he had had many, sometimes three or four a week. The attacks began by smells, which he declared to be horrible, but he could give no particular description of them; his wife said that he had likened them to the smell of phosphorus. There was no loss of smell (tested November 17) as there sometimes is in epileptics who have paroxysms beginning with such so-called " subjective " smells. (There was no organic disease of the nose.) The patient had another preluding sensation—one seeming to him to start from the epigastric region. No doubt both these crude sensations were concomitant with the onset of the central discharges causing the fits—of the cells of that part of the cortex risen into that high degree of instability which I call a " discharging lesion." His wife said that for a day or two before an attack he felt drowsy and stupid. In the attacks the patient would become " vacant," and would sometimes lose consciousness altogether for a short time. But besides negative affection of consciousness (that is, when consciousness was only defective), there was at the same time the diametrically opposite, the super-positive, state, " increase of consciousness," that is, there was the so-called " intellectual aura," what I call the " dreamy state." Thinking it very likely, because he had a " warning " of smell, that he had this super-positive state, I urged him to tell us all that he felt in his paroxysms, asking no leading questions. He said that he " began to think of things years gone by," " things intermixed [like all the rest on this matter, these were his own words] with what had occurred recently," " things from boyhood's days." Another account is " peculiar sensations passing through his memory and appearing before his eyes." " He thinks of things he has, might, or will do," " he mentally sees people whom he has not seen for some years." He had also in the paroxysms left-sided movements (he was, it is necessary here to say, right-handed). They were described as " trembling." According to the patient's wife, the movements began after the other paroxysmal symptoms; according to him, with them. He said they began either in the leg or in the arm; according to his wife, they always began in the leg. All that is certain is that they were left-sided, but I have little doubt but that they did, most often at least, start in the leg. On January 12, to anticipate, the following note was made: " Another fit this morning early. Tremor began in the left leg and then ' went up ' the side of the body and into the left arm. Trembling was very rapid, and lasted on and off quite an hour. He tried to put bread to his mouth with the left hand, but the trembling prevented him from doing it without using his right hand as well. He tried to walk, and in doing so he says he felt as if he must go to the left, and it was only by dint of a good deal of effort that he could walk at all straight. In some attacks beginning in the left toes there occurred flickering in the left side of the face, and when the arm was gained it was affected after the face." That these attacks should last so long as mentioned in the foregoing note does not invalidate the assertion, that they were owing to central discharges. It is well known that even some severe epileptiform seizures of the common kind last for hours, there being not a mere succession of fits, but one continuous seizure. The " reflexes," superficial and deep, were considered to be normal.

For more than twenty years I have urged the routine examination of the fundus oculi in all cases of nervous disease. But in this case at the first visit I stupidly omitted using the ophthalmoscope. On November 17, Mr. Wholey, my then house physician, discovered double optic neuritis. On that day I for the first time saw double optic neuritis in a case of this variety of epilepsy.

As is exceedingly common in physicians' practice, there was no defect of sight to careful testing. A few days later Mr. Couper examined the patient's fundi, and reported as follows :

" *Left eye.*—Considerable capillary redness of disk, with œdematous swelling amounting to 2½ *D*. The choroidal boundary of the disk is concealed from view. The optic nerve fibre bundles are faintly visible above and below. There are radial streaks ; they show no blood-staining. The œdema and greyish opacity extend a short way from the disk into the retina. The veins are large and prominent, and slightly varicose.

*Right eye.*—There is more œdema of this disk, the swelling amounting to 3 *D*, also more greyish opacity ; the choroidal margin is concealed. The veins are large, very slightly varicose, and this latter change extends far towards the equator throughout several ramifications. There are no visible hæmorrhages or blood-staining of the disk, but there is considerable capillary engorgement, the disk being as red as the adjoining part of the fundus."

Finding double optic neuritis, the conclusion was that all the symptoms were dependent (mostly indirectly) on tumour of the cerebrum, its right half as the left-sided motor symptoms showed. No conclusion was at first come to, as to the nature of the tumour ; it was not considered likely to be a syphilitic one.

Under mercurial inunctions the optic neuritis passed off. The fundi were examined again by Mr. Couper, January 5, 1885 ; the swelling was less. Details of this examination need not be given. On February 19, Mr. Couper examined for the third time, and reported that if he had then examined for the first time he could not have said that there had been neuritis ; the disks had become again normal in appearance.

The patient, rid of his optic neuritis, did not seem much better in general. He was slightly bemazed, slightly hesitating, slow rather in speech and suffered from headache. He was, however, up and about, and to an ordinary non-medical observer no decided mental or physical defect would have been at most times observable. But, as often happens in cases of optic neuritis, or, as in this case, in patients who have had it, death occurred rapidly. Mr. Wholey noted, March 25, that the patient had been complaining very much of pain in the head. About 7.30 p.m. the patient went to the lavatory and was no doubt sick there, as some yellowish fluid came from his mouth and nose. He became suddenly pale and fell down unconscious ; there was left hemiplegia. He died about six hours after the attack. Necropsy was forbidden.

*Commentary on Case* 1.—The things to be remarked on are : (1) double optic neuritis and its existence without defect of sight ; (2) rapid death in cases of double optic neuritis (from the intracranial disease it signifies) ; (3) treatment of cases of brain disease with optic neuritis ; (4) the left-sided motor paroxysms ; (5) crude sensation warnings (smell and the " epigastric sensation ") ; (6) (*a*) negative affections of consciousness with (*b*) super-positive affection of consciousness (" dreamy state ").

Of 1, 2, 3, and 4 I intend to say little here. I have written on 1, 2, and 3 many times since 1865, and at very great length in the *Transactions Ophthalmic Society*, vol. i, 1881, pp. 60 *et seq.* The double optic neuritis is clinically the most important thing in the case, certainly a thing of most importance in prognosis as regards life. It is accepted doctrine nowadays that it is (*a*) the *best* evidence (which means that it is not decisive evidence) of local gross organic disease (tumour, etc.) within the cranium ; that (*b*) it is of no localising value beyond that it points to disease " within the cranium ; " that (*c*) it very often exists with good sight [1] ; that (*d*) under treatment it may pass off, sight remaining good.

It is certain that double optic neuritis may pass away under treatment when the organic disease within the skull causing it remains, sight continuing good. It is an error to suppose, when a patient is rid of double optic neuritis, of headache, and all other symptoms pointing to intracranial tumour, by anti-syphilitic treatment, that a syphilitic tumour of the brain has been got rid of. No doubt the organic disease in A. B. (Case 1) remained when the optic neuritis had disappeared, and that this disease afterwards caused his death. I always treat optic neuritis in the same way as I should intracranial syphilis ; the cause of it is sometimes a syphilitic tumour of the brain ; but could I know that the lesion was not syphilitic I should give mercurials and iodides. (Of course, cases in which the neuritis occurs in Bright's disease and cases of swelling of the disks in tubercular meningitis are excepted.) I believe that there would be fewer blind people if the ophthalmoscope were used by routine in cases of severe headache ; optic neuritis, discovered in its præ-amaurotic stage, presumably the stage most amenable to treatment, would very often yield to treatment. I do not, however, say that optic neuritis will not pass away without drug treatment. For after removal of tumour from the brain (Horsley), optic neuritis has disappeared when no medicines have been given. Ferrier narrates a case of cerebral abscess (*Lancet*, March 10, 1888) in which optic neuritis passed off after operation by Horsley ; no drugs were given. Horsley trephined and evacuated a cerebral abscess, the position of which Ferrier had very accurately diagnosed. The patient is now quite well. Yet I should not dare to omit treatment of the kind mentioned in ordinary cases of optic neuritis. If it does nothing for intracranial tumour, it often, I am convinced, prevents blindness. To return to the case of A. B.

It is well known that patients with double optic neuritis often die suddenly or rapidly, as A. B. did. A. B. probably died by hæmorrhage from a vascular tumour of the right cerebral hemisphere (temporo-sphenoidal lobe ?). In some cases, as Hilton Fagge has pointed out, patients who have cerebral tumour die by rapid respiratory failure. This may happen when there is no hæmorrhage from the tumour. It is possible that cerebral tumour, besides producing optic neuritis, sometimes produces similar pathological changes in centres in the medulla, the respiratory among others.[2]

The attacks of one-sided tremor (" diluted convulsion ") such as A. B. had, occur, in my opinion, in cases of disease behind the so-called motor regions ;

[1] I very well remember my astonishment on finding for the first time, that a patient with double optic neuritis could see well (" Case of Tumour at the Base of the Brain," *Medical Times and Gazette*, June 17, 1865 ; *Royal London Ophthalmic Hospital Report*, vol. iv, 1865). But nowadays the young medical men I am acquainted with are astonished that anyone doubts that marked optic neuritis often exists with good sight. For all that, although well known, it is not sufficiently known that patients with very striking abnormal changes in the disks may have no visual defect.

[2] Some time ago (*Transactions Ophthalmic Society*, vol i, 1881, p. 98) Dr. Buzzard said : " Was it possible . . . that the vomiting and slowing of the pulse might represent an affection of the pneumogastric brought about by the same cause as that which produced optic neuritis, and that the sudden or rapid death Dr. Hughlings Jackson had mentioned as one of the possible contingencies of optic neuritis from intracranial disease, might also be explained by a more severe influence on the same nerve ? "

if so, there is some little evidence towards showing that the supposed sensory districts are not purely sensory. They were not epileptiform seizures, I mean not like fits I have seen dependent on disease of the so-called motor region. I shall speak of these " diluted convulsions " elsewhere.

Saying again that the topics 1, 2, 3, and 4 are clinically of vast importance, I shall go on to speak of cases of epilepsy with the " dreamy state " more generally.[1] I have only seen three cases (Dr. James Anderson's patient, A. B., and that of a woman [2]) in which with this variety of epilepsy there were strong symptoms of local gross organic disease within the cranium. Before speaking further of the (5) crude sensations and (6) abnormal affection of consciousness (*a* and *b*), I will narrate other cases of this variety of epilepsy in which there is no reason to suppose that there exists local *gross* organic disease. I say local *gross* organic disease, meaning such as tumours, abscesses, cysts, etc. That there is some local disease in every epilepsy I have no doubt whatever ; there is, beyond question, some *pathological* process productive of high instability, which is a functional change (abnormal physiological change) of a few cells of some part of the cortex. I would here refer to remarks I made on the use and misuse of the term " functional " (*Brain*, vol. x, January 1888, p. 312).

The case next to be related is unusual, in that the severe fits preceded, for some years, the slight attacks. It is, I think exceptional in other ways.

*Case 2.—Severe epileptic fits without " warning " for twenty-five years.—Slight seizures for the last eighteen months* (*true vertigo ; smells ; " dreamy state "*).

William B., aged 47, was an out-patient under the care of Dr. Beevor, National Hospital for the Epileptic and Paralysed.

My colleague, knowing my interest in this variety of epilepsy, told me the particulars of the patient's fits and permits me to report the case. It may be well to give first what the patient, at my request, wrote down of his own case, exactly in his own words. " W. B., who for twenty-five years suffered from occasional attacks of epilepsy, has now for the last eighteen months (on and off) been subject to [attacks of] violent giddiness and headache, accompanied with strange smells and tastes, the more prominent being that of chloride of lime ; he also has at the same time, the sensation of walking or moving in space and

[1] The question whether fits of epilepsy are produced by tumour or not is, however, I think, important with regard to the epilepsy itself. I imagine that the pathology of most cases of epilepsy proper is that the " discharging lesion " is the consequence of plugging of arterioles (such arterio-cortical pathology is certainly the pathology of some epileptiform seizures). Whether the discharging lesion is produced by an encephalitis about a tumour or by plugging of vessels, the physiological condition (the " discharging lesion ") is the same. I am suggesting that there is another sort of difference. Centres for taste and smell lie, according to Ferrier's localisation, in the region of the posterior cerebal artery, whilst, still according to his localisation, the centres for hearing and part of the centre for sight (angular gyrus) lie in the region of the middle cerebral. Hence, if arterial plugging be the pathology, it may be that we have different varieties of epilepsy proper, according as arterioles are plugged in different vascular regions. The variety of epilepsy I am remarking on in the text may be owing to morbid changes in the district of the posterior cerebral. But tumours would grow regardless of vascular regions. I suggest that cases of epilepsy with mixed warnings (of smell or taste along with warnings of noise or colour) are more likely to be owing to tumour or other gross organic disease, than to have the minuter pathology I have mentioned—that of arterial plugging and its consequences. However, doctrines as to the sensory localisations are in an unsettled state. Ferrier thinks that another part of the visual centre is the occipital lobe, and this region is supplied by the posterior cerebral artery. Schäfer (*Brain*, April 1888) says that the visual area " comprises the whole of the occipital lobe," and that it " perhaps includes a part or the whole of the angular gyrus."

[2] See footnote, p. 386.

being brought into close contact with prominent buildings, such as churches, railway stations, etc., although a long distance from them, and not having seen them for a length of time."

I now give a fuller account, which I got by inquiry, although it involves some recapitulation. For twenty-five years the patient had been subject to fits, in which he became unconscious and was convulsed; his tongue was not bitten. Of these attacks he had no immediate warning, but was drowsy six or eight hours before their onset. He would not go to town on business when he felt drowsy, taking this as evidence that a fit was coming. He had at that time no slight fits. For eighteen months he has had slight fits only, and it is to the peculiarities of these that I wish to draw attention.

The first thing is a giddy feeling; it is true vertigo. This case is the only one investigated by myself in which I have been certain of the occurrence of this variety of vertigo—apparent movements of external objects—in epileptic fits with the dreamy state. He said "things were all of a move," and was quite sure that they moved to one side; he was not absolutely certain to which side they moved, but was almost certain that they passed to the left (apparent movement of real external objects is meant, not of ideal objects, *vide infra*). With or just after this came "strange smells and tastes," the "most prominent" being like chloride of lime; he said it was odd to speak of the taste of chloride of lime as he had never tasted that substance. He knew nothing of chewing, etc., movements, and had not been told of them. The next thing was his "dreamy state." He seemed to actually see large buildings which he had once seen; it might be that he seemed near a church, "close to its wall." In the last attack he "saw" certain alms-houses, "all in a moment saw that building and could actually see the clock." The things he "saw" seemed of a natural colour. He did not always lose consciousness; when he did it was just after "seeing" the buildings. Indeed in one, since the above was written, he had "had the smell," but no movements of external objects and no visions. The general feeling in the fit was disagreeable; he said there was no fear. There was no epigastric sensation. He did not pass urine in the attacks. There was no tendency to evacuation of the bowels after them. He had no one-sided symptoms, beyond the feeling of displacement of external objects to one side. He was not left-handed.

His smell, each nostril, was tested by Dr. Beevor and was found present. His taste was not defective so far as he knew. He was, he said, always sniffing; I observed that he was always doing it when with me; it was like someone strongly inhaling a scent. He had a sensation of trickling in the left nostril, but there was no unusual secretion from the nose. His optic disks were normal. He could not hear quite so well with the left ear as with the right, but the defect was trifling.[1]

Dr. Ferrier has given me the notes of a case of epilepsy, in which there was a crude sensation of smell with the "dreamy state." In the letter accompanying his report, he writes, "I send you the notes of the case of 'reminiscence' which I promised you. I think you will find it interesting in reference

[1] As said, warnings by crude sensations of smell occur in epileptics who have no "dreamy state." Recently Dr. Beevor has drawn my attention to the case of a woman (L. E.) who has that warning and no "dreamy state"; she has another crude sensation, a peculiar feeling in the two ulnar fingers of the left hand.

to your views of 'dreamy states.' The patient described the stages of her condition with great lucidity, and without any suggestions from me." The following is the account which Dr. Ferrier has sent to me. The case is, I think, unusual in that the smell comes last.

*Case* 3.—*Attacks of le petit-mal, etc.; crude sensations of smell and the "dreamy state"; reminiscence.*

X., married, the mother of three children, had a convulsive attack (said to have been uræmic eclampsia) about a year ago, which came on while nursing her husband in an attack of scarlet fever. Since then she has been subject to attacks of *le petit-mal*, without convulsions. These attacks coincide with her monthly periods, and always begin in the night and continue for a day or two. They vary in frequency; occasionally as many as seventeen occur in one day. They are always of the same character, and the patient describes them as going through three distinct stages. The first stage is a dreamy state or reminiscence, in which everything around her seems familiar or to have happened before. The second stage is a pain in the stomach; and the third is a "terrible" smell in the nostrils, associated with a similar taste and occasionally nausea, but without vomiting. Then she feels tired and sleepy. She never falls during the attacks, but says her husband knows when she has an attack by a kind of imploring look on her face, as if she were asking for help.

When the attacks occur in the night she knows of their occurrence and their number by being awakened each time by the terribly offensive smell.

The patient is spare (formerly robust) and rather anæmic. There are no indications of organic disease anywhere. The urine is free from albumen; there are no indications of local affections of the nostrils.

*Case* 4.—*Slight epileptic attacks for many years* ("*dreamy state*," *etc.*), *before severe fits; onset of severe attacks by feelings like those of the slight fits—certain movements of lips.*

A woman, M. W., 42, consulted me, 1881. Since the age of 13 or 14 she had been subject to the frequent occurrence of slight "nervous attacks"; with each of them was "reminiscence." She also called them "flashes of unconsciousness"; the two descriptions showing that the mental state was duplex, of two opposite elements. For many years she took no notice of them, never mentioned them, nor did any other person observe anything wrong. At length she consulted a medical man, who said that her case was one of hysteria. As the sequel showed, this was not so. Two years before I saw her, when her age would be about 40, she had two severe epileptic attacks with tongue-biting, and a third later on. Of course it may be said that she may have had the two severe epileptic attacks quite independently of the "nervous attacks," and that the two things were quite different. But she continued to be subject to the "nervous attacks," and that they were slight fits of epilepsy, or, if anyone likes, abortive fits, is shown by the fact that each of the severe attacks began by her having in a slight degree the feelings she had in the slight attacks.

The slight attacks might occur two or three times a day, or she might miss a month. They are very slight. As said, no one, early in the case, noticed anything of them. Of recent years, only once has anyone, other than her intimate friends, noticed anything wrong, nor do they always. If walking, she goes on walking ; only once or twice have they been so bad that she has had to stop. If at tea, she would go on pouring out, but would pour out wrongly. She may go on with her sewing, and may thread a needle. These things show that her attacks are very slight. (*Vide* p. 387, on negative affection of consciousness.) The feeling she describes in the slight attacks used to be pleasant, but is not so now : there is, however, she says, no fear with it. The attack is " over in a moment." Her " dreamy state " is variously described as " like some scene or dream," " as if you remember that again." The feeling is vivid, and yet she cannot say what the particulars of the " dream " or " scene " are. It is not of anything which has happened in real life, but is like what has happened (I suppose she meant that the " dreamy state " was as vivid as if it were a memory of something which had actually happened). So much for the positive, or rather super-positive, element of her mental condition in the seizures. She speaks of a negative element, " a withdrawal from the present ; she hears people talking, but does not know what they say."[1] She may, she is told, reply, but gives random answers. There is clear evidence of defect of consciousness ; her expression " withdrawal from the present " is a popular expression, meaning the same thing as " defect of (object) consciousness " ; I say *defect*, because I take it that the withdrawal was, considering the facts stated when dealing with the slightness of her attacks, partial only. As a rule she does not lose consciousness altogether.

She does not pass urine in the slight attacks ; there is no tendency for her bowels to be moved after them.

As to crude sensations. Sometimes when the attacks " are about " (occurring frequently) she has a sensation either of smell or of taste at the back of the throat, *but not in connection with the seizures*. A friend who came with her said that M. W. would make, in the seizures, a peculiar movement of her lips, slightly like a tasting movement. There was no evidence of one-sided symptoms, that is, no account of spasm, numbness, etc., on one side of the body.

I ask a similar question to that I asked when giving some details of the case of H. (in the introductory remarks, p. 389), what would have been thought of this patient's " nervous attacks " if she had consulted one for them before she had the severe fits ? If they were like those she has had since the severe ones, one could have concluded that they were epileptic. But such a diagnosis, say it had been made when she was 14, would have been accepted by few medical men, and by some the non-occurrence of ordinary epileptic attacks for years would have been taken as proof that the " nervous attacks " were not epileptic. That she was epileptic from the age of 13 or 14 I have no doubt whatever.

*Case 5.—Slight attacks of epilepsy with the " dreamy state " for some years before severe attacks—mouth movements—automatic actions during unconsciousness (which continued after the slight fits).*

The following is a very important case. It is that of a highly educated medical man, who reports it himself. Names of places are omitted or altered

[1] It is easy to say of this one part of the condition (common in slight attacks of epilepsy) that it is " word-deafness." If it be, it is, or, rather, is part of, a negative affection of consciousness.

from his original report, the alterations being endorsed by the patient; the alterations make no difference in the medical import of the case. He had first very slight attacks, then severe attacks at long intervals also. I shall comment on the slight attacks only.

What he calls " recollection " is what I have called " reminiscence." I retain his term " aura," putting it between commas, although I do not use it myself for any form of the " dreamy state." The report shows clearly that he has some attacks without *loss* of consciousness (see his remarks on reading poetry and on his glacier expedition). In other attacks he had loss of consciousness, and during unconsciousness continuing after them he acted automatically. The actions related in the closing paragraphs show very complex, special, etc., actions after a fit which was presumably slight. I may refer to remarks on this matter in my part of the discussion on Dr. Mercier's paper on " Inhibition." [1]

He had no crude sensation, but the words I have italicised in his account of his physical state, p. 402, during the slight paroxysms imply, I consider, discharge of cortical elements, serving during taste. (The report was finally sent in July 1888.)

" I first noticed symptoms which I subsequently learnt to describe as *petit-mal* when living at one of our universities, 1871. I was in very good general health, and know of no temporary disturbing causes. I was waiting at the foot of a College staircase, in the open air, for a friend who was coming down to join me. I was carelessly looking round me, watching people passing, etc., when my attention was suddenly absorbed in my own mental state, of which I know no more than that it seemed to me to be a vivid and unexpected ' recollection '—of what, I do not know. My friend found me a minute or two later, leaning my back against the wall, looking rather pale, and feeling puzzled and stupid for the moment. In another minute or two I felt quite normal again, and was as much amused as my friend at finding that I could give no distinct account of what had happened, or what I had ' recollected.'

" During the next two years a few similar but slighter attacks occurred, involving mental states which struck me as like to the first and to each other, but of which I can now recollect no details. I asked medical advice, but gathered no explanation, received no treatment, and regarded the matter playfully as of no practical importance. I have been in the habit of dreaming very little all my life, but during these years noticed a few occasions when I woke in the night with an impression that I had succeeded in recollecting something that I wanted to recollect, but was too sleepy to give any attention to it, and had no definite idea of it in the morning. These feelings were slightly uncomfortable, and usually, I think, accompanied by a slight involuntary escape of saliva found on the pillow in the morning, and once or twice by a soreness of the edge of the tongue, due, I should presume, to its having been slightly bitten. They did not recur after about 1875.

" In 1874 I first had a *haut-mal*, preceded by the mental condition I had felt in *petits-maux*, and after medical advice from a physician in London learnt the nature of the disease, and began to attend a little more carefully to the symptoms, which interested me more, as I had then begun to turn my attention to medicine.

" I had a severe attack of pneumonia with pleurisy, and perhaps empyema,

[1] *Brain*, vol. xi, p. 312.

beginning in October 1875, and during slow convalescence (December 1875—March 1876) was more frequently affected. The character of the *petits-maux* gradually became more stereotyped, and during the period 1876–1886 varied only within comparatively narrow limits. I will attempt to describe the features which I think were common to all, or nearly all.

" *Mental condition.*—In a large majority of cases the central feature has been mental and has been a feeling of Recollection, *i.e.* of realising that what is occupying the attention is what has occupied it before, and indeed has been familiar, but has been for a time forgotten, and now is recovered with a slight sense of satisfaction as if it had been sought for. My normal memory is bad, and a similar but much fainter feeling of sudden recollection of a forgotten fact is familiar. But in the abnormal states the recollection is much more instantaneous, much more absorbing, more vivid, and for the moment more satisfactory, as filling up a void which I imagine at the time I had previously in vain sought to fill. At the same time, or perhaps I should say more accurately in immediate sequence, I am dimly aware that the recollection is fictitious and my state abnormal. The recollection is always started by another person's voice, or by my own verbalised thought, or by what I am reading and mentally verbalise ; and I think that during the abnormal state I generally verbalise some such phrase of simple recognition as, ' Oh yes—I see,' ' Of course—I remember,' etc., but a minute or two later I can recollect neither the words nor the verbalised thought which gave rise to the recognition. I only feel strongly that they resemble what I have felt before under similar abnormal conditions. I re-enter the current of normal life, as a rule, quickly—sometimes, as far as I can judge from my own movements or other people's evidence, within ten or fifteen seconds ; there is never, however, as sudden a rush of returning normal consciousness as there has been of incipient abnormal consciousness ; it is more gradual, and it is hard to say when it is complete, as it almost always leads up to a passive and non-critical mental attitude in which I feel no originative mental impulse. One point which I almost always feel a tendency to avoid, though I am generally dimly aware of a previous wish to attempt it, is to go over my previous abnormal mental state critically and to give my attention to all its details. But attention seems not to be completely under my control ; I sometimes put it off, and delude myself with the impression that remembrance will be just as complete after another five minutes, sometimes let it slip with a feeling of indifference, and sometimes, if I am in company or in any active employment, I have no distinct recollection of any desire for self-criticism or analysis. Accompanying this want of control over reflection I often notice a temporary loss of memory for habitually familiar names or facts, which lasts a minute or two, or sometimes more, after my consciousness seems otherwise normal. This may co-exist, indeed, with so normal a state of consciousness, that I can hardly believe I shall find any difficulty in saying what I want to say, and so I fall now and then into the mistake of beginning without hesitation a sentence which I cannot finish. I have found myself just after a *petit-mal* at a London Railway Booking Office, meaning to go to K——, and asking without hesitation for ' Second return to—to—that school, don't you know—' (or some such words) and being a good deal startled at my forgetfulness.

" A *petit-mal* has two or three times come on when I have been reading poetry aloud—the line I am reading or just going to read seems somehow familiar, or just what I was trying to recollect, though I may never have seen or heard it before. I recognise my morbid condition and stop, though I have generally sense enough to finish the line or even sentence, and remain silent for a minute or so; then go on again where I left off, recovering my sense of rhythm and metre sooner than my capacity of giving attention to or understanding the words. I do not remember to have made any deliberate effort to go on reading aloud, *coûte que coûte*, throughout a *petit-mal*. I have made several rude attempts to go on writing, and have kept four or five specimens of what I have written. They were made in very slight *petits-maux*. The writing was done slowly and in a fairly normal hand. I was in the main occupied with the usual impression of recollection, but was dimly aware that I was morbid, and attempted to criticise what I was writing. My impression at the time that I was writing was that the words and sense were quite reasonable, and that I had kept within very familiar and prudent limits of expression. I had found, I thought, just the words I was seeking for. A minute or two later I could see that some of the words were grotesquely *mal à propos*, though I think the grammatical forms of sentence were always preserved. I could not trace any undercurrent of thought or recollection from which the irrelevant words had come.

" *Physical conditions.*—As to the physical conditions accompanying these mental states I can gather a little from my own consciousness, and have learnt a little more from friendly observers. At the onset I can rarely notice any physical change in myself, my attention being chiefly occupied with my mental condition; but once or twice when I have been standing near a mirror I have noticed pallor of the face, and I have learnt from others that this is common, and that my eyes have a somewhat staring vacant look as if they were not directed to anything near me, or indeed taking notice of anything particular. In this condition I am told, and in fact occasionally remember, that I often say 'yes,' with an air of complete assent to any remark made to me, whether it is a pertinent answer or not; and further, that I occasionally make a slight half-vocalised sound, whether addressed or not. This latter, I have been told, *is somewhat like a modified and indistinct smacking of the tongue like a tasting movement, and is generally accompanied by a motion of the lower jaw*, and sometimes by some twitching of the muscles round one or both corners of the mouth or of the cheeks, but by no sense of taste in my recollection. I have no clear evidence that one side of the face is affected more than the other, and no clear evidence against it; from what little I can learn, if it is at all unilateral it is rather more on the right side than the left; but the evidence is very scanty. I never notice it myself. I also never notice myself, but learn from others, that sometimes, specially if sitting, I give one or two light stamps on the floor with one foot; and in the only cases where this has been accurately observed it has been with the right foot.

" With the returning normal consciousness I generally feel some superficial flush over the skin, especially over the face, and a slightly quickened and more thumping heart-beat which does not go beyond causing me very slight *malaise*. A very constant symptom is increased urinary secretion, which sometimes makes itself felt in as short a time as five or ten minutes, but usually after a longer interval. The water, if soon passed, is very light in colour, of low specific gravity, once or twice as low as 1005, and contains no albumen.

" The *petits-maux* have not been accompanied or followed by hallucinatory sensations of sight, sound, taste, smell, or feeling. There has been, I think, no loss of balance. I well recollect in 1878 running across a Swiss glacier, and jumping across many small crevasses when the initial stage of ' aura ' came on, and a reflection shot through my mind, that if ever I was likely to pay dearly for the imprudence of going on, it would be then. But I had insufficient control to stop myself and felt no fear, but only a slight interest in what would happen. I went through the familiar sensations of *petit-mal* with such attention as I had to give concentrated on them, and not on the ice, and after a few minutes regained my normal condition without any injury. I looked back with surprise at the long slope of broken ice I had run over unhurt, picking my way, I know not how, over ground that would normally have been difficult to me. In the same way a *petit-mal* when I was playing lawn tennis did not in the opinion of my adversary make my strokes or judgment of pace and position of balls to be struck any worse than normal. I had no recollection of the strokes during a minute or two.

" I had no *haut-mal* before 1874, and since then such attacks have recurred mostly at long intervals, sometimes of as much as eighteen months ; during slow convalescence from pneumonia, however, in 1875–6 I had as many as seven or eight in two months. The ' aura ' of recollection has preceded all of them, more or less, but is less vivid in my subsequent memory than after a *petit-mal*. My evidence as to the subsequent phenomena of the *haut-mal* is very incomplete. My loss of consciousness has not seemed longer to those who watched me than five or ten minutes as a rule, but my loss of memory has been longer and my return to consciousness more gradual. I have not heard that there has been any epileptic cry ; the muscular spasms have been variable but generally slight, and not specially localised (except that once I was told of a constant grasping motion of my right arm and hand). In one or two cases the spasms have not been noticed, and the state has been at first supposed to be one of syncope ; but some snoring has almost always been noticed before recovery. My subsequent mental condition has been one of indifference and a sense of fatigue ; my bodily sensation is, as a rule, of having been lightly bruised all over.

" During the past year (1887), and more especially during the last four months, there has been some change in the symptoms of the *petits-maux*, which may be shortly summed up by saying, that there has been less vivid sense of recollection and there have been longer periods of automatism without memory. I think I had best attempt to explain what I mean by two or three instances.

" (1) In October 1887 I was travelling along the Metropolitan Railway, meaning to get out at the fourth station and walk to a house half a mile off. I remember reaching the second station, and I then recollect indistinctly the onset of an ' aura,' in which the conversation of two strangers in the same carriage seemed to be the repetition of something I had previously known—a recollection, in fact. The next thing of which I have any memory was that I was walking up the steps of the house (about half a mile from the fourth station), feeling in my pocket for a latch-key. I remembered almost at once that I had had a *petit-mal* coming on at the second station, and was surprised to find myself where I was. I recollected that I had meant to reach the house not later than 12.45, and had been rather doubtful in the train whether I should be in time. I looked at my watch and found it within a minute or two of 12.45. I searched my pockets for the ticket, which was to the fourth station, found it gone, and concluded that I must have passed the third station, got out at the fourth, given up my ticket and walked on as I had previously intended, though I had no memory of anything since the second station some ten or twelve minutes previously. I imagine that I had carried out my intention automatically and without memory.

"(2) Again, in November 1887, after dark—about 6 p.m.—I was walking westwards in a London street, when I felt a *petit-mal* coming on of which I can remember no particulars. My intention was to walk westwards for about half a mile; my thoughts were occupied with some books I had been reading in a house which I had just left. With my return of memory (which was incomplete and indistinct I found myself in a street I did not at first recognise. I was somewhat puzzled, and looked up at the street corners for information as to the name of the street. I read the name 'P—— St.' which crossed my path at right angles, and with some difficulty realised that I was walking not westwards, as I had been intending, but eastwards, along the street by which I had come, and had, in fact, retraced my steps some three hundred or four hundred yards. I felt no purpose in doing this, no aim at going anywhere in particular, and to save further difficulty, and because I was puzzled, I got into a hansom which was standing still close by me. I have no recollection of giving the driver any orders, and was in a very unreflective state. My impression is that the cab-driver drove quickly to the right house, and I distinctly remember some slight surprise I felt at his knowing the house, and at finding myself giving him a shilling, when I doubt if I could have explained where he came from. Immediately after entering the house I realised tolerably distinctly what had probably happened, and looking at my watch, I calculated that I had not lost more than five minutes by this, if so much.

"(3) About a fortnight later I was walking by the same route about 10.30 p.m., and again felt a *petit-mal* at a point within a hundred yards or so of the one described above. I cannot be certain that a memory of the previous attack recurred to me, but I think it is very probable. My memory again was a blank until I found myself facing eastwards and looking up at the name 'P—— St.' Then the memory of the previous retracing of my steps recurred to me at once. I more quickly than before gathered together full consciousness, felt a cab unnecessary, walked home, and had no difficulty in writing steadily for about three hours without fatigue.

"In the earlier of this pair of cases (2 and 3) I had no thought whatever of going back to the house where I had been reading, or to any point in that direction; but I believe I am correct in saying that I was thinking of what I had just been reading there. As far as I know, this is the first instance of my changing my intended action *ex proprio motu* in a mental state of which I have no memory. In the companion case (3) I cannot feel sure how much I was influenced by recollection in the earliest stages of the *petit-mal*.

"(4) A fourth occasion is perhaps worth record. I was attending a young patient whom his mother had brought me with some history of lung symptoms. I wished to examine the chest, and asked him to undress on a couch. I thought he looked ill, but have no recollection of any intention to recommend him to take to his bed at once, or of any diagnosis. Whilst he was undressing I felt the onset of a *petit-mal*. I remember taking out my stethoscope and turning away a little to avoid conversation. The next thing I recollect is that I was sitting at a writing-table in the same room, speaking to another person, and as my consciousness became more complete, recollected my patient, but saw he was not in the room. I was interested to ascertain what had happened, and had an opportunity an hour later of seeing him in bed, with the note of a diagnosis I had made of ' pneumonia of the left base.' I gathered indirectly from conversation that I had made a physical examination, written these words, and advised him to take to bed at once. I re-examined him with some curiosity, and found that my conscious diagnosis was the same as my unconscious—or perhaps I should say, unremembered diagnosis had been. I was a good deal surprised, but not so unpleasantly as I should have thought probable."

# CASE OF TUMOUR OF THE RIGHT TEMPORO-SPHENOIDAL LOBE, BEARING ON THE LOCALISATION OF THE SENSE OF SMELL AND ON THE INTERPRETATION OF A PARTICULAR VARIETY OF EPILEPSY[1]

(With Dr. C. E. Beevor.)

Emily M., a widow, aged 53, was admitted under our care (National Hospital for the Epileptic and Paralysed), November 25, 1887; she died December 31, 1887. For nearly all the notes of the case we are indebted to Dr. Hull. There is nothing very noteworthy in her family history, nor, until this illness, in her personal history. She said that she had had a polypus removed from the uterus some years ago. The first thing in her present illness, about thirteen months before admission, was the occurrence of epileptic fits. As these attacks were very odd, independent accounts of them were obtained by Dr. Beevor, Dr. Hull, and Dr. Hughlings Jackson; there was no essential variation, if indeed any, in the several accounts.

The first account given is by the patient's sister; some of the facts stated were of course obtained by her from the patient. The patient was a cook. In the paroxysm the first thing was tremor of the hands and arms; she saw a little black woman who was always very actively engaged in cooking; the spectre did not speak. The patient had a very horrible smell (so-called "subjective sensation" of smell) which she could not describe (*vide infra*). She had a feeling as if she were shut up in a box with a limited quantity of air (probably this was only her way of speaking of a feeling of suffocation; see Dr. Hull's note of the paroxysm). She would stand with her eyes fixed and directed forwards for a few moments, and then say, "What a horrible smell!" The patient did not, so her sister reported, lose consciousness, but remembered everything that happened during the attack; she turned of a leaden colour. The patient told us that she passed her urine in the seizures. There was no struggling, and the tongue was not bitten. She never believed the spectre to be a real person. After leaving her kitchen work she had paroxysms with the smell sensation, but no spectre. She had had these paroxysms ever since, sometimes three a day, sometimes one in two days.

The patient herself gave to Dr. Beevor, before her admission, and to Dr. Hughlings Jackson and Dr. Hull afterwards, essentially the same account of the paroxysms with the spectre and smell. The following is a redescription in essential features.

Dr. Hull writes that she said that in the paroxysms she used to see a little black woman who was rather agreeable and was always flitting about the kitchen; she always saw the same woman in every paroxysm. She never thought it was anything but a vision, but was much worried about it. When she had a fit, she used to have a very nasty smell—"burning dirty stuff"; the smell rising after the fit made her feel *suffocated*.

The patient's memory had been getting worse for six or seven months, but

[1] Read before the Medical Society, February 18, 1889. *Brain*, vol. xii, 1890, p. 346.

no other mental symptoms were noted except those which were paroxysmal—those already stated. It is to be particularly noted that she had not complained of headache during her illness—a noteworthy fact in a case of large cerebral tumour ; she had pains in the neck for the last week or two. Her illness had been preceded by trouble, loss of money—not a likely thing to have been the cause, or, at any rate, more than the exciting cause, of any such symptoms as she had. A week before admission she was noticed to get gradually weak of the left side, and it was observed that the face was " lop-sided," and the left eye was noticed to close. She complained of a leathery feeling on the left side of the body.

*On admission, November* 25.—A very fat woman ; she lay mostly in a torpid condition. After a good deal of rousing she could be made to walk, and could walk fairly well when urged along, yet without decided paralysis of the limbs there was a tendency to go to the left. The patellar, triceps and wrist jerks were equal on the two sides ; there was no ankle clonus ; the right plantar reflex was greater than the left, but both were active. There was a little dropping of the left side of the face, especially seen when she spoke. The tongue was protruded slightly to the left ; it was not tremulous. There was no ocular paralysis, no nystagmus ; the pupils were of equal size and their reactions were normal. There was no hemianopia. Sensation, tested by light touches and by pin pricks, appeared to be normal and equal on the two sides of the body. The optic disks were normal. A few days later (December 1), it was found that she could read fairly well with spectacles, but did so as if it were a great trouble, and spoke in a slipshod, slovenly kind of way. (There was never any aphasia, nor any real difficulty in articulation ; nothing more in her speech than inertness, as in all else.) Taste and smell were normal. To return to the account of November 25 : there was no obvious defect of hearing, she being able to hear on both sides. No trustworthy comparison between the ears could be made on account of her condition. There was no visceral disease discovered, and the necropsy revealed none. It may be well to say that she kept her bed until death, except that she was occasionally got up, as will be mentioned, to test her legs ; as will be seen, she had the delusion that she got up to walk at other times.

*November* 27.—She disturbed the other patients in the night for some time by calling out for chops. In the morning she did not remember anything about it.

*December* 1.—It was to-day that her reading was tested and that hemianopia was excluded. She walked half the length of the ward, but had to be supported ; she leant heavily against the table and chairs, and would, unhelped, have fallen ; she made no attempt to save herself. She took food well : she said she had no pain anywhere.

*December* 8.—She said that this morning she had a fit, and that it consisted in a suffocating feeling ; she had also a " nasty dreadful smell," but she could not describe it more.

*December* 9.—This morning, at 7 a.m., she said she wanted to get up and go out. She said she was convinced that she was perfectly able to walk, and said that she did walk yesterday. She said that she sometimes got up, and she complained that she was flung back on her bed ; she spoke in an aggrieved way. When got up it was found that she did walk a little better than when last tested ; she still has a marked tendency to fall to the left, and would fall to that side if not supported. She says, notwithstanding, that she is quite able to walk.

*December* 19.—She says that she thinks she went for a walk yesterday. Is very lethargic this morning and can scarcely be got to say anything. No optic neuritis. Urine acid, no albumen.

*December* 23.—The patient has been getting into a still more torpid condition the last few days. The left arm and leg are almost perfectly powerless ; passive movements of the leg causes pain. Sensation not absent, but difficult to estimate on account of the patient's condition. No optic neuritis.

*December* 27.—Is still very drowsy. Her left side seems to be quite paralysed, but no loss of sensation is made out. To-day Mr. Gunn examined the patient's eyes. The examination was difficult on account of the patient's condition, and from mucus on the cornea. She was asleep when the examination was begun, and her pupils were contracted to a small (normal) size ; shortly afterwards she became partially aroused, and then the pupil suddenly dilated to the same size that it had been some hours previously under atropine. It did not contract to light. There was well-marked double optic neuritis ; the edge of the right disk was undefined ; the outer edge of the left was still determinable ; there was not much swelling, and there were no hæmorrhages.

*December* 31.—After only a gradual worsening, she died to-day at 3 a.m.

Necropsy, January 2, 1888 (thirty-five hours after death). There was a small subperitoneal fibroid, about the size of a hen's egg, of the uterus. Beyond this nothing noteworthy was found except in the head. The brain and cord were given to Dr. Beevor for investigation.

### Examination of the Brain by Dr. Beevor

The patient, a description of whose case Dr. Hughlings Jackson has just read, first came under my care as an out-patient at the Queen Square Hospital. She there described to me the aura which Dr. Jackson has detailed, the nasty smell followed by a sense of suffocation, and the vision of the little black woman who was very busy about the kitchen. The combination of these two things sounds so fantastic and almost absurd that I feel pretty sure that one would be very liable to overlook their importance, or to consider them to be merely the utterances of an hysterical patient, if Dr. Jackson had not impressed upon us in his writings the absolute necessity of accurately recording all the details which a patient gives of the warning preceding an epileptic seizure, however trivial they may seem.

It is interesting to note with regard to the co-existence of the visual aura and the sense of suffocation with this sense of a horrid smell, that Dr. Gowers, in his work on *Epilepsy*, p. 62, states, " that the only associations noted (with the olfactory aura) were, with a visual aura (two cases) and with a feeling of suffocation (two cases)."

After the patient had been an out-patient for a few weeks she became worse, and was admitted under Dr. Jackson.

As the case has been so fully described from its clinical aspect by Dr. Jackson, I need not further allude to it. On examination of the brain, it was seen that the right temporo-sphenoidal lobe was the seat at its most anterior extremity of a tumour of the size of a tangerine orange. The growth was seen to involve the extreme tip of the temporo-sphenoidal lobe, and especially the part of it which is in front of the uncus of the hippocampal or uncinate convolution, and which contains the structure known as the nucleus amygdalæ.

This extreme anterior end of the temporo-sphenoidal lobe is called the pyriform or hippocampal lobule, and has been found by Broca to be very much developed in animals with a keen sense of smell, such as cats, dogs, and rabbits, and to be quite rudimentary in animals, like the dolphin, which have very little powers of smelling.

According to Dr. Ferrier's experiments (*Functions of the Brain*, p. 320), he states that the " affections of smell and taste are evidently related to lesions of the hippocampal lobule and the neighbouring regions."

The exact position of the growth will be more clearly shown by describing the appearances seen when frontal (*i.e.* transverse vertical) sections are made across the brain.

On making a frontal (transverse vertical) section through the brain at the level of the optic chiasma the whole of the anterior end of the temporo-sphenoidal lobe of the right side was found to be occupied by a tumour ; it involved the nucleus amygdalæ and the central white matter of the temporo-sphenoidal lobe ; but it did not affect the grey cortex of the uncinate convolution (hippocampal convolution), or of the first temporo-sphenoidal convolution. The nucleus lenticularis was much compressed and flattened by the growth, and the internal capsule seemed to share in the compression. On making a frontal section of the brain at the level just in front of the pons, all the central white matter of the right temporo-sphenoidal lobe was seen to be involved. The lesion lay just outside the descending cornu of the right lateral ventricle. The cortex and white matter of the hippocampal and first and second temporo-sphenoidal convolutions were not affected ; the cortex of the third temporo-sphenoidal convolution was not involved, but its central white matter was partly invaded by the growth.

At the level of a frontal section through the middle of the pons, the lesion is seen about the size of a threepenny piece just outside and below the descending cornu of the lateral ventricle and the cornu ammonis ; it involves the interior part of the central white matter of the temporo-sphenoidal lobe, but it does not extend to the convolutions or their central white matter.

Behind this point the lesion rapidly diminishes in size and was hardly visible in the next section, which was made about ½ inch behind the preceding one.

On microscopic examination by Dr. Colman, the resident medical officer to the hospital, the growth was found to be a small round-celled sarcoma.

It will thus be seen that we have here a tumour which is localised in one spot, namely, the extreme anterior end of the right temporo-sphenoidal lobe, the part which is called the hippocampal lobule and which contains the nucleus amygdalæ. This region is largely developed in animals with a keen sense of smell, and in his experiments Dr. Ferrier has found in monkeys that this part of the brain is associated with the sense of smell. I think we are therefore justified in thinking that the sensation which the patient complained of, *viz.* " the horrid smell," was produced by the irritation of the grey matter of the olfactory centre in the right hippocampal lobule, and it is interesting to note that this centre was probably not entirely destroyed, as is shown by the fact that the sense of smell was not abolished on that side, and that had the whole olfactory centre been destroyed, there would not have been any cells remaining to register the irritation caused by the growth, and to produce in the mind of the patient the sensation of a " horrid smell."

The growth had also pressed upwards upon the right lenticular nucleus and the internal capsule of the same side, and this would account for the weakness of the left side of the tongue and the protrusion of this organ to the left, and also for the drooping of the left side of the face—symptoms which were noticed on the patient's admission. It is important to note that although on admission there was no absolute paralysis of the left arm and leg, they subsequently became completely paralysed, due, no doubt, to the gradual growth of the tumour. The fibres in the internal capsule which pass down from the cortex for the face and tongue are more anterior in the horizontal line than those for the limbs, and this would perhaps account for the face being affected before the limbs.

*Remarks by Dr. Hughlings Jackson*

This case interests me especially as presenting epileptic fits with what I call the "dreamy state" (commonly called "intellectual aura"), in association with a crude sensation of smell. It is one of a group of epilepsies on which I remarked in a paper in *Brain*, July 1888 ("On a Particular Variety of Epilepsy : Intellectual Aura") (see p. 385). The case is referred to in a footnote on the first page of that article.

The case is of great value as evidence bearing on localisation in the cortex of the anatomical basis of the sense of smell ; it confirms Ferrier's researches. I leave this aspect of the case for my colleague, Dr. Beevor, to comment on. I would, however, remark, that had there been no crude sensation of smell (physically no paroxysmal discharge of olfactory nerve elements the case might have been thought of as discountenancing Ferrier's localisation. But the case shows that not only the effects of destructive lesions, but those of discharging lesions also have to be considered with regard to sensory localisation, just as both are considered with regard to motor localisation.

I refer to my paper in *Brain*, July 1888, p. 385, for further remarks on the variety of epilepsy, of which this case is one example. I once more draw attention to Dr. James Anderson's report of the case of one of his patients, who had this variety of epilepsy and a crude sensation of taste (*Brain*, October 1886).

*Remarks by Dr. Beevor*

Besides the case reported by Dr. James Anderson, to which reference has already been made, Dr. Ferrier has referred us to two cases in which there were olfactory symptoms during life due to intracranial growths. The first case is one by Sander,[1] described as "Epileptische Anfalle mit subjectiven Geruchs Empfindungen bei Zerstorungdes linken Tractus olfactorius durch einen Tumor." Here the patient had fits which were preceded by the warning of a "dreadful disagreeable smell," and he then had chewing movements of the jaws and spitting of saliva,[2] and latter on he had convulsions about the face but not in the limbs. The patient became blind, and his mental condition very obtuse, so that it was never possible to test his sense of smell on the two sides. On post-mortem examination there was found, in the middle fossa of the skull, a tumour (glioma) the size of half a large apple, situated on the under surface of the brain, at the border of the left frontal and temporal convolutions. Half the growth involved the anterior part of the temporo-sphenoidal lobe,

[1] *Arch. f. Psych.*, vol. iv, 1874, p. 234.

[2] Dr. Hughlings Jackson has frequently drawn attention to the occurrence of the "dreamy state" with chewing movements and with spitting. In Sander's patient, and in the other cases referred to in my remarks in the text, there is no mention of a "dreamy state" (intellectual aura).

the other part reached anteriorly across the fissure of Sylvius, so as to involve completely two gyri of the frontal lobe (which two gyri is not stated) ; inwards the growth reached the middle line. The important point was that the left tractus olfactorius was intact only at its anterior part, but posteriorly it was involved in the growth with the left optic nerve and tract. Part of the growth affected the base of the left temporal lobe and grew into the brain substance below the lenticular nucleus, and another part on the inner surface of the lateral ventricle involved the left ammon's horn.

In the above case, although the anterior end of the temporo-sphenoidal lobe seemed to have been involved, the growth was so large as to have destroyed the left olfactory tract, so that it would be impossible to say whether the attacks were not caused by pressure of the growth on this tract ; it was also impossible to ascertain whether the sense of smell was intact on the two sides.

Sander refers to other cases by Lockemann,[1] Westphal,[2] Schlager,[3] in which olfactory auræ preceded the fits, but in all these cases the olfactory bulb or tract was affected by tumours growing either in them or from the over-lying frontal lobes.

In none of these cases did the lesion occur in the temporo-sphenoidal lobe without involving the olfactory nerves, and they do not afford any direct evidence of the localisation of the olfactory centre in the tip of the temporo-sphenoidal lobe.

The second case referred to by Dr. Ferrier is one by Dr. McLane Hamilton—" On Cortical Sensory Discharging Lesions (sensory epilepsy).[4] Here a woman, aged 40, had attacks dating from her tenth year, when she had a fall on to her head. In the attacks she frothed at the mouth, became livid and was convulsed for a great time, but before the fits she nearly always had a peculiar aura : " She suddenly perceived a disagreeable odour, sometimes of smoke, sometimes of a fœtid character, and quite uncomplicated by other sensory warnings. She compared it to the smell of burning rags or the smell of a match, and ' it sometimes rose up her head and choked her.' " Two years later she died from phthisis, and in the brain a low grade of hæmorrhagic pachy-meningitis was found about the base of the brain. The most marked changes were found in the lower part of the right temporo-sphenoidal lobe, where a decided shrinkage of tissue was seen, with depression and adhesion of the pia mater, the induration involving the uncinate gyrus and parts of the adjacent convolutions. The olfactory nerves were not involved, nor was the third frontal convolution. From the sketch of the brain given in this paper, the lesion seems to have involved the inferior surface of the temporo-sphenoidal convolution extending to the anterior end, and affecting especially the third temporo-sphenoidal and the uncinate convolutions ; but to what extent this latter was involved is not mentioned, nor is it stated whether the disease involved the uncus itself, the cornu ammonis, the hippocampal lobule, or the inner surface of the temporo-sphenoidal lobe.

The last case is exceedingly good for the purpose of localisation, as the lesion, as far as it is described, was very definite, and the olfactory nerves were found to be intact. Unfortunately, however, there is no mention as to the condition of the sense of smell on the two sides during life.

[1] *Zeitschr. f. ration. Med.*, vol. xii, p. 340.
[2] *Allg. Zeitschr. f. Psych.*, vol. xx, p. 485.
[3] *Zeitschr. der Gesellsch. d. Aerzte zu Wien*, 1858, Nos. 19–20.
[4] *New York Medical Journal*, vol. xxxv, 1882, p. 575.

# ON CONVULSIVE SEIZURES[1]

## Lumleian Lectures Delivered at Royal College of Physicians

### Lecture I

*Definition of Terms—Classification of Convulsions—the Three Evolutionary Levels in the Nervous System—Middle Level Fits—" Epileptiform "—Highest Level Fits : " Genuine Epilepsy "—Lower Level Fits : " Ponto-bulbar "—Varieties of Lowest Level Fits—Abnormal Affections of Consciousness in different kinds of Fits—the Discharging Lesion in Epileptic and Epileptiform Fits—the Interconnecting Fibres—the Kinetic Route—Representation of Movements—the Right Motor Region—the Cerebellar System.*

There are two pleasant preliminaries, the sole parts of my address I can enter upon with a light heart. The first is most earnestly to thank you, Mr. President, for the honour you conferred on me in asking me to deliver the Lumleian Lectures. There is one thing for which I cannot blame myself. I have, as was my duty, taken all the pains I could over the task you were so good as to assign to me. The second preliminary is to mention my great obligations to Dr. Ferrier. There are very few men of the day by whom both the art and science of medicine have been so greatly helped. It is only since his remarkable researches that medical men in this country have studied convulsions in a thoroughly realistic way. Without further particular acknowledgments I make the general one, that all over the field of neurology I am profoundly indebted to Ferrier.

Convulsions and other paroxysms are owing to (1) sudden, (2) excessive, and (3) temporary nervous discharges.[2] The term " nervous discharge " (used before me by Spencer) has been much objected to ; when I say that it is used synonymously with " liberation of energy by nervous elements," it will mislead no one. There are nervous discharges in all the operations of health. I should use the term " explosive discharge " for the abnormal liberation of energy in convulsions were it not that physiologists speak of " explosive decomposition of the muscle's substance," which gives rise to contraction of the muscle in health ; and thus it may be that normal nervous discharges, those in the operations of healthy people, are " explosive." So then I use the word " excessive " for the discharges which have the three characters mentioned, the words " sudden " and " temporary," or the word " paroxysmal," being understood ; when dealing with convulsions, it will not be always necessary to add the term " excessive." I shall, however, occasionally use " explosive " for states of cells of a discharging lesion, qualifying it by the word " highly," and sometimes the term " high instability." I do not speak of " disorderly discharges," for if

[1] *British Medical Journal*, vol. i, 1890, pp., 703, 765, 821 ; *Lancet*, vol. i, 1890, pp. 685, 735, 785.

[2] A term introduced by Dr. Edward Liveing in his masterly work *On Megrim* is " nerve storm." This term has met with much favour, and the conception it stands for has been of great value in elucidating some very complex problems in neurology.

in some ways the expression be correct, it hides from us the fact that the most brutal-looking convulsion is only the sign of a departure by a vast excess and by a caricature from normal nervous discharges.

I have always assumed, and shall continue to suppose, that convulsion results from excessive discharges of nerve cells, meaning, of course, liberation of energy during rapid decomposition (katabolism) of some matter in, or of part of, those cells. I shall frequently speak of cells concerned with excessive (primary) discharges as constituting a "discharging lesion," and sometimes of them as making up a "physiological fulminate," or occasionally, using Horsley's term, of their being together an "epileptogenous focus." Some material of the cells which make up the discharging lesion has, by morbid nutrition, become of very high tension and of most unstable equilibrium (briefly of high instability), and occasionally discharges excessively. I do not assert that excessive (primary) discharges producing convulsions always depend on a persistent state of high instability of cells; to give but one example to the contrary, excessive discharges beginning in a healthy rabbit's respiratory centres are induced by rapidly bleeding the animal to death, or by quickly asphyxiating it.

The discharging lesion, though I speak of it as persistent, meaning that it is of the same locality throughout each case, yet varies in its condition.[1] The discharges are occasional. After their excessive discharge the cells are no doubt far below the degree of stability (properly comparatively slight instability) of normal cells; they will reattain a highly abnormal degree of instability—again become highly explosive—by further morbid nutrition. These qualifying remarks should be borne in mind, and especially when the discharging lesion is spoken of as a fulminate—it is occasionally fulminant.

I make three classes or kinds of convulsions. Convulsions, or I will say, fits, differ in kind, according as centres discharged differ in rank; or, speaking more definitely, as the centres first engaged in paroxysms make up different evolutionary levels of the central nervous system. I have several times suggested that there are three levels of the cerebral (central) nervous system; each is sensori-motor, and each represents impressions and movements of all parts of the body. I speak briefly of what I suppose to be the hierarchy of centres of the nervous system as a basis for the classification of fits.

(1) The lowest or first level is roughly and incompletely defined as consisting of cord, medulla, and pons,[2] and more completely, and yet still roughly, as being that sensori-motor division of the central nervous stystem, to and from which pass nerves (all cranial and all spinal nerves) for every part of the body. This level, speaking of its motor elements, represents simplest movements of all parts of the body by a series of lowest motor centres (lowest motor centre being a proper name for a centre of the lowest level) from those in the aqueduct of Sylvius for simplest movements of the ocular muscles to those of the sacral cord for simplest movements of the muscles of the perineum. This universally representing level is cerebro-cerebellar; it is at once the lowest level of the cerebral system and of the cerebellar system. For the present I ignore the higher levels of the cerebellar system, and go on to speak of two higher levels of the

[1] The rapid reader must not take "persistent discharging lesion" to be "persistently discharging lesion."

[2] I have spoken briefly on what I believe to be the importance of reckoning the cord, medulla, and pons, or, rather, certain elements of these morphological divisions, as one, the lowest level—I believe it is the "spinal system" of Marshall Hall (see p. 349). I do not pretend to be able to define the upper limit of this level.

cerebral system. These levels are, as the lowest level is, sensori-motor, but I find it possible to illustrate by motor centres only, not, however, believing that these so-called " motor centres " are purely motor. (2) The middle or second level (its motor province) of the cerebral system is composed of centres of the Rolandic region (so-called " motor region " of the cerebral cortex), and, possibly, of the ganglia of the corpus striatum also. It represents complex movements of all parts of the body from eyes to perineum (re-represents). (3) The highest or third level (its motor province) of the cerebral system is made up of centres of the præfrontal lobes (highest motor centres, motor division of the " organ of mind "). It represents most complex movements of all parts of the body from eyes to perineum (re-re-represents). The highest centres (sensory and motor divisions of the highest level)—the " organ of mind," or anatomical substrata of consciousness—are the acme of the evolution ; they have the same kind of constitution as lower centres ; they are sensori-motor as certainly as the lumbar enlargement is. (Of course each level is bilateral.)

That the lowest level is a very distinct division of the central nervous system will, I think, be granted. The separation of the frontal lobe into middle motor centres (" motor region "), making up the motor province of the middle level, and highest motor centres (præfrontal lobe) making up the motor province of the highest level, is, of course, hypothetical ; there is no obvious morphological separation. I do not suppose that the evolutionary distinction is so abrupt or so decided as that between the middle and lowest levels. I will mention some differences in the two regions of the frontal lobes. (*a*) It seems certain that the middle motor centres (" motor region ") are those cerebral centres directly connected with the lowest motor centres, as the facts of " Wallerian wasting " show ; there is, however, possibly some " wasting " of fibres from the præfrontal lobes as low as the pons. This wasting has been differently interpreted. (*b*) The middle motor centres contain most large cells. (*c*) The middle motor centres are experimentally " excitable," and the præfrontal lobes are not. This is a very important difference ; it may be taken to mean that the præfrontal lobes are not, as I suppose, motor. The distinction currently made is vastly greater than the one I have submitted. Believing that the whole central nervous system (the organ of mind included—the mind, of course, not included) is a sensori-motor mechanism of three levels, the distinction I make is not of kind but merely of degree—it is that the præfrontal lobe is only greatly more complex, etc., than the " motor region." But, according to the received doctrine, whilst the latter alone is motor, the former differs from it in two ways ; the præfrontal lobe has no motor constitution, and is part of the " intellectual centres." Distinguishing the psychical from the physical, I would say that psychical states are not functions of any centre, but are simply concomitant with functioning of the most complex, etc., sensori-motor nervous arrangements—those of the highest level (" organ of mind ") of which level the præfrontal lobe is the motor division.

There are, I submit, three kinds of fits corresponding to the three evolutionary levels. It is convenient to speak of the three kinds in an order different from that used in stating the levels. (2) I mention epileptiform seizures first because their localisation is not doubtful. (They were first described by Bravais in 1824.) They are " middle level fits " —that is, they are produced by excessive discharges beginning in parts of the middle level (motor province) of the cerebral system (" motor region "). My hypothesis is that (3) fits of epilepsy proper (" genuine epilepsy " of some nosologists) are " highest level fits," and that many of them, not all, are produced by excessive discharges beginning in parts of the præfrontal lobes, highest level (motor province) of the cerebral system. Although the præfrontal lobes are not experimentally excitable, I suppose it will not be denied that their cells katabolise and liberate energy in their normal activities, and it is not unreasonable to suppose that cells of parts of them may, by pathological changes, become highly explosive, so that they occasionally discharge excessively. So that, if the præfrontal lobes are divisions of the " intellectual centres," as no doubt they are, and not, as I think, motor too, excessive discharge beginning in parts of them may produce epileptic fits.

Of course, this is speculative. I am not aware that anyone pretends to know the seat or the pathology of cases of " genuine epilepsy." I do not use the term " cortical epilepsy," because both epilep*tic* and epilep*tiform* seizures are, to my thinking, cortical fits. (The difference in meaning assigned to the two terms " epileptic " and " epileptiform " must never be lost sight of.) (1) I think that there are " lowest level fits." These are fits produced by excessive discharges beginning in parts of the lowest level, a level which is common to the cerebral and the cerebellar systems. I suppose that most of them are owing to excessive discharges beginning in centres of the bulbar and pontal regions of the level, hence I sometimes use the term " ponto-bulbar fits." With regard to epileptiform and epileptic fits, I deal almost exclusively with cases of patients subject to fits—with, so to speak, " chronic cases."

I have so far spoken only of three Kinds of fits. No doubt there are Varieties of each kind. Whilst the kind answers to the level, the variety of each kind answers to the particular part of the level in which the excessive discharge begins. It is certain that there are varieties of (2) epileptiform seizures ; each is marked by a particular place of onset of the convulsion. There must be at least as many varieties of (3) epilepsy proper as there are different " warnings " of the paroxysms. Presumably there are varieties of (1) ponto-bulbar fits.

Then, of course, there are Degrees of each variety dependent directly on degree of the primary discharge, and indirectly on that of the secondary discharges. (2) For example, there are degrees of that variety of epileptiform seizures marked by the first spasm being of the thumb. There are many ranges of it, from convulsion almost limited to a thumb, thence onward to universal convulsion. (3) Everybody recognises that epileptic attacks occur in two vastly different degrees, *les petits-maux* and *les grand-maux*, and there are subdegrees of each of these degrees. (1) There are degrees of convulsion in lowest level fits produced by Brown-Séquard's method in guinea-pigs. There are, no doubt, degrees of respiratory fits produced in certain lower animals by rapid bleeding, by ligature of the great arteries of the neck, and by sudden stoppage of respiration.

To repeat, " fit " is a term used to include convulsive paroxysms of all kinds dependent on excessive discharges beginning in any part of any one of the three levels, the epileptic and epileptiform beginning in one half[1] of a level. There are three kinds of fits, (1) ponto-bulbar, (2) epileptiform, and (3) epileptic. There are, the supposition is, varieties of each kind, and degrees of each variety of each kind.

I have used the wide term " fit " advisedly because my method is not merely

[1] It is convenient to use the word " half " (lateral) for nervous system and " side " for body.

an empirical or clinical one. It is not only an endeavour to find out whether a convulsive paroxysm a patient has is like or unlike that of the type " genuine epilepsy " of nosologists or any other type, but is also an endeavour to discover how it shows a particular departure from normal states of his nervous system.

Is there any difficulty in recognising the difference in the two mental attitudes, or, as I shall now say, the distinctness of the two view-points ? From the empirical or clinical view-point we look to see how this or that fit approaches this or that nosological type. From the scientific view-point we look to see how these or those paroxysmal manifestations are produced, asking ourselves, " What is the level and what is the particular part of it in which the excessive discharge producing this or that set of manifestations begins ? " or, regarding all kinds of fits, the more general question, " What different effects can an excessive discharge 'get out of' the different levels ? "[1] The use of the general term " fit " compels careful segregation of kinds and analysis of individual cases. In this frame of mind we note the manifestations whether they have " the characters of an ordinary epileptic fit " or not. Whilst for purely scientific purposes I care very little for an answer to the question, " Do excessive discharges beginning in ponto-bulbar centres produce paroyxsms resembling those of the epilepsy of nosologists ? " I care very much for one to the question, " What effects do excessive discharges beginning in ponto-bulbar centres produce ? " This question is, as yet, only to be replied to by experimenters who artificially produce fits in lower animals. I should be very much astonished if it turns out that excessive discharges beginning in any centres of the lowest level do produce convulsions having the same characters as those produced by such discharges beginning in centres of the higher levels. It would be marvellous if excessive discharges beginning in centres lowest in rank produced fits like those (epileptiform seizures) which are produced by excessive discharges beginning in parts of the more evolved centres, the middle motor cerebral centres (" motor region ").[2]

As I shall not have time to deal with lowest level fits, I will here mention what I think are some fits of this kind, not classifying them, but making a rough arrangement into three groups : 1. *Respiratory fits* (respiratorily beginning from primary discharge of the main (medulla) respiratory centre.[3] I think that fits of laryngismus stridulus come in this category, but Semon thinks they are cortical seizures.[4] Respiratory fits are easily induced in animals, and are

[1] I formerly used the term " epilepsy " generically for all excessive discharges of the cortex and their consequences. At that time I did not think there were any fits depending on excessive discharges beginning in any part of the ponto-bulbar centres. Using then the term " epilepsy " generically, I submitted that any part of the cerebral cortex might become highly over-unstable and discharge excessively. So that under the term " epilepsy " used generically there were epilepsy proper, epileptiform seizures, and migraine (the last mentioned being then spoken of as a sensory epilepsy), and, indeed, any paroxysmal symptoms attributable to sudden excessive discharges of any part of the cortex. I now use the term " epilepsy " for that neurosis which is often called " genuine " or " ordinary " epilepsy, and for that only. Of course in all quotations I preserve the term " epilepsy " when used regarding any class of fits.

[2] Long ago (*St. Andrews Medical Graduates' Transactions*, vol. iii, 1870) I had the same mental attitude. After speaking of observations of the local onset and march of spasm in cases of fits from cerebral tumour, at a time when the cortical " motor region " had not been defined, I wrote : " We do not care to say that a tumour of the brain (or minute changes near it) had 'caused epilepsy,' but that changes in a particular region of the nervous system—say in the region of the middle cerebral artery—led to convulsions in which the spasm began in the right hand, spread to the arm, attacked next the face, then the leg, etc." (See p. 8.)

[3] *Brain*, April 1886.

[4] See an able paper by Dr. Gay in *Brain*, January 1890, for much valuable information on laryngismus stridulus, and for arguments against the view I take of the causation of the paroxysms.

described in all works on physiology when asphyxia is considered. Kussmaul-Tenner fits are respiratory fits.[1] It is said that convulsions occur in new-born animals after division of the cord below the medulla when they are asphyxiated; if so, these are certainly lowest level fits if not respiratory; it is possible that they are owing to discharge of subordinate (spinal) respiratory centres. 2. *Fits produced by convulsant poisons* (fits from nitrous oxide and curara are respiratory fits). Fits are experimentally produced in animals by absinthe and camphor. According to Magnan, convulsions are produced in animals by absinthe when the cerebrum has been removed. Many years ago Dr. George Johnson showed that convulsions occur in man from poisoning by camphor. Possibly some fits in renal disease (some so-called uræmic fits), and, it may be, fits occasionally part of a constitutional disturbance after urethral lesions, are ponto-bulbar fits from home-made poisons, as those just mentioned are supposed to be from foreign poisons. 3. *A condition for fits consequent on certain injuries of the cord or sciatic nerve* in guinea-pigs (Brown-Séquard). These are so well known that mere mention will suffice. There are often fits attending the onset of infantile paralysis; these are very difficult of explanation. I submit the hypothesis that they are lowest level fits produced by action on the ponto-bulbar centres of ptomaines, the result of disintegration of nervous matter of anterior horns; if so, they come in Group II.

In all severe lowest level fits it is supposed that the primary discharge of ponto-bulbar centres not only induces discharge of other lowest motor centres, but also that by intermediation of sensory ("ascending") fibres it discharges centres of higher levels. (I never thought of implication of higher centres in these or any other fits by intermediation of sensory nerves until after consideration of the researches of Victor Horsley and Binswanger.)[2]

It is necessary now to speak of abnormal affections of consciousness with regard to kinds of fits. I presume that there is loss of it in severe fits of all kinds. Consciousness is not a function of the highest cerebral centres; it is simply concomitant with their functioning. There is no physiology of the mind any more than there is psychology of the nervous system. On the basis of mere concomitance, mental symptoms (synonymously abnormal states of consciousness) are, strictly speaking, only signs to physicians of what is not going on or of what is going on wrongly in part of a patient's material organisation. Thus cessation of consciousness at, or close upon, the onset of an epileptic fit is of value to physicians as a sign that the correlative physical process, the excessive discharge, begins in some part of the "organ of mind," or equivalently, highest centres of the cerebral system; the physical process in these and all other kinds of fits is our proper concern as medical men. Con-

[1] The fits produced in lower animals by rapid bleeding, by ligaturing the great arteries of the neck, and by asphyxia, are alike respiratory fits; they all depend on stimulation of the respiratory centres by lack of oxygen. Asphyxia experimentally produced in animals does not produce cerebral convulsions, but, on the contrary, renders the cortex inexcitable, whilst at the same time it increases the excitability of the ponto-bulbar centres. Again, as Franck says (*Fonctions Motrices du Cerveau*, pp. 86, 87), "l'anémie soit totale, soit partielle de l'encéphale, n'est nullement la cause des convulsions épileptiformes." Arrest of the heart by excitation of the vagus stops these fits.

[2] Horsley (*Lancet*, December 25, 1886, abstract of Brown Lectures) believes that "all the convulsive, tonic, and clonic phenomena may originate from the ordinary bulbo-spinal centres such as exist for carrying out normal mechanisms. Tonic or clonic spasm, then, may be produced by any motor centre, but the combination and sequence of tonic-clonic could originate only from the cerebral motor cortex." This is important with regard to the question of ponto-bulbar fits.

sciousness is lost late in epileptiform seizures, and in those of but little range there may not be even defect of consciousness ; this agrees with the empirical evidence that the excessive discharge begins in lower (middle motor) centres ; probably excessive discharges are induced (upwards) in the highest sensori-motor centres by intermediation of sensory fibres when consciousness begins to cease in an epileptiform seizure. Availing ourselves of abnormal affections of consciousness as signs of states of the central nervous system, we next, so to speak, put them on one side in order to study the process in fits in a purely materialistic manner.

We must bear in mind that not only is consciousness absent in negative functional states of the highest centres, but also that it ceases during the diametrically opposite functional state, excessive discharge beginning in those centres ; there is loss of consciousness not only during, but also for some time after, a severe epileptic fit ; in post-epileptic states there is temporary exhaustion of elements of the highest centres, and, corresponding to that exhaustion, there is absence of consciousness. There are, however, degrees of negative affection of consciousness. There are degrees from that slight defect in some fits of epilepsy (*les petits-maux*) to seemingly entire loss of it in severe epileptic paroxysms ; and there are degrees from that existing with trivial confusion of thought after a very slight epileptic fit to seemingly loss of all consciousness in deep coma after a very severe one. I now return to the physical process of fits.

It will be observed that I have spoken of the excessive discharge productive of fits beginning in this or that level ; further, of its beginning in some part of a level. In recapitulation, the primary discharge in all kinds of fits is of some part of but one of the levels. And now I add that in epileptic and epileptiform seizures, of which alone I speak in the remainder of this lecture, the excessive discharge begins in some part of one half (lateral) of a level ; thus, so to say, in these two kinds of fits the discharging lesion is " doubly local." If the discharging lesion be, as I suppose, of but a few cells, very little of a convulsion is directly due to it. Most of the convulsion is produced by intermediation of fibres between the cells of the discharging lesion and other cells of its own level and of other levels ; there are induced, consecutive discharges of normal stable cells. Hence the interconnecting fibres of each level and the fibres connecting the several levels with one another, and the fibres connecting the lowest level with all parts of the body (lowest level of the whole organism), have to be considered. (I am straining the meaning of the word " fibre," making it stand for any kind of nervous pathway ensuring physiological union, definite or indefinite.) Consideration of these connections is essential for clear ideas of the full process in fits, the only visible part of which is convulsion ; it is especially important with regard to the way by which in epileptiform seizures a very local (a " doubly local ") discharging lesion causes widespreading and even universalisation of convulsion. Again, the study of the interconnections of the levels is a necessary preliminary to the comparison and contrast of the effects of " discharging lesions " and of " destructive lesions," an essential thing in the scientific investigation of diseases of the nervous system, as I urged in my Gulstonian Lectures.[1] I speak only of connections of motor centres of the levels.

Each level being bilateral is a twin series (right and left) of centres. There are connections (commissures) between " identical " centres and between

[1] *Lancet*, 1869, i. 307, 344, 379.

" non-identical " centres of its two halves—presumbly between centres of the two halves as they correspond for co-operation of the parts of the body they represent in joint operations by the two sides of the body. There are also connections between the centres making up the lateral half of each level. The fibres of the two connections spoken of are Intrinsic fibres of levels. I speak next of Extrinsic fibres—that is, of those interconnecting levels. Considering for a moment all the levels, the motor path,[1] or, as I shall say, kinetic route, extends from the highest motor centres to the muscles, which in a certain regard, being dischargeable, are centres too. This route (strictly the three series of motor centres are parts of the kinetic route) is in three segments : from highest to middle centres, first segment ; from middle to lowest, second segment ; and from lowest to muscles, third segment. I can, however, consider in detail only the second segment of the kinetic route, that connecting the middle and lowest levels. I shall, for convenience, speak of the motor centres of the right half of the middle level. There are three sets of motor fibres, kinetic lines of the second segment, uniting all right middle motor centres to all lowest motor centres—at least to all motor centres of the left half of the lowest level, if not, as I imagine, to those of the right also.

*First Set of Fibres of the Second Segment.*—Those which have been traced (on the Wallerian method by Charcot and others) from the right " motor region " along the right corona radiata, right internal capsule, through the right crus cerebri, right halves of pons and medulla into the (left) lateral column of the cord as low, Sherrington has found in one case, as the origin of the coccygeal nerve roots. These fibres are (and so are the second and third sets) extrinsic of the levels ; they belong to neither level, and yet they belong to both in the sense of interconnecting the two.

*Second Set of Fibres.*—Those of the direct pyramidal tract. They have been said to be traceable no lower than the mid-dorsal region. Tooth has traced them by the Wallerian method in one case as low at least as the second lumbar ; these are fibres of the inner part of the right anterior (Turck's) column.

*Third Set of Fibres*, comparatively recently (1884) discovered by Pitres, and seen by Schäfer, Sherrington, Hadden, Tooth, France, and others.[2] These fibres have been traced, on the Wallerian method, into the right lateral column.[3] The degeneration in the (right) lateral column in cases of (left) hemiplegia is recognised by Charcot. So we see that the interconnection of the middle and lowest motor centres is very complex.

[1] Dr. Gowers (*Diseases of Nervous System*, vol. i, p. 116) gives a diagram of the " motor path." He makes two segments, " cerebro-spinal " and " spino-muscular." The kinetic route is a modification of his scheme.

[2] Mr. E. P. France, (*Philosophical Transactions*, B 48, 1889) has not found after lesions of the marginal convolution in monkeys (made in some very important researches by Schäfer, Horsley, and Sanger-Brown, *Philosophical Transactions*, B, 1888), nor in any other case in these animals degeneration of the direct pyramidal tract ; but in all cases in which the degeneration in the crossed pyramidal tract was well marked he found degeneration much less in amount, but in the same position, in the other half of the cord (side of lesion). Horsley and Schäfer have, so to say, completed the " motor region " by their discovery of trunk centres in the marginal convolution.

[3] They were called by Sherrington " re-crossed fibres " ; but he now thinks (*Journal of Physiology*, January 1890) that this name is unsuitable. Sherrington, in a case of small and superficial lesion of one half of the brain at the lower end of the fissure of Rolando has traced degenerated fibres into both halves of the pons and medulla.

Some years ago[1] I inferred from the then known connections of the right corpus striatum (internal capsule) with both halves of the cord (by the first and second set of fibres) that both sides of the body are represented in the right half of the brain (I still say "right" for convenience), but the degenerated fibres being of different columns (the left lateral and the right anterior), that the left and right sides of the body were differently represented in the right half of the brain. (This, I have since stated, seems to me to be but an expansion and modification of the principle of Broadbent's well-known hypothesis as to the double representation of the bilaterally acting muscles.) I should have thought the discovery of the third set of fibres rendered my hypothesis more tenable. But there are serious difficulties. The second set of fibres (those found in the right anterior column) are supposed by some great neurologists to cross to the left half of the cord.[2] The same has been said of the third set of fibres found in the right lateral column. So that it may be that all three sets of fibres pass from the right middle to the left lowest motor centres. It is, however, not really known where the second and third sets of fibres end. No wasted fibres are found in the anterior commissures. Hence, I provisionally keep to the hypothesis mentioned, and now say regarding it that the three sets of fibres may show that the right middle motor centres are connected with lowest motor centres of the left and right halves of the lowest level, and thus that the right middle motor centres represent, by intermediation of the twin lowest motor centres, movements of muscles of both sides of the body. The expression "movements of muscles" introduces a matter which must be considered before I can illustrate the hypothesis.

Having considered the whole central nervous system with the rest of the body represented by it to be a sensori-motor mechanism, I now wish to urge that the motor centres of every level represent movements of muscles, not muscles in their individual character. The same muscles, that is, all the muscles, are represented in Simplest, in Complex, and in Most Complex movements by respectively the lowest, middle, and highest motor (better "movement") centres. If so, it is possible, as I believe happens in hemiplegia, to lose one series of movements of muscles, and to retain another series of movements of the very same muscles. Thus, to take a case of left hemiplegia in which the right middle motor centres, if not destroyed, are cut off from lowest motor centres (to neglect the second and third sets of fibres), the condition is not properly described as "loss of power of the muscles" of the left arm and leg, but as loss of complex movements of the muscles of those limbs. The simplest movements of the very same muscles remain represented by the left lowest motor centres. The muscles certainly are unaffected, and when rigidity comes on the simplest movements of them are developed by over-activity of their lowest motor centres. To repeat, there are, in cases of hemiplegia with rigidity, the double opposites, loss of complex movements and over-development of simplest movements of the very same muscles. The fixed rigid state

[1] *Medical Times and Gazette*, October 23, 1869. In the abstract of one of my Gulstonian Lectures (1869), after reference to Broadbent's hypothesis, there appears: "Taking one side of the brain, the right, the lecturer thinks the muscles acting unilaterally, both of the left and of the right side of the body, are represented in the right side of the brain, but that the muscles of the left side of the body are especially represented there. First, more in quantity, for they are more affected when the hemisphere discharges. Secondly, first in time (instability), for they are affected before those of the right side.

[2] Gowers, *Diseases of Nervous System*, vol. i, p. 114.

of the left arm and leg, which clinically we speak of as a symptom, as if it were something *sui generis*, is only the algebraical sum of the co-operating and antagonising " pulls " of the simplest movements of the muscles of these limbs. If the hemiplegia be very slight, we may say that the muscles of the left arm and leg " are only a little weak," but the strict description is that there is then loss of but a very few complex movements of all the muscles of these limbs, with persistence of the rest of the complex and of all of the simplest movements of those same muscles. Similarly, convulsion is not to be looked on as convulsion of muscles ; in an epileptiform seizure the convulsion is a contention of complex, and also of simplest, movements. In this contention the individuality of each movement is lost. I will consider a more complex case, that of a man imperfectly hemiplegic permanently, and yet subject to occasional epileptiform convulsion of the region paralysed ; the paralysis is loss of but some of the complex movements of all the muscles of the arm and leg, and there is persistence of the whole of the simplest movements of all those muscles ; when the fit comes there is a temporary contention of the remaining complex movements and of the simplest movements of all those muscles.[1]

The distinction between muscles and movements of muscles is exceedingly important all over the field of neurology ; I think the current doctrine of " abrupt " localisation would not be so much in favour if it were made. The occurrence of convulsion of a muscular region which is already imperfectly and yet permanently paralysed is unintelligible without that distinction. And without it we shall not understand how it can happen that there is loss of some movements of a muscular region without obvious disability in that region. This bears closely on the realistic study of the physical conditions in aphasia and insanity. We are concerned with both these morbid affections in this inquiry. The anatomical loss in cases of aphasia is of certain complex movements of the tongue, palate, etc. ; there is a paralysis in that sense. In cases of insanity (post-epileptic states, for example) there is, I submit, corresponding to the negative element of the psychical symptomatology, paralysis in the sense of loss of some of the most complex combinations of impressions or of most complex movements, or of both ; for one example of those most complex, etc., movements of the hands, which are represented in the anatomical substrata of tactual ideas. In brief, a negative lesion of any part of the nervous system (" organ of mind " included) causes, and always causes, paralysis in the sense spoken of, sensory or motor, or both, and causes nothing whatever else.

It may seem absurd to say that when there is no obvious disability in a muscular region, there may be loss of some movements of that region. This is, however, what I do affirm confidently. We shall be particularly concerned with this dictum when dealing with post-epileptiform aphasia. An eminent physician, referring to a previous statement I made [2] of the dictum, described my aim as being to prove two things—that a motor centre does and also that it does not represent movements. I never consciously attempted that very

[1] The distinction between movements and convulsion is of extreme importance, and is not always made. In some slight epileptic fits there are mixed up, so to say, with convulsion movements properly so-called, as those of chewing, spitting, clutching the throat, etc. It is very necessary not to mistake writhing movements of the arms with suspended respiration for convulsion of those limbs. I regret that time will not allow me to consider this part of my subject, for the question raised bears closely on the interpretation of post-epileptic mania, and thus indirectly on the study of insanity in general.

[2] *Journal*, May 10, 1873.

marvellous feat. Then, as now, I am content with the supposition that the non-disability of a muscular region when some movements of it are lost by destruction of part of a centre is accounted for by that muscular region being represented by other movements in other parts of the centre or in other centres. On this supposition of Compensation, we can explain recovery from hemiplegia (without relying altogether on the hypotheses of subsidence of "shock" or diminished pressure) dependent on very small destructive lesions; there is recovery when a few movements are permanently lost. That the seeming paradox holds for some cases is undeniable, as the experiments of Semon and Horsley on the cortical representation of the vocal cords show. These experiments give a crucial verification of Broadbent's well-known hypothesis for one case. Moreover, France[1] has found degeneration in the lateral column of the cord after lesions of the gyrus, fornicatus in monkeys. This shows, by the way, that the gyrus although no doubt (Horsley and Schäfer) mainly sensory, is not purely sensory. Although in the monkeys mutilated as mentioned, there is no discoverable disability in any muscular region, I submit that the degeneration France describes is proof of loss of some movements, skeletal or visceral, or possibly of negative movements (inhibitory). It would be remarkable if there were any conspicuous disability, considering the enormous compensation given by the intact "motor region." I can now return to the question of representation of both sides of the body in each half of the brain.

I suppose that the right "motor region" represents complex movements of muscles of both sides of the body (1) as they serve in bilateral actions, (2) as they serve in alternate actions (or, I should say, with preponderance of activity on one side), and (3) as they serve in unilateral actions. But I suppose, too, that those movements which are "bilateral" are represented most nearly equally in right and left halves; that those which are "alternate" are represented less equally in the two halves (those of the left side more in the right half), and that those which are "unilateral" are represented most unequally in the two halves (those of the left side most in the right half). We must bear in mind that movements are spoken of, for the so-called alternate muscles may serve in bilateral movements; they may serve with a great degree of preponderance on one side approaching unilateral movements; and the most unilateral muscles may serve in bilateral movements.

It may, however, be asked, Where is the paralysis corresponding to abrogation of the second and third set of fibres from the right "motor region"? The existence of some weakness of the right side (the so-called non-paralysed side) has been urged by Brown-Séquard, Pitres, Freidlander, and Gowers; but when in the difficult circumstances attending investigation of the state of the right side no disability is demonstrable, there may yet be loss of some few movements of the muscles of that side. The loss of these few movements is masked by the compensation given by the left half of the brain, which represents most numerous movements of the right side. If we take the case of excessive discharge beginning in some part of the right middle motor centres, we find that, in severe epileptiform fits, both sides of the body are convulsed. In this case compensation is "inverted," that is to say, centres which would compensate a loss are compelled to co-operate in an excess. The comparison and contrast of hemiplegia and an epileptiform seizure are, however, by no means simple, as

[1] *Philosophical Transactions*, B 41, 1889.

we shall see when the process of universalisation of an epileptiform convulsion is considered.

Although when speaking of the hierarchy of nervous centres I excluded from consideration the higher divisions of the cerebellar system, it is necessary to say something of them. There are in some cases of tumour of the median lobe of the cerebellum, seizures very like, if not quite like, those of ordinary surgical tetanus. I have suggested that the convulsion of surgical tetanus is owing to cerebellar discharges ; but no doubt the poison causing that morbid affection affects lowest centres too. It has been suggested that the tetanus-like seizures in the cases of cerebellar tumour mentioned are owing to pressure upon, or to changes induced in, the corpora quadrigemina or medulla oblongata, or both. But surgical tetanus is, at all events, in order of development of spasm over its regional distribution the " complementary inverse " of epileptiform seizures. And when we consider nervous diseases each as a flaw in a whole nervous system, the study of " corresponding opposites " is most important. There is a more direct reason for taking note of the cerebellum in the present inquiry. What the structures are connecting the cerebellum with the lowest motor centres I know not. If there be a connection—if the lowest level is at once the lowest level of the cerebral and of the cerebellar system—we may expect the higher levels of the cerebellar system to be concerned in post-epileptiform states ; the question is important, especially with regard to increased tendon reactions in post-epileptiform paralyses. I have suggested [1] that the cerebellum is concerned with the rigidity and exaggerated tendon reactions of (left) hemiplegia [2] when that paralysis is the result of a destructive lesion of the (right) internal capsule, that there is not only exaltation of function of the (left) lowest motor centres from loss of control, but also that the cerebellar influx upon them is no longer antagonised. This hypothesis has been objected to on the ground that in transverse lesions of the upper dorsal or cervical cord (the cerebellum being thus excluded) there is nevertheless rigidity of the legs with exaggerated knee jerk and foot clonus. I was obliged to admit that the cerebellum is not necessary for the production of the exaggerated jerk and rigidity.[3] But Charlton Bastian,[4] who has advanced proof where I only speculated, has found that, in man, on complete transverse lesion of the regions of the cord mentioned, the muscles of the legs are flabby and the knee jerks absent ; what is very striking, he finds that the condition of rigidity of the legs and exaggerated knee jerk in cases of incomplete transverse lesions changes to one of flaccidity with no tendon reactions when that lesion becomes completely transverse. If Bastian be correct, as I think he is, the hypothesis of cerebellar influx, on which we are in fundamental agreement, is supported.

[1] *Medical Examiner*, April 5, 1877, and March 29, 1878.

[2] Not rarely both knee jerks are exaggerated ; this perhaps helps to show that the third set of fibres ends in the right lowest motor centres.

[3] *Medical Times and Gazette*, February 12, 1881.

[4] Quain's *Dictionary of Medicine*, p. 1481.

## LECTURE II

*Epileptiform (Middle Level) Fits—Varieties—Diluted Convulsions—Crude Sensations—Locality and Order of Convulsive Movements—Degrees and Ranges of Fits—Hyper- and Hypo-physiological States—a Discharging Lesion—the "Buttoning Centre"—Physiological Fulminate—the March of the Convulsion—Compound Order—Cells of a Discharging Lesion Quasi-parasitical—Nutrition of Cells—Summary*

I TAKE for most particular consideration the second kind of fits, epileptiform seizures (middle level fits); they were first described by Bravais in 1824. There are many reasons why we should study them first. (1) Their investigation is comparatively easy. We can, if present at a paroxysm, ascertain the place of onset and trace the march of the convulsion; and if we witness no attacks, since consciousness is not lost or is lost late in the seizures, the patient can tell us the place of onset and much more about his fits. (2) They have permanent paralytic counterparts in monoplegias and hemiplegias from destructive lesions of the "motor region." (3) There is after them, at least in many cases, temporary paralysis of the parts first and most convulsed. (4) There is not rarely permanent paralysis of the parts which are occasionally convulsed, this showing —a very important thing with regard to doctrines of localisation—that in the same case there is coexistence of a destructive lesion and a discharging lesion of different elements of the same centre. (5) Because there is after some seizures temporary defect of speech ("partial aphasia"). (6) Because, if we can find the condition of centres answering to paralysis and aphasia after these seizures, we shall be greatly helped in our investigation of the state of the highest centres in insanities after epileptic fits. (7) Because epileptiform seizures often depend on gross organic disease, such as tumour (syphilitic or non-syphilitic); hence, we may at post-mortem examinations obtain proof or disproof of any notions on localisation and gross pathology we had from a study of the patient's symptomatology during his life. (8) It is in epileptiform seizures that operations have been done by Macewen, Godlee, Horsley, Barker, and others. Hence, very precise study of fits of this kind is necessary. In this regard, as well as in many others, the minute investigations of the "motor region" by Beevor and Horsley are of great value.

It would be very unmethodical to begin the scientific study of the more complex (epileptic) kind of fits before the study of the epileptiform kind.

There are Varieties of epileptiform seizures. The convulsion begins in some part of one side of the body. Varieties are distinguished by the particular place of onset ("signal symptom" of Seguin) of the convulsion. The fit may begin in some part of either right or left side of the body; I call that on which it does begin the "first side," and the corresponding (opposite) half of the brain in which the discharge begins the "first half." If the fit begins on the left side, that is the first side, and the right half of the brain is the first half; suppose that the convulsion becomes universal, then the right side of the body is the second side, and the left half of the brain (if it discharges after the right) is the second half. Whether the onset be right- or left-sided is a very important matter, because there is often defect of speech after right-side-beginning fits; moreover, on account of the "speech centre," operations on the left half of the brain are more serious than operations on the right.

The three commonest varieties of epileptiform seizures are—(1) fits starting in the hand (most often in the thumb or index-finger or in both); (2) fits starting in one side of the face (most often near the mouth) or in the tongue, or in both these parts; (3) fits starting in the foot (nearly always in the great toe). (Of course one always means convulsive development of movements of muscles belonging to the several parts mentioned.)

Of necessity the three varieties depend on the fact that the local discharging lesion is of cells of different parts of the "motor region"—of hand, face, and foot centre respectively. The starting-point is almost invariably the same in each patient, but not always. A patient whose fits commonly begin in the hand may sometimes have the face of the same side slightly and solely affected; or a patient may tell us that his fits "fly about"—that is, leaving the face for the hand, or vice versa.

We sometimes meet with paroxysms of one-sided tremor—what looks superficially like tremor, really a "diluted convulsion"—dependent, I think, on discharges beginning in motor elements of the so-called sensory centres behind the motor region.[1] I do not call these epileptiform seizures.

Often enough there is "tingling" or some other crude sensation in the place of onset before convulsion starts; this is part of the proof that the so-called motor region, although mainly motor,[2] is not purely motor. Sometimes there is at or near to the onset of an otherwise ordinary epileptiform seizure excessive development of colour, or of sound; these also are Crude Sensations. Epileptiform seizures with crude sensations deserve very careful attention, but time will not allow me to consider these complications.[3]

It is worth mentioning that some patients have a feeling as if a part were convulsed when it does not really move; one of my patients subject to veritable convulsions beginning in his left thumb had sometimes what he called "convulsions not to be seen" of that part. Another patient had the feeling of convulsion of one side of his face, but looking in a glass he saw that it did not move. He died of brain tumour (necropsy), but its exact position I did not learn. A patient who has fits starting in the hand will say that he feels "it" in the face, when, however, the face does not move; this "it" may be owing to very slight discharges of sensory or motor elements, or of both.[4]

Epileptiform fits begin in the animal parts of the body and commonly in those of them which are the most animal. Thus the majority begin in the

[1] I have never believed that any part of the cortex is purely motor or purely sensory. If the elaborate visual projections in some cases of migraine occur during discharge beginning in a "sensory centre," then the elements of that so-called sensory centre are only chiefly sensory; the fortification outline and the vibrations of parts of the migrianous visual spectre imply discharge of motor elements as certainly as the colours imply discharge of sensory elements.

[2] See remarks (Lecture I) on France's *Researches on Degeneration of Fibres of the Lateral Column of the Cord, consequent on Lesions of the Gyrus Fornicatus*, p. 419.

[3] Of course crude sensations (psychical) and convulsion (physical) are in no way comparable: the comparisons and contrasts are of excessive discharges of sensory elements *during which* crude sensations arise, with such discharges of motor elements *from which* convulsion arises.

[4] When a healthy person thinks of doing something ("has an idea of a movement"), I consider that what occurs physically is slight discharge not only of sensory but also of motor nervous arrangements of his highest centres; there is "nascent movement"—slight discharge of the very same motor nervous arrangements of the highest centres which, if more strongly discharged, would be intermediation of middle and lowest motor centres, produce the actual movement. It is probable that a similar explanation (the middle motor centres being here primarily concerned) applies to the "ideas of convulsion" spoken of in the text. No doubt if a man subject to fits beginning in his right thumb were to lose the right arm by amputation his fits would still *seem* to him to begin in this thumb—to begin in his spectral thumb, for some time at least.

arm, and nearly all these in the most animal part of that most animal part, the hand, and most of them in the thumb or index-finger or both—the most animal parts of the whole organism. Perhaps the term "animal" is awkward in this connection; it is convenient in contrast to "organic." We can, however, use other terms, and say that epileptiform seizures most often begin in those parts which, speaking popularly, have the most "voluntary" uses; in those parts which have great independence of movement; in those parts which have the greater number of different and more special (definite) movements, at the greater number of different intervals. The foot in man has, however, few *different* movements; the hallux in him is much less specialised than in the monkey. It is, then, a very striking thing that epileptiform seizures beginning in the leg almost invariably start by spasm of the great toe, in the most, and yet but little, differentiated part of the whole lower limb.

It may be objected to the principle stated that, to take an example, convulsion in an epileptiform seizure may begin in the shoulder, the least "voluntary" part of the arm, and spread down the limb.[1] I have considered this objection in the *Journal* of August 17, 1889. We have, as I continually insist, in strictness to speak not of representation of parts of the body (muscular regions), but of representation of movements. Movement of any part of the body done with intention is a "voluntary" movement. Evidently when a card-sharper shrugs his shoulder as a sign to a confederate to play a trump, that is his then most voluntary movement. In so far as any part of the body has a movement independent of the rest, in so far that movement has, I suggest, a degree of localness of representation in the middle and highest motor centres. Horsley and Beevor assign a point of the "motor region" for the primary movement of each segment of the upper limb. It may, however, be taken that epileptiform seizures most often begin in the most "voluntary" parts, and that admitting many varieties the three commonest are selected for comment.

Epileptiform seizures illustrate Dissolution—dissolution in process of being effected—in which the order is from "voluntary" towards automatic. *In normal development of movements the order is the opposite—is that of Evolution; it is from automatic to "voluntary."* [2]

The "motor region" (motor province of the middle level) presumably represents at least motorily the whole of the body, demonstrably nearly all parts organic as well as animal. Hence, as the discharging lesion may theoretically be of any part of the "motor region," it is a legitimate hypothesis that there are fits starting by excessive discharges of cells of nervous arrangements of the "motor region" which especially represent parts in the organic field, and that some fits called *epileptic* are such seizures. I do not hold that hypothesis. There are parts—for example, the vocal cords—which we may speak of as organico-animal.

Munk and Krause[3] in the dog, and Horsley and Semon in the monkey, have investigated the cortical representation of the movements of the vocal

[1] I have recorded a case of this kind, *Medical Times and Gazette*, June 5, 1875.

[2] Properly from most automatic to least automatic in evolution; the opposite in dissolution. "Most voluntary movement" is objectionable because it is a mixture of psychological and anatomico-physiological language; it is a popular expression, equivalent to what is scientifically "least automatic movement."

[3] *Sitzungsberichte der Königlichen Academie der Wissenschaften und Archiv für Anatomie und Physiologie*, 1883.

cords. Krause in the dog, Horsley and Semon in the monkey,[1] produced convulsive seizures by excitation of the cortical "laryngeal centre." Semon thinks that laryngismus stridulus in man (the infant human being) is a cortical fit; but if so there is not an exception to the statement that epileptiform fits begin in the animal parts, if we adopt Semon's views of, and inferences from, the kind of representation of the vocal cords in the motor cortex (" purposive or volitional, since it is adduction, that is phonation ").

Although epileptiform seizures most often begin in the three most animal parts of the animal parts mentioned, yet as the fits go on the organic field becomes involved. In a dog poisoned by curara (respiration being artificially kept up) the animal parts are excluded, and then we see that by excessive discharges experimentally induced in its "motor region," effects are produced in, and are then limited to, the organic field.

There are Degrees of each variety corresponding to degrees of the "severity" of the excessive discharge. Degrees are to be considered with respect to two factors, (1) amount of convulsion, and (2) range of convulsion. I illustrate here quite arbitrarily by range only, and take the case of an epileptiform fit starting in the thumb. Admitting that there are many ranges, it is allowable to make arbitrary divisions (they must not be taken for real distinctions) into four ranges: (1) Terminal[2] fit—the spasm involves, say the hand, or some part of it only; (2) monospasm—the arm becomes involved; (3) hemispasm; (4) bilateral convulsion—the second side being gained, the fit becomes universal. Observe the use of the word "become." In the range (4) there is a march of spasm from the part first seized all over the body, answering to increased spreading of the central excessive discharge beginning in some particular part of the motor region of the first half, and may be extending to the second half, of the brain. The second side of the body (in 4) is affected later, and commonly less, than the first side.

From (1) to (4) there is but a single variety of epileptiform seizure in four different degrees. Otherwise stated, a man who has had convulsion of the range (1) or (2) does not become subject to another variety of epileptiform seizure when he has also fits which, beginning in the same terminal part (hand, we are supposing), have a more extensive range however much more extensive it is; so to speak, that patient is subject to *a* fit, and has it in different degrees on different occasions. However limited or however wide the range of convulsion, the corresponding discharge begins in the very same centre of the motor region of but one, the opposite half of the brain. This means that it is the place of onset (" the signal symptom " which localises)[3]; it points to the particular part of the "motor region" of the cells of which part the discharging lesion is made up. When a man's epileptiform fits "get worse"—when we are supposing they become of greater range—there is the same discharging lesion, but it has become of more cells, or the cells of it have become still more highly

[1] *B.M.J.*, December 21, 1889.

[2] It may be well said that a fit beginning by spasm of the cheek does not begin in a *terminal* part; but the meaning of the word "terminal" may, for my present purpose, be used to include that onset. Peripheral would have too wide a meaning. I would suggest acro-epilepsy as a name for epileptiform seizures were it not that it might mislead some to think that there are epileptiform seizures which begin in the nose.

[3] The term "aura" is, I suppose, never used now in its original sense. When a medical man speaks of an aura in an epileptic fit starting from the epigastric region, he is understood to mean that some sensation is referred by the patient to that part of the body, and to believe that the sensation arises during the incipience of a discharge of some central sensory elements.

unstable, or perhaps there are both kinds of change ; in consequence of this purely local ingravescence, the induced discharges (compelled discharges) of normal stable cells are more numerous.

Were A and B to be universally convulsed, they would have different varieties of epileptiform seizures if in A the onset was by spasm of the hand, and in B by spasm of the foot, however much alike the fits looked at the acme of each ; the discharging lesion in A would be of some cells of his " arm centre," in B of his " leg centre." To note the " signal symptom "—to use Seguin's term again, and therefrom to infer the seat of the discharging lesion—is more important, obviously for " brain surgery," than anything else about the paroxysms.

It has been implied, but it may be well to say explicitly, that an epileptiform seizure does not, when become universal, turn into the other *kind* of fit—the epileptic. I mention this because I think a rapidly universal epileptiform seizure superficially resembles an epileptic one, and a slowly developed epileptic seizure superficially resembles an epileptiform seizure.

I have often urged that the clinical problem in every nervous malady is of three elements : (1) anatomical, (2) physiological, (3) pathological. In other words, we have in every case to seek : (1) the seat of the lesion, the structure damaged, (2) to infer the kind of functional change of structure, and (3) to discover the nature of the abnormal nutritive process by which the alteration of composition of nervous matter producing the abnormal functional state of structure is effected (*vide infra*).

It may be properly said that structure, function, and nutrition never exist separately. It is quite obvious, taking for comment normal conditions, that there would be no persistence of function without continuous nutrition ; that function is not conceivable apart from some structure, and that structure without function is nothing for an organism. It is, however, convenient, if not necessary, for clear exposition of nervous maladies, to consider for a time each of the three separately. It will, however, be impossible to consider one without frequent explicit and always implicit reference to the others. Perhaps I use the term " anatomy " regarding the nervous system in an unusual sense ; I do not use it convertibly with " morphology." A knowledge of the anatomy of any centre is *a knowledge of the parts of the body which that centre represents, and of the ways in which it represents them.*

*Anatomy* (Localisation).—I shall say very little under this head. The patient A is subject to fits, every one of which begins in his right thumb ; there is a lesion of the thumb centre of the left middle level (" motor region ")—this is the anatomical diagnosis. (According to Beevor and Horsley, " the middle third of the ascending parietal convolution is the focus of representation of the movements of the thumb.")

*Physiology.*—Physiology deals with the dynamics of the organism—that is, with its function. I use the term " function " with regard to nervous diseases in a strict sense, and never in the way it or its adjective is used when applied to the symptoms of an hysterical woman, or to minute or transitory changes of structure.[1] I must now define the term. The function of organic matter and *par excellence* of nervous matter, to which I confine further remarks, is to store up energy,[2] to liberate that energy (nervous discharge) at different rates

[1] See an able paper by Dr. Allchin, *Westminster Hospital Reports*, vol. ii.

[2] Assimilation of material having potential energy (anabolism) ; decomposition of material (katabolism) with liberation of energy.

against resistances of different amounts : the energy liberated is dissipated or does work, or there are both consequences according as the resistances encountered are or are not overcome, or are only partially overcome. We have here to deal with abnormalities of this function—that is, with abnormal physiological states (I need not always add the adjective abnormal).

There are two kinds of physiological or functional states in cases of disease of the nervous system. (1) Function may be exalted, and is, sometimes, as that of cells of a discharging lesion, very greatly exalted ; these are super-positive functional changes—that is, hyper-physiological states. (2) Function may be diminished or lost ; these are negative physiological or functional states—they are hypo-physiological states. Destructive lesions come in this category, although there is in them loss, not merely of function, but of functionable material also.

The two kinds of functional changes—the hyper- and the hypo-physiological—are opposites ; there are no degrees from one to the other ; so to say, they depart from normal function, the one upwards, the other downwards. We shall have to speak later of a negative functional change in temporary post-epileptiform paralysis ; that negative change (there is temporary exhaustion of nervous elements) is a direct result of the excessive discharge in the prior paroxysm ; the two opposite functional states of the same nervous elements occur in immediate sequence.

Now I consider the inclusion of negative functional states in cases of mere temporary exhaustion of nervous elements in the same category with destructive lesions when nervous elements and function are gone together. I dare say the former would be called functional, because the alteration in the composition of the material of nervous elements, whatever its nature, is no doubt slight and is certainly temporary. But I call it a negative functional change, *because function is lost* ; the slight and temporary alteration of composition is a pathological change. For the time being fibres exhausted are not in effect nerve fibres at all ; with a morphological plenum there is a functional vacuum as certainly as there is when they are destroyed. Whether nervous elements are functionless or gone altogether, the situation *for the time being* is the same. I shall speak of both as " negative lesions." And saying that the exhausted fibres recover soon is recognising fully the vast difference in their condition from that of fibres destroyed—properly, absence of fibres.

There are degrees of negative function from defect to loss. Of these I will say nothing. There are two greatly different degrees, if indeed we may not say two kinds, of super-positive (hyper-physiological) function. We are concerned with both in this inquiry ; it is imperative to distinguish them clearly.

There is (*a*) the vast exaltation of function of cells of a discharging lesion : this degree is always produced by some pathological process—that is, by morbid nutrition, a nutrition which alters the composition of nervous matter.[1] This, the

[1] This is the definition I would suggest of a pathological process (morbid nutrition) or of its result. I suppose that such poisons as strychnine alter the composition of nervous elements, in consequence of which morbid nutrition (a substitution nutrition) there is a functional change of the degree (*a*). It seems more likely that strychnine enters into the very composition of matter of nerve cells than that it stands outside the cells and " irritates " them. When a rabbit's respiratory centres discharge excessively on withdrawal of blood, one must suppose that before that discharge there is an abnormal metabolism (pathological process) whereby matter of the cells of the centre becomes more explosive. Certain " pathological processes," such as cerebral hæmorrhage, are really injuries ; hemiplegia resulting from clot is, so far as destruction of fibres goes, like that caused by the prong of a pitchfork ; there is no real pathological process in either of these modes of destruction.

first degree of functional change, is of a highly explosive character ; it issues in paroxysmal discharges.

There is (*b*) a comparatively slight exaltation of function with which we shall be particularly concerned when we consider post-epileptiform conditions. In these conditions, besides paralysis answering to a negative functional state of fibres of the second segment of the kinetic route, there are increased tendon reactions answering to a hyper-physiological state of this degree (*b*) of cells of anterior horns (lowest motor centres). I believe that the second degree of super-positive functional state is not—certainly not in the case just alluded to—the direct result of a pathological process, but that it is the *indirect* result of a negative functional state of *other*, related nervous elements. (Here is, essentially, an application of a principle long ago put forward by Anstie and Thompson Dickson). This, the second degree of functional change, does not issue in paroxysmal discharges, but in continuous discharges ; or discharge can at any time be evoked by appropriate slight excitations. Returning to post-epileptiform conditions, the negative functional state answering to the paralysis is alone produced by a pathological process ; the abnormal condition of anterior horns implied by increase of the tendon reactions is one of over-activity of perfectly healthy nervous elements. There is simply the proper activity of certain lowest motor centres, which is manifested at its maximum when an obstacle has been removed, when control has been taken off. I think, too, that cerebellar influx is no longer antagonised (see Lecture I) ; and if so, the cerebellum is simply unhindered in its activity, and is doing, now that an obstacle is removed, what it was always " trying to do." Here, again, we come across the principle that parts of the symptomatologies of nervous maladies are owing to activities or over-activities of perfectly healthy nervous arrangements. If this principle be valid, it is evidently important to distinguish between the physiological and the pathological factor in nervous maladies. Of course increased activity of any nervous elements implies increased nutrition, but there is not, I submit, in the case of elements answering to the second kind of functional change, morbid nutrition. There is not, then, what I call a pathological process ; the composition of the matter of the cells concerned is not altered. For the present I shall speak only of the first degree (*a*) of super-positive functional states—that which is of a highly explosive degree—and is produced by a pathological process.

The hyper-physiological state (degree *a*) in the case of A—(*vide supra*) is what I call a " discharging lesion." It is a crude hyper-physiological state just as its diametrical opposite, loss of function, is a crude hypo-physiological state. I continue to speak of healthy cells as stable ; they are naturally unstable, of course, but I mean by using the term " stable " that they are so *in comparison with* those of discharging lesions, which I speak of as being *highly* unstable. The discharging lesion is of a few cells which have got far above the rest of the cortical cells in degree of tension and instability of equilibrium. That lesion is made up of cells of nervous arrangements which represent some most special movements of a particular muscular region ; the sudden and excessive development of these movements from discharge of those cells is the convulsion incipient (" signal symptom " of Seguin), or, if there be no spreading of the spasm, it is the convulsion total.

The hyper-physiology of epileptiform seizures is the element of the three-fold clinical problem of which we are sure. We are quite certain that normal movements are the results of liberation of energy attending katabolism ; thus the inference is irresistible that that sudden and excessive development of many movements at once, which we call convulsion, must be a result of an excess of the same physiological process—of a sudden and excessive energy-liberation attending great and rapid katabolism. I will give illustrations of the different effects of discharges of stable cells (cells of comparatively low tension and of comparatively stable equilibrium) in normal operations, and of those of cells of a discharging lesion (cells of very high tension and very unstable equilibrium) in a convulsion.

It would be most absurd to say that there is a Buttoning Centre, but for convenience of illustration we may imagine such a centre. I illustrate by motor elements only, although, of course, sensory elements are concerned in all operations. In the operation of buttoning there are slight and slow discharges of normal stable cells (fibres are understood) of different nervous arrangements of our supposed centre (lower centres and muscles being understood) simultaneously and successively ; in consequence there is a harmony and a melody of the different movements of the hand and arm by which the button is got into its hole. There is Harmony by Contemperation [1] of different movements, and there is Melody in that the compound contemperated movements follow one another at proper time intervals ; there is what is commonly called co-ordination, although the time element (melody) is not much considered in most accounts of the process of co-ordination. So much for the discharges of stable cells in the operations of health.

Now let us suppose that the cells of the buttoning centre become by some, any, pathological process so highly unstable as to constitute a discharging lesion. (For the present we shall speak as if the excessive discharges of the highly unstable cells did not provoke similar discharges of stable cells of collateral centres.) The discharges are sudden and rapid,[2] and of all the cells nearly at once ; they do not cause a speedy and vigorous act of buttoning, but a short, severe, and rapid contention of all the movements of that operation ; this contention is convulsion of the hand and arm. There is no harmony and melody ; on the contrary, in the tonic stage, all contemperation is lost and all time intervals are merged, so that there is but one rigid state of the musculature of the hand and arm, and, in the clonic stage, there is but a succession of such rigid states. There are no movements properly so-called in this convulsion ; but, if I may use the word for once, there is first but a single big useless movement, and next a series of such so-called movements which do nothing but " mark time."

The illustration, although the supposition of a buttoning centre is grotesque, may render clear what presumably occurs when A is " attacked by his convulsion." The convulsion is a brutal development of that man's own movements. I make this odd remark because I do not think that it is always vividly realised that an ordinary severe epileptic " attack " (to take that kind of fit for a moment's illustration) is nothing more than a sudden excessive and temporary contention of very many of the patient's familiar normal movements—those of smiling, masticating, articulating, singing, manipulating, etc. A

[1] " Contemperation " is, says the *Imperial Dictionary*, an obsolete word. One of its meanings given op. cit. is, " The act of reducing a quality by admixture of the contrary."

[2] I do not mean by using the word " rapid," here or anywhere, that nerve impulses travel more rapidly in the case of excessive discharges, but that more occur in a given time than is normal—that there is a greater quantity of motion in a given time.

convulsion is not something altogether *sui generis*. Speaking figuratively and more generally, and still of an epileptic paroxysm, there is the mad endeavour of the highest centres to develop the maximum of function of every part of the body, animal and organic, and of all parts at once ; the phenomena of a very severe epileptic fit show that this endeavour is nearly successful ; the patient is almost killed by the paroxysm, and is nearly dead (deeply comatose) after it.

The cells of a discharging lesion are not to be thought of only as occasionally discharging excessively ; we have also to consider their aspect of too easy dischargeability, otherwise their highly unstable equilibrium. In health the cells of the " buttoning centre " are made to discharge slightly on special excitations of definite force, so that their discharges are in particular relations, and in some degree of community with those of cells of other centres (I will call them " collateral stable cells ") with which they are connected. The cells of the " buttoning centre," when they have become highly explosive, are still integral parts of the nervous system, and have the very same connections they had before some pathological process so altered their nutrition that they became highly explosive (and then, metaphorically speaking, " mad parts "). Their equilibrium can be upset, they can be made to discharge, and to discharge excessively, by less special excitations of less definite force coming to them from collateral stable cells—that is, their discharge depends on their own easy dischargeability rather than on the particularity of the excitation reaching them. Possibly their discharge is spontaneous when tension is very great, and equilibrium very highly unstable.

I repeat that the cells which have become very highly " explosive " (those of the discharging lesion) continue to be elements of the same nervous arrangements, and that these nervous arrangements are still connected in the very same ways with the remainder of the nervous system [1] as when their cells were stable. Hence I do not speak of the highly explosive cells as being *in* any motor centre, but as being *of* that centre. I submit that the highly " explosive " cells of a discharging lesion will on their fulminating discharge overcome the resistance of, and thus produce excessive discharge of, collateral stable nervous elements. The epileptiform fit (excepting, perhaps, some slight terminal fits) is not the result only of the discharge of the cells of the discharging lesion, as was supposed for a limited illustration, when speaking of the imaginary " buttoning centre." Making a purely abitrary limitation, we may imagine that the primary excessive discharge, that of the fulminate of A's thumb centre, only produces directly the initial spasm, that of his thumb (the " signal symptom ") ; all the rest of his convulsion will be indirectly produced by it, by *compelled* excessive discharges of stable cells. Of these compelled discharges I shall speak again later.

It will now be seen why the term " physiological fulminate " is occasionally used. I use it in almost a literal sense ; the discharging lesion is supposed to be a detonator of collateral stable cells, just as a fulminate (in the artillerist's use of the term) is of the comparatively stable gunpowder in a cannon. I believe that the only thing persistently physiologically abnormal in A is that some few cells of his thumb centre have become fulminant. To speak figuratively, this " mad part " compels many collateral " sane " cells and cells of

[1] There is the obvious qualification that some nervous elements may have been destroyed by the same pathological process which caused high instability of other elements, and thus that some connections of the latter are cut.

middle and lowest motor centres, and ultimately the muscles, to co-operate in its occasional and sudden excesses—makes them " act madly " for a time. If the few highly explosive cells, those of the discharging lesion, could be destroyed, the patient would be rid of his fits ; he would lose nervous elements which are doubtless never of value for co-operation with the collateral stable cells in normal operations ; he would lose cells of negative value and of positive injury—cells like those of an animal poisoned by strychnine, which, on their discharge, " run up " movements into useless contentions. The cells of A's fulminate, when called on to co-operate with normally stable cells in any operation, function excessively, and so as, after the manner of a detonator, to cause wide excessive discharges of many stable cells. It is a pity that A cannot be rid of these worse than useless cells ; but I know of no way of effecting this riddance. There is the surgical question of cutting out part of the cortex.

I have, in the foregoing, used, regarding hyper-physiological discharges, the term "excessive," and, regarding the resulting convulsion, the term " severe " ; the more excessive the discharge the severer the fit. I now use more precise terms, and consider this part of the subject as it was in effect, so it seems to me, long ago considered by Herpin. I regret greatly that my ignorance of physics renders me unable to deal with it adequately.

With regard to nervous discharges, or, as I shall here say, liberations of energy by nervous elements, we have to consider two aspects—quantity of energy liberated, and the rate of its liberation ; the two varying factors both in normal and in " excessive " nervous discharges. With regard to the convulsion, we have to consider its degree, and the rate at which it is produced.[1] We have to study the amount of convulsion, the range of convulsion, and particularly the " deliberate " or " sudden " rate of onset. In two liberations of equal quantities of energy at different rates there is the same momentum or quantity of motion. But the force of the more rapid but shorter liberation of energy will be greater than that of the slower and longer liberation. Force only exists while it lasts ; there is no doctrine of conservation of force. The more rapid the liberation of energy by a discharging lesion the greater resistances will be overcome, the more numerous collateral stable elements will be compelled to discharge, and thus the more the amount of convulsion and the greater its range.

I suppose that there are degrees of instability of the cells of the fulminates in different cases of epileptiform seizures and at different periods of the same case. When A's fits " get worse " (greater amount of convulsion and greater range of convulsion), more cells may have then become highly unstable, or those already highly unstable may have become still more so ; his fulminate becomes more fulminant, but that fulminate is made up of cells of the same part of the " motor region," if not of the very same cells. I now consider it must be taken hypothetically, the differences of fulmination of discharging lesions. Let me suppose two cases, in each of which there is a discharging lesion constituted by cells of the thumb centre. In the patient A the cells are (I am only able to distinguish vaguely) of lower degree of high instability (his fulminate is much less of a fulminate) than in the case of AA. In both the first spasm is of the

[1] Herpin, in his valuable work on *Epilepsy*, sums up several propositions as follows (italics in original) : " En résumé : *plus le début est long, moins la crise est violente, plus il est instantané, plus l'accès est intense*."

thumb. I shall mention the cortical discharges only ; the sequent discharges of the lowest motor centres and of the muscles are to be taken for granted.

In A the primary discharge, that of the fulminate, is deliberate, produces (secundo-primary) discharges of few collateral stable cells, and produces them slowly one after another ; the corresponding convulsion sets in deliberately and spreads slowly ; is of little range (very local ; for example, of the arm only), is of long duration, and there is an easily traceable distinct sequence over the range (all this, of course, comparatively with what occurs in the next case). In AA the primary discharge is sudden, produces (secundo-primary) discharges of many collateral stable cells, and produces them rapidly and more nearly at the same time ; the corresponding convulsion sets in suddenly and spreads rapidly ; it is of great range, is of short duration, and there is a less easily traceable distinct sequence over the range.

The more rapid, though the shorter, of the two primary liberations, by the discharging lesions—supposing an equal quantity of energy to be liberated by each—will overcome greater resistances, and will thus compel discharges of a greater number of collateral stable elements ; the convulsion produced will be both of greater amount and of greater range. Lines of many different degrees of resistance will be overcome by such a primary liberation more nearly at the same time ; the convulsion will more quickly attain its maximum at every part affected, and will be more nearly of the same degree in all parts affected.

We have not only to note how much of the body is ultimately involved, but also the order in which the several parts involved are affected—the march of the convulsion. There is not a simple, but a compound sequence of spasm ; the convulsion does not cease in one part when another is involved. To observe, to give a simple example, how much of the arm has been involved when convulsion appears in the face will, I think, help us to clearer notions of localisation of movements of those two separate parts of the body in the centre discharging (anatomical localisation) ; or if not, at any rate as to the time relations of different elements of different centres (physiological localisation). From increasing discharge of a motor centre there is a double effect ; there is not simply " more convulsion," there is (1) greater amount of convulsion of the part first seized, and there is (2) extension of convulsion to the next part of the same muscular region, or to some other part represented in the centre discharging (or in another centre connected with the one primarily discharging by particular time relations). Most generally, the progress of the two dissolutions—convulsion from increasing discharge of a motor centre, and paralysis from increasing destruction of a motor centre—may be rudely (and without the least pretence at exact quantification) symbolised as (1) $x$, (2) $x^2y$, (3) $x^3y^2z$ ; the order $x$, $y$, $z$, implies the representation in the centre supposed of the time relations, and of the degree of speciality of movements of the three parts. Horsley and Beevor find Compound Order in their development of " simple movements " by very slight excitations of small parts of a monkey's " motor region." After developing what they call the Primary Movement of a part, say one of the shoulder, there follow, on increasing the excitation, secondary and tertiary movements—that is, there is produced a sequence of movements of segments of the arm. But when the secondary movement comes the primary has not ceased ; on the contrary, it is intensified : the development may be roughly symbolised as $p$ and then $p^2s$.

Returning to epileptiform seizures, compound order is observed on a small scale in fits involving limited regions of the body (very well seen in the face), and on a large scale when such seizures become universal. There is a very intricate compound sequence from the beginning of the fit to its universalisation. I shall, however, make artificial separations, and say of a fit which becomes universal, that excessive discharge beginning in some cells of a part of the right middle motor centre produces convulsion (1) starting in the left hand and spreading up the arm and down the leg (first side), (2) involving both sides of the trunk, and (3) finally gaining the limbs of the right (second) side when all parts of the body are in convulsion together. That the left limbs are convulsed from discharge of the right middle motor centres, by intermediation of the first set of fibres of the second segment, is not doubted. I used to suggest that convulsion of both sides of the trunk and of the right limbs is also produced by discharge of that half by the second and (or rather as I should now say) third sets of fibres. This was rash, for supposing that some convulsion of the second (right) side *is producible* by discharge of that one half (right), it does not follow that the convulsion which actually occurs *is produced* by it alone. For my hypothesis of representation of both sides of the body in each half of the brain, it would suffice if there were any degree of tonic or clonic convulsion of the right (second) side, for I only suppose that the right side is represented less than and subordinately to the left side, and also second in time in the right half. The subject is a difficult one. Horsley finds that when the corpus callosum is divided, excitation of the right (I continue to say " right " for convenience) middle motor centres produces epileptic convulsion of the left limbs only.[1] In the case of dogs, Franck and Pitres found that artificially induced discharges of the right " motor region " caused universal convulsion when the left motor region had been extirpated and the corpus callosum divided. I quoted them to this effect in my third Croonian Lecture.[2] They, however, as I then said, attribute the universalisation of the convulsion to the pons, medulla and cord (which together I call the lowest level).

Considering, then, the opinions of those who hold that the second and third sets of fibres, as well as the first set (all the fibres of the second segment of the kinetic route interconnecting the right middle motor centres with the lowest motor centres), end in the left lowest motor centres, the researches of Franck and Pitres and those of Horsley, and also the great complexity of the subject, I ought not to be dogmatic as to the process by which universalisation of an epileptiform convulsion is produced. Most likely in severe seizures the left middle motor centres are discharged, as Horsley supposes, after the right by intermediation of callosal fibres, although possibly some slight convulsion of the right limbs is produced from discharge of the right half alone by intermediation of the second and third sets of fibres. And most likely, too, the anterior commissure of the pons, medulla, and cord (intrinsic fibres of the lowest level interconnecting left and right lowest motor centres) are concerned. Probably the loss of consciousness answers to excessive discharges of the highest centres caused by the medium of sensory (upward) fibres. The process of universalisa-

[1] In the abstract of Brown Lectures, *Lancet*, December 25, 1886, Mr. Victor Horsley is reported : " The conclusions . . . all round, therefore, were very emphatic, to the effect that convulsions due to cortical discharge are evoked in various groups of muscles by nerve energy proceeding from that centre in each hemisphere which is in relation to each group of muscles, and that in generalised epileptic convulsions both cerebral hemispheres are involved."

[2] *B.M.J.*, March 29, 1884.

tion of epileptiform seizures is a very intricate one, and deserves more precise analysis than I am capable of making.

I stay here to say that, taking the case of A in illustration, when we have located his lesion we have done anatomical work only ; when we have noted all we can about his convulsion (therefrom inferring that the lesion is a " discharging lesion " and the effects of its discharge direct and consecutive), we have done physiological work only. The experimenters on animals do the anatomico-physiological work thoroughly well.

Taking up again the case of A, we have now the third element, pathology, to consider. Here is the great difficulty. Being sure that A has a discharging lesion of his thumb centre, there may be no evidence to show whether that lesion is produced (indirectly) by tumour or not. Here I urge again the necessity of distinguishing between the physiology and pathology of cases of nervous disease.[1] Having urged that there is a degree or kind of functional change (*b*) which is not the result of any pathological process, I am all the more wishful to urge the distinction. I continue to speak of the first degree (*a*), and urge the distinction from this point.

It may be epigrammatically said, and with truth, that an epileptiform seizure is " only a symptom." Nevertheless, it is always symptomatic of one *physiological* thing, a " discharging lesion." Otherwise put, an epileptiform seizure is not a symptom of tumour, of " softening," or of meningitis ; it is a symptom of the one thing—high instability of certain cortical cells, *however produced*—produced by any pathological process. Physiologically speaking, there is but one " cause " of epileptiform seizures, namely, high instability of some cells of some centre of the Rolandic region ; but there are many " causes " of them if we mean pathological processes leading to that instability. So that in the case of A (he being *subject to fits*), the question in pathology is not the vague one : " What is the *disease* of a certain part of his cortex ? " but " What abnormality of the nutritive process has produced such an alteration in the composition of the material of cells in that part as to render them highly explosive, and how was that abnormality set up ? " Or, more generally and regarding all cases of epileptiform seizures (and epileptic too) we put the question : " How are local persistent discharging lesions established and kept up ? "

The first question is : " What is the most general nature of the abnormal nutritive process of cells of discharging lesions in epileptiform seizures ? " This we ask ourselves, whatever the particular gross pathology or morbid anatomy, tumour, " softening," etc., may be in any case.

The cells of the discharging lesion, although *quasi*-parasitical, are not strictly parasitical ; for another purpose I urged that the nervous arrangements into which they enter remain integral parts of the nervous system, and now I urge that they are nourished along with the rest of the body. Their nutrition does go on in some base fashion as certainly as that that of their stable neighbours goes on in a proper way. By nutrition of some kind the cells of the discharging lesion attain high tension and very unstable equilibrium, and occa-

[1] I have urged this many times for at least twenty years. " Functional changes must not be confounded with pathological changes, although of course the two necessarily co-exist " (" Study of Convulsions," *St. Andrews Graduates' Reports*, vol. iii, 1870, p. 29). I mention this as I am said to have put forward the " theory of discharges " as the *pathology* of epilepsy—a thing I earnestly repudiate. In 1870 I did not make two degrees of functional changes, and spoke only of what I now call the first degree (*a*).

sionally discharge suddenly, excessively and temporarily; their stability is after their discharge below normal; by continuance of this abnormal nutrition they reattain high tension, or no more fits would ensue. What is the " base fashion " of nutrition of these cells? It does not follow that the cells are *more* nourished, although they are certainly *worse* nourished. So to put it, they may be less nourished in quantity and worse nourished in quality. The nutrition must be such that it alters the composition of nervous matter of the cells, and in such a way that it becomes more explosive.

I have so often spoken on this subject that I will only mention the hypothesis that the nutrient fluid bathing the cells is comparatively stagnant, and that in consequence there is inferior nutrition. I suggest that there is " substitution nutrition," phosphorus compounds becoming more nitrogenous, or nitrogenous compounds more nitrogenised. I may illustrate by the well-known case of glycerine becoming explosive (nitro-glycerine) when some of its hydrogen is replaced by nitric peroxide. The composition of this substance is altered, but its constitution remains the same. It may possibly be that the mass of the explosion of nerve cells, both of health and convulsion, is of non-nitrogenous matter, as is the case in the normal discharges of muscle. But the suggestion is that a nitrogenous substance is the " pivot " of the metabolism of nervous matter both in physiological and in hyper-physiological states.[1] I suppose the greater nitrogenisation of the material of nerve cells makes it highly explosive, but that the constitution of that material and the morphological structure of the cells remain the same. If this hypothesis be valid, there are presumably degrees of substitution (as there are in the three chloracetic acids, for example), and consequently degrees of high explosiveness. It may be that when a patient's fits " get worse," the original fulminate becomes more fulminant by still greater nitrogenisation, as well as that more cells become part of his fulminate. The abnormal nutrition leading to change of composition is a pathological process, whilst the high explosiveness it produces is a functional change. Surely it is the change of function which should be called a functional change. Whether these speculations be valid or not, it is a warrantable inference that the nutrition of the cells of the discharging lesion goes on, that it goes on wrongly, and that some material of the cells does become highly explosive.

Now I consider differences in sizes of cells with regard to their normal and morbid nutrition.

For theoretical reasons, and after the observations of Betz and Mierzejewsky, I suggested[2] that those centres of the motor region which especially represent small muscles (eyes, face, and hands) will have a greater number of small cells than those which especially represent the large muscles of the limbs. I think this is generally true of the " motor region." And I suggest that it accounts for the great frequency of onset of epileptiform fits in the hand and face, for reasons to be given presently. The " leg " centre contains many large cells, but it also contains some small cells. Bevan Lewis's researches, to which I am very greatly indebted, show that the parts of the motor region representing small muscles have most small cells. He says—and this bears on the remark

[1] " Whether the chief product of the metabolism of any tissue be a proteid substance, or a fat, or a carbohydrate, proteid substance is the pivot, so to speak, of the metabolism, and nitrogenous bodies always appear as the products of metabolism " (Foster, *Physiology*, pt. ii, p. 828).

[2] *Medical Press and Circular*, August 23, 1876, p. 262.

I made on the leg centre—" that alongside the largest pyramidal cells are numbers of others of the *smallest* dimensions " (italics in original)[1] so that the discharging lesion of the " leg centre " may be made up of small cells.

Although it is convenient for some purposes to say " small muscles," the expression is not exact. For I urge once more that nervous centres do not represent muscles, but movements. I will substitute the expression " small movements " for " small muscles," and that of " large movements " for " large muscles." As these terms, the best I can think of, are vague, their meaning must be taken as defined here. Most of the movements of the hand are " small " according to the definition I now give of " small movements." The parts moved have little mass, and in most of the operations they serve in there is little more added mass. The muscles are small and numerous, and in most operations by the hand their movements are of little excursion, of short duration, and rapidly changing. Short, prompt, and frequent liberations of small quantities of energy will be required for these successions of " small " different movements ; I submit that the nervous arrangements for these movements of the hand have small cells, and very many small cells. Most of the muscles of the shoulder are " large movements," according to the following definition. The muscles are large and few ; there is much mass to move, the whole arm to lift, and the added mass is often great in some of the operations they serve in, as in lifting weights the hand takes up. In most operations they serve in, the movements are of large excursion, of comparatively long duration, and are comparatively little changing. They will require persisting and slow liberations of large quantities of energy by, I suggest, comparatively few and large cells. We may have " large " and " small " movements of different parts of one limb in a single operation. When the arm is put forth there are " large movements " of the shoulder, upper arm, and forearm ; and when the fingers, thus put forward, elaborately explore an object, there are " small movements " of the hand.

But although parts which most often engage in " large movements " have large muscles, yet there may be " large movements " of parts having small muscles. If we grasp an oar and pull a boat, the whole of the musculature of the arm serves in a succession of similar large movements (and then subordinately to other movements). For these, I suppose, will be discharges of large cells, even for the movement of the hands grasping the oar ; there is, indeed, then but one unchanging movement of the whole hand, a large movement *as defined*, all the small muscles serving together as if one muscle.

A principle of representation is here in question ; we have not only to do with sizes of cells, but also with numbers of cells, and therefore with the volume of different centres. Schroeder van der Kolk, illustrating by the case of the sturgeon, which has large muscles and few cells in its spinal cord, pointed out that there is not a mere relation between quantity of grey matter and size of muscles, but that the grey matter is greater in proportion to the complexity of movements of muscles. This shows that we have never to forget that centres represent movements of muscles, not mere muscular masses. I have several times drawn attention to Herbert Spencer's statements bearing on this question.[2] One remark he makes is : " In proportion to the number, extensiveness, and complexity of the relations, simultaneous and successive, that are formed among different parts of the organism, will be the quantity of molecular action

[1] *A Textbook of Mental Disease*, p. 106. [2] *Psychology*, 2nd ed., vol. i, pp. 35, 55, 67.

which the nerve centres are capable of disengaging." Spencer takes count of both impressions and movements ; I am illustrating by movements alone. The much greater volume of the middle motor centres is in accord with the fact that they represent vastly more numerous different movements than the lowest motor centres do ; the muscles represented by both levels are, of course, the same, being in each case all the muscles of the body ; hence the middle motor centres contain many more cells and fibres than the lower centres do. Presumably the same principle applies in detail. According to Horsley and Beevor, the thumb and index-finger, which have a great number of different movements, chiefly " small movements," have a large area of representation in the motor region. As to the trunk area of the cortex, I quote what Horsley and Schäfer say[1]: " It certainly is not a little remarkable that the numerous and powerful muscles of the spine should be governed from so small a portion of the cerebral cortex, *but it is to be remembered that the movements of which the spine is capable are comparatively few and simple* " (no italics in original). The supposition is that parts having many small and greatly changing movements are especially represented by small cells and by many small cells, and that parts having but few and little changing (" tonic ") movements are represented by large cells and by few large cells.

The size of cells is a very important matter with regard to their nutrition. Both in health and in disease small[2] nerve cells will be nourished more quickly than large ones when both are bathed in the same nutrient fluid. (From diminished nutrient supply the small cells will atrophy sooner than large ones.) The smaller cells will become highly unstable sooner than large ones during morbid nutrition. It certainly is the fact that most epileptiform seizures begin in parts having " small movements," in parts represented by areas of the cortex having most small cells. As I have pointed out, they may begin in the large muscles of the upper arm ; it would be begging the question to say that in these cases the smallest cells of the " shoulder centre " are those which first become highly unstable. The size of cells bears also on rates of discharge.

Four hot iron balls will become cold much sooner than the same mass of iron in one ball having the same quantity of heat as the four balls together have. From discharge of four small cells, which are together equal in mass to that of one large cell, there will be, I submit, a liberation of energy in a shorter time than by the large cell, supposing equal quantities liberated in the two cases. Hence another reason for fulmination of the highly unstable cells of discharging lesions if these cells are small. As being somewhat illustrative, I may refer to different sizes of grains of powder used as ammunition ; slowly burning (pebble) powder is required for large cannons, quickly burning (fine-grained) powder for firearms.

To repeat the several hypotheses, epileptiform seizures begin most often

[1] *Philosophical Transactions*, vol. clxxix, 1888, B.

[2] " Other things equal, the smallest cells will soonest become unstable. A mass of nervous matter in many small cells will ' present a much larger surface to the contact ' of nutrient fluid than the same mass in a few large cells " (Harveian Lectures, *Medical Times and Gazette*, January 11, 1879) (see p. 280). My attention was first directed to this subject on reading Spencer's *Biology* where he expounds his theory of growth. A brief statement of Spencer's theory will be found on p. 220 of *The Evolution of Sex*, by Geddes and Thomson, from which I quote. " In spherical and all other regular units the mass increases as the cube of the diameter, the surface only as the square." I refer the reader to Ross's great work, *Diseases of the Nervous System*, vol. i, p. 13, where he deals with the significance of differences in sizes of nerve cells with regard to normal and abnormal nutrition and its consequences.

in parts of the body having "small movements"; these movements are represented by nervous arrangements having many small cells.[1] Small cells present a more extensive surface to nutrient fluid than the same quantity of grey matter in large cells, and will be more quickly nourished than large ones are. Nerve cells become highly unstable from an abnormal nutrition, such that, although their structure and the constitution of their material are unaltered, that material becomes of more nitrogenous composition, and thus more explosive. Small cells become highly unstable more readily than large ones do; thus discharging lesions are supposed to be especially of small cells. A rapid liberation of energy overcomes greater and more numerous resistances than a slower liberation of an equal quantity of energy. Small cells liberate their energy in a shorter time than large ones; hence the currents developed by fulminates of small cells overcome greater and thus more numerous resistances than would fulminates of large cells, and hence produce more convulsion and greater range of convulsion.

We have assumed that the nutrition of the cells of the discharging lesion is continuous, and have supposed in effect that the nutrient fluid is comparatively stagnant. But how is this comparative stagnation brought about? This brings us to pathology, commonly so-called. We have to distinguish between what I may call the coarse pathology of a case and its immediate pathology.

[In the remainder of the lecture the production of discharging lesions by tumours and by arterial occlusion was considered.][2]

## Lecture III

*After-effects of Epileptiform Fits—Paralysis due to Cortical Exhaustion—Analysis of a Case—Variations in Degree and in Range of Post-epileptiform Paralyses—Hemiplegia, Post-epileptiform and from Destruction of Motor Part of Internal Capsule contrasted—Post-epileptiform Defects of Speech—the Negative and Positive Elements of these Defects—the Psychical and Physical—the Concern of the Right and of the Left Half of the Brain in Speech.*

I HAVE now to consider the after-effects of excessive nervous discharges in cases of epileptiform seizures. This part of our subject is of extreme importance; the presumption is that from the study of the comparatively simple post-epileptiform conditions we shall obtain a basis for the interpretation of post-epileptic conditions. It is for this reason that I go into some detail as to the former.

There is not rarely after epileptiform seizures local temporary paralysis;[3] and sometimes aphasia with it. For the present I speak of paralysis only. In this inquiry we have no direct concern with paralysis, temporary or permanent,

[1] The movements, speaking most generally, represented by the cerebrum are, I suppose, numerous different punctuated movements (many and different "small movements"). Presumably those represented by the cerebellum are, in comparison, few and little different movements, movements as it were gliding into one another (few and similar "large movements"). It is interesting to observe that the structure of the cerebellum is more uniform than that of the cerebrum, and that those cells of the cerebellum which are presumably motor are large and of nearly equal size. The movements for bracing up the spine in standing or walking, and the separate movements of the legs and arms in walking, will require comparatively continuous supplies of large quantities of energy. (I believe, however, that the cerebrum and cerebellum are both engaged by contemperation in at least all extensive operations.)

[2] See *B.M.J.*, July 21, 1888.

[3] This paralysis was long ago described by Todd under the name "Epileptic Hemiplegia."

owing to destruction (by clot, softening, or any other pathological process) of any part of the brain, not even if the malady set in with a convulsion.

I must particularly mention cases in which there are both (1) permanent paralysis—for example, imperfect hemiplegia ; and (2) occasional epileptiform seizures, the convulsion beginning in some point of the muscular region paralysed and involving part or the whole of it, and sometimes also parts beyond that region. In these cases the two opposite functional states—destruction of some nervous elements which represented complex movements, and high instability of some others which still represent other complex movements of the same muscles—are side by side in one part of the cortex (or the latter of cortex and the former of fibres passing down from it). After a paroxysm in such a case there may be temporary increase of the paralysis. For my present purpose, which is only an attempt to explain the nature of the sequence (paralysis after convulsion), I shall exclude these cases, and deal only with what I may call uncomplicated cases—that is, with those in which there is only paralysis immediately when epileptiform seizures have ceased, such paralysis being temporary (unless, of course, the fits recur at short intervals). Something has to be said, however, regarding certain of the so-called uncomplicated cases.

In some cases in which there is no *discoverable* paralysis in the intervals of the fits, except for a short time after one, there may be indirect evidence of a negative functional state of a few fibres of the second segment of the kinetic route. That evidence is foot clonus and exaggerated knee jerk on the same side as that in which the convulsion occasionally starts. I mean, of course, cases in which these abnormal tendon reactions are producible at all times, although in a greater degree just after a fit. It may be that severely careful tests would show some *quasi*-trifling paralysis—loss of a very few complex movements. I shall here ignore this slight inferential paralysis, and speak of such cases as " uncomplicated."

The term " post-epileptiform paralysis " will be used to include all paralyses the immediate sequels of epileptiform seizures. Arbitrary divisions may be made, speaking of range only. (1) Terminal paralysis, as of a hand ; (2) monoplegia, as of an arm ; (3) hemiplegia ; and (4) a range which is not generally admitted—some degree of slight universal paralysis. I hold the hypothesis (essentially that of Todd and Alexander Robertson) that there is exhaustion of central nervous elements, including fibres of the second segment of the kinetic route, and that this is produced by the sudden and excessive discharge in the prior paroxysms. These nervous elements are exhausted, not otherwise injured, so that recuperation is prompt, and the corresponding paralysis is temporary. There is a sequence of two opposite functional states, super-positive of the first degree ; (*a*) in the paroxysm, and then, after the paroxysm, negative. But there is often more than a negative functional state in the post-epileptiform condition. We may find increased tendon reactions implying a super-functional state of the second degree (*b*) of lowest motor centres. The duplex nature of these post-epileptiform conditions must be borne well in mind.

The term " exhaustion " has been objected to ; general bodily prostration is, of course, not meant ; but, as said, exhaustion of nervous elements in a particular part of the central kinetic route. There are, I suppose, degrees of exhaustion, and no doubt of different numbers of nervous elements of the kinetic route in different cases. But illustrating by the extremest degree, the supposition is that nervous elements of the route, after their excessive " exercise" in the fit, are left " fatigued " to the degree of utter impotence. The nervous elements exhausted in post-epileptiform paralysis are, I suppose, in the same state as are the motor nerve fibres of the sciatic nerve going to the cut-off leg of a frog after strong faradisation of that nerve trunk ; the leg is convulsed by the faradisation (stage analogous to epileptiform seizure), and is next paralysed (stage analogous to post-epileptiform paralysis) because its motor fibres are exhausted by the unnaturally high functioning they have been artificially compelled into. A closer analogy may be stated, although the case to be instanced is a complicated one. The motor nerves of a frog, poisoned by a very large dose of strychnine, lose function partly by the direct action upon them of that poison, but partly (this is what is relevant) through exhaustion—" the exhaustion of over-use due to the intense activity of the nerve during the stage of spasm." [1]

Not only the term, but the hypothesis itself is objected to. I will consider other hypotheses. The paralysis has been ascribed to cerebral congestion consequent on arrest of respiration in the preceding seizure. It is difficult to see how cerebral congestion, even if we grant that it can produce paralysis, could be so exquisitely local as to produce what we sometimes observe, paralysis of one arm only, or even of but part of one. Again, absolute paralysis of a limb is found after seizures nearly limited to that limb, in which seizures there was no arrest of respiration and (if that is thought to bear on the question) no loss nor even defect of consciousness ; the patient may talk throughout an attack in which an arm is involved, and after which it is temporarily paralysed. There is the hypothesis that the temporary post-epileptiform paralysis is owing to a small extravasation of blood in the brain, caused, I suppose it is meant, by congestion consequent on arrested respiration in the preceding seizure. I admit that very small clots may cause local paralysis, and that such paralysis may be transitory. But the post-epileptiform paralysis is—that is, in my experience—always of the parts which were first and most convulsed in the prior fit ; it would be marvellous if a small hæmorrhage happened locally in one half of the brain, so as to produce temporary paralysis of the parts first and most convulsed, and happened in the same place in every fit the patient had. Besides, if arrested respiration could cause cerebral hæmorrhage by leading to sudden great congestion of the brain, we should find very local paralysis after fits of the epileptic kind, and we do not ; according to current opinion there is no paralysis at all after seizures of this kind. I shall exclude the two hypotheses just dealt with.

Post-epileptiform paralysis has been ascribed to inhibition by some medical men whose hypotheses deserve respectful consideration. Gowers believes that discharges in epileptic fits sometimes inhibit ; he thinks that temporary paralysis is found in some cases after a purely sensory discharge which does not next discharge motor centres, but inhibits them. In some cases of epileptiform seizures the patient tells us that his arm " falls dead," there being no spasm in it, whilst the face of the same side is being convulsed. This, so far as I can learn, is a paroxysmal, not a post-paroxysmal paralysis, but possibly it remains for a short time after the convulsion of the face has ceased. I express no decided opinion as to the validity of the inhibition hypotheses. I think it possible that there may be discharge spreading slowly in a motor centre of the middle level,

[1] See Wood's *Therapeutics*, 7th ed., pp. 258–9.

excessive enough to cause slight after-exhaustion of some of its elements, although not one strong enough to overcome the resistance of lowest motor centres, and thereby to produce actual convulsion. I have spoken of " feelings of convulsion " in which there is no actual convulsion, but do not know whether there was any degree of post-paroxysmal paralysis of the parts " ideally convulsed." I go on to consider how far the hypothesis I hold, essentially that of Todd and Robertson, accounts for the facts of different cases.

There is exhaustion of the cortex after artificially induced epileptiform fits in some lower animals, as Franck and Pitres [1] have shown ; they use the term " épuisement cortical post-épileptique." They write : [2] " Le phénomène de l'épuisement cortical consécutif aux accès d'épilepsie partieille [what I call epileptiform seizures] est très facile à constater." The " épuisement " is transitory ; it lasts a quarter or half an hour. By artificial excitation of the part of the cortex in question, as the exhaustion diminishes, simple movements are first producible, and later epileptiform seizures, but not, for some time, is an attack provoked so intense as before the " épuisement." I think that the researches of these distinguished physicians countenance the inference I have drawn that the exhaustion in post-epileptiform conditions, although local, is yet widespread in the " motor region " ; that besides " running down " of the cells of the fulminate there is also running down of the collateral normal (stable) cells which were compelled by the fulminate to discharge excessively. Franck writes : [3] " Cet épuisement est tout *local*, non point qu'il se borne exclusivement à la portion circonscrite du champ moteur excité en premier lieu, mais il est limité à la zone motrice de ce côté." Exhaustion in the sense of general bodily prostration is not meant, for Franck and Pitres point out that excitation, without effect on the exhausted part of the motor region, when transferred to the motor region of the opposite hemisphere, produces severe convulsions.

I will here mention an objection to the hypothesis of exhaustion made to me by a physician whose opinion I respect highly, that during post-epileptic coma there may occur a convulsion affecting all parts of the body, which I say are then paralysed. But what I mean by paralysis in post-epileptic coma is loss of some most complex movements, represented by the highest centres of all or very many parts of both sides of the body ; there is retention of other most complex movements represented by those centres ; most of the complex (middle centres) and simplest movements (lowest centres) being also retained. Further, it is quite certain that an arm which the patient is quite unable to move in the slightest degree after an epileptiform seizure may be suddenly seized with another severe convulsion (I am supposing a case in which neither in nor after the paroxysm consciousness is lost). This, however, is only reasoning by analogy, and I admit that the interpretation of the last-mentioned case is to me most difficult.

I will now give an illustration of post-epileptiform paralysis. It may be taken to be an artificial one, but it is essentially that of a patient whose case I reported.[4]

A man, B., was *seemingly* (1) quite well when he arrived at my house after a walk of about a mile. (It is convenient to speak of this as the " first stage," not, of course, of the fit, but of the dramatic occurrence I am relating.)

[1] *Arch de Phys.*, 1883.
[2] Op. cit.
[3] *Fonctions Motrices du Cerveau*, pp. 90, 91.
[4] *Medical Times and Gazette*, February 12, 1881.

(2) (*a*) A fit began in the toes of his left foot.[1] (*b*) The whole leg was gradually involved, the spasm passing up the limb. In about eight or ten minutes the convulsion ceased, when (3) the leg was found to be (*a*) paralysed, and (*b*) there was exaggeration of its knee jerk and clonus of the foot. (4) In six hours or less he was *seemingly* well again, certainly he was then rid of his paralysis ; and next day (I did not test his tendon reactions before) his knee jerks were normal and there was no foot clonus. Let me consider the four acts of this drama.

(1) The patient was not really well when he arrived at my house. He had a persistent discharging lesion, presumably of a few cells of his leg centre (perhaps only of some of those of the hallux centre) ; so to say, he always carried it about with him, or, to speak more precisely, it was a persistent *quasi*-parasitical hyper-functionable part of himself.

(2) (*a*) The discharging lesion did function and that excessively, and possibly produced the initial spasm (of the toes) by its sole discharge ; but (*b*) next, as a fulminate, by overcoming the resistance of (discharging) other cells of the leg centre it compelled these normal stable cells to discharge—compelled them to co-operate in its excess.[2] So much for the discharges (primary and secundo-primary) of the cortex (middle motor centres). That there was a super-normal activity from cortex excessively discharging to and of the muscles of the leg convulsed is certain. The route of the numerous and rapidly succeeding nerve impulses from the hyper-physiological cortical process would be certain fibres of the corona radiata, of the internal capsule, of the crus cerebri, pons and medulla of the right side, then of fibres of the left lateral column (possibly also of the second and third sets of interconnecting fibres, both of which I shall ignore here) up to the anterior horns (some lowest motor centres) ; so far the second segment of the kinetic route is concerned. The resistance of the cells of these lowest motor centres would be overcome (secondary discharges), and the impulses (presumably increased in number) would then be of fibres of the nerve roots from those centres, thence of the continuing fibres of nerve trunks and their branches to the end plates of the muscles (third segment of the kinetic route) ; the resistance of the muscles would be overcome, and there would finally be great " explosive decomposition " of muscle substance (tertiary discharges).

(3) The paralysis signified exhaustion of nervous elements previously ex-

[1] Referring to the real case (op. cit.), the patient said that in all his seizures the first " sensation " was to the outer side of the ball of the great toe ; very likely I missed a very earliest stage, one possibly of spasm limited to the big toe.

[2] In the real case (op. cit.) the left arm was slightly convulsed. The current hypothesis would be that, in causing this part of the fit, the discharge spread from the leg centre to the arm centre. This I cannot disprove. Yet I think it an equally legitimate hypothesis that the discharge causing the slight movements of the arm in this case was of those elements of the " leg centre " representing subordinate movements of the arm. No doubt, of course, in a severer fit other centres of the motor region would be discharged. As implied in several parts of these lectures, I do not accept the current doctrine of localisation. The minute investigations of the monkey's cortex by Horsley and Beevor go strongly against it. To me the " leg centre " is only a part of the " motor region " where most special movements of the leg are represented, and where subordinate movements of the arm and of other parts of the body are also represented (the same, *mutatis mutandis*, for other centres). The researches of Sherrington (*Journal of Physiology*, vol. x, No. 5) seem to me to be counter to the current doctrine. He writes : " . . . After lesion in the leg area, encroaching little if at all upon the cortex of the arm area, the degeneration of the cord stopped short in great part in the cervical region, especially in the cervical enlargements. Again, after lesion in the arm area, encroaching little if at all upon the cortex of the leg area, the degeneration of the cord extended down through the dorsal into the lumbar and even throughout the sacral region of the cord." He suggests, however, that the fibres descending from the arm area into the lumbar region are visceral.

cessively functioning in the paroxysm. There would be exhaustion of cells of the cortex, not only of those of the discharging lesion, but also of those collateral stable cells which it, as a fulminate, compelled to discharge excessively. There would be exhaustion, too, of the fibres passing down from both sets of cells. The hyper-kinetic route, or at least part of it, would now be a hypo-kinetic tract. There would be exhaustion as low down as certain lowest motor centres ; these centres were therefore exalted in function (second degree of super-positive functional change), hence the increased tendon reactions.

(4) The paralysis had passed off ; the patient could walk well. Next day the knee jerks were normal. There was recuperation of the exhausted nervous elements. No doubt the cells of the discharging lesion (after the fit, stable below normal) began at once by gradual morbid nutrition to reattain high tension and very unstable equilibrium—" began to prepare for the next fit."

So far as I have seen, post-epileptiform paralysis is always most of the parts which were first and most convulsed in the preceding paroxysm, as in the case of the patient B. This correspondence is denied by some eminent physicians ; further observations will settle the matter. It is an important one, for according to the view I take, post-epileptiform paralysis adds no evidence to that afforded by the prior convulsion as to the seat of pathological changes in the cortex. If, however, there is not the correspondence I suppose, the case is very different and the situation is a most difficult one.

I think there is a relation of proportionality between the severity of the epileptiform fit (severity of the discharge) and the subsequent temporary paralysis (amount of exhaustion). I should have thought this a truism if it had not been expressly denied. It is averred that whilst after the epileptiform kind of seizure there is often decided paralysis, there is not, as a matter of fact, any whatever after the severer fits of the epileptic kind. I demur to the " fact," believing that whilst after a limited epileptiform seizure there is often great *local* paralysis, loss of *many movements* of a small part of one side of the body, there is after a severe epileptic fit *widespread* paralysis, loss of *few movements* of most, if not of all, parts of both sides of the body. Indeed, I submit that the whole condition of bodily impotence after a severe epileptic fit is paralysis, and that, speaking generally, there is really more paralysis than is found after severe epileptiform seizures.

The relation of an epileptiform fit to the sequent paralysis, or, more exactly, the relation of the two opposite functional states, discharge, and subsequent exhaustion, is not a simple relation.

According to the hypothesis I hold, there should always be some, however little, paralysis after an epileptiform seizure, at least some in the parts first and most convulsed, however slight the attack may have been. Trifling degrees of paralysis are easily overlooked. This deserves remark. Once more I urge that more or less paralysis from negative central lesions is always loss of more or fewer *movements* ; it is not to be thought of merely as *loss of power in muscles*. There may, for example, be loss of the most special (the most " delicate ") movements of the muscles of the hand with retention of other, the next special (the " coarser ") movements of those muscles. I will illustrate by a case of imperfect post-epileptiform paralysis.

After a slight epileptiform seizure starting in the hand, the patient may have difficulty in picking up a pin, and may yet be able to grasp strongly. There is clumsiness of movement, or perhaps some may say " loss of muscular sense."

These terms must not let us overlook the fact that the slightly abnormal motor condition of the hand is a double condition, one of two opposite elements. There is in the case supposed difficulty in picking up the pin, because a few most special movements of the hand are lost (so far paralysis, negative element); the pin has to be picked up by the next most special movements remaining, which are *now* the most special of the movements (positive element); they do not serve so well as the most special would have done; hence the operation is "clumsy."[1]

From such *quasi*-trifling paralysis as that indicated, loss of a few most special movements of the muscles of the hand, there are met with after severer epileptiform seizures beginning in the hand degrees of loss of next and next most special (or, equivalently, of the next and next more general) to loss of all movements of the muscles of it, and of some movements of the rest of the arm too; there is then no "clumsiness," for no movements of the hand remain to do anything.

The last remark introduces another part of our subject. It implies that post-epileptiform paralysis varies in a double way, (*a*) in degree (number of movements lost) and (*b*) in range (number of parts of which movements are lost). I think, in harmony with what was said in Lecture II, on compound order of spreading of convulsion, that degrees of difference between what may be called little and great paralysis after epileptiform seizures are not simple degrees of more or less amount of paralysis, nor simple degrees of more or less range; there are degrees of both, there are differences of compound degree. After the slight epileptiform seizure alluded to in the foregoing, there was slight paralysis limited to the hand. If that patient had had a somewhat severer fit, he would have had after it more paralysis of the hand (loss of more movements of it) and greater range of paralysis (loss of some movements of the next part, say the forearm).

That there was exhaustion lower than the cortex in B.'s case, exhaustion also of fibres of the second segment of the kinetic route, that is, up to the lowest motor centres, is signified by the exaggerated tendon reactions. I have spoken of the lowest motor centres and of the third segment of the kinetic route (fibres from them to the muscles) and of the muscles as not being exhausted in B. at the time when his leg was paralysed. It would, however, be remarkable if a few elements of these lowest parts of the kinetic route were not hypo-kinetic to some trifling degree after the hyper-kinesis during the convulsion—if there were not after their excessive exercise some exhaustion of a few of their elements. No doubt, being more strongly organised structures, the lowest motor centres and the muscles are less easily exhausted by the discharge, and, if exhausted, recuperate soonest of all parts of the route. After some epileptic fits (Westphal, Gowers, Beevor) the knee jerks are temporarily lost; in these cases some

[1] Here is an illustration of the principle of duplex symptomatology of nervous maladies, and that the positive element is often owing to activity or to over-activity of nervous arrangements untouched by any pathological process. The movements by which the pin is picked up are the outcome of activity of healthy nervous arrangements. To blame these, to speak figuratively, for the clumsiness of the operation is to ignore that they are doing their best in the evil circumstances. The principle is most important, if it applies, as I think it does, throughout the nervous system, from the symptomatology of a case of paralysis of an ocular muscle to that of cases of insanity; in the former case it is quite certain that most of the symptomatology answers to activity of perfectly healthy nervous arrangements of the highest centres; the negative mental symptoms in cases of insanity alone correspond to disease; they signify dissolution of part of the highest centres; the coexisting positive mental symptoms signify evolution going on on a lower level of those centres. The very same principle is displayed in cases of aphasia.

lowest motor centres, the lumbar nuclei (as Gowers suggests) are probably temporarily exhausted. For my part, I think it likely that during the post-epileptiform paralysis in B., although his knee jerks were exaggerated, there was some trifling hypo-kinesis of the lowest part of the route, that the hypo-kinetic tract was from cortex up to and of the muscles, although, no doubt, elements of the cortex and of the first segment of the kinetic route were most exhausted. The muscles in such cases act to faradisation (I did not test B. this way) as well as do those of the fellow leg. But if we were to take a case of paralysis, such as that of a man a few years ago under my care who had nineteen hundred and forty-five fits—each beginning in his left thumb, involving the left arm, fixing his chest, and turning his head to the left—in about fourteen days, and whose left arm was absolutely paralysed in the intervals, we might find by fine testing (what we did not find in that patient by ordinary testing) some slight degree of reduction of faradic reaction of the muscles, or, if not, of reduction of faradic or galvanic reaction in their nerve trunks, of the part paralysed. In B. the exaggeration of the knee jerk would not show that *all* the cells of the anterior horn which is concerned with that jerk were intact; a few of the smallest cells may have been exhausted.

In a case of amyotrophic lateral sclerosis there is wasting of some cells of anterior horns (hence the atrophy of some muscular elements) and increased activity of other cells of the same horns (hence the increased tendon reactions of the same muscles). This case shows that the functional condition of different cells of the same anterior horns may be diametrically opposite, and that the symptomatology in the muscular region which the horns supply may be of two correspondingly opposite elements. I shall put aside the hypothesis of exhaustion of a very few elements of the lowest motor centres, and of the third segment of the kinetic route, and of the muscles in such cases as that of B. for the present, but yet do not abandon it. I shall speak of the hypo-kinetic tract in such cases as that of B., as if it extended no lower than fibres of the lateral column, and as not involving any cells of the lowest motor centres in which they end. It would be reasonable to grant that it was at least of that depth in B.'s case.

It will be well to draw attention to resemblances and differences between post-epileptiform hemiplegia and the hemiplegia which is the result of destruction of the motor part of the internal capsule; for the moment assuming that the explanation given of the former is correct, and that the statements accepted by most physicians as to the latter are accurate. I will call the former Hemiplegia E, the latter Hemiplegia D.

First, for resemblances, taking to begin with, for comparison and contrast, *recent* Hemiplegia D. The regional (paralytic) affection is the same as in Hemiplegia E, and in each depends on a negative state of the same strand of fibres, those interconnecting the right middle motor centres and the left lowest motor centres. (I shall speak only of what I call the first set of fibres.) Now for differences. In Hemiplegia E (as in the case of the patient B.) there is exaggeration of the tendon reactions, in Hemiplegia D they are, we shall suppose, normal. Correspondingly for the negative lesions; in Hemiplegia E the negative lesion is of the whole length of the interconnecting fibres mentioned (and spoken of before as the second segment of the hyper-kinetic route become a hypo-kinetic tract) up to, but not involving, the lowest motor centres. In recent Hemiplegia D the negative lesion is quite local, a breaking up of the capsular part of the interconnecting fibres; the rest of the segment, its whole extent below the capsular break, being normal.

Now for *old* cases of Hemiplegia D; in these there are increased tendon reactions; in them a negative lesion secondary to the capsular one has been established; there is then a negative state (destruction) of the fibres (lateral sclerosis) below, and added on to, the local capsular lesion;[1] that is to say, in the case of Hemiplegia E there is established at once the state of things which only occurs late in Hemiplegia D. So long as the exhaustion lasts (so long as the central kinetic route is hypo-kinetic) in Hemiplegia E, the situation is the same as in old cases of Hemiplegia D; it is the same for the time being whether the nervous elements in question are functionally dead, as in the former, or actually dead (broken up and wasted away), as in the latter.

In a popular use of the word "cause," these negative conditions may be said to cause the increased tendon reactions, just as, popularly speaking, opening floodgates is said to cause water to flow. But using the word "cause" properly, it is an impossibility that the negative functional state in either Hemiplegia E or D can cause anything; a nothing cannot cause the something, the super-positive condition for exaggeration of the knee jerks. If Bastian be right in his conclusions as to the effect of absolutely complete transverse lesion of the dorsal or cervical cord (see Lecture I), the hypothesis of a change in the anterior horns, produced by any sort of pathological process, is no longer tenable, as he has pointed out. I shall, however, consider other arguments against that hypothesis, which are supplied by cases of post-epileptiform paralysis.

It is agreed upon that the increased tendon reactions in cases of hemiplegia depend on exalted "excitability" (a super-positive functional state) of nervous elements of some anterior horns. There are different hypotheses as to the process by which that exaltation is produced, and thus as to the exact state of the cells of the anterior horns concerned. Two questions may be asked. Is the abnormal condition of the cells the result of any pathological process involving the horns themselves, or are the cells healthy although in greater activity? I reply to the first question negatively, and to the second affirmatively.

I take, for further consideration, an old case of Hemiplegia D, one in which lateral sclerosis is established. And now I consider rigidity as well as increase of the knee jerk (limiting illustration to that one tendon reaction), both of which super-positive phenomena it is agreed upon imply exaltation of function of cells of anterior horns. One hypothesis as to the production of exaltation of function of the anterior horns (some of the lowest motor centres) is that the same process which leads to destruction of fibres of the lateral column produces, when come to the horns with which they are in physiological union, increased "excitability" of their cells; the same process, on this hypothesis, produces loss of function (destruction) of fibres and its physiological opposite super-function of cells. The hypothesis of Charcot deserves to be received with profound respect. Referring to the condition of the cells of the anterior horns, as it corresponds to rigidity in hemiplegia, he considers it the theory which best accounts for facts we daily witness in cerebro-spinal diseases, that there is a purely dynamic lesion of their ganglion cells—a state analogous to that produced by strychnine. If this state of the cells be produced by an extension to them of the same process as that which has destroyed fibres, it

[1] Sherrington has traced the "descending wasting" in the lateral column of the cord of the monkey as low as the coccygeal nerve roots.

(however slight the alteration affected may be, and however insusceptible of microscopical demonstration the change may be) must be considered to be the result of a pathological process.

This hypothesis cannot apply to Hemiplegia E ; in this case it is not likely that there are caused by the excessive discharge a negative state of fibres, and a super-positive one of cells. All the more that after some epileptic fits there is found exaltation of the knee jerk, and after others loss of it ; differences, explainable on differences in the severity of the discharge in the paroxysm, and on the different " depths " of exhaustion after it ; there is a negative functional state in both, but lower down in the kinetic route, of cells of anterior horns, when the knee jerks are absent.

My hypothesis is that both in Hemiplegia E and in *old* cases of Hemiplegia D the cells of the anterior horns are perfectly healthy. They are, I submit, untouched by the pathological process causing the lateral sclerosis or by any other, and are simply over-active, partly from loss of control, and partly from non-antagonised cerebellar influx (second degree (*b*) of super-positive functional change). But I do not state the hypothesis of loss of control as I used to do. There is sometimes exaggeration of the knee jerk in recent cases of hemiplegia, and this may be owing to sudden loss of cerebral (middle motor centres) control. I shall, however, speak as if the current opinions were correct—that both the increased tendon reactions and rigidity " wait for " the descending degeneration in cases of Hemiplegia D. I now adopt an hypothesis put forward by Gowers, which is to the effect that close upon the anterior horns there are small inhibitory centres, the anterior horns being, in his nomenclature, " muscle centres."

In cases of recent Hemiplegia D, before the degeneration in the lateral column, these local inhibitory centres are intact, and the knee jerks are not exaggerated. But I suggest that in such cases of Hemiplegia E as that of the patient B., they are exhausted as well as are fibres of the lateral column ; after those epileptic fits, when the knee jerks are lost, both the inhibitory centres and the muscle centres are exhausted. Now taking old cases of Hemiplegia D, and dealing with rigidity as well as with the exaggerated knee jerk, I would say that the " descending " process, when it reaches the anterior horns, destroys the small local inhibitory centres ; the anterior horn proper, " the muscle centre " now bereft of its inhibitory centre, in uncontrolled. The cells of the " muscle centres " are not invaded by any pathological process ; they are healthy, but yet over-active from loss of control. This hypothesis as to old cases of Hemiplegia D invokes but one mode of action—destruction. That hypothesis brings the facts of Hemiplegia E into harmony with those of long-standing cases of Hemiplegia D ; it accounts for the absence of increased tendon reactions in recent cases of Hemiplegia D. Certainly cases of Hemiplegia E have to be considered as well as cases of recent and old Hemiplegia D in all hypotheses as to the nature of increase of the knee jerk in cases of brain disease.

Of any degree of rigidity of muscular regions paralysed—during the paralytic stage or part of it I mean of course—after epileptiform seizures I know nothing. Possibly I have overlooked it. But Franck and Pitres have made very important observations on a muscular rigidity after epileptiform seizures produced in dogs and cats. Of course it might be said that this active muscular condition is owing to a slighter degree of the same cortical discharge which produced the obvious fit—that it is not post-paroxysmal, but a great attenuation of the paroxysm itself. But these distinguished observers tell us that the rigidity is altogether different from the convulsion in the attack itself. And what is decisive is that ablation of the whole motor zone does not cause disappearance of the rigidity.[1] It seems to me that the hypothesis I have taken from Gowers, exhaustion of inhibitory centres, and consequent over-activity of the muscle centres of the anterior horns to which they belong, best explains these phenomena.

Although beyond mentioning it I have not in this lecture spoken of cerebellar influx, I believe it to be a factor in the causation of the exaggerated tendon reactions in Hemiplegia E, and of these and the rigidity in old cases of Hemiplegia D—that in both there is loss of control and unantagonised cerebellar influx, and thus that the two positive symptoms are owing to the unhindered activity of perfectly healthy structures.

In some cases of epileptiform seizures at, or close upon, their onset, there is loss or, at least, defect of speech with very little local spasm. (We have, of course, no concern in this inquiry with any cases of *le petit-mal*.) I shall, however, speak only of temporary abnormal affections of speech, not in, but after the paroxysms—of what is present when all convulsion is over.[2] I explain post-epileptiform defects of speech in the same way as I did post-epileptiform paralyses, supposing there to be in the former exhaustion of nervous arrangements of " Broca's region."

Just as there are cases of epileptiform seizures with permanent paralysis of the side of the body in some part of which the convulsion starts and in which there is more paralysis, temporarily, of that side after a paroxysm, so in some cases of epileptiform seizures there may be permanent defect of speech and a temporary increase of that defect after a paroxysm. I shall omit consideration of these important cases. So far as I have seen, abnormal affections of speech are found after fits with right-side " signal symptoms." They certainly occur after left-sided fits, as Dr. Herman Weber has pointed out.[3]

I have only once known abnormal affection of speech to occur after a fit beginning in the foot (right); that case is of no particular value in localisation, as at the necropsy two large blood cysts were found, causing extensive compression of each cerebral hemisphere. Temporary defect of speech after epileptiform seizures beginning in the (1) right hand or (2) right side of face or tongue, or both, is not rare.

The " abnormal talking " after some epileptiform seizures has long seemed to me [4] not to be what could commonly be called aphasia; it often sounds like a *mélange* of an articulatory defect and of a speech defect. It may be that in these cases there is not only exhaustion of some elements of Broca's region, but also of elements of the corresponding lowest (bulbar) motor centres; if so, the situation is analogous to cases where, after epileptic fits, the knee jerks are absent, from, presumably, exhaustion of (lumbar) lowest motor centres. I think the " abnormal talking " referred to most likely to occur after epileptiform fits beginning in the cheek or tongue. What may be distinguished as " pure aphasia " is itself, physically regarded, a paralytic affection in the sense of loss

[1] *Les Fonctions Motrices du Cerveau*, by François Franck, pp. 88, 89.

[2] " There is a peculiar class of cases of epileptic hemiplegia in which the exciting cause of the epileptic fit at the same time damages or greatly injures voluntary power and speech " (Todd, *Nervous Diseases*, Lecture xv).

[3] *Transactions International Medical Congress*, 1881, vol. ii, p. 19.

[4] " Study of Convulsions," *St. Andrews Medical Graduates' Association*, vol. iii, 1870, p. 20; Reynolds's *System of Medicine*, vol. ii, 2nd ed., p. 287; see also Gowers's *Epilepsy*, p. 101.

of complex (" articulatory ") movements of the tongue, palate, lips, etc. ; so the *mélange* spoken of, if the hypothesis suggested be valid, is physically a mixture of loss of some complex (middle level) and some simplest (lowest level) movements of those parts. The subject is not a simple one, because along with right hemiplegia from destructive lesions we sometimes meet with a difficulty of articulation (I used to call it " ataxy of articulation ") when there is no obvious disability in the tongue, palate, lips, etc.[1] There is one thing which must be mentioned in this connection. We should not consider that the inability of a patient who is more or less aphasic after an epileptiform seizure to put out his tongue when told is evidence of implication of lowest motor (bulbar) centres ; for in these cases the tongue moves well in other and simpler operations. Moreover, this inability is often found in cases of aphasia from destructive cerebral lesions, and lasts too long in those cases for the easy explanation of " shock " ; in them implication of bulbar centres is out of the question. This curious symptom is loss of a most special movement from a cortical or sub-cortical lesion ; in that sense it is paralysis. It is no way regarded as speech or articulatory defect. To put out the tongue when told is what is called a " voluntary " movement, just as lifting the arm when told, or the card-sharper's shrug (p. 426, Lecture II) is.

I shall ignore the hypothesis mentioned, and deal only with cases which would be admitted by all to be defects of speech proper, that is, to be " of an aphasic character "—cases in which much speech of an imperfect kind remains, the utterances being clearly articulated. In most of these the prior convulsion starts in the right hand, and, I have thought, most often, not in the thumb or index-finger, but in the hand generally or in the ulnar fingers. Of course there are many degrees of abnormal affection of speech of this kind, and it varies according to the time elapsed since the cessation of the fit.

I have not observed post-epileptiform *loss* of speech, but only defect of speech (" partial aphasia "). I shall use the term Defect of Speech E, or Partial Aphasia E. The term " defect of speech " is equivocal, as is also the term " partial aphasia " ; it really covers two opposite elements, negatively loss of some speech, and positively retention of the rest of speech.[2] The patient gets words out clearly, and may even get out simple appropriate replies, such as " Very well," and may answer correctly by " Yes " or " No," or both. This is the positive element : it is the inferior speech to which the patient is reduced. But he is *not* able to reply correctly except by " Yes " and " No," and by other simple and very general expressions ; he is *not* able to converse properly on simple subjects ; he is *unable* to explain anything at all complex. These statements give the negative element : the speech lost. It is of extreme

[1] Dr. Charles K. Mills, of Philadelphia, relates, *University Medical Medicine*, November 1889, a very important case of " Softening of the Face-area with Oro-lingual Monoplegia."

[2] My present concern with aphasia is only a very limited one. I need not always supply the obvious qualifications to statements made in the text. The expressions " loss of some speech " and " retention of the rest of the speech " must not be taken literally as if they meant that the patient had lost certain words or propositions of the (his) English language altogether, and had retained the rest of them intact. Such is an impossible condition of things when an aphasic patient corrects his mistakes. But the statements may be taken literally for the mere purpose of a limited illustration. I do not suppose that there are fixed nervous arrangements—some for these words or syllables (properly movements corresponding to syllables) only and some for those only. I would rather than hold this mechanical doctrine go to the other extreme, and say that there are no nervous arrangements for movements in any centres except at the time when these and those motor nervous elements are functioning together in a particular temporary grouping.

importance to distinguish the two opposite elements of the symptomatic condition. It is plainly impossible that the post-epileptiform exhaustion (*vide supra*), which I suppose there is of part of Broca's region, can answer to the patient's utterances—to the positive element: that negative functional state of nervous elements of the region answers to the patient's loss of some speech. His utterances, positive element, however inferior as speech, answer to activities of nervous arrangement of Broca's region which are healthy—which are in all ways normal except possibly for slight "loss of control." Here is another illustration of the statement that part of the symptomatology of nervous maladies is the outcome of activity of healthy nervous arrangements.[1]

We must bear well in mind that speech is a psychical process. Nowhere is it more important to distinguish the psychical from the physical. I say once more that psychical symptoms are to medical men only signs of what is wrong in a material system. Our task as physicians is to ascertain the nature of the physical process correlative with speech, or more exactly the nature of the anatomical substrata of words (syllables). No one denies that the physical basis is of cells and fibres, but this is a morphological account of it. The anatomical basis is, I submit, of morphological elements so grouped as to form certain sensori-motor nervous arrangements. These, I presume, are audito-articulatory—that is, they are nervous arrangements representing certain auditory impressions along with certain corresponding complex (articulatory) movements of the tongue, palate, lips, etc. We suppose the *motor* elements of these *sensori-motor* arrangements to be of Broca's region. In the case of Defect of Speech E our ultimate concern is with the two opposite functional states of these motor elements which answer respectively to the two opposite psychical elements of the double symptomatic condition, which is unfortunately named (defect of speech or partial aphasia) after the negative element only. The motor elements alone of the sensori-motor substrata of speech are damaged. I submit that in Defect of Speech E there is, *correlative with* its negative psychical element, exhaustion of some nervous arrangements of Broca's region, which is productive of loss of some of the complex movements of the muscles of the tongue, etc. ("articulatory muscles"). And I submit that the speech remaining possible is correlative with integrity of other nervous arrangements of that same region for other complex movements of the same muscles; these healthy nervous arrangements function during the inferior speech remaining possible to the patient, and produce the corresponding articulatory movements. I have now to support the conclusion that the inferred exhaustion of some elements of Broca's region in Defect of Speech E produces paralysis in the sense of loss of complex movements of the tongue, etc.

There is often with Defect of Speech E some temporary decided paralysis of (loss of many movements of) the right arm. This statement, however, although allowable clinically, is not a scientific one. We should not in a realistic

[1] It is one thing to locate the negative lesion which destroys speech (renders a person unable to speak aloud), and quite another thing to say that "speech resides" in any particular part of the cortex. Words, or some other symbols, serve us during thought; when a man is thinking "gold is yellow," words in propositions are as certainly concerned as they are when he says that aloud. I submit that the highest centres ("organ of mind") must be engaged during speech, whether external or internal, notwithstanding that a negative lesion of a part of the middle motor level produces aphasia. Not believing in abrupt localisations, I do not mean by using the term "Broca's region" to limit the negative lesion productive of aphasia to that part of the lowest frontal convolution which enters into the "motor region." As is the custom, I shall neglect the concern which the highest centres must have with speech.

inquiry group together a psychical symptom and a physical one as if when so considered they were symptoms of the same order. In harmony with what I have said, the things really comparable are respectively loss of some complex movements of the muscles of the tongue, etc. (corresponding to the negative element in the defect of speech), and loss of some complex movements of the muscles of the arm (in both of movements represented by the middle motor centres). In this sense the two coexisting things are paralyses. On this basis alone is their concurrence intelligible and their comparison and contrast possible. With regard to the defect of speech, it is to be vividly kept in mind that the fellow part of the right middle motor centres (centres of the left half of the brain) for other complex movements of the muscles of the tongue, etc., and the right and left lowest (bulbar) motor centres for simplest movements of those muscles are intact.

Those who do not follow me in distinguishing the psychical from the physical will, perhaps, think that I am confounding difficulty of articulation, a physical symptom, with a mental symptom (with " aphasia "). The fact is that I am making an absolute distinction between speech, which is a psychical process, and its correlative anatomico-physiological process, which is purely physical. It is only the *physical bases* of words (or properly of syllables) which I assert to be sensori-motor nervous arrangements representing complex movements of the muscles of the tongue, etc., in association with complex combinations of auditory impressions. I only say that *correlative with* the negative psychical element in defect of speech there is the *physical loss* of some complex movements of the tongue, etc. Still, it may be thought that I have no clear ideas on the difference between aphasia, a mental defect and, for example, " bulbar paralysis." In reality I have said that the " bulbar centres " (some lowest motor centres) are quite intact in Defect of Speech E. In bulbar paralysis there is loss of the simplest movements of the tongue, etc., and the negative lesion is bilateral (of certain motor centres of both halves of the lowest level), whereas in all cases of aphasia there is loss of complex movements of the tongue, etc., and the negative lesion is of motor centres of but one (left) half of the middle level, and the lowest motor (bulbar) centres are intact. Is not this difference enough ?

The objection may be made that, whilst in the case of post-epileptiform paralysis with partial aphasia there is obvious paralysis of the arm, there is, as a matter of fact, none of the tongue, palate, lips, etc. It will be well in further exposition to stop speaking of Defect of Speech E, and to take in illustration a simpler (although much more serious) case, one of *loss* of speech (" complete aphasia ") from a destructive lesion, say from softening of Broca's region. I shall suppose, however, that there is retention of " yes " and " no."[1] Here the negative element is loss of nearly all speech ; the positive element being only retention of " yes " and " no." I shall call this case Loss of Speech D, or Complete Aphasia D ; but the word " loss " is to be taken as qualified by " except for retention of ' yes ' and ' no.' " We shall suppose there to be, as there nearly always is, right hemiplegia.

[1] To speak is not merely to utter words, but *to propositionise*. The patient spoken of in the text, although not absolutely speechless, is so, except that he has only the use of the two most general of all propositions ; I say " the use of " supposing that in the case taken for illustration the patient can assent and dissent by them. If he only uttered them at random, or if they were only signs of emotion, they would not serve propositionally, they would then be of no speech value.

To say that the patient Aphasia D is speechless because he has lost the memory of words is to give no explanation of his inability to speak, any more than it is an explanation of the paralysis of his right arm and leg to say that it is owing to loss of volition. All psychological explanations of physical inabilities are merely verbal. Admitting for the sake of argument only that loss of memory of words is a correct *description*, our concern as physicians is with the physical condition correlative with that psychical loss. A part of the patient's brain has disappeared, probably the hinder part of the lowermost (left) frontal convolution (and no doubt more brain adjacent) has been changed to diffluent stuff which is brain no longer ; we shall speak of this as " destruction of Broca's region." I repeat that the lesion causes paralysis. I admit that there is no disability in the muscles of the tongue, palate, lips, etc., in their commonplace services, as in eating, drinking, swallowing, etc. ; I admit it readily, because I only mean that there is loss of the complex articulatory movements of those muscles. There is nothing discoverably wrong with these muscles except for the slight facial and lingual paralysis which is a part of hemiplegia, right or left. The case illustrates that we may have loss of some *movements* of certain *muscles* without discoverable disability of those muscles. The seeming paradox in the particular case under remark is easily explained by Broadbent's well-known hypothesis.

In our speechless patient, not only are the lowest motor centres of *both* halves of the bulbar part of the lowest level for simplest movements of the muscles of the tongue, etc., intact, but also, what is most important, complex movements of these muscles of both sides remain represented in the right half of the brain (middle motor centres). Hence, on account of those remaining representations, there is no obvious disability of the muscles of the tongue, etc., in their commonplace services. Taking the simple representation by the lowest level for granted, the assumption is that the muscles of both sides of the tongue, palate, lips, etc., are represented by complex movements in each half of the brain, though no doubt more especially in Broca's region than in the fellow region of the right. Here is an exemplification of Broadbent's hypothesis. Horsley and Schäfer write : The *face area*, although we have so called it for convenience' sake, actually gives rise to movements not only of the facial muscles but also of the whole of the upper part of the alimentary tube (mouth, throat, and larynx). . . It is physiologically remarkable from the fact that many of the movements which result from its excitation are apt to be executed bilaterally, which is only exceptionally the case with excitation of the other areas (except that for the head and eyes.)"[1] Hence destruction of neither Broca's region nor its fellow part of the right middle motor centres produces disability in the commonplace services of the muscles of the tongue, etc., although beyond all question some movements of them are lost. But destruction of part of both halves does,[2] as some cases of double hemiplegia show, notably one recorded by Dr. Thomas Barlow.[3]

So that, so far from " confounding cases of aphasia with cases of bulbar paralysis," I am making a very definite distinction. So far am I from comparing loss of speech, considered as a negative psychical symptom, with the physical

[1] *Philosophical Transactions*, 1888.

[2] Such cases are sometimes called cases of cortical bulbar paralysis ; they are double cortical ; the bulbar centres are intact.

[3] *B.M.J.*, 1877.

symptoms of bulbar paralysis, that I urge that there is not even a basis for any reasonable contrast of the two ; psychical symptoms and physical symptoms are " not on the same platform." Regarding the physical condition correlative with the aphasia and that of the case of bulbar paralysis, the cases are alike in that there is in each loss of movements of the same muscles ; on this basis I urge their resemblance as cases of paralysis. At the very same time I urge the differences between loss of complex movements of the tongue, etc., represented by certain *middle* centres of but *one* half (left) of the brain in cases of Loss of Speech D, and loss of simplest movements of those parts represented by certain *lowest* (bulbar) centres of *both* halves of the lowest level in cases of bulbar paralysis.

Furthermore, the tongue, palate, and lips not only act well in eating, drinking, swallowing, etc., in Loss of Speech D, but also when the patient says " Yes " and " No." He may have a stock utterance, as " Awful," " Oh, my God ! " etc. He may when excited swear or get out other elaborate ejaculations ; none of these are speech proper—they are not propositions, but compound interjections ; the patient cannot repeat (" say ") what he ejaculates. The articulation of all these utterances is perfect, and I presume that no one would deny that the articulatory movements are effected by perfectly healthy nervous arrangements. They are effected, I submit, by those of the undamaged right half of the brain, of course with sub-agency of lowest (bulbar) motor centres of both halves. Still neglecting, as everybody else does, the concern of the highest centres with speech and with morbid affections of it in disease, I submit that as regards speech the right half of the brain is the automatic half, and that the left is that half in which automatic action ceases into what we call voluntary action.

The positive condition of our patient, Loss of Speech D, is that he retains the propositional use of " yes " and " no," physically two complex articulatory movements of the tongue, etc.

Now I draw attention to the fact that the patient who never speaks, never does make (with the exceptions stated) the complex movements of articulation, which I say are lost. Instead of explaining that he does not do so *because* he has lost " the memory of words," I submit that he never makes them because the nervous arrangements for those movements have disappeared—that he has not got those complex movements. Once more I urge that what is psychically aphasia is physically paralysis.

Moreover, the part destroyed in the case of aphasia is motor ; no one denies since the researches of Hitzig and Ferrier that the homologous part in lower animals is motor. Hence, there is nothing for destruction of it to produce in these animals except paralysis. Mark that although destruction of that part of the " motor region " on the left in man produces no disability of the muscles of the tongue, etc., of either side (beyond the slight right facial and lingual paralysis spoken of as part of hemiplegia), discharge of that part develops movements of these muscles of *both* sides ; by sub-agency, of course, of certain lowest motor centres of both halves of the lowest level, develops a contention of complex and of simplest movements of those muscles. From discharge of the part on the left are revealed the movements, the loss of which, upon destruction of that part, is masked by compensation by the fellow part of the right half of the brain. Yet there may be discharge (impulses passing by *route* of the callosal fibres) of the fellow part on the right consequent on the primary discharge of the left. I mention again that Sherrington has traced degenerated fibres from a unilateral lesion of the lower end of the fissure of Rolando into both halves of the pons and medulla.

Hence I conclude that the patient hemiplegic and speechless (aphasic) has not only lost very many complex movements of the muscles of the right arm and leg, but that he has also lost many complex movements of muscles of both sides of the tongue, lips, etc.; the conclusion is that his whole physical condition is, and is nothing else than, paralysis *in the sense of loss of movements*.

The condition is fundamentally the same in the Defect of Speech E, but the negative element (loss of some speech) is less, and the positive element (retention of much speech) is greater. Here, again, it will be well to illustrate by the case of a destructive lesion (a much smaller one than in Loss of Speech D), by softening, destroying but little of Broca's region; I will call this case Defect of Speech D. There is not rarely from such a pathological process a condition essentially like that in some cases of Defect of Speech E. Let us suppose that in the case of Defect of Speech D the patient frequently makes mistakes when he talks, either by using wrong words or by being reduced to very "automatic" utterances, such as "Very well," or that he often uses roundabout expressions, such as "It won't come out here" (which, eked out by appropriate pantomime, meant "I can't make water"). And yet, to simplify exposition, I will take the patient's saying "hat" for "carpet" only, that to be a sample of the whole of his condition. Here we see the necessity of distinguishing the two elements, negative and positive. It is certain that the softened brain (really what is brain no longer but a hole filled with detritus of nervous elements) cannot be the cause of the patient's saying "hat"; that is the speech left, and is owing to activity of the part of Broca's region which remains perfectly healthy.[1] This, his positive condition in speech, is sampled by his saying "hat." His negative condition is alone owing to "disease" and is sampled by his inability to say "carpet."

The negative element in Defect of Speech D is a minor degree of that in Loss of Speech D; the positive element is a major degree of the positive element ("Yes" and "No" only) in Loss of Speech D; in the former the dissolution of Broca's region is shallow and the level of evolution high, whilst in the latter the dissolution is very deep and the level of evolution very low, if there be any in that region. The two cases differ in double degree. In the Defect of Speech D there is much speech left, and there are very many mistakes; in the Loss of Speech D there is very little speech left, and there are no mistakes, the patient correctly assenting to and dissenting from (by "Yes" and "No") all statements made to him.

Now for the physical condition in Defect of Speech D. Answering to the slight negative element, there is loss of but a few complex articulatory movements represented in Broca's region; answering to the positive element there is retention of many other such movements; or we may say, limiting illustration to the samples, there is loss of the complex movements answering to inability to say "carpet," and retention of the complex movement answering to saying "hat." If anyone says that a word (properly a syllable) is not a

[1] To give another example, surely it is impossible that when the patient referred to in the text said, "It won't come out here," there was engagement of nervous arrangements which were "diseased" in any way whatever; the "disease" was the cause of his inability to say "I can't make water."

movement he is agreeing with me ; for I am contending that activity of nervous arrangements representing certain complex movements (with, of course, corresponding impressions) of the tongue, etc., is only the anatomico-physiological process going on during the appearance of what are the psychical things—words. I need only say that the softening in Defect of Speech D is the negative lesion equivalent to the exhaustion in Defect of Speech E. The utterances both in Defect of Speech E and D are the outcome of activities of perfectly healthy nervous arrangements. The negative lesion in both is dissolution ; in each the speech, however imperfect, as certainly signifies evolution going on on a lower level, as the speech of healthy persons does evolution going on on the normal level.

I have admitted that the patient in Defect of Speech E and D may correct his mistakes—that after saying the wrong word " hat " he may immediately say the right word " carpet "—and I will here admit that when he says " hat " he knows that the word is not the right one. But this does not invalidate the principle of the explanation. For convenience of exposition I made the arbitrary assumption that there are fixed and unalterable nervous arrangements for particular movements, in this case for complex movements of the tongue, etc., corresponding to syllables. I think the seeming difficulties could be met if, abandoning that assumption, I were to go into detail as to the constitution of nervous centres. At any rate, the attempt is to give a materialistic explanation of the physical condition in aphasia, without confounding the concomitant psychical states with that physical condition. I submit that the explanation is, at any rate, as good as the psychological explanation. If we do invoke the latter so-called explanation, we have not only to account for, to take the samples again, " loss of memory " for " carpet," but also for the " over-memory " for " hat." When the patient cannot say " carpet," why does he utter anything ? Why does " hat " come out instead ? And admitting that the " loss of memory " for " carpet " is only temporary, and that next moment the patient can say " hat," we have to account for the temporary defect of " memory " and for its sudden restoration for that case. Moreover, if the patient says " hat " and knows that it is wrong, he can only know it by there being revived in him the word " carpet " at the very same time ; certainly these two words must be revived mentally ; there is then " verbal diplopia." If it is admitted that the psychological statements as to the aphasic conditions are correct descriptions, those who make them are just as much bound as anyone else to seek the abnormal material conditions of the several phenomena of " amnesic aphasia." And bearing in mind the proof given by Ferrier, Horsley, Schäfer, Beevor, Sherrington, and many others, that the region damaged is motor, a merely morphological account of the physical condition in aphasia will not suffice. If anyone says that he cannot understand how activities of motor nervous arrangements can correspond to words, I would remind him that, except the popular psychologist, no one pretends to understand how any material conditions correspond to any psychical states.

# CASE OF EPILEPSY WITH TASTING MOVEMENTS AND "DREAMY STATE"—VERY SMALL PATCH OF SOFTENING IN THE LEFT UNCINATE GYRUS[1]

(WITH DR. WALTER S. COLMAN.)

## PART I[2]

IN this article are given further particulars of a case of epilepsy which I published[3] about ten years ago. I will call the patient Z. There was in this patient's slight attacks the "dreamy state" (commonly called "intellectual aura"). With at least some of his seizures there were certain movements of the mouth and tongue, tasting movements; these were, I suppose, the indirect "reflex" results of an epileptic discharge beginning in gustatory elements of a certain region of the cerebral cortex (taste region of Ferrier). After Z's slight attacks, or after some of them, there were very elaborate actions during "unconsciousness." The patient died, January 1894, from an overdose of chloral. Dr. Walter Colman found at the necropsy a very small lesion of the left uncinate gyrus. A report of Dr. Colman's examination of the brain will be found in the second part of this article.

### *History of the Case of Z*

I first saw the patient, a medical man, whom I call Z, in December 1877. He was then 26 years of age. He began to have slight epileptic attacks in 1871; they were so slight at first that he, to use his own words, "regarded the matter playfully and as of no practical importance." In 1874 he had a *haut-mal*, and then for the first time knew the evil meaning of the slight seizures he had disregarded. He afterwards wrote out for me an account of his case, which, with his consent, I published (*Brain*, Pt. xlii, July 1888, pp. 201 *et seq.*) (see p. 400). I may remark at once that there were no such signs of local intracranial gross organic disease (such disease as tumour, I mean) as optic neuritis and severe headache in any part of the patient's illness. I now give some details I obtained from Z in 1877.

He had that variety of the dreamy state I call "reminiscence"; he called it "recollection." In his slight attacks there was, he told me, a sentence in his mind which was as if well remembered. For example, if anyone was at the time speaking to him it would be as if he (Z) were trying to remember it, as if it were familiar, but yet he could not remember it. Again he said—I give the words I hastily wrote in my case-book, here intercalating other words in square brackets—"Attending to what was going on in [my] mind because [it was] interesting, and dim to what [was] going on outside." He could not,

[1] *Brain*, vol. xxi, 1898, p. 580.
[2] This part is written by J. H. J.
[3] *Brain*, July 1888, "On a Particular Variety of Epilepsy (Intellectual Aura); One Case with Symptoms of Organic Brain Disease." Case V of that paper, pp. 200 *et seq.*, is the case of Z. (See p. 399.)

on recovery, remember what the "interesting matter" was. (See p. 400, for further particulars of his dreamy state.) According to a report Z gave me in 1890, the reminiscence had disappeared, and from this report I gathered that he had had another kind of dreamy state with the reminiscence, and that this other kind occurred in his later fits. After the severe fit in 1874, in which he bit his tongue, he was subject both to slight and to severe attacks.

There was no evidence of any crude sensation warning of smell, taste, hearing, or sight, nor did I ever afterwards hear of any; there was no epigastric sensation. There was no vertigo. Although there was no crude sensation warning of taste at any time, there were certain movements which, I think, imply an epileptic discharge of gustatory elements of the cortex cerebri. I did not, when I first saw the patient, obtain any information as to such movements. He wrote of them as being, he had been told, "*something like a modified and indistinct smacking of the tongue like a tasting movement and is generally accompanied by a motion of the lower jaw* [italics in original] and sometimes by some twitching of the muscles round one or both corners of the mouth or of the cheeks, *but by no sense of taste in my recollection.*" (My italics.)

I ought here to say that several observers, one of them a highly accomplished medical man, who saw many of Z's attacks, never noticed any such movements as I have mentioned. They were very slight; in an attack (*vide infra*) which I witnessed, the noise made was only just audible. That they occurred in at least some of Z's slight attacks I do not doubt, because of the observation I made, and because he reported that some others had noticed them. It may be that the patient had, during the period this medical man knew him, ceased to have such movements. Z wrote to me, May 1890, a report in which, among other things, he says, comparing with previous years: "Although I have often asked observers to describe such a sound as I have made, and which in former notes I described as a smacking of the tongue like a tasting movement, I have not found it so described, but rather as some indistinct attempt to speak."

He had a slight feeling of dread. It was not a fear of the fit; the dread came first, and then the fit, or rather the rest of the fit. He said the fit seemed somewhat within his control; he made a rule when it set in to try to do something definite, for instance, to speak. He gave, as another example, that he once made an excuse to pick up a ball. In August 1880 he was still subject to slight fits. When a clinical clerk, he would have them in the wards of the hospital, but they were so slight that no one noticed anything particularly wrong. One medical man observed something peculiar, and so did several friends. Z was told that he appeared anxious to answer, but seemed to have lost the drift of the conversation—used in the connection some wrong word, and yet appeared to search about for another word. This is not very definite, but serves to show how slight the slight attacks were at that time.

In the remainder of this article I shall speak only of Z's slight seizures. I witnessed but two of them, and these I saw years after his first visit to me. In one he stopped talking to me, remained standing, and made slight, very slight, just audible (*vide supra*) smacking movements of his lips. I have no further details of this seizure; it occurred at the meeting of a Medical Society, and I had no opportunity of watching him throughout the attack. I knew that he was quite safe; no one but myself noticed anything amiss with him. On another occasion he was sitting in a room consulting me; he stopped talking—I have no remembrance of any smacking movements of his mouth on this occasion—his head was bent forward, but in a second or two, the paroxysm being then, I suppose, over, he looked up, and next (post-paroxysmal stage of actions) he leaned over one arm of his chair and felt about on the floor as if searching for something : next he did the like on the other side. Shortly, having a pin in his hand (how he got it I know not, perhaps from the floor) he made a feint of pricking my hand ; the action was as if in fun, for he stopped well short of my hand and was smiling. This little affair was exactly after the manner of joking with a child, as if one said playfully to a child, " Now I'm going to prick you," and smilingly pretended an attempt to do so. Z, however, did not accompany his playful-seeming feint by words. Soon, perhaps a minute, afterwards, his actions, or I should say the irrelevant-seeming actions, ceased ; he replied correctly to simple questions, and told me that it was not necessary for me to go home with him. He, however, looked confused and seemed strange. When we got to his house a few yards away, I thought he was fully recovered, and, as I was thinking of making another room on the ground floor of my house, I took the opportunity of speaking to him about a third room there was on the ground floor of his house. Among other things he said he used to breakfast there. I was surprised when he afterwards, next day, told me that he remembered nothing from the time of being in my room consulting me (before the fit) to a little time after I left him at his own house.

These post-paroxysmal actions during what we clinically call unconsciousness were as elaborate and purposive-seeming as any of those of his normal self ; such post-paroxysmal actions are very important in a medico-legal point of view. On another occasion there were post-epileptic actions by Z during " unconsciousness," of a kind which in a man fully himself would be criminal, and must have led to very serious consequences had not, fortunately, his condition been known. What he did was overlooked by those concerned.

In Z's report of his case (see p. 404) he speaks of examining and prescribing, when temporarily unconscious after an attack, for a patient. I now give a specimen of what he wrote—notes of a patient's case—in such circumstances. The words I have put in curved brackets were crossed out by Z : those in square brackets are my words. " For six or seven (years) weeks he has felt very discomfort of the throat and also for the swelling of the throat and (legs) arms and —— " [The word for which I have put a mark signifying a blank I cannot decipher]. Here is another specimen : " For the last few days his beginning (starting to walk ?) is more difficult for his tenderness of speechlessness and quick power of talk light swolleness of feet last three days." The words " starting to walk " in the brackets were inserted later. Here is another specimen with Z's remarks on it : " I had written the above [*i.e.* he had filled up the form for name, age, etc., of the patient] correctly and ascertained that the man had had gradually increasing œdema of the legs lately, when a *petit-mal* came on with no overpowering impression, or indeed any distinct impression that I can recollect. I wrote the words below [below the heading] slowly and with difficulty, wishing to be correct ; on reading them over they seemed to me correct ; but I could not go on ; I turned over the page and tried to describe the man, stared at him and felt too undecided to write more than ' A rather ' ;—could easily copy what I saw before me written down over the man's bed already as to the urine.

Altogether it took two or three minutes. I remained undecided and disinclined to write, but able to talk for five minutes more." This is what Z wrote on this occasion : " For about the last fortnight about the legs are about the gradual for several debts of the " (Z adds, " no connection in thought traceable for the word ' debts ' ").

Still one more specimen of Z's writing. He wrote the following in a state which, at the time, he thought was full consciousness, but afterwards knew to have been defective consciousness : " There [then a word obliterated] was constant repetition of sickness for the last twenty-four hours. Abdomen [this word crossed out]. The sick [a word like " neck," joined to sick, crossed out] on the grateful rightnessness has felt a large knowfulness." Z wrote down when well what he thought this should have been : " The sickness has left a painful feeling on the right side : she has felt much fullness there."

The following specimen of Z's writing (it was written as notes of a case) was not corrected : " For the last 18 mos [mos, no doubt, is for months] years there has been some decided indefinite on R. side in dress circle." Moreover in the heading of the case in the part for occupation he made a mistake—" Hairdresship " for, I presume, " Hairdresser." The patient was a woman, but this may have been for her husband's occupation.

For localisation of the lesion I relied entirely on Ferrier's researches. I say this not only because credit should be given to the right man, but also because, having said what I have said, I can without immodesty put some facts more strongly than I otherwise should like to do. Let the following four statements be considered.

(1) Ferrier found that certain movements of the lips, tongue and cheek-pouches follow on artificial excitation of a certain region of a monkey's cortex. From the nature of these movements he inferred that that region contains gustatory nervous elements—that the movements were " reflex " consequences of the artificial excitation of those elements. (2) I suppose that similar, or analogous, movements in human beings subject to certain epileptic fits, as in the case of Z at the onset of their seizure, are " reflex " effects of epileptic discharges beginning in some gustatory elements of that cortical region which, according to Ferrier, is for taste. (3) I begged Dr. Colman to call on me before he went to make the necropsy on Z, in order to ask him to search the taste region of Ferrier on each half of the brain very carefully. (4) Dr. Colman (see Part II) found a very small focus of softening in that region (in the uncinate gyrus) of the left half of the brain.

There was no trustworthy evidence to point to the half of the brain affected. Z wrote (*Brain*, July 1888, p. 204) : " I have no clear evidence that one side of the face is affected more than the other, and no clear evidence against it ; from what little I can learn, if it is at all unilateral it is more on the right side than on the left ; but the evidence is very scanty. I never notice it myself. I also never notice myself, but learn from others, that sometimes, especially if sitting, I give one or two light stamps on the floor with one foot, and in the only cases where this has been accurately observed it has been with the right foot."

There are many points for comment in Z's case. I refer to " Lectures on Epilepsy " (*Medical Times and Gazette*, vol. i, 1879, p. 295 ; *Brain*, July 1888) (see p. 385) for remarks on the group of cases to which this case belongs. In those papers I consider the dreamy state in its associations with crude sensations of smell and taste, and with the epigastric sensation and with chewing and tasting movements. In *Brain*, October 1889, (see p. 406) Dr. Beevor and I record a case of epileptic attacks with a crude sensation of smell and a dreamy state; there was tumour of the right temporo-sphenoidal lobe. In that paper Dr. Beevor refers to cases previously recorded of epileptic attacks with warning of smell. In the *Lancet*, January 14, 1899, I published a note on what I call the Uncinate Group of epileptic fits. I there consider the asphyxia in slight fits of some cases of this group, and suggest, having regard to some researches of Mr. W. G. Spencer (*Transactions of Royal Society*, vol. clxxxv, 1894 B, pp. 609–57), that the asphyxia may be owing to inhibition of the respiratory (medulla) centre by discharge spreading from a discharge lesion of the uncinate gyrus to the cortical centre for arrest of respiration; this arrest centre is close in front of the uncinate gyrus.

## Part II[1]

### Pathological Report

The autopsy was made thirty hours after death. The weather was very warm and damp. Post-mortem lividity was extreme and decomposition was rather advanced.

*Examination of Head.*—The scalp was unusually thick and firmly bound down to the periosteum. The *skull cap* was natural except for two symmetrical, flat, rounded elevations about half an inch in diameter situated on the outer table, on each side of the bregma. The *dura mater* was unusually adherent to both parietal bones, but not elsewhere. The surface of the pia arachnoid was normal, except beneath the bony prominences at the bregma, where there was some adhesion. Pacchionian bodies were large and numerous in this region, but inconspicuous elsewhere. There was no adhesion between the pia mater and the surface of the convolutions at any part.

Both hemispheres were fully convoluted, especially in the frontal and occipital regions, the convolutions following the usual arrangement. Their surface was perfectly normal in appearance, and the consistence of the brain was natural except in the left uncinate gyrus, where it could be felt that there was a patch of softening beneath the surface. On a section being made through the patch it was found to be a small cavity, collapsed and almost empty, with indefinite walls, situated in the uncinate gyrus $\frac{5}{8}$ inch below the surface just in front of the recurved tip of the uncus. The existence of the patch and its position were verified in the fresh specimen by Dr. Hughlings Jackson, Dr. Dawtrey Drewitt, Dr. James Taylor, and Dr. Guy Wood. The cavity was like those seen long after softening from thrombosis or embolism; there was no surrounding inflammation nor any indication that it was of recent origin. Search was made for an occluded artery in the neighbourhood, but without success. The other vessels of the brain did not show any signs of atheroma to the naked eye.

Unfortunately, the uncinate region became so soft and friable during the hardening process that it was impossible to make satisfactory sections, and the microscope did not throw any further light on the cause of the lesion.

The urine contained a small amount of albumen, and there were early interstitial changes in the cortex of the kidneys.

[1] This part is written by W. S. C.

There were many pulmonary infarcts apparently produced during the prolonged coma which was present for twenty-four hours before death, and the lungs themselves were extremely œdematous.

With these exceptions the organs were healthy.

A localisation of the lesion in this situation had been suggested by the presence of the "dreamy state" or "intellectual aura." In a paper read before the Medical Society of London in 1889 and afterwards published in *Brain*, Drs. Hughlings Jackson and Beevor published the case of a woman, 53 years of age, who had a tumour, the size of an orange, at the anterior extremity of the temporal lobe. During life she had numerous fits, with an intellectual aura and with "a horrid smell." A very instructive case recorded by Sander [1] is quoted in the paper by these authors. The patient had fits which were preceded by the warning of a "dreadful disagreeable smell," and he then had "*chewing movements of the jaws and spitting of saliva*." Later on he had convulsions about the face, but not in the limbs. He became very dull mentally, so that few subsequent observations on his sense of smell or of taste could be made. On post-mortem examination a gliomatous tumour the size of half a large apple was found on the under surface of the brain, at the junction of the left frontal and temporo-sphenoidal lobes. Half the growth involved the anterior part of the temporo-sphenoidal lobe, the other part reached across the fissure of Sylvius involving the lower convolutions of the frontal lobe. Inwards the growth reached the middle line.

[1] Sander, "Epileptische Anfälle mit subjectiven Geruchs Empfindungen bei Gerstorung des linken Tractus olfactorius durch einen Tumour," *Arch. f. Psych.*, vol. iv, p. 234.

# EPILEPTIC ATTACKS WITH A WARNING OF A CRUDE SENSATION OF SMELL AND WITH THE INTELLECTUAL AURA (DREAMY STATE) IN A PATIENT WHO HAD SYMPTOMS POINTING TO GROSS ORGANIC DISEASE OF THE RIGHT TEMPORO-SPHENOIDAL LOBE[1]

(WITH DR. J. PURVES STEWART.)

THE patient, A. B., a member of the medical profession, was 51 years of age, married, and of excellent health until three and a half years ago. He then had a severe attack of septicæmia, during the course of which an abscess formed in his anterior chest wall and required to be opened surgically. From that illness he recovered and remained well until October 1898, when he had a fresh septic infection in his right hand, which required several incisions. At that time his temperature was over 105° on several days and he was occasionally delirious. Since his second attack of septicæmia his general health has never been quite so good. There was no history of specific disease nor of any exposure to it. He never had any head injury, nor had he, at any time, suffered from otorrhœa.

Ever since his second attack of septicæmia the patient had been subject to occasional attacks of excitement, without sufficient apparent cause. He used to come home from his rounds in a state of excitement. His general manner became different; his memory also became impaired, so that on several occasions he forgot important appointments. On one occasion he called to inquire for a patient who had long been dead.

About eight weeks before he came under our observation he began to have occasional attacks of nausea and what he called "giddiness" with frontal headache. In these attacks there was a strong sensation of smell, which he described as being "like camphor or ether." This smell was succeeded by what is commonly called an intellectual aura (dreamy state), in which—to use his own words—he "felt as if he was saying, doing and looking at things which he had experienced before." He also stated that surrounding people seemed to have strange expressions on their faces, and that "people and things seemed to be far away" (he meant in physical distance). The average duration of each attack was about a minute; the patient's face, according to the account of a competent eye-witness of several seizures, one of which was very carefully observed throughout, was pale and his expression was that of one "facing an expected horror," but he was not apparently unconscious. No twitchings of face or limbs were observed. There was no vomiting either during or between the attacks.

After four weeks of such attacks, the crude sensation of smell ceased to occur, but there were numerous attacks, sometimes three in a day, of a slightly different type, in which he had nausea and vertigo. External objects did not appear to move, but the patient himself felt giddy, and he had a sense of fear and of

[1] *Brain*, vol. xxii, 1899, p. 534.

impending death. Occasionally, during such an attack, he became momentarily unconscious and fell backwards. His face was always pale during an attack, and his pupils were dilated.

He never had diplopia, though six weeks after the commencement of his "attacks," when lighting a cigarette one day, he applied his lighted match to the cigarette-holder, apparently owing to some mental confusion.

His headache gradually became almost constant, the pain being both frontal and occipital, but within a week or so before he came under our observation the headache became less severe, and he seemed rather drowsy. Three weeks before, his left foot was noticed to drag a little in walking, but he could walk fairly long distances until he took to his bed, a week before we saw him.

His condition, on examination on September 11, 1899, was as follows: he is a very intelligent man, able to answer clearly all questions put to him, though he seems somewhat drowsy; speech and articulation are normal. He can smell asafœtida and cloves in both nostrils, and names them. He can taste sugar and salt equally on both sides of the tongue, back and front. He hears a watch better in the right ear than in the left, and Mr. Ballance, on applying Weber's test, finds that the tuning-fork on the vertex is heard louder on the right side, all wax being previously removed from the right ear. The visual fields are normal on rough testing. There is no hemianopia on careful testing with small objects moved at the periphery of the visual fields, nor is there any obvious defect of sight.

On ophthalmoscopic examination there is found well-marked neuritis of the right eye, with + 2D of swelling; there are no hæmorrhages; the left optic disk is red but not swollen. The pupils are equal is size, and react normally to light and during accommodation. The external ocular movements are normal. There is no squint, no diplopia, and no nystagmus.

There is slight but distinct weakness of the left facial muscles, more marked in the lower than the upper part of the face. The left angle of the mouth is less energetically retracted and the left naso-labial fold shallower than on the right side. The left eye is less tightly "screwed up" by the orbicularis palpebrarum than on the right side when he is told to close both eyes as strongly as he can.

The palate rises normally on phonation. The tongue comes out straight on protrusion, but can be pushed better into the left cheek than into the right.

There is no anæsthesia anywhere on the face, trunk, or limbs to the lightest touches or pricks, but when the fingers of the left hand are touched and the patient is asked to point with his other hand to the exact point touched, his eyes being closed, he is several inches wide of the mark in every instance. There is no constant relation between the point touched and the position to which he refers the sensation.

The sense of position on passive movement is normal at all joints of the upper and lower extremities.

As to motor power, the patient can move all parts of the head, trunk and limbs as he lies in bed, but the left grasp is much weaker than the right. (L. = 30, R. = 63, with dynamometer.) There is no ataxia of the limbs and no tremor on voluntary movements.

The patient cannot stand alone; when supported he tends to fall backwards and slightly to the left side; in walking he scrapes the left foot very slightly on the ground.

The knee jerks are normal and equal. There is no ankle clonus. The right plantar reflex constantly shows flexion of the hallux. The left side is sometimes flexion, at other times extension of the hallux. The sphincters are normal.

The lungs and heart are normal on physical examination ; the pulse is 70, regular, and of moderate tension. There is a scar of an old abscess on the front of the chest. The abdomen and urine are normal. The temperature is normal.

To-day, for the first time, he complains of unilateral headache, and indicates the right temporal region as the seat of pain. There is no tenderness on pressure or percussion over any region of the skull.

*September* 12.—During last night the respiration was of Cheyne-Stokes type, and the patient passed urine and fæces unconsciously. To-day he feels better and talks with perfect intelligence. The headache is less severe. His appetite is extremely good, and he can smoke cigarettes. The left facial weakness is more evident than yesterday. The pulse is 72, respiration 20 per minute. The knee jerks are very faint, and can only be elicited by Jendrassik's method.

*September* 13.—During the night patient's temperature rose to over 100° F. He rapidly became comatose, and was observed to have occasional clonic spasms, confined to the left arm and hand. Death occurred at 1 a.m. from failure of respiration. The temperature at the time of death was not taken.

Unfortunately no autopsy could be obtained.

*Summary*.—To sum up the history of the case : the patient had gradually increasing mental dullness, followed nine months later by attacks of headache and nausea with a sensation of smell and a " dreamy state." Later the attacks changed in type. The paroxysmal smell ceased to occur, but there was occasional momentary unconsciousness. A few days before his death slight left hemiplegia developed, most marked in the face, without hemianopia or hemianæsthesia, but with some " cortical anæsthesia " of the left hand. There was some impairment of hearing in the left ear and optic neuritis in the right eye. Two days before death the headache became more localised and was referred to the right temporal region. The patient rapidly became worse and died from failure of respiration, slight jerking being observed in the left arm and hand just before death.

### *Remarks by Dr. Hughlings Jackson*

I saw A. B. with Sir William Gowers about September 9, 1899. We concluded that there was disease, probably tumour, of one temporo-sphenoidal lobe. Sir William, from the right-sidedness of the optic neuritis, suggested, before the setting-in of the left hemiplegia, that the right lobe was the one implicated. I saw A. B. again a day or two later, this time with Mr. Ballance and Dr. Purves Stewart. Mr. Victor Horsley also saw the patient. The question of operation was considered ; it was decided not to operate.

It is very unfortunate that necropsy was not permitted, but the case is clinically a very important one, especially, I think, as exhibiting the association of a warning of a crude sensation of smell with the " dreamy state," and with the emotion fear, in slight epileptic seizures. The notes were taken by Dr. Purves Stewart. Dr. Stewart will remark on the question of localisation of the lesion, on the olfactory and paralytic symptoms, and on some other points.

I have published a case somewhat like that of A. B. (*Brain*, July 1888, Pt. xlii, p. 191) (see p. 385), but unfortunately necropsy was not permitted; that case,[1] however, is one of great clinical interest. Dr. Stewart will mention other cases already published of epileptic fits with crude (warning) sensations of smell, cases completed by necropsies.

I have several times [2] written on the group of cases of epilepsy to which that of A. B. belongs; and have (*Lancet*, January 14, 1899), suggested for these cases the name of Uncinate Group of Fits; this was on the hypothesis that the discharge lesions in these cases are made up of some cells, not of the uncinate group alone, but of some cells of different parts of a region of which this gyrus is part—a very vague circumscription, I admit—the uncinate region. In cases of this group there is at the onset of the paroxysms a crude sensation of smell or one of taste, or there are movements of chewing, smacking of the lips, etc. (sometimes there is spitting). In some cases of this group there is a warning by what is known as the epigastric sensation, a crude development of a systemic sensation; this warning sometimes occurs along with a crude sensation of smell or with the chewing, etc., movements. Different varieties of this group of cases, depend, I suppose, on discharge lesions of different parts of what I call the uncinate region. As will have been inferred, it is supposed that especially in this cortical region, not confined to this region, are the physical bases of some of the systemic sensations—the physical bases of those systemic sensations which, to speak very roughly, especially appertain to the digestive system.

Many of the symptoms of even slight paroxysms of uncinate fits depend, of course, on discharges widespread beyond, some far beyond, the uncinate region—depend on discharges *secondary* to the *primary* discharge, that of the discharge lesion.

There is the dreamy state in the paroxysms of many, not of all, cases of the uncinate group of epileptic fits.

I hope soon to be able to write more fully on the uncinate group of epileptic fits. I shall then consider exceptions to the statements made in the preceding paragraph, and shall reinquire particularly as to the relation in slight epileptic paroxysms of crude auditory sensations to the dreamy state.

A. B. had only slight epileptic attacks, *le petit-mal*, and two degrees of them; in the slightest of his slight attacks he had crude sensations of smell and the dreamy state; in the severer of his slight attacks there was "unconsciousness" without the crude sensation and without the dreamy state.

The dreamy state in the uncinate group of epilepsies varies very much in different cases.[3] In A. B. it was the peculiar intellectual state which many healthy people or people slightly out of health have occasionally—Reminiscence. It is quite evident that in some slight epileptic paroxysms with the dreamy state —in all of them, I believe—there is a kind of double consciousness—a "mental

[1] The title given to the report of the case is a short summary of its symptomatology: "Epileptic Attacks with Crude Sensation Warnings, by Smells and the 'Epigastric' Sensation, 'Intellectual Aura' or 'Dreamy State.' Double Optic Neuritis. Attacks of Left-sided Tremor. Apoplexy and Left Hemiplegia. No necropsy."

[2] *Medical Times and Gazette*, vol. i, 1879; *Brain*, July 1880, July 1888, (With Dr. Beevor) October 1889 (see p. 406), (With Dr. Colman) Winter Number, 1898 (see p. 458); *Lancet*, January 14, 1899.

[3] I have said the dreamy state does not occur in the paroxysms of every case of the uncinate group, and I now say, too, that the dreamy state may, according to statements of patients and their friends, occur without any one of the crude sensations I have mentioned in the text, and without the chewing, etc., movements.

diplopia." In a quotation from Herpin (*vide infra*) will be found clear evidence of " mental diplopia " in several of the cases he mentions. I think, too, that there is probably some defect of consciousness in every paroxysm with the dreamy state ; certainly there is in some of them. The psychical condition, therefore, is a very complex one. There is defect of consciousness, so far negatively. Positively, there is (1) the quasi-parasitical state of consciousness (dreamy state), and (2) there are remains of normal consciousness ; and thus (1 and 2) there is double consciousness. To discover the physical conditions correlative with this complex psychical condition is a very difficult task. There was also an abnormal [1] emotional state in some at least of A. B.'s severer attacks —fear, *and a sense of impending death* ; in the slighter of his slight attacks there was an expression of " one facing an expected horror " (see Herpin, *Des Accès*, etc., p. 111, quoted at the end of these remarks). I have said (*Medical Times and Gazette*, March 1, 1879) that the epigastric sensation in epileptic paroxysms is often accompanied or quickly followed by the emotion of fear. Sir William Gowers thinks that this association is very rare. A. B. had no epigastric sensation warning.

We must not, in this part of our investigation of epileptic paroxysms, limit inquiry to the symptom fear ; we have to take heed of all departures from the patient's " ordinary state of feeling." And it must be well borne in mind that the departure in uncinate paroxysms is in some cases towards a more pleasurable, although more often towards a more disagreeable, state. Further, what is obviously equally significant, early in the course of a case of epilepsy the feeling in the slight paroxysms may be pleasurable, and, later, disagreeable—differences depending probably on the degree and rate of the discharge of the discharge lesion.

The symptom at the onset of A. B.'s attacks—that external objects seemed to be far away—deserves careful attention.

In, or before, or after some slight paroxysms of cases of the uncinate group, there are gastric or intestinal symptoms, or both.

To speak very roughly, much of the symptomatology of uncinate fits refers very especially to the digestive system ; the crude sensations, smell, taste, and the epigastric sensation are, to speak with brutal disregard of psychological propriety, crude developments of " digestive sensations." [2] In what, for reference, I will call Herpin's " third smell case " (*vide infra*), there were in the patient's paroxysms crude sensation of smell, abnormal intellectual and emotional states, and gastric spasm. The dreamy state, an abnormal intellectual state, is not a " digestive symptom," nor is an abnormal emotional state. But the occurrence in healthy people of gastric and intestinal states, things physical, along with the psychical states, pleasure and pain, is known to everybody (" bowels of mercy," etc.). The occurrence of gastric and intestinal symptoms in some cases of uncinate fits with abnormal emotional states is obviously significant.

[1] I say abnormal because, of course, I do not mean the natural fear of the fit itself, but a fear which " comes by itself "—the *symptom fear*.

[2] Although smell takes low rank as it serves as a " digestive sensation," it has very high rank in another way. It has been called the most suggestive of all the senses ; and smells have remarkable power in calling up remembrances of past scenes. We must, however, for several reasons, not be hasty in concluding anything from this with regard to explanations of the nature of the association of crude sensations of smell with the dreamy state in slight epileptic paroxysms.

I take this opportunity of advising the younger medical neurologists to study carefully Herpin's writings on Epilepsy. I have long known his valuable work, *Du Pronostic et du Traitément Curatif de l'Epilepsie*, 1852, but I have only recently heard of his still more valuable work, *Des Accès Incomplets d'Epilepsie*, 1867. I give, from the latter work, a quotation which mentions one case of the association of an intellectual aura (" dreamy state ") with a crude sensation warning of smell in epileptic paroxysms (" third smell case ").

Among three hundred cases of epilepsy observed by Herpin there were three, the paroxysms of which began by a warning of smell. In the report of only one of these three (I called it Herpin's " third smell case ") is what I take to be a " dreamy state " (" tristes souvenirs "—" un trouble intellectuel ") mentioned ; the patient's emotional state in her paroxysms, from the description Herpin gives in the words I italicise, was similar to that A. B. had (" sense of fear and of impending death ") in those of his paroxysms in which he lost consciousness. Herpin writes, *Des Accès Incomplets d'Epilepsie*, 1867, pp. 115 and 116 :

" L'un de trois maladies à début par de fausses perceptions d'odeurs perdait si vite connaissance qu'il ne pouvait que rarement avertir. Un autre sentait l'odeur descendre dans la gorge ; alors toute perception se perdait. La troisième éprouvait une sensation qui de la gorge descendait dans l'estomac où elle se convertissait en inquiétude et en tortillements ; pendant ce spasme, de tristes souvenirs assiégeaient la patiente ; *il lui semblait qu'elle allait mourir* ; aussi, quoique l'odeur fut agréeable, l'impression qu'elle en éprouvait (était) des *plus pénibles*, mais bientôt elle perdait ses sens.

" Dans les débuts par l'organe olfactif, l'abolition de la conscience suivait donc le plus souvent le prelude ; dans un cas, celui-ci était suivi d'un *spasme gastrique précédant un trouble* intellectuel pendant lequel la connaissance se perdait."

In the following quotation, from p. 140 op. cit., Herpin mentions a case so similar to the third case mentioned in the foregoing quotation from pp. 115 and 116, that I think it is the same case—that there is, in one of the two reports (pp. 115 and 140), some mistake in the words which indicate sex.

" De trois patients a début par de fausses perceptions d'odeur, deux n'avaient pas d'accidents moindres que les vertiges. Le troisième avait quelque fois de simples préludes ; la mauvaise odeur ne s'étendait pas au de la des fosses nasales (tandis que dans le vertige la sensation descendait dans la gorge) ; bientôt tout était fini ; il n'y avait pas trace de trouble intellectuel ; il appelait ces accidents légers ' ses mauvaises odeurs.' " In this third case (supposing it to be the same as the third case Herpin mentioned, pp. 115 and 116), the paroxysms were sometimes very slight indeed, simple preludes ; there were then crude sensations of smell without the " trouble intellectuel " ; in somewhat stronger slight fits there was the " trouble intellectuel " ; also—differences due to differences in the degree of " intensity " of the primary discharge, that of the discharge lesion, and consequent differences in the range of the induced (secondary) discharges of the normal nervous element with which the fulminant cells of the discharge lesion were connected.

I have several times drawn attention to the importance of taking careful note of chewing, etc., movements in the epileptic paroxysms ; they occur in one variety of uncinate fits, and sometimes there is, as in the other varieties, the dreamy state with them, and sometimes, as in the other varieties, there are elaborate actions during so-called unconsciousness after such seizures. There were no such movements in A. B.'s paroxysms.[1] I published (with Dr. Colman) (see p. 458) a case in which there were such movements in the epileptic paroxysms of a patient who had the dreamy state, small focus of, or relics of, softening in the left uncinate gyrus. As I have several times mentioned, I consider, in accord with certain of Ferrier's inferences from experiments on the monkey, that these movements signify—are indirect consequences of—epileptic discharges of cortical gustatory elements. I quoted an account of an epileptic paroxysm with these movements (machillement, etc.), *Lancet*, January 14, 1899, from Herpin's *De l'Epilepsie*, p. 275, 1852; there is in Herpin's report of that case no mention of a dreamy state. I now give a quotation from Herpin's other work, Des Accès, etc. I do so to impress on the younger medical neurologists the great importance of observing a symptom which at first thought may seem to be of little value.[2]

Herpin wrote (*Des Accès Incomplets d'Epilepsie*, pp. 150–1): " En étudiant les débuts des attaques, nous avons décrit les symptomes qui se lient a ce spasme (le spasme pharynge) sous les noms de machonnements, de mastication, de gustation, de déglutition, nous ne répéterons pas cette description, mais nous devons insister sur le fait *que ces signes sont précieux pour le vertige comitial qu'ils distinguent du vertige ordinare d'une syncope légere*, d'un faible accès hysterique, etc. [No italics in original.] Ces phénomènes sont, chez quelques épileptiques, tellement caractérisés et constants, que les patients, au lieu de donner aux accès incomplets dans lesquels il se montrent, les noms, en quelque sorte génériques, d'absences, d'étourdissements, de fausses attaques, etc., les appellent *mouvements de bouche*, *machonnements*, *machillements*, *rincements de bouche*." [Italics in original.][3]

I give also part of what Herpin wrote on " perturbations de l'intelligence " (commonly called intellectual auræ), which I call dreamy states. It is a pity that he did not mention the particular " hallucinations " some of the patients had; I imagine these " hallucinations " were what I call crude sensations.

" Pour dix patients le début consistait en des *perturbations* de l'intelligence, avec ou sans hallucinations. Des exemples peuvent seuls donner une idée juste de ces aberrations; une malade d'un esprit tres-distingué nous disait:

[1] Most neurologists will have read the report of a very remarkable case published by Dr. Mesnet (L'Union Médicale, juillet 21 et 23, 1874), a case of what he calls " Pathological Somnambulism." I draw attention to the words of Dr. Mesnet, which I have italicised in the subjoined quotation.

He writes of his patient: " Sa démarche est facile, son attitude calme, sa physionomie paisible; il a les yeux largement ouverts, la pupille dilatée; le front et les sourcils contractures, avec un mouvement incessant de nystagmus accusant un état de malaise, de souffrance vers le tête; *et un machonnement continu.*" There is no mention of a dreamy state, and it appears that the " machonnement " was not at the onset of the paroxysms only.

This case is remarked on by the late Prof. Huxley in an article " Animal Automatism " (*Collected Essays*, vol. i). The case has also been remarked on by Azam (Tuke's *Dict. of Psych. Med.*, article, " Double Consciousness "), and by the late Hack Tuke, in his work on *Somnambulism*. Huxley alone mentions the " chewing motion of the jaws."

Without expressing any opinion as to the nature of the case Dr. Mesnet reports, I may say that I have notes of cases in which after epileptic fits which began by chewing, etc., movements or by a crude sensation of smell, there have been post-epileptic actions of great elaborateness during so-called unconsciousness.

[2] I do not think, I may say here, that Herpin distinguishes between what we now call the epigastric sensation warning and warnings by gastric spasm.

[3] One of my patients who had such movements at the onset of slight epileptic attacks (no dreamy state, but a temporary very elaborate quasi-somnambulistic state after his seizures), in a letter to me, spoke of his fits as " champing fits."

'Il s'agit d'un trouble purement intellectuel ; je n'ai ni éblouissements, ni vertiges, je puis lire encore les mots, mais je n'en comprends plus le sens. C'est un des plus pénibles ; il me semble qu'une partie de mon intelligence assiste a l'égarement de l'autre.' . . . Un jeune prêtre de grande espérance s'exprimait ainsi : 'Ce sont des idées sans suite et cependant contradictoires ; si j'entends une conversation, elle me suscite deux idées qui se combattent ; je perds la tête et non pas la connaissance ; j'entends, je comprends, mais mon esprit est ailleurs.' Autre version d'un autre patient : 'Il y a en moi deux personnes dont l'une jouit de la raison et l'autre déraisonne.' Un épileptique parlait d'une idée fixe, toujours la même, mais qu'il n'a jamais pu se rappeler. Un autre mentionnait seulement un agarement de la raison. Une jeune personne d'un esprit tres-observateur racontait ainsi le début de ses attaques : 'Je suis prise, sans cause, d'une tristesse subite, et à l'instant même mes yeux restent fixés sur un objet et ma pensée sur une idée qui me rapelle l'image tres-nette d'un ancient rêve ; l'idée fixe m'absorbe tellement que, quoique je regarde toujours vers le même point, je ne vois plus l'objet'" (*Des Accès Incomplets d'Epilepsie*, 1867, p. 111).

One reason for giving these quotations is that some of the symptoms I have mentioned here and in other papers as occurring in some slight epileptic paroxysms, seem so odd that the reports of the cases may appear to some medical men more like collections of scientific curiosities than things with practical bearing. I wish to show by the quotations from Herpin that statements essentially the same as those I make were made by a great authority long ago. I will here quote from a former article (*Brain*, July 1888, p. 187).[1] (See p. 390.)

"Before leaving this part of my subject, I remark, by way of recapitulation, that he who neglects the 'dreamy state,' because it is indefinite and 'merely curious,' and such symptoms as chewing, etc., movements, and apparent alteration in the size and distance of external objects, because they seem trifling things, may not even surmise that his patient has the serious disease, epilepsy, in a rudimentary form, until a severe fit comes to tell him so."

*Remarks by Dr. Purves Stewart*

In the above case the history of gradual mental impairment followed by attacks of unconsciousness, together with the presence of headache, of optic neuritis, and of slight hemiplegia, pointed to the existence of gross intracranial disease. The left-sided weakness, most marked in the face, but also distinct in the arm and leg, indicated clearly as the site of the lesion some part of the motor tract, or of its vicinity, in the right cerebral hemisphere. The absence of hemianæsthesia and of hemianopia showed that the lesion was probably not in the neighbourhood of the internal capsule, but that it was situated more towards the cortex of the brain, a view which was strengthened by the presence of "cortical anæsthesia" of the left hand. The occurrence of Babinski's extensor plantar reflex—extension of the hallux instead of the normal flexion on tickling the sole of the foot—was not sufficiently constant to be of much significance.

The peculiar nature of the paroxysms, and especially their association with a sensation of smell, pointed to some abnormal condition of the temporo-sphenoidal lobe.

[1] "On a Particular Variety of Epilepsy ('Intellectual Aura'): One Case with Symptoms of Organic Brain Disease."

Drs. Hughlings Jackson and Beevor[1] (see p. 406) record the case of a sarcoma, the size of a tangerine orange, situated at the most anterior extremity of the right temporo-sphenoidal lobe. During life the patient had left hemiplegia without hemianopia, hemianæsthesia, or affection of smell, taste, or hearing. She also had numerous fits with an "intellectual aura" and a "horrid smell of dirty burning stuff."

Drs. Hughlings Jackson and Colman[2] (see p. 458) also record a case of a small subcortical patch of softening in the left uncinate gyrus. The patient had been subject to epileptic attacks accompanied by a "dreamy state," with smacking movements of tongue, lips and jaw, but without crude sensations of taste or smell.

Dr. James Anderson[3] published a case of a large basal cystic sarcoma arising from the pituitary body and spreading into the left temporo-sphenoidal lobe. It had given rise to attacks of peculiar sensation in the right hand, preceded by a sensation of a bitter taste in the mouth, with occasionally also a peculiar smell, and accompanied by the "dreamy state." There were never any chewing or smacking movements of the lips. Smell was impaired on the left side, and there was slight defect of taste on both sides, especially the left. From affection of the left optic nerve, optic chiasma, and optic tract, the patient had blindness of the left eye with temporal hemianopia in the right.

Mr. Nettleship[4] also records a case of tumour of the pituitary body implicating the left optic nerve, chiasma, and tract, as well as the left temporo-sphenoidal lobe. In that case there had been paroxysmal sensations of suffocation in the nose and mouth. There is no mention of a dreamy state in that case.

Sanders[5] records a case of a large glioma on the under surface of the brain, involving the anterior part of the left temporo-sphenoidal lobe and the lower convolutions of the left frontal lobe, and destroying the left olfactory tract. The patient had fits, preceded by a warning of a "dreadful disagreeable smell," also chewing movements of the jaw and spitting of saliva. Later he had convulsions affecting the face, but not the limbs. No dreamy state was recorded in that case.

Dr. McLane Hamilton[6] also published a case of a localised chronic pachymeningitis affecting the right uncinate gyrus and part of the adjacent convolutions, but without involvement of the olfactory bulbs. The patient had been subject to attacks, preceded by a peculiar disagreeable odour, either of smoke or of a fœtid character. No mention was made of any dreamy state.

In our case of A. B. the view as to the localisation of the disease in the right temporo-sphenoidal lobe was further supported by the impairment of hearing in the left ear without any discoverable cause in the ear itself, and, therefore, possibly referable to some slight affection of Ferrier's auditory centre on the side of the lesion.

The slight "cortical anæsthesia," the slight hemiplegia, most marked in the face, together with the occurrence of localised fits in the left arm and hand before death, are facts which, so far as they go, indicate either that the lesion

[1] *Brain*, vol. xii, 1889, pp. 346–7.
[2] Ibid., vol. xxi, 1898, pp. 580–90.
[3] Ibid., vol. viii, 1886.
[4] *Ophth. Society Transactions*, vol. iv, p. 285.
[5] *Arch. f. psychiat.*, vol. iv, 1874, p. 234.
[6] *New York Medical Journal*, vol. xxxv, 1882, p. 575.

was not confined to the temporo-sphenoidal lobe alone, and extended to the lower central convolutions so as to affect the face and arm centres, or, more probably, that it pressed upwards in that direction.

The absence of an autopsy unfortunately leaves undetermined the exact nature and limits of the lesion. On the whole, the slow course and progressive march of the symptoms indicate that it was a new growth of some sort. The history of septicæmia rendered it conceivable that a chronic abscess might have been present. Mr. Ballance informs us that he had known a brain abscess to lie latent for fifteen months after an attack of septicæmia, without previous otorrhœa or other apparent local exciting cause, at the end of which period symptoms appeared for the first time, and rapidly proved fatal. But in A. B.'s case the symptoms were those of a lesion involving not only the temporo-sphenoidal, but also the lower central region, and this with very slight motor weakness, less in amount than an abscess of such size would have been likely to produce. It is, therefore, more probable that there was an infiltrating growth involving the temporo-sphenoidal lobe and the adjacent part of the "central" region. This, however, is mere hypothesis, and the absence of an autopsy is much to be regretted.

Amongst other points of interest in the case is the unilateral optic neuritis present on the side of the cerebral lesion. Mr. Marcus Gunn,[1] in a discussion on the diagnosis of brain tumours, states that unilateral, or preponderatingly unilateral, neuritis is, on the whole, in favour of the tumour being on the same side as that on which the neuritis is more intense, if other reasons exist for localising the tumour far forward in the brain. Our patient's case, so far as it goes, seems to bear out Mr. Gunn's views. But the rule is not an invariable one, for I have seen a case of a large frontal tumour in which the optic neuritis was both earlier and more intense on the opposite side from the lesion.

The remarkably large appetite, which our patient exhibited up to the last, is of interest when considered with a case of temporo-sphenoidal abscess and a series of cases of head injuries published by Mr. Stephen Paget,[2] in which voracious hunger and thirst were outstanding symptoms.

[1] *Brain*, vol. xxi, 1898, p. 337.

[2] *Essays for Students*, 1899, pp. 92–100.

# OBSERVATIONS OF A CASE OF CONVULSIONS (TRUNK FIT OR LOWEST LEVEL FIT)[1]

(With Dr. Douglas Singer.)

The following case is of interest from two points of view: (1) the association of " epileptic fits " with congenital syphilis, and (2) the kind of convulsion. That the convulsions occurred in a patient the subject of inherited syphilis is, of course, of great importance. It does not, however, necessarily follow that the patient's attacks were owing, directly or indirectly, to syphilitic changes in some part of her nervous system. In this paper we remark almost solely on the patient's fits.

The state of the respiratory apparatus in " epileptic " paroxysms has received little special attention, even in cases of so-called cortical (Bravais) epilepsy fixation of the chest may be overlooked. In a case of this kind of epilepsy observed by one of us there was—along with the convulsion starting in one hand and affecting the whole of the arm, with turning of the head and eyes to the same side—complete fixation of both sides of the chest; this occurred in paroxysms of the range mentioned, during which the patient was not unconscious.

One of us (J. H. J.) has suggested that, besides what are commonly called epileptic fits, there occur, in the human subject, bulbo-pontal (lowest level) fits, analogous to those experimentally produced in some lower mammals. With regard to proving or disproving this hypothesis, it is, among other things, particularly important to note where the first spasm is, or what the very first symptoms are. Are there seizures, such as would be commonly called epileptic, which *begin by* fixation of the chest, or in which the chest is involved before

[1] *Brain*, vol. xxv, 1902, p. 122.
The above note in Dr. Jackson's writing and signed with his initials is on the reprint of the paper from *Brain* which is in the Editor's possession.

the limbs, if these are involved in the seizures ; or, speaking more generally, are there fits which begin by convulsion of respiratory muscles ?

The case we are about to report is an example of fits of this sort ; it is clear that, in many of this patient's attacks, the first symptoms were involvement of muscles of both sides of the neck (back and front), soon followed by fixation of both sides of the chest. The neck muscles may have been engaged by discharge of central nervous arrangements representing them as they serve respiratorily—that is to say, as they serve in difficult respiration. And, what is particularly significant, in many of this patient's attacks, those during what we shall call the First Period, the limbs were not affected at all, although the trunk muscles of both sides were strongly engaged. Were this patient's attacks bulbo-pontal fits ? There is another possibility : the seizures may have been owing to a discharge lesion of some part of Horsley and Schäfer's trunk centres. There is yet another possibility. Recently Sherrington and Grünbaum have discovered, in the chimpanzee, a trunk centre in the external surface of the Rolandic cortex, between the arm area and the leg area. They write (*British Medical Journal*, December 28, 1901), that they " find between the representation of shoulder and hip an area which, next to the shoulder, yields unilateral movement of the chest muscles, and, next to the hip, yields unilateral movement of the abdominal muscles." If there be a trunk centre in the Rolandic region of the human brain, the discharge lesion in our patient may have been of some elements of it. It is true that the movements Sherrington and Grünbaum produced were unilateral, but possibly an intense (" an epileptic ") discharge beginning in their Rolandic trunk centre of but one half of the brain might produce bilateral convulsion of the parts they mention.

There are difficulties in the way of each of the hypotheses we have stated ; we prefer, whilst giving in great detail particulars of the attacks our patient had, to refrain from speculations on the localisation of the lesion causing them. We may, however, say what the question is.

It is of little moment whether the fits are to be labelled " epileptic " or not. Admitting that the slight fits (*vide infra* 4) in which there was movement of the eyes and no fixation of the chest, offer a difficulty, the question as to the severe fits is, " Where is the lesion (discharge lesion) which, on its occasional " intense " discharge, produces a convulsion *beginning* in muscles of the trunk (that is, in muscles of two sides of the body, the normal action of which may be and often is bilateral) and beginning in those muscles of the two sides of the body simultaneously—a convulsion in some paroxysms (first period) not involving the limbs at all, and in others (second period) involving both arms *after* the trunk, involving these limbs simultaneously ; also, what is very significant, involving the muscles of the arms from above downwards, thoracico-humeral muscles to those of the hand.

We have considered it advisable to describe the fits under two headings, for two periods, because as the seizures diminished in number they became modified in character. We wish particularly to lay stress upon this division, because, although there were some slighter fits of somewhat different nature common to both periods, no attacks such as those which formed the main feature of the Second Period occurred as far as our observations went, and they were numerous, in the First Period. The following order will be followed : (1) The history of the case ; (2) the results of the general examination of the patient ; (3) a description of the fits occurring in the First Period ; (4) a description of the slighter attacks occurring in both periods ; (5) an account of the seizures in the Second Period.

## (1) History

J. K., aged 17, is the eldest of a family of nine. Her father, mother, brothers and sisters are all living and healthy ; the mother had no miscarriages until the last nine months, during which time she has had two. Most of the children are said to have a " narrow bridge " to the nose and several of them had snuffles in infancy, but none of them, as far as the mother can remember, had any rash. None have had any troubles with their eyes.

The patient was born at full term and without instrumental help ; she had snuffles, but no rash as an infant ; she has always had a squint which is said to have been worse since the onset of the fits. She was backward in walking, not beginning to do so until 3 years old, but she began to talk at the same age as her brothers and sisters, *viz.* 12 months. She has suffered from whooping cough, measles and scarlet fever. During the first dentition for about two years she had " teething convulsions " at intervals, in which she is said to have been quite quiet and " looking dead " ; there were never any twitchings in these attacks.

The present illness began at the age of 9 years ; the fits at first occurred about once a month, gradually increasing in frequency at the onset of puberty at the age of 15 years, to about one a week. After this they rapidly increased in number up to several daily. In March 1901 she was in a condition of *status epilepticus* for ten days, followed by a period of complete freedom from fits for a month ; after this time the fits again increased in number until four days before she came under our observation on December 20, 1901, when she once more passed into *status epilepticus.*

## (2) General Examination

When first seen she was having a fit about every ten minutes, with recovery of consciousness but not of much mental power in the intervals. The general examination was not completed until December 22, the time being devoted to the observation of her fits. At this time she had had no fit for half an hour and would obey simple orders and answer simple questions. She was, however, extremely fatuous, with very bad memory, and had difficulty in fixing her attention.

She is dark, with muddy, coarse skin ; the forehead is large, square and overhanging, the bridge of the nose flattened and the nostrils thick and snub. The lips are coarse, thick and habitually parted, the upper teeth projecting over the lower lip. The lower part of the face is thin with pointed chin and forms a striking contrast to the large forehead. She breathes habitually through the mouth, but can blow down her nose. The tonsils are not enlarged and neither they nor the fauces show any scars of past ulceration. The palate presents a high, narrow arch. The left upper median incisor tooth shows a well-marked notch and narrows gradually from base to cutting edge (the kind of teeth described long ago by Hutchinson). The pupils are large, equal, and react to light and in convergence ; they dilate well under homatropine and show no iritic adhesions. There is a well-marked convergent strabismus due to weakness of the right external rectus muscle ; Mr. Marcus Gunn agreed with us in this observation and inference. The fundi were examined under a mydriatic by Mr. Gunn after the fits had ceased. He reported as follows : " The corneæ are hazy and there are remains of vessels running into both—undoubted evidence of old interstitial keratitis. The fundi show numerous patches of choroidal atrophy of typical syphilitic nature, and the optic disks show the usual atrophy secondary to that condition of the choroid."

The patient's *power* generally is feeble, but except for the weakness of the right external rectus muscle there is no paralysis and certainly no unilateral weakness, all *movements* are present and well co-ordinated. *Respiration* is of the type normal in her sex—that is to say, her inspiration is mainly upper thoracic ; there is some widening of the costal angle and slight protrusion of the abdominal wall. In the act of drawing a deep breath, that is, when told to do so, the movement is mainly upper thoracic at first, the sterno-mastoids being used ; but towards the end of this voluntary act the diaphragm descends and the abdominal walls are pushed forward. *Sensation* appears to be normal in every way. The knee jerks, when the patient was first seen, were well marked but not exaggerated, equal on the two sides, but when examined two days later and at some considerable time after a fit, they were obtained only with difficulty ; this was also the case after complete cessation of the fits for three weeks. There was no ankle or rectus clonus. The *plantar reflexes*, both feet, were definitely extensor in type, but after complete cessation of the *status epilepticus* they were flexor in character. The *feet* show a high arch with some extension at the metatarso-phalangeal joints and flexion of the distal joints. This was said by the mother, in answer to questions, to have always been the same.

The *lungs* showed no sign of disease ; it was particularly observed that there was no emphysema and no deformity of the chest. The heart sounds were everywhere clear and without murmurs, but tended to approximate to the fœtal type, that is to say, the character of the two sounds were very similar and the intervals were nearly equal. The *pulse* was regular, soft and easily compressible, its rate being about 100. Nothing abnormal was found on examination of the abdomen.

### (3) Fits occurring in the First Period

The duration of each fit was very brief, and their frequency being very great, particular attention was paid to different points in different seizures. We shall first give accounts of some of the individual attacks copied almost verbatim from the notes made immediately after each observation, and shall then describe an attack compounded from the notes taken of numerous fits.

#### *Descriptions of Individual Fits*

(1) At the moment when first noticed there was tonic spasm of the muscles of the neck on both sides, back and front, of the jaws and of both sides of the face, while the thorax was fixed in a position of partial expiration. The jaws were separated so that there was an interval of about half an inch between the teeth while both masseters and both mylo-hyoid muscles could be felt to be firmly contracted, contending against one another. The eyebrows were raised and the eyes, still maintaining the convergent strabismus noted above, were directed upwards. After a few seconds the tonic was replaced by clonic spasm affecting the whole face (the angle of the mouth being drawn a little more to

the left than to the right), also the muscles of mastication, the sterno-mastoids, and the muscles at the back of the neck on both sides. Here is to be mentioned a point of great importance. *No movement or spasm of any kind occurred in the arms ; they remained quite flaccid and loose.* The legs were not specially observed in this fit, but there was no obvious movement. As the fit passed off several deep inspirations were taken. Immediately afterwards the patient was asked to draw in her breath voluntarily, but appeared not to understand, and merely replied, " Yes, thank you."

(2) This fit began while I (H. D. S.) was auscultating the chest, and consequently it was observed from the beginning. The stethoscope was retained over the heart and attention was also directed more particularly to the face and neck. The patient was lying at the time on her back with her head turned to the left. The first motion consisted in a slow rotation of the head to the middle position with a little drawing down of the occiput by the muscles at the back of the neck, whilst at the same time both sterno-mastoids were seen to stand out prominently. Almost at the same moment, but I think a little later, the face muscles were contracted in tonic spasm, the eyebrows raised, the angles of the mouth were retracted a little, somewhat more to the left than to the right. The eyes, with the convergent strabismus still present, were rotated upwards, the right being mesial while the left was rotated inwards. The teeth were separated by about three-quarters of an inch, the jaws were rigidly fixed and the mylo-hyoid muscles were felt to be firmly contracted. The tongue could be seen and did not appear to be contracted in tonic spasm, and certainly was not involved in clonic spasm later.

*Respiration* had ceased from the time the earliest motion was observed ; and as the head moved round towards the middle line, a moaning noise was produced by, as proved by holding the hand in front of the nose and mouth, air being forced out of the chest.

After a few seconds clonic spasms replaced the tonic contraction in all the affected muscles, *viz.*, face, neck and mylo-hyoids ; at this time air was sucked into the chest with a grunting noise, as if through an almost closed glottis, by each clonic jerk. The spasm in the thoracic muscles then ceased and several deep breaths in succession were taken. The clonic spasms of the face and jaw muscles continued for a few seconds after the onset of the deep breathing and ceased last in the orbiculares palpebrarum and the frontales muscles.

The heart sounds were listened to occasionally through the binaural stethoscope ; at the height of the tonic stage, just before the clonic spasms began, the heart was beating at a rate which I (H. D. S.) estimated at 60 per minute. When counted shortly before the fit the pulse rate was 102 per minute. When the clonic spasms began the noise of the contracting muscles and of the indrawing of the breath prevented the heart sounds from being heard, but immediately after the fit the rate was 120 per minute. The arms and legs were not watched in this attack.

(3) The patient was lying on her right side apparently asleep. As I (H. D. S.) approached the bed there was a slow conjugate movement of the head and eyes to the left. The limbs being covered nothing could be seen of any movement or spasm, but through the clothes there did not appear to be any movement of them. The corneal reflexes were present when I (H. D. S.) reached her and the head slowly came back to the original position and the patient began to mutter inarticulate sounds. A few seconds later one of the

attacks similar to those described above began. Attention was at once directed to the pulse and to the erector spinæ muscles, which could easily be observed as she was lying on her right side. At the moment of feeling the *pulse* the tension seemed higher than when examined at other times and it distinctly increased, while the pulse rate became slower until the clonic stage was reached, when the tension markedly dropped and the rate became much more rapid.

Although the muscles at the back of the neck could be felt to be in a state of tonic contraction and later in the seizure were seen to undergo clonic spasm, I (H. D. S.) was unable to satisfy myself that there was any spasm in the muscles lower down the spinal column.

In other fits attention was directed specially to the condition of the limbs, the abdominal muscles, the degree of expansion of the thorax, the colour of the lips, and the presence or absence of sweating about the forehead.

### *Description of the Character and Course of the Fits compounded from all the Observations made at Different Times during the First Period*

For convenience the fit may be divided into three stages : the tonic, the clonic and the stage of recovery, although the three merge into one another and in part overlap.

STAGE I.—Tonic spasm occurred first in the muscles of the neck, followed almost at once by spasm of the muscles of respiration, causing complete fixation of the thorax. Then followed spasm of the face, the jaw, the mylo-hyoid and the abdominal muscles ; and for all these it was impossible to determine any definite order. It is to be understood that the spasm of all the regions involved was of both sides at once and, except for the muscles of the face, of both sides equally. These several muscular regions will now be considered seriatim.

*Neck.*—The head was rigidly fixed in the mesial position, with the occiput drawn a little downwards and backwards as a result of the contraction in the muscles in the back of the neck, while both sterno-mastoids stood out prominently.

*Respiratory Muscles.*—As the spasm involved these muscles there was a brief moaning expiration, evidently through an almost closed glottis, ending with complete fixation of the thorax, and thereby arrest of all respiratory movement. The degree of expansion of the chest when this arrest occurred was in most observations below the mean between full inspiration and full expiration, but on two or three occasions it was noted that the thorax was expanded rather more than the mean.

*Abdominal Muscles.*—These were found to contract and to become firmer and more resistant, but the degree was never great.

*Face.*—The eyebrows were raised and the angles of the mouth drawn outwards ; generally, if not always, more towards the left than the right side.

*Jaws.*—The masseters were felt to be strongly contracted, but the teeth were separated by about half an inch, indicating powerful spasm in the depressors of the lower jaw. No deviation of the mandible was noted, although on one occasion there was some doubt as to whether it was not directed a little to the left. The mylo-hyoid muscles were rigidly contracted.

*Eyes.*—The internal strabismus due to weakness of the right external rectus muscle was always maintained, and the eyes were strongly rotated upwards, the upper lids being also elevated.

STAGE 2.—Typical clonic spasms followed the tonic contraction in all the affected muscles, including in some attacks, but not in all, the respiratory muscles ; when they were so affected air was sucked into the chest by each spasm, causing a grunting noise. The abdominal muscles were never observed to undergo clonic spasm.

STAGE 3.—*Recovery.*—As the fit passed off, the spasmodic fixation of the thorax ceased first and there then ensued one or more deep breaths ; it was considered probable that the depth of inspiration was greater at this time than when the patient was asked to draw a deep breath during an interval between two attacks. On several occasions she was told to draw a deep breath immediately after a fit was over, with a view to determining whether or not there was any weakness of the respiratory muscles as a sequence of the previous spasm—such weakness as is seen in a limb after a seizure due to (remaining after) some local cortical discharge. But on no occasion could she be induced to draw in her breath when told ; the shortest interval between a fit and the performance of this voluntary act was about five minutes. The non-compliance with this request was probably due to the mental state, as she made no attempt to make the movement and generally answered " Yes," or " Yes, thank you." With regard to the order in which cessation of spasm occurred in the other muscles, the only observation on this point is recorded above when the last muscles to relax completely were the frontales and orbiculares palpebrarum.

The *pulse* was observed to become slower in rate but of higher tension up to the time when the tonic spasm of the thoracic muscles gave way ; there was then a notable and rapid fall in the tension and a marked increase in the frequency leading to a more rapid rate than had been present before the seizure.

*Reflexes.*—The corneal reflex was definitely lost and probably unconsciousness was complete. The knee jerks became a little more marked during a fit, but were never much exaggerated. The plantar stimulation yielded extensor responses which continued to obtain between the attacks until the *status epilepticus* ceased.

So far we have dealt entirely with the positive results of the observations, but there still remain the equally important negative results. The *limbs* were very carefully examined, the sister examining the thighs both with hand and eye in many attacks, and we are confident that *there was no spasm of muscles and no movement of the limbs of any kind whatever at any time during the attacks* ; both arms and both legs remained absolutely flaccid throughout the seizures. *No definite change of colour* in the face or lips could be determined, although frequently looked for, and there was *never any sweating* of the head or face either to be seen or felt.

The duration of the fits varied a little, but may be stated roughly to have been forty to sixty seconds. When the fit was over the patient remained in a heavy, stupid condition for some minutes and often until the onset of the next attack. She would, however, sometimes obey simple commands, but never spoke rationally, her almost invariable reply to any remark being " Yes " or " Yes, thank you."

### (4) SLIGHTER FITS OCCURRING IN BOTH PERIODS

On the fourth day after we first saw the patient some very short fits were observed for the first time ; they continued to occur with considerable frequency from that time onwards. One of these is briefly described above as occurring just before the onset of fit 3 in our account of the individual fits of the First Period. These slighter seizures were very brief, lasting only a few seconds and consisted in a slow conjugate deviation of the head and eyes; this movement was generally towards the left side, but on several occasions it was towards the right and then the convergent strabismus was still maintained, the right eye moving only a little beyond the median position, whilst the left well into the inner canthus. A very fine symmetrical rotatory nystagmus was seen in the eyes in some of these slight attacks; and flushing of the conjunctival vessels with some lachrymation was also noted. There was no fixation of the thorax in these attacks, although on one or two occasions it was thought that respiration became a little slower, but of this we are not certain. No spasm was observed in any other muscles.

### (5) Fits of the Second Period

The first of this series of attacks was seen on the sixth day after the patient came under our observation, and even at the risk of being accused of too much repetition we must reiterate that no attack such as that described below, that is, with convulsion extending to the limbs, was observed during the First Period. The seizures in the Second Period differed from one another only in severity, hence it will be unnecessary to do more than give one description compounded from all our observations, which were not nearly as numerous as in the case of the fits in the First Period because the frequency became progressively less.

The first change observed in these attacks was a sudden and complete fixation of the thorax with arrest of all respiratory movement; this was followed by spasm, on both sides of the body, of the muscles of the face, jaw, neck, and upper extremities, and in some cases, but not in all, also of the muscles of the lower extremities. The spasm, at first tonic, very shortly became clonic. The head was retracted and there was sometimes conjugate turning of the head and eyes to the left, although both sterno-mastoids contracted. The upper extremities were not affected until the tonic contraction in the muscles of the face, jaw, and neck had given place to clonic spasm; *the order in which the muscles of the arms were involved was from the large thoraco-humeral muscles to the smaller forearm and hand muscles.* The trapezii seemed to be the first to contract, and this was followed almost at once by contraction of the deltoid and the remaining muscles of the shoulder girdle. Next followed spasm of the upper arm muscles, and finally those of the forearm and hand were involved. The spasm was at first tonic and resulted in adduction with slight flexion of the shoulder and slight flexion at the elbow and wrist with pronation of the forearm. The fingers were flexed at all joints and closed over the thumb, which was bent into the palm of the hand. In some attacks the left arm appeared to suffer more than the right. This tonic stage was rapidly replaced by clonic spasm of small range and brief duration. The lower extremities were unfortunately never very carefully observed, but the movement in them was never great. Spasm was felt in the thighs and in some attacks slight flexion of the hip and knee occurred. The position of the feet we are unable to describe owing to imperfect observation.

# FURTHER OBSERVATIONS ON A CASE OF CONVULSIONS (TRUNK FIT OR LOWEST LEVEL FIT?)[1]

(With Dr. Stanley Barnes.)

## Part I[2]

This is a further report of a case published (*Brain*, 1902, Pt. xcvii) (see p. 474) by Dr. Douglas Singer and myself. Although it is convenient, following custom, to use the term *status epilepticus*, the important question, as we then said, is not whether the fit the patients had are to be called epileptic or not. The really important question is, to reproduce part of what we wrote (op. cit.), " Where is the lesion (discharge lesion), which, on its occasional ' intense ' discharge, produces a convulsion *beginning* in muscles of the trunk (that is, in muscles of two sides of the body, the normal action of which may be, and often is, bilateral) and *beginning* in those muscles of the two sides of the body simultaneously ? " It will be seen that in the " first period " of the *status* Dr. Stanley Barnes describes, the convulsion did not affect the extremities in the slightest degree. In the " second period " the limbs were affected, but after the trunk ; Dr. Barnes carefully describes " a march " of the spasm *down* the arms. As ought always to be done, he distinguishes between movements proper, in two attacks of the first period, and spasm (contention of many movements). I think now, considering especially the observations Dr. Stanley Barnes made on the " inspiratory cry " in a certain part of the march of some of the patient's attacks, that her fits are probably Lowest Level (Ponto-Bulbar) Fits and not fits of ordinary epilepsy (Higher Level Fits).

I draw particular attention to Dr. Barnes's observations on the reflexes in and after the fits ; these observations seem to me worthy of great attention. It is very striking that the knee jerks were lost *in* attacks when there was not the least spasm of any limb.

## Part II

### History

The patient, J. K., is the eldest of a family of nine children, all of whom are alive. Most of the other children are said to have a " narrow bridge " to the nose, but no history of any other sign of syphilitic taint can be obtained.

The patient has always had a squint, and in childhood suffered from measles, whooping cough, and scarlet fever. For about two years during the first dentition she suffered from " teething convulsions."

The present illness began at the age of 9 years ; the fits at first occurred about once a month and gradually increased in frequency. After the age of puberty, their number rapidly increased to several daily. In March 1901 she was in *status epilepticus* for ten days, followed by a period of complete cessation for a month ; the fits then recurred, and in December 1901 she

[1] *Brain*, vol. xxv, 1902, p. 286.
[2] The first part is by J. H. J., and the second by S. B.

again passed into *status epilepticus* for sixteen days. At this time she was admitted to the National Hospital, and many of the fits were observed (*vide Brain*, 1902, Pt. xcvii, "Observations of a Case of Convulsions," by Dr. Hughlings Jackson and Dr. Douglas Singer) (see p. 474). She remained in hospital for three months longer, and during this time only had one slight attack. The patient then went to the Convalescent Home at Finchley, where she remained for nearly two months, a few slight seizures occurring there. During the second week after her return to her own home a few severe attacks came on, and these continued to occur and increase in number until the fifth week, when for the third time she passed into *status epilepticus* and was readmitted to the National Hospital on June 13, 1902.

### *General Examination*

As in the previous attack of *status epilepticus*, the general examination was deferred until consciousness was regained on June 27. No material change in her general condition had occurred since her previous admission in December 1901, so that it is unnecessary to repeat here the description given in the previous paper (see p. 474).

### *The Fits*

The first ten days after admission some 200 fits a day were seen to occur ; it is highly probable that the actual number was even larger. The maximum recorded was on the second day, when 394 were observed. After the tenth day the number rapidly diminished, and on the fifteenth day no fit occurred. From that day (June 27) until September 2, only one severe and three slight attacks occurred at irregular intervals.

In describing the attacks it will be convenient to classify them as in the previous paper, according as they occurred in the earlier or the later stages of the *status epilepticus*.

### *Fits occurring in the First Period*

The attacks occurred at intervals of about three minutes, each attack lasting about forty seconds. She was unconscious between the attacks.

Before the attacks, the patient was lying on her back in bed with her head resting on a pillow, the arms lying, as a rule, in front of her. The breathing was quiet and regular, both chest and abdomen moving about normally for a girl of her age ; the accessory muscles of respiration were not in action during inspiration.

In every instance in which the onset was particularly watched a bilateral deepening of respiration with action of the sterno-mastoids and scaleni was the first sign of an approaching fit. These accessory muscles of respiration did not at once go off into tonic spasm, but contracted in inspiration and relaxed in expiration ; after two such inspirations, in the second of which the contraction was more marked than in the first, the sterno-mastoids and scaleni failed to relax completely in expiration, so that the chest remained unusually expanded although respiration continued for several seconds afterwards.

The contraction of the accessory muscles of respiration appeared to be equal on both sides ; it was not very powerful, and the head was never lifted off the pillow ; at times a slight rotation of the head occurred, sometimes to the left, occasionally to the right.

Usually at the end of the second inspiration mentioned above, the next movement occurred ; this was a contraction of the frontales and levatores palpebrarum of both sides symmetrically. The eyes then turned jerkily to the left, the elevators of the eyebrows and eyelids being at this time in tonic spasm.

The lower segment of the face was next affected, both sides at the same time, but as a rule, the left side slightly more than the right ; the angles of the mouth were drawn downwards and the lips separated. Tonic spasm here rapidly gave way to clonic spasm, but before the latter was fully established the jaws were separated by a tonic spasm of the depressors of the mandible overcoming the contracting masseters and temporals. The teeth, as a rule, were separated about ½ inch, and the jaw always opened strictly in the middle line.

Up to this point respiration had continued at the usual rate, although the salceni and sterno-mastoids were contracted apparently as much in expiration as in inspiration. Just as the jaw opened, the chest being full, respiration ceased, but not all respiratory movement. The abdomen swelled slowly forwards (diaphragmatic action), and at the same time the chest slowly sank in and diminished in volume, no air either entering or emerging from the glottis. This complex movement continued for about twelve seconds, and then ensued a long-drawn crescendo inspiratory cry ; at the beginning of this cry the pitch was high, and gave the impression of air entering the chest through a very narrow glottis owing to great inspiratory effort ; later the spasm of the glottis appeared to give way, and allow air to enter more and more freely. The cry lasted about five seconds, and as it occurred the abdomen remained fixed in its inspiratory position whilst the chest again filled out. After the cry the respiration was resumed almost at once, and, as usual in her sex, was of the costal type. The eyes before the cry were turned to the left ; after it, as they slowly returned to their usual position, the conjunctivæ became suffused and much lachrymation occurred, the tears usually rolling down both cheeks just at the end of a fit.

In the majority of the fits very little cyanosis occurred ; in one that was carefully observed there was very marked blueness just before the cry. No noticeable sweating occurred.

In none of the fits did the slighest spasmodic hand or arm movement occur. In two of them, just as the fit was beginning, an irregular purposive-seeming movement was going on in the right upper extremity, the elbow being flexed and the forearm pronated as though she were going to rub her eyes—a thing she often does between the attacks. There was no spasm about the movement, and it was of an absolutely different nature from the face and neck movement ; it never occurred whilst the fit was in progress after the corneal reflex was lost. Apart from this movement, not a trace of muscular contraction occurred in the upper extremities, which were loose and slack at all their joints. The lower extremities were also carefully observed repeatedly, but no movement or muscle contraction could be felt here.

During the attacks the patient was quite unconscious, and she often micturated in or after them. The reflexes were carefully observed in many of the attacks, and deserve mention in some detail.

*State of Reflexes in the Fits*

The *corneal reflexes* were only lost at the height of the fit ; they began to diminish as soon as the elevation of the eyebrows occurred, and were lost at the time when the jaws were separated. They returned before the face had ceased to twitch, and quickly reached their normal intensity.

The *supra-orbital* reflexes disappeared during the attacks, during, speaking roughly, the same period as the corneal reflexes.

The *jaw jerk* between the attacks was unusually brisk ; it remained so during the attacks, except when the jaw was fixed by spasm of the mandibular muscles.

The *knee jerks* were carefully and repeatedly tested during several attacks. The method adopted was to support the thigh so that the leg hung down at an angle of about 120°, and the ligamentum patellæ was then tapped with a percussion hammer about once a second, beginning before the commencement of the fit and ending after the end of the fit. Each knee jerk was tested in several fits. Between the attacks the knee jerks were brisk, and no alteration occurred at the beginning of a fit until the lower part of the face went into spasm, and breathing had ceased ; at this stage the knee jerk rather suddenly completely disappeared, and remained absent until the cry occurred ; it now at once began to return, and just at the end of the fit was more brisk than usual, resuming its usual slightly brisk condition a few seconds later. This observation was confirmed by Dr. Hughlings Jackson and by Dr. Risien Russell on separate occasions. At the risk of appearing tautological, I would reiterate that in these attacks in which the knee jerks were lost not the least movement of spasm of any limb occurred.

*Fits of the Second Period*

On June 22, for the first time, fits were observed in which limb movements occurred. On this day these fits to a large extent alternated with those previously described as " fits of the first period," and in which no limb movement occurred. It was noticeable that the fits in which limb movements occurred were of longer duration and apparently of greater severity than those in which no such limb spasm was present. Repeated and careful observation convinced me that the fits of the two periods began in exactly the same way, the difference being that during the second period, in many instances, the fit spread from the trunk to the limb muscles, so that in the most severe attacks the spasm became general.

The first limb movement to occur was always at the proximal end of one of the upper extremities ; usually the left, sometimes the right shoulder group was first affected, the point of the shoulders being shrugged upwards, the arm elevated forwards, then the elbow was flexed, the wrist extended, and the fingers were strongly flexed over the thumb, which was adducted into the palm ; in this way the fit could be observed to spread from the proximal to the peripheral terminal muscle groups. The movements were at first tonic and afterwards clonic.

In the lower extremities the extensors of the knee appeared to be first affected ; beyond this I was unable to trace the order of involvement of muscle groups, as only two fits were observed in which the legs went into spasm. When in full spasm, however, the legs were, in these two attacks, in the fully extended position, *i.e.* with extension at hip, knee and ankle. The first lower extremity movement appeared to begin a little later than the first upper extremity movement, but before the whole upper limb was involved. I cannot say whether the left or right leg was the more frequently affected.

None of the above-described limb movements ever occurred until after the " cry " (*vide* " Fits of the First Period ").

*Slighter Fits*

Beyond the two kinds of fits already described, many slighter attacks were frequently occurring during both periods. In their onset these fits exactly resembled those described as " fits of the first period," but instead of going on until the jaw was depressed, they died away as soon as the upper part of the face had become involved ; there was no cry with these attacks. Every gradation was observed between these slighter attacks and the more severe ones in which the limbs were fully involved.

*Mental Condition*

Until June 27, the day on which the fits ceased, no reply in answer to a question could be got from the patient ; nor did she utter any sound which would lead one to suppose that she was at all conscious. On that day she first began to speak, but it was evident that she was only dimly conscious, and her ideas appeared to be much distorted. At times also she appeared to be suffering from hallucinations of vision and hearing. By June 28 she could reply sensibly to very simple questions, and thereafter she gradually resumed her usual mental state, so that by July 18 she could write letters passably well.

Incontinence of urine and fæces continued for nearly a week after all fits had ceased, but is now (September 8) no longer troublesome.

END OF VOL. I

# INDEX

*The letter 'n' after a number indicates that the reference occurs in a footnote.*


Abnormal talking, post-epileptiform, 450–451
Actions, post-epileptic, 295, 298–300, 305, 316
Adamûk, on ocular movements, 61, 76, 88
Addison (W.), on absence of insensibility in convulsions, 18
Albertoni, on nervous system in infants, 352
Allbutt (Sir Clifford), on effect of blow in syphilised patients, 340
Amaurosis, associated with convulsion, 102
Anæmia, local, caused by plugging of middle cerebral artery, 98
Anatomical investigation of epilepsy, example of, 206
Anatomy of nervous system, 49, 238 *et seq.*
— — — use of term, 428
Anderson (James), case of brain tumour, 341, 343, 344, 345
— — case of dreamy state in epilepsy with sensation of taste, 410
— — case of dreamy state with auditory sensations, 386–387
— — case of large basal cystic sarcoma, 472
Andrews (T. H.), case of destruction of part of cerebral hemisphere without symptoms, 24 *n.*
Aneurism, relation to epilepsy, 31, 234
Anger at onset of fit, 315
— in post-epileptic actions, 304, 305
Animals, nervous centres of, comparison with man, 113
Anstie (F. E.), on cellular changes caused by lesions, 226 *n.*
— — on lack of inhibition in higher centres, 176 *n.*
— — on nutrition of nerve tissue, 96
— — on over-action of lower centres, 123 *n.*, 184
Anterior part of cerebral hemisphere, function of, 178, 189
Aphasia, Broca's, 3
— cases of, localisation of movements revealed by, 77–89
— cause of, 38, 39
— epileptic, as after-effect of discharges, 142
— epileptiform, use of term, 168
— from lesions in left corpus striatum, 60
— hysterical, 20 *n.*
— loss of movements in, 64–66
— nature of, 50
— partial, use of term, 451
— post-epileptiform, 83, 338, 451 *et seq.*
— principle of dissolution in, 38
— study of, method of, 84
— use of words in cases of, 302 *n.*
— *See also* Speech.
Apoplexy, method of distinguishing from drunkenness, 88 *n.*
Arrangement, distinction from classification, 192
Arsenic, use in epilepsy, 237
— — nervous affections, 224
Arterial disease as origin of neuroses, 232
— relaxation, causes of, 236
— system, relation to nervous action, 236
Arteries, cerebral, aneurism of, as cause of convulsions, 31
— — sequence of movement developed through, 36
— contraction of, cause of paroxysm, 36
— plugging of, influence on nutrition of parts supplied, 233
— representation in brain of, 46, 47, 249
Artery, middle cerebral, aneurism of, 234, 234 *n.*
— — — plugging of, 98
— — — region of, liability to disease, 182
— — — relation to convulsions, 36, 147, 148 *n.*
— sylvian, 9
Articulation, ataxy of, 83–85, 451
— — cases without paralysis, 84 *n.*
— centre for, 51
— difficulty of, in cases of convulsion, 22
— movements of, loss of, 455
— suppressed, 51
Articulatory muscles, effect of epileptic discharge of " memory " centre on, 57
— — in speech, 452
Asylum cases of epilepsy, 157
Asymmetry of convolutions, 73
Ataxic affection of speech, use of term, 65
Atkinson (Richard), on case of brain tumour, 341–342
Auditory nerves, association with movement, 238
— — relations with hemispheres, 33 *n.*, 148 *n.*
— sensations, rarity of association with dreamy state, 385–386
Aura, stopping of, arrest of convulsions by, 6–7
— of thumb, in case of epileptiform convulsions, 1–2
— of tongue, in case of epileptiform convulsions, 3
— use of term, 427 *n.*
Automatic, use of term, 63 *n.*, 68 *n.*, 72 *n.*, 116
— action, continuance during unconsciousness, 124, 125
— — relation to voluntary, 64, 66
— condition, reduction to, as result of disease, 64–66
— — *See also* Dissolution.
— movements, compared with voluntary, 261
— — effect of convulsions on, 27, 28
— — order of loss of, compared with voluntary, 90

Automatic movements, relation of right side of brain to, 65
— part, definition of, 91
Automatism, mental, cases of, 124–134
— — use of term, 122
Axenfield, on uniformity of epileptic attacks, 100

Baillarger (J. G. F.), on crossed development of the brain, 60
Bain (A.), debt to, 167
— — on effects of emotion, 138
— — on muscular consciousness, 53
— — on " out-going " current, 55 *n.*, 171
— — on sensations, 152
— — on subject and object consciousness, 244 *n.*
— — on the organ of the mind, 47
— — on word memory, 51
Ballance (C. A.), on brain abscess, 473
Barlow (Sir Thomas), case of double hemiplegia, 454
Barnes (Stanley), observations on case of convulsions (lowest-level fit), 482–486
Barrel-organism, use of term, 305 *n.*
Bastian (H. C.), on Bain's opinions, 168 *n.*
— — on transverse lesions of cervical cord, 423
— — on word memory, 51
Beale (Lionel), on contraction of arteries in the frog, 235–236
— — on growth of bioplasm, 224
— — on order of attack in disease, 228
Beevor (C. E.), case bearing on localisation of sense of smell, 406–411
— — on epilepsy with dreamy state, 385 *n.*, 386
— — on epileptic attacks with warning of smell, 406, 462
— — on post-epileptiform reflexes, 337
Bell (Sir Charles), influence of debility on muscles, 71 *n.*
Belladonna, in treatment of fits, 358
Bemazement, as symptom of epilepsy, 388
Bernard (Claude), on reflex excitability, 184
Bilateral convulsions, caused by discharge of one hemisphere, 109
Bleeding. *See* Hæmorrhage.
Blindness, in case of convulsions, 33
— internal sight in cases of, 86
— relation to disease of hemisphere, 32 *n.*, 58
Blisters, arrest of convulsions by, 16
Blood, loss of, relation to convulsions, 222–223
— venosity of, relation to fits, 356, 357 *n.*, 359
Blow, relation to brain tumour, 346
Bloxam (C. L.), details of case of convulsions, 34
Boucher, on localisation of epilepsy, 164
Brain, aneurism of arteries of, as cause of convulsions, 31
— anterior part, as chief motor centre, 139
— blood supply of, 222
— composition of, anatomical expression of, 49
— constitution of, 48
— destruction of part of one hemisphere without symptoms, 24, 24 *n.*, 44, 46
— differences of two sides of, 153, 154
Brain, diseases of, eye symptoms in, 87–89
— — importance of study of tissues in, 229
— duality of, 73
— grey matter of. *See* Grey Matter.
— hemispheres, as centre for movements, 39
— — effects of disease of, 59
— — functions of, 162 *n.*, 178, 189
— — nature of, 40, 42, 43, 48
— — relationship of lesions to hemiplegia, 25
— — representation of body in, 326 *n.*
— — results of disease in, 24–25
— left side, function of, 39, 311
— — — relation to words, 65
— local lesion of, as cause of unilateral spasm, 24–29
— — — relation to universal convulsion, 71
— localisation of discharging lesions in, 102
— — of function in, 27, 29, 145, 242
— — — from nature of convulsions, 248 *et seq.*, 331
— — of movements in, 37 *et seq.*, 62–89, 168, 185
— posterior part, as chief sensory centre, 139
— right side, function of, 39, 65
— surface of, relation to organic functions, 137
— — *See also* Cortex Cerebri.
— tubercle in, case of, 115
— tumour of, case of, bearing on localisation of sense of smell, 406–411
— — as cause of convulsion, 208
— — — of hemiplegia, 144, 145
— — — of instability of nerve tissue, 94
— — — of paralysis, 320
— — case of localised convulsions from, 341–347
— — hæmorrhage from, 347
— — relation to epilepsy, 396 *n.*
— *See also* Arteries, Artery, Cerebellum, Cerebrum, Convolutions, Medulla Oblongata.
Brain-cells. *See* Cells.
Bravais, on epileptiform seizures, 414, 424
— on hemiplegic epilepsy, 148 *n.*
Bridgman (Laura), case of, 86
Broadbent (W.), hypothesis of representation of muscles, 28, 71, 104, 105, 150, 164, 265–266, 266 *n.*, 277, 333, 334, 420, 454
— — on use of phosphorus, 237
Broca's aphasia, 3
— convolution, involved in cases of loss of speech, 22
— region, relation to speech, 452, 452 *n.*, 454, 456
Brown-Séquard (C. E.), debt to, 167
— — on experimental production of fits in animals, 16, 348, 362
— — on heredity of artificially produced epilepsy, 231
— — on methods of arresting convulsions, 16
— — theory of production of paroxysm, 36
Browne (Sir James Crichton), on aura in epilepsy, 251
Browne (W. A. F.), on injury to intellect after convulsions, 158
Brunton (Sir Lauder), on asphyxia fits in animals, 359
— — on cerebral centre for movements of stomach, 249

Brunton (Sir Lauder), on irritation of sensory nerve, 243
— — on the medulla oblongata, 352
Bucknill (J. C.), on relation of mental diseases to epilepsy, 119
Budge, on cerebral centre for movements of stomach, 249
Bulbar paralysis, relation to aphasia, 453, 454 *n.*, 455
Bulbo-pontal fits, 474
Burdon-Sanderson (Sir J.), experiments of, 43
" Buttoning centre," 431–432

Callender, " The Anatomy of Brain Shocks," 24 *n.*
— on epilepsy due to aneurism, 234
Cause, use of term, 112, 206
Causes, of epilepsy, use of term, 218–219
— exciting, of epilepsy, 293
Cazauvielh, on localisation of epilepsy, 164
Cells, brain-, abnormal, nutrition of, 436–437
— — of discharging lesion, nature of, 432, 436 *et seq.*
— — size of, 262 *n.*, 288 *n.*
— — — relation to instability, 320 *n.*
— — — relation to nutrition, 439–440
Centre, use of term, 357
Centres, highest, use of term, 279 *n.*
Cerebellar influx, in hemiplegia, 450
— system, 423
Cerebellum, impressions of, as estimating properties of bodies, 53 *n.*
— movements represented by, 440 *n.*
— relation to co-ordination in space, 62, 76
Cerebral centres, relations of, 306–307
" Cerebral fever," relationship to arterial regions, 36
Cerebrum, anterior region of, seat of motor aspect of mind, 58–62
— as seat of convulsions, 348
— disease of, effect on movement of eyes, 62
— lobes of, effects of discharge of, 248 *et seq.*
— movements represented by, 440 *n.*
— nature of, 26 *n.*, 42, 138, 291
— posterior region of, seat of sensory aspect of mind, 58–62
— relation to eye processes, 76
— representation of organic parts in, 290
— *See also* Brain, Convolutions.
Charcot (J. M.), on Bravais's study of epilepsy, 148 *n.*
— — on corpus striatum, 148–149
— — on range of paralysis dependent on destruction of tissue, 144, 145
— — theory of dynamic lesion of ganglion cells, 448
Chest, movements of, character of, 91
Chewing movements, as symptom in epilepsy, 470
Children, convulsions in, 222
— young. *See* Infants.
Chloral in treatment of fits, 359
Chlorides, importance of, 224 *n.*
Chorea, cause of, 37
— fright as cause of, 24
— hyperæmia as cause of, 98
— in dogs, 100 *n.*
— localisation of movements revealed by, 77–89, 114 *n.*
Chorea, pathology of, 93 *n.*, 219 *n.*
— principle of compensation in, 44–46
Church (Sir W.), " Contributions to Cerebral Pathology," 31 *n.*
Circus movement, from injury of encephalus, 273
Clark (Sir Andrew), on diet in nervous debility, 97, 225
Classification, nature of, 190 *et seq.*
— of diseases, 276
Clinical entities, nature of, 165 *n.*, 166, 190, 195
— types of consciousness, 187
Clonic spasm from epileptic discharge, 272
Clouston (T. S.), on mental symptoms after fits, 379
Coarse disease of brain, definition of, 19 *n.*
Coates (Joseph), case of brain tumour, 343
— — — of epilepsy with intellectual aura, 386
— — — of fits preceded by giddiness, 313 *n.*
— — on mental states in epilepsy, 298
Colman (Walter S.), case of epilepsy with tasting movements, 458–463
Colour, loss of power of recognition, 146
— relation to sensory impressions, 54–55
Coloured vision, associated with epileptic discharges, 59, 59 *n.*
— — as beginning of fit, 302
— — case of, 1–2, 130
— — rarity of association with dreamy state, 385
Coma, post-epileptic, 380
Comatose, use of term, 158
Compensation, principle of, 44–46, 59, 144, 145, 148 *n.*, 149, 173, 210, 212, 215, 422
Compound order of movements, 434–435
Confusion of thought, post-epileptic, 380
Congestion, cerebral, supposed cause of post-epileptiform paralysis, 319, 442
Consciousness, affections of, relation to fits, 339, 417–418
— defect of, in epilepsy, 285
— degrees of, 187–188
— double, 298 *n.*, 467–468
— loss of, distinction of cases by, 185, 204, 205
— — in epilepsy, 18, 47, 142, 156–160
— — nature of, 99, 136, 221
— — post-epileptic, 380
— — relation of local lesion to, 252
— — study of, 172
— — symptoms preceding, 247–248
— — use of term, 193–194
— modes of, 61
— motor substrata of, 154
— nature of, 158–160, 186, 187, 204, 205 *n.*, 242, 288–289, 323, 417
— physical basis of, evolution of, 376–377
— relation to nervous states, 136, 139
— — of time to, 143
— seat of, 107, 110, 172
— substrata of, 47, 152, 239 *et seq.* 289
— use of term, 221
Contact, use of term, 241 *n.*
Contemperation, use of term, 431
Contemporaneous, use of term, 217 *n.*

Control, loss of, in epilepsy, 123 *n.*, 293, 370
— — of, principle of, 146 *n.*, 149
Convergence, relation to cerebellum, 88
Convolutions, discharge of, relation to movements, 68–70, 77
— movements represented in, 81, 115, 115 *n.*
— nature of, 27, 42, 43, 45
— relation to corpus striatum, 67–68
Convulsion, march of, importance of, 434
— nature of, 331
— of ideas, relation to epilepsy, 122
— region affected in, method of study, 251
— relation to consciousness, 186–187
— relation to "organ of mind," 58
— universal, cause of, 155
— — in cases beginning respiratorily, 357–358
— — question of, 263–264
— — relation to discharge, 185 *n.*
Convulsions, association with paralysis, 211–213
— causes of, 4
— definition of, 8
— effect on consciousness, 242
— epileptiform, 1–7, 8–36, 424–440
— — after-effects, 440 *et seq.*
— — anatomical investigation of, 112–117
— — arrest by pressure, 6–7, 13–14, 15, 16
— — association with hemiplegia, 94
— — attended by defects of speech, 19–23
— — case of, attended by aura of thumb and coloured vision, 1–2
— — — attended by defect of sight, 1
— — — from injury to head, 2–3, 33
— — — starting in the face, 21
— — — starting in foot, 23
— — — starting in left hand, 12, 32
— — — starting in right hand, 12, 13–14, 17–18
— — — starting in right thumb, 14–15
— — causes of, 37, 38, 412–413, 436
— — from cerebral disease, 330–340
— — classification of, 350, 413 *et seq.*
— — comparative study of, 79, 348–361
— — degrees of, 100, 103, 200–201, 281–282
— — dependent on instability of nerve tissue, 30
— — evidential value for localisation, 62–63, 77–89, 185
— — isomeric, 23
— — locality and order of, 425–427
— — mental disorders after, 119–134
— — mode of onset, importance of, 90, 263
— — nature of, 354
— — — of discharge in, 57, 66–67
— — relation to syphilis, 474
— — slight, patients' names for, 284
— — treatment of, 340
— — unilateral, 256–268
— — — causes of, 23–36
— — — place of onset, 68
— — — relation to hemiplegia, 67
— — — — to middle cerebral artery, 147, 148 *n.*
— — — result of post-mortem examination of cases, 25
— — — varieties of, 10
— — varieties of, 350, 413 *et seq.*
— — warning sensations in, 137, 153
— — warnings, intellectual in, 274–275
— — *See also* Epilepsy.
Convulsions, epileptiform, localised, from brain tumour, case of, 341–347
— lowest level, case of, 474–486
— regarded as experiments by disease, 168
— scale of, 349
— slight, significance of, 213 *n.*
— *See also* Fits.
Convulsive seizures, 412–457
Co-operation in motor centres, 157
Co-ordination, disorders of, nature of, 371
— — use of term, 210
— in nervous centres, evolution of, 107
— nature of, 36, 82
— of movements, 49, 49 *n.*, 272
— space, 154, 155
— time, 154, 155, 261 *n.*
— varieties of, 204 *n.*
Corpus striatum, "containing" movements of, 26
— — lesions of, as cause of unilateral spasm, 25, 28
— — — effects of, 27, 72, 103
— — relation to adjacent convolutions, 67–68, 82
— — — to convulsions, 221
— — — to loss of speech, 22
— — — to unilateral convulsions, 38
— — representation of eye-movements in, 88
— — — of movements in, 64, 114–115, 212–213
— — — of muscles in, 17, 150. *See also* Broadbent.
— — symptoms of disease of, 9
— — units of, 148–149
Corpus striatum epilepsy, use of term, 257
Correlations of movements, 75–76
Cortex cerebri, constitution of, 277
— — *See also* Brain, Surface of.
Cortical epilepsy, use of term, 415
Cotard on local hyperæmia of brain, 98, 233
Crichton-Browne (Sir James), on asylum cases of epilepsy, 157, 158
— — on pallor as phenomenon of fit, 138
Criminal aspect, in cases of mental automatism, 127–134
Crude sensations. *See* Sensations, crude

Day (Dr.), criticism of views on loss of movement, 144
Deaf mutes, nature of mental operations in, 86
Deafness, relation to disease of cerebral hemispheres, 32 *n.*, 58, 148 *n.*
Decussating fibres, 72
Degrees of nervous discharge, 254–255, 256
Delirium, ideation of, 181 *n.*
— nature of, 26 *n.*, 43, 115 *n.*
— post-epileptic, 121 *n.*
Destroying lesions, use of term, 208
Deviation, conjugate, of head and eyes in post-epileptic hemiplegia, 149–150
Diagnosis in cases of convulsions, 195
Dickens (Charles), on feeling of reminiscence, 389
Dickson (Thompson), on over-action of lower centres, 123 *n.*, 146 *n.*
Diet, in epilepsy, 15, 97, 225, 237
Difference, principle of, in motor centres, 154

Diluted convulsions, 395–396, 425
Diplopia, mental, 467–468
Discharge, epileptic, 180, 181, 182, 185
— — relation to healthy discharges, 180
— nervous, 29, 35–36, 178, 179, 182, 193, 254–255
— — rate of, relation to paralysis, 328–329
— — *See also* Nervous Discharges.
Discharging lesions, as cause of epilepsy, 94–95, 203
— — difficulty of discovery of, 220, 222
— — doubly local, 418
— — localisation of, 102
— — nature of, 97, 136, 276, 354, 369, 371
— — relation of spasm to, 108–109
— — use of term, 92, 208, 318 *n.*, 391 *n.*, 430
Disease, cerebral, use of term, 331
— coarse, as cause of nervous instability, 234–235
— investigation of, methods of, 191–192
— use of term, 279
Disorientation, in case of paresis of external rectus, 87
Disposition, alteration of, 66 *n.*
Dissolution, law of, 38, 116, 149, 173–174
— — in convulsions beginning unilaterally, 260–262
— — in insanity, 197, 299
— of nervous system, degrees of, 147, 324 *n.*, 380–381
— — — study of, 318–329
— use of term, 318 *n.*
Distance, estimation of, 62, 76, 87 *n.*
Donders (F. C.), on affection of orbicularis pulpebrarum associated with affection of limbs, 75
— — on movements of the eyes, 61, 88
Double consciousness, 298 *n.*, 467–468
Down (Langdon), on singing of imbeciles, 73 *n.*
Dreamy state in epilepsy, 295–298, 303–304, 313, 385–405
— — — associated with tasting movements, case of, 458–463
— — — associated with warning smell, case of, 464–473
— — in uncinate group of fits, 467–468
— — *See also* Intellectual Aura.
Drunkard, increase of power in, 71 *n.*
Drunkenness, method of distinguishing from apoplexy, 88 *n.*
Duality of brain, nature of, 73
Duchenne (G. B.), on co-ordination, 62
— — on movements of muscles, 67, 178
— — on the thumb, 116, 261
Duplex symptomatology of nervous maladies, 370–372, 446 *n.*
Dupuy (Eugène), experiments of, 43
— — on localisation of epilepsy, 164
Duret (H.), on " seats of election " of disease, 156
Dyspepsia, relation to convulsions, 15, 35, 291, 361
— — to melancholy, 118

Ear, diseases of, associated with convulsions, 21 *n.*, 105, 234
— noises in, as beginning of fit, 302
Effort, degrees of, 64
Effort, order of movements in, 69–70, 74, 271–272
Ejaculations, relation to speech, 455
Elective affinity of remedies in epilepsy, 306
Embolism, as cause of aneurism, 234 *n.*
— — of chorea, 93 *n.*
— — of epilepsy, 4, 30
— — of nervous instability, 232–234
Emotion, bodily manifestations of, 47, 138
— nature of, 173, 244 *n.*
— relation to highest nervous centres, 289, 290
Emotional, use of term, 175 *n.*
Endarteritis, nature of, 236
Environment, action on consciousness, 152 *n.*
— use of term, 311 *n.*
Epigastric sensation in epilepsy, 118, 285, 301
— — relation to dreamy state, 386
Epilepsies, anatomy of, 112–117, 238–255
— causes of, 203–207
— classification of, 199–202, 279–280, 362
— investigation of, 90–111, 162–273
— nervous discharges of, effects of, 247
— pathology of, 217–237
— physiology of, 208–217
— symptoms of, 182
Epilepsy and epileptiform convulsions, contributions on, 1–7
— case of, with tasting movements, 458–463
— cases of, characterised by dreamy state, 392–405
— — value of analysis of, 392
— cause of premonitory symptoms, 47
— causes of, use of term, 218–219
— characterised by intellectual aura, 385–405
— degrees of, 281–282
— definition of, 4–5, 81, 92, 94, 99–101, 120–121, 135, 137, 165, 166, 177 *et seq.*, 416 *n.*
— diagnosis of, 276–307, 387–388
— diet in, 97, 225
— " genuine," cause of, 155, 156
— — differences from convulsion, beginning unilaterally, 257–258
— — nature of fits, 415
— — use of term, 78, 79, 278
— idiopathic, bilateral convulsions in, 109
— — nature of, 200 *n.*
— — universal convulsion in, 185 *n.*
— — use of term, 66, 163, 165
— importance of mode of onset, 90, 91
— localisation of lesion in, 249 *et seq.*
— masked, 122
— paralysis after, 321 *et seq.*
— relation of local lesion to, 252
— — to insanity, 230 *n.*
— — to nervous diseases, 294
— systemic sensations in, 118
— treatment of, 226, 306
— varieties of, 121, 391
— — relation to warnings, 309
— " vital " symptoms of, 110, 115 *n.*
Epileptic discharges, after-effects of, 135–161
— — nature of, 181, 182, 185
— hemiplegia, use of term, 337, 347
— paroxysms, importance of study of, 391
— — unilateral spasm at onset of, 308–317
— seizures, brought on by touching head, case of, 362–365
— vertigo, use of term, 286

Epileptiform, use of term, 99
— fits, nature of, 415
Epileptogenous zones, 361, 362 *n.*
Esquirol (J. E. D.), on injury to intellect after convulsions, 158
Evolution of nervous centres, 106–111, 171–174, 215–217, 324, 349, 353, 372–377, 413–415
— principle of, 38, 116, 367
Excitement as cause of convulsions, 35
Exhaustion, cortical, as cause of paralysis, 322, 318–319, 441–443
— of substrata of consciousness, effects of, 246
— use of term, 441–442
Explosive cells, 432 *et seq.*
Expression, in cases of epilepsy, 283
Eye, lateral deviation of, 88–89
— movements of, estimation of distance by, 76
— — relation to tactual movements, 58, 75, 88
— — representation of, 61–62
— paralysis of external rectus, 87
— symptoms in brain disease, 87–89
— voluntary closing of, in cases of hemiplegia, 104
— *See also* entries under Ocular, Visual.

Face, convulsions beginning in, 19, 21, 70
Faculties, theory of, 245
" Faculty " of co-ordination, use of term, 36
Fagge (Hilton), on death from cerebral tumour, 395
Falret (J.), on coloured vision in epilepsy, 130 *n.*
— — on delirium, 121 *n.*
— — on epileptic insanity, 122
— — on mental states in epilepsy, 298
— — on uniformity of attacks of epilepsy, 250–251
Farinaceous diet, in epilepsy, 237
Fatigue, of central nervous system, post-epileptic, 145
Fear, effects of, 290
— feeling of, in epilepsy, 301, 315, 468
— in post-epileptic actions, 304
Ferrier (David), debt to, 167, 177, 277, 281, 412
— — experiments on brains of animals, 38, 39, 43, 44, 54 *n.*, 62, 77, 91, 96, 112, 113, 114, 145, 162 *n.*, 260
— — on bilateral convulsions, 334
— — on blindness produced in animals, 58 *n.*
— — on case of reminiscence, 397–398
— — on cerebral localisation, 59
— — on localisation of sense of smell and taste, 409, 461
— — on movements of the eyes, 62
— — on reflex movements of lips in monkeys, 310
— — on visual centre, 396 *n.*
— — on word memory, 51
Fibre, use of term, 418
Fibres, nerve, 9, 27, 47, 72, 211, 270, 419–420
Finger, little, convulsions beginning in, 19
— *See also* Index-finger.
Finger-language, use of by Laura Bridgman, 86
Fiske (John), on infancy, 352
— — on relation of consciousness to molecular motion of nervous centres, 375
Fits, classification of, 387 *n.*, 414
— degrees of, 427
— use of term, 415
— *See also* Convulsions, Inward Fits.
Flatulence, as cause of convulsions, 35
Foot, start of convulsions in, 23
Force, use of term, 328
Foreign body, in brain, as cause of convulsions, 31
— — — definition of, 19 *n.*
Foster (M.), on the brain surface, 137
— — on metabolism, 437 *n.*
Fothergill (Milner), on relation of visceral states to mental conditions, 292
Fournie, definition of idea, 50 *n.*, 51
France (E. P.), on degeneration of pyramidal tract, 419 *n.*, 422
Franck (F.), on bilateral convulsions, 334
— — on cortical exhaustion, after fits, 443
— — on experimental epilepsy in animals, 280
— — on muscular rigidity, 449
— — on nervous system in infants, 352
Fright, as cause of chorea, 24
— — of convulsions, 35, 254
Fritsch (G.), experiments on brains of animals, 77, 96, 112
Frontal lobe, divisions of, 414
Fulminate, physiological, use of term, 432
Function, modifications of, 217
— post-epileptic loss of, 143 *et seq.*
Functional, use of term, 29 *n.*, 92–93, 143 209, 252
— units, hypothesis of, 236

Gairdner (W. T.), on barrel-organism, 305 *n.*
Galvanism, movements of single muscles produced by, 67
Gamgee (A.), on results of excitation of nerves, 223 *n.*
Ganglia, hemispherical, functions of, 47
Ganglion cells, nature of, 26, 27, 211
Gastric disorder as exciting cause of convulsions, 15
Gay (W.), on laryngismus stridulus, 416 *n.*
Gee (S. J.), on injection of apomorphia into a dog, 249
Giddiness. *See* Vertigo.
Gowers (W. R.), on associations of olfactory aura, 408
— — on case of tumour of right cerebral hemisphere, 312
— — on examination of brain in case of fits, 116
— — on inhibition, 442, 449, 450
— — on mode of convulsion of second side, 151
— — on post-epileptiform reflexes, 337–338
— — on sequence of spasm, 271
— — on the motor paths, 14 *n.*
— — reference to Sir Charles Bell, 71 *n.*
— — reports of cases of convulsion, 40
*Grand-mal*, use of term, 282, 283
Gratiolet (L. P.), on the hemispheres, 59–60, 73
Gravity of lesion, use of term, 71 *n.*
Grey matter of brain, blood supply of, 222
— — instability of, as cause of epilepsy, 204
— — — causes of, 68 *n.*
— — — results of, 46

Grey matter, nature of, 108
— — variation of quantity of, 262
Griesinger (W.), on effects of imperfect nervous system, 176
— — on migraine, 278 *n.*
Grünbaum (A. S.), on a trunk centre, 475
Gunn (Marcus), on diagnosis of brain tumours, 473

Hæmorrhage from brain tumour, relation to hemiplegia, 347
— as cause of convulsions, 96
Hamilton (McLane), on case of epilepsy with olfactory symptoms, 411
— — — of localised chronic pachymeningitis, 472
Hamilton (Sir William), on sensation and perception, 245
— — on time as factor of consciousness, 143 *n.*
Hand, importance of, 68, 117 *n.*, 268 *n.*
— movements of, 91
— — relation to movements of eyes, 58
Handfield-Jones (M.), on classification of epilepsy, 278
— — on epilepsy, 202–203
— — on nutrition of nerve tissue, 96
Harmony of movements, nature of, 272
Haughton (E.), on effect of meat diet, 225
— — on relation of food to work, 15, 97
Head, case of fits brought on by touching, 362–365
— injury of, in case of convulsions, 33
— pain in, symptomatic of foreign body, 19
— turning of, significance in epileptic paroxysms, 308
Health, good, relation to epilepsy, 293
Hearing. *See* Auditory, Ear.
Heart, diseases of, in infants, relation to fits, 360
— ganglia of, action of, 95, 213
— valvular disease of, associated with epilepsy, 3–4
Helmholtz (H.), on case of paralysis of right external rectus, 87
Hemichorea, analogy of, to defects of speech, 22 *n.*
— relation to hemiplegia, 79
Hemikineses, use of term, 79, 273
Hemiopia, in case of hemiplegia, 75
— lateral deviation of eyes in, 87
Hemiplegia, case of, caused by blow, 2–3
— complicated with hemiopia, 75
— contrasted with convulsions, 8
— — definition of, 9
— degrees of, 64, 264, 266
— epileptic, 13, 24–25, 33, 94, 135, 142
— — compared with mania, 196
— — tumour as cause of, 144
— loss of movements from, 63–64
— ocular symptoms in, 87
— relation to convulsions beginning unilaterally, 67
— — to corpus striatum, 221
— — to hemi-chorea, 79
— — to loss of speech, 19, 22
— study of, 229–230
— symptom of destruction of motor tract, 29
— varieties of, 447–450
Hemiplegic epilepsy, use of term, 257
Hemispasm, case of, 104
— ocular symptoms in, 87
Hemisphere. *See* Brain, Hemisphere of.
Henoch (E. H.), on inward fits, 351, 353, 356, 360
Heredity, facts of, importance in legal enquiry, 134
— in disease, 176 *n.*, 236
— in epilepsy, 294
— in nervous diseases, 175, 230–232
Hering (Ewald), on movements of the eyes, 62, 88
Herpin (J. C.), on chewing movements, 470
— — on dreamy states, 468–471
— — on symptoms of convulsions, 138
Hilton (J.), hypothesis regarding nerve trunks, 17 *n.*
Hitzig (E.), debt to, 167, 277, 281
— — experiments on brains of animals, 39, 43, 44, 54 *n.*, 77, 96, 112, 145, 162 *n.*
— — on galvanising the cerebral hemisphere, 194
Horsley (Victor), on convulsions due to cortical discharge, 435 *n.*
— — on force-area of brain, 454
— — on representation of movements, 439
— — on tonic spasm, 417 *n.*, 422
— — researches on epilepsy, 362
Hull (S. E.), case bearing on localisation of sense of smell, 406–411
Hunger, as sensation of ill-nutrition, 305, 311
Huxley (T. H.), on the thumb, 116, 261
Hyperæmia, as cause of instability of nerve tissue, 94
— local, caused by plugging of middle cerebral artery, 98
— relation to nervous symptoms, 233
Hyper-physiological states, 429, 430
Hypo-kinesis, in post-epileptiform paralysis, 446, 447
Hypo-physiological states, 429

Idea, definition of, 50
Ideas, degrees of, 56
— latent, 56
— method of acquirement of, 240–241
— nature of, in epileptic discharges, 57
— relation to energising of cells and fibres, 55
— — to movements, 52
— — to perception, 246
— seat of, 81
— substrata of, 82, 171
— *See also* Convulsion of Ideas, Tactual Ideas, Visual Ideas.
Images, objectivity of, 383 *n.*, 384
Imbecility, relation to disease in right optic thalamus, 60
Imperception. *See* Recognition, Defect of.
Impression, use of term, 238
Index-finger, importance of, 91, 261
Infants, convulsions in, due to morbid affections, 360
— nervous system of, 351–353
Inhibition, as supposed cause of post-epileptiform paralysis, 442
Insane, personality of, 383
Insanity, classification of, 196–199, 366–384
— defect of consciousness in, 323

Insanity, double condition in, 123 *n.*, 198–199
— epileptic, nature of, 174, 175, 176
— — violence in, 120
— equivalence to dissolution, 38 *n.*
— heredity of, 230 *n.*
— relation to epilepsy, 230 *n.*
— study of, 366–384
— *See also* Mental Diseases.
Insensibility, absence of, in convulsions, 18–19
Instability of grey matter, as cause of convulsion, 208
— nervous, 226, 227, 232–235, 280
— use of term, 214, 218
Intellectual aura of epilepsy, 274, 380 *n.*
— — use of term, 296, 386
— — variety of epilepsy characterised by, 385–405
— — *See also* Dreamy State.
Intensity, electric, 227
Internal Evolution of highest nerve centres, 376
Inward fits, 351, 353, 355–358
Iodide of potassium, use in epilepsy, 237
Ireland (W. W.), on diet in epilepsy, 225
— — on taste for music in idiots, 73 *n.*
Irritations, eccentric, as cause of nervous instability, 235
Isomeric convulsions, 23

Jaccoud (S.), on effects of excitation, 109
— — on epilepsy, 81, 254 *n.*
— — on injury to intellect after convulsions, 158
Jellett, on velocity of chemical reactions, 227
Johnson (George), on convulsions produced by camphor, 417
Johnson (Metcalfe), use of term "mentation," 180
Jones (Handfield). *See* Handfield-Jones.

Kinetic route, 419
Kirke, on ganglia of heart, 95
Kussmaul (A.), on epilepsy, 220
— — experiments on brains of animals, 109, 348

Landouzy (L.), on range of paralysis dependent on destruction of tissue, 144, 145
Laryngismus stridulus, 351
Laryngitis in children, relation to convulsions, 358
Latham, on migraine, 153 *n.*
Laycock (T.), doctrine of reflex cerebral action, 37, 38 *n.*, 40, 47, 61, 122, 123, 167, 176 *n.*, 179
Left-sided convulsion, relationship to defect of speech, 20
Leg, paralysed, use of for walking, 34
Lepine, on range of paralysis dependent on destruction of tissue, 144, 145
Lesion, in epileptiform seizures, localisation of, 339
— — — pathology of, 340
— — — physiology of, 339
Lesions, local, cause of local symptoms, 252–255
— destroying, movements lost from, 63–64
Lesions, discharging, movements developed by, 66–76
Lewes (G. H.), debt to, 168
— — on distinction of mental and physical, 41
— — on sensations, 152
— — on sensibility, 48, 188, 239 *n.* 243 *n.*
— — on systemic sensations, 118
— — on words, 40, 193
Lewis (Bevan), on cells representing small muscles, 320 *n.*
— — on motor region representing small muscles, 437–438
Ligature, arrest of convulsions by, 6, 15, 16, 34
Limbs, association with orbicularis palpebrarum, 75
Liveing (Edward), on migraine, 153 *n.*
— — use of term "nerve storm," 412 *n.*
Local symptoms, relation to local lesions of brain, 24–29
Localisation, anatomical, use of term, 69
— doctrine of, 444 *n.*
— of lesion, in epileptiform seizures, 339
— physiological, use of term, 69
— *See* Brain, Localisation.
Locomotor, use of term, 62 *n.*
Loring, experiments on external recti, 62
Lumleian Lectures, 412–457

Mackenzie (Stephen), on case of brain tumour, 345
Magnan (V.), on convulsions produced by absinthe, 417
Malnutrition. *See under* Nutrition.
Mania, epileptic, 122, 135, 174, 175, 176, 183–184, 196
Masked epilepsy, 122
Mastication, movements of, relation to epileptic discharge, 310
Materialism, scientific, 52, 325 *n.*, 330, 367
Meat, in diet of epileptics, 97, 225
Medicine, nomenclature of, 190
Medulla oblongata, disease of, effects on speech, 86
— — supposed seat of epilepsy, 95, 203, 207, 218, 250, 348
Meigs, on inward fits, 351
Melancholy, relation to dyspepsia, 118
Melody of movements, 272
Memory, failure of, 124 *n.*, 305 *n.*
— loss of, relation to disease in right optic thalamus, 60
— of words, centre for, 49–53
— — — effect of epileptic discharge of, 57
Menial, use of term, 139
Meningeal hæmorrhage, violence due to, 120
Mental automatism, cases of, 124–134
— — use of term, 122
Mental diseases, order of loss of faculties in, 64–65
— — methods of study, 89
— — relation to dissolution of highest centres, 381
— — — to epilepsy, 119–134
— disorders of epileptics, occurrence after fits, 379
— operations, nature of, 64 *n.*
— pathology, use of term, 53 *n.*
— physiology, relation to psychology, 84
— — study of convulsions in, 81

Mental physiology, value of motor symptoms for, 77
— states, in epileptic discharges, comparative elaboration of, 141
— — relation to consciousness, 289
— — — to molecular movements, 55
— — — to physical states, 41–42, 48, 49, 137, 169
— — — to visceral states, 292
— symptoms, ascribed to "organ of mind," 81
— — causes of, use of term, 382
— — distinction from motor symptoms, 83
— — positive, significance of, 382
— — relation to order of loss of movements, 66
— — — to sensori-motor processes, 43, 58, 115
Mentation, nature of, 199
— relation of nervous discharges to, 180
— sensori-motor processes in, 41
— use of term, 41 *n.*, 180 *n.*
— words in, 39, 40
Mercier (Charles), case of self-mutilation in epilepsy, 131-133
— — case of spasm in left arm, 271
— — on coma, 368
Merson, on diet in epilepsy, 233, 237
Mesnet, on pathological somnambulism, 470 *n.*
Metaphysical explanation of consciousness, 160
Mickle (Julius), case of post-epileptic hemiplegia, 149–150
Middle centres, use of term, 151
Migraine, nature of, 153 *n.*, 166 *n.*
— ocular symptoms in, 140 *n.*, 142, 425 *n.*
— relation to epilepsy, 278, 416 *n.*
— symptoms of, 249 *n.*
Mill (James), on ascertaining correspondencies, 191
— — on primary qualities, 171
— — on use of term "sensation," 55
Mills (Charles K.), on case of oro-lingual monoplegia, 451 *n.*
Mind, diseases of, classification of, 196–199
— experimental investigation of, 197
— organ of, 26 *n.*, 43, 45, 47, 48, 49, 140, 215 *n.*, 290–291, 330, 350, 372, 414
— — constitution of, 115 *n.*, 169, 277
— — relation to speech, 452 *n.*
— — symptoms of disease of, 58, 81
— — use of term, 367
— relation to body, 159–160, 325
— *See also headings under* Mental, Psychology.
— and matter, 169–170
Mitchell (Weir), case of fits preceded by giddiness, 314
— — on faradising stumps, 171 *n.*
— — on injuries of nerves, 55 *n.*
Molecular movements, relation to mental states, 55
Monro (Alex.), on double condition in insanity, 123
Morphology, use of term, 239 *n.*, 428
Motor aspect of mind, localisation of, 58–62
— centres compared with cerebrum, 26 *n.*, 42
— — epileptic discharge of, effects of, 155
— — evolutionary levels of, 414
Motor centres, localisation of, 139
— — partial destruction of, effect on movements, 373
— — principle of difference in, 154, 156–157
— — subordinate, use of term, 142
— processes, complexity of, 45
— — substrata of visual ideas, 53–57
— — — of words, 39, 49
— region, right, 422
— sensation, physical basis of, 305
— symptoms, ascribed to medulla oblongata, 81
— — distinction from mental symptoms, 83
— — value for mental physiology, 77
— tract, involved in cases of unilateral palsy, 24
Movement, relation to ideas, 54
Movements, bilateral, relation to brain, 71–74
— convulsive, locality and order of, 425–427
— co-ordination of, 272
— correlations of, 75–76
— development of, 114
— localisation of, 37–76, 77–89, 168
— loss of, 26, 27, 371
— of mastication, relation to epileptic discharge, 310
— of muscles, distinction from muscles, 421
— relation to nervous centres, 372–373
— representation of, 113, 115 *n.*, 269, 270 *n.*, 330, 440 *n.*
— size of, relation to size of representation cells, 438
— *See also* Automatic Movements, Simultaneous Movements, Succession of Movements, Voluntary Movements.
Moxon (W.), on muscle, 353 *n.*
— — on nomenclature, 190, 278, 278 *n.*
Müller (Franz), case of tumour of brain, 341
Muscle centres, use of term, 449
Muscles, action of, bilateral, 265, 266 *n.*
— condition of, value for localisation, 251, 252 *n.*
— effects on, of exciting nerve, 223 *n.*
— involved in convulsions, order of, 70
— paralysis of, use of term, 323
— relation to nervous centres, 113–114, 372–373
— representation of, in brain, 28, 45, 61, 71, 150, 263. *See also* Broadbent.
— — in nervous centres, 263
— — relation to movements, 420–421
— sequence of spasm in, 268–269
— size of, relation to size of brain-cells, 288 *n.*, 320 *n.*, 437–438
Muscular consciousness, 53
Music, automatic nature of, 73 *n.*
Mutilation. *See* Self-mutilation.

Neatby, on post-epileptiform reflexes, 337
Negative lesions, use of term, 429
Nerve fibres, destruction of, 9
— — nature of, 47, 211, 270, 419–420
— — passage into corpus striatum, 72
— storm, use of term, 412 *n.*
— tissue, discharge of, 35–36
— — function of, 25, 93
— — functional changes in, 29–30, 94, 179
— — instability of, cause of convulsions, 30
— — nutrition of, 96, 223, 224

Nerves, conductivity of, 226
Nervous centres, composition of, 136
— — discharge of, in health, 96
— — evolution of. *See* Evolution.
— — highest, whole organism represented by, 326
— — independence of, effect of evolution on, 375–377
— — middle, 151
— — movements represented by, 113
— debility, 97
— — diet in, 225
— discharges in epilepsy, 287–289
— — relation to bodily phenomena, 143
— — theory of, 354
— — *See also* Discharge, Nervous.
— diseases, heredity of, 230–232
— — relation to epilepsy, 119, 294
— matter, unstable, nature of, 97, 98
— organs, constitution of, 227–228
— — order of attack in disease, 228, 232
— processes, results of increase in complexity, 26, 27, 45
— symptoms, duplex condition of, 370–372
— — non-nervous pathology of, 230
— — physiological divisions of, 331
— system, anatomy of, 49, 238 *et seq.*
— — — use of term, 368–369
— — differences of lowest and highest levels, 374
— — diseases of, causes of, 229
— — — clinical study of, 368–370
— — — importance in study of epilepsy, 172
— — — methods of study, 377–378
— — dissolution of. *See* Dissolution.
— — duality in, 245
— — fatigue of, post-epileptic, 145, 146
— — in epilepsy, 294
— — of infants, 351, 353
— — pathology of, 369–370
— — physics of, distinction from psychology, 48
— — physiology of, 369
— — relation to psychology, 372
— — "seats of election" of disease in, 156
— — unit of action of, 64 *n.*
Nettleship (E.), case of tumour of pituitary body, 472
Neural physiology, use of term, 52 *n.*
Neuralgia, continuance after division of nerve, 17
Neuritis, double optic, symptomatic of foreign body in brain, 19
Neuroses, use of term, 209
Niemeyer (F.), on intermediate stages in epilepsy, 193 *n.*
— — on inward fits, 351
— — on relationship of hemiplegia to lesions of hemisphere, 25
— — on use of pressure to arrest convulsions, 16 *n*
Nitrogen, substitution for phosphorus in nerve cells, 97, 224
Nitrogenisation of cells, effect of, 437
Nitrogenised substances, 227
Nitrogenous diet in epilepsy, 237
Nomenclature, nature of, 190
Nothnagel (H.), on Broadbent's hypothesis, 150, 151
Nutrition, abnormal, of brain, as cause of discharge, 213, 218, 222
— — of cells, nature of, 436–437
— altered, nature of, 223–224
— morbid, 429 *n.*
— of nerve tissue, 96, 99

Object consciousness, nature of, 244, 244 *n.*
— — substrata of, 245, 246
Objective, use of term, 310
Occlusion of vessels, as cause of nervous instability, 232–234
Ocular movements, relation to orientation, 311
— — — to visual impressions, 54 *n.*
Ogle (John W.), on aneurism by embolism, 31, 31 *n.*, 234 *n.*
Olfactory aura, associations of, 408, 411
Optic nerves, atrophy of, in case of convulsions, 34, 35
— — relations with hemispheres, 33 *n.*
— neuritis, caused by clot, 33 *n.*
— — double, as evidence of syphilis, 32
— — relation to arterial regions, 36
— — — to epilepsy, 387, 393, 394–395
— thalamus, right, symptoms from lesions of, 60
Orbicularis palpebrarum, association with limbs, 75
Organ of mind. *See* Mind, Organ of.
Organic disease, diagnostic value of absence of insensibility, 18–19
— sensations, nature of, 241
Orientation, relation to ocular movements, 311

Pagenstecher, ophthalmoscopic examination in case of convulsions, 34
Paget (G. E.), on diet in epilepsy, 292
— — on gastric epilepsy, 15
Paget (Sir James), case of convulsions, 33
— — on case of neuralgia, 17, 235
— — " On the Chronometry of Life," 35 *n.*
— — on rhythmic processes, 213
Pain, use of term, 305
Pallor, in epileptic convulsions, 138
Palsy, cause of, 9
— regional, compared with spasm, 5–6
Parallelism. *See* Psycho-Physical Parallelism.
Paralysis, association with convulsions, 211–213
— bilateral, after lesion of one side of brain, 267
— effect on convulsions, 34
— evidential value for localisation, 62–63, 335
— in post-epileptic insanity, 368
— post-epileptiform, 210, 318–329, 336–337, 440 *et seq.*
— — case of, 443–445
— — degrees of, 147, 445–446
— recovery from, dependent on size of lesion, 92
— relation to epileptic discharges, 146–147
Parenth (Joseph), on nervous system in infants, 352
Paresis, of second side, 150, 151
Parkes, on influence of diet on the heart, 237
Paroxysmalness of symptoms, importance of, 387–388
Pathology of epilepsies, 206, 217–237
— relation to clinical study, 112

Pepper, on inward fits, 351
Perception, nature of, 244, 244 *n.*, 245
— relation to idea, 246
— seat of, 59
Peripheral effects of epileptic discharges, grouping of, 288
*Petit mal*, cases of, inferences from, 47
— — cause of, 66
— — discharging lesions as cause of, 203
— — loss of consciousness in, 157, 158
— — symptoms of, 172 *n.*
— — use of term, 282, 283
Phosphorus, replacement by nitrogen in nerve cells, 97, 224
— use in epilepsy, 237
Physiological, use of term, 208
— fulminate, use of term, 432
— unit, use of term, 89
Physiology of epilepsy, 206, 208–219
— neural, distinction from psychology, 48
— of mind, use of term, 52 *n.*
— relation to medicine, 81
Pitres, experiments on muscular rigidity, 449
— on bilateral convulsions, 334
— on cortical exhaustion after fits, 443
— on experimental epilepsy in animals, 280
— on nervous system in infants, 352
Poisons, fits produced by, 417
Pontobulbar fits, nature of, 415, 416, 417
Post-epileptic states, 366–384
Posterior part of cerebral hemisphere, function of, 178, 189
Poumeau (Ivan), on the effects of plugging of vessels, 233
Power, loss of, after convulsions, 158
Powerlessness, universal, how caused in convulsions, 71
Presentation of ideas, 56
Pressure, arrest of convulsions by, 13–14
Prévost, on the effects of plugging of vessels, 233
— on lateral deviation of eyes, 71 *n.*, 87, 88 *n.*
— on local hyperæmia, 98
— on movements of the eyes, 62
Prostration, after-effect of epileptic discharges, 142
Psychical process, relation to physical, 43, 452–453, 455, 457
— medicine, use of term, 53 *n.*
— states, at onset of fits, 312–317
— — relation to nervous discharges, 300
— — — to physical states, 322, 325, 330, 366
Psychologico-materialistic method of explanation, 52
Psychology, distinction from physiology, 41–42, 48
— importance of, in study of brain disease, 330, 366
— relation to mental physiology, 84
— — to physiology of nervous system, 168, 198
— use of term, 53 *n.*
Psycho-physical parallelism, 52, 139, 169, 239 *n.*, 367 *n.*
Pulse, effect of convulsions on, 248

Rachitis, relation to fits, 353, 355
Radcliffe (C. B.), on causes of convulsions, 4
— — on chorea, 79
Radcliffe (C. B.), on localisation of choreic lesions, 273
— — on nutrition of nerve tissue, 96
Rapid, use of term, 431
Reading, as test of defect of speech, 20
Recognition, defect of, cause of, 59, 60
— nature of, 180
Recollection, 26 *n.*, 43, 56
Recoverability from paralysis, 210
Reeling, nature of, 192–193, 371
Reflex action, 60–61, 122–123, 179
Reflexes, post-epileptiform, 337
Reminiscence, cases of, 398, 400, 458
— in epilepsy, 467–468
— sensation of, 274, 297, 385, 389
— use of term, 296 *n.*
Remorse, relation to nerve exhaustion, 302
Representation in motor centres, 154
— of ideas, 56
— of movements, 420–421
Respiration, suspension of, in epilepsy, 288, 290
Respiratory convulsions, 355–357, 416
Retino-ocular action, 180
Retino-ocular processes, use of term, 56
Reynolds (Russell), on cause of convulsions, 99
— — on eccentric irritations, 235
— — on epilepsy, 220
— — on relation of nervous diseases to epilepsy, 119
Rhythm of consciousness, 245, 246
Rhythmic action, 95
— processes, 213
Ribs, rickety, relation to fits, 355
Rickets. *See* Rachitis.
Right third nerve, paralysis of, in case of convulsions, 33
Rindfleisch (G. E.), on causes of diseases of the nervous system, 229
Rivington, case of self-mutilation in epilepsy, 131–133
Robertson (Alexander), case of colour aura in epilepsy, 146
— — — of epilepsy, 154
— — — of right-sided convulsion, 312
— — hypothesis of dissolution, 135–161, 318, 321
Rokitansky (C.), on local hyperæmia, 98
Ross (J.), on sizes of nerve cells, 439 *n.*
Russell, paper on "Hemiplegic Epilepsy," 36
Rutherford (J.), on nerve conductivity, 226
— — on over-action of lower centres, 123 *n.*

Saliva, increased flow in epileptic convulsions, 138
Sander, case of epilepsy with olfactory symptoms, 410, 463
— — case of large glioma on under surface of brain, 472
Satanic possession, theory of, 252
Satisfaction, as sensation of nutrition, 305
Savage (G.), on relationship between epilepsy and insanity, 379
Schäfer (Sir E.), on face area of brain, 454
— — on representation of spinal muscles, 439
— — on visual centre, 396 *n.*

Schrœder van der Kolk (J. L. C.), on epilepsy, 95
— — on relation between grey matter and size of muscles, 438
— — on seat of convulsions, 214
Seizures. *See* Convulsions.
Self-mutilation, in epilepsy, case of, 131–133
Semon (Sir Felix), on laryngismus stridulus, 416, 422
Sensation, use of term, 55–56, 140, 177 *n.*, 243 *n.*, 244 *n.*, 245, 287
Sensations, crude, relation to fits, 286, 425
— — relation to psychical states, 300–301
— nature of, 312
— systemic. *See* Systemic.
— use of term, 152, 170
— warning, in epilepsy, 137, 153
Sensibility attending lowest nervous centres, 48
— doctrine of, 239 *n.*
Sensori-motor nature of highest centres, 323, 325, 330, 367–368
— use of term, 170, 171
— process, definition of, 178
— — nature of, 238–239
— processes, as substrata of consciousness, 42, 110, 162 *n.*, 186
— — — of ideas, 82
— — — of mental states, 49
— — — of mentation, 40–41
— — discharge of, effects of, 57
— — — importance of mode of onset for localisation, 91
— — relation to visual ideas, 53, 54
— — results of disorderly development of, 26 *n.*, 43, 58
Sensorium, definition of, 188
Sensory, use of term, 140
— aspect of mind, localisation of, 58–62
— centre, localisation in posterior part of brain, 139
— sensation, physical basis of, 305
Shape, visual idea of, 53, 54
Sherrington (C. S.), on degeneration of the cord after lesion, 444 *n.*
— — on re-crossed fibres, 419 *n.*
— — on a trunk centre, 475
Shock, influence on nerve of, 223
Shoulder, movements of, 91
Sight, defect of, in case of epileptiform convulsions, 1
— failure of. *See* Blindness.
— internal, in cases of blindness, 86
— *See also* Vision.
Simultaneous, use of term, 217 *n.*
Simultaneous movements, how effected, 36
— — loss of, in hemiplegia, 26, 27
Singer (Douglas), case of convulsions (lowest-level fit), 474–481
Singing, relation to speech, 73 *n.*
Size, visual idea of, 53, 54
Sleep, 124 *n.*, 356 *n.*, 376, 383
Smell, sensation of, associated with epilepsy, 127, 303, 464–473
— sense of, importance of, 468 *n.*
— — localisation of, 406–411
Smith (Eustace), on congenital heart disease, 360
— — on convulsions in children, 222
— — on treatment of fits, 358
Sneeze, nature of, 96
Soltmann, on nervous system in infancy, 352, 353
Soul, belief in, does not affect study of anatomy, 52
Soutter, case of fits limited to right arm, 116–117
Space co-ordination, 26, 26 *n.*, 27, 272
Spasm, case of, in right arm, 11
— compared with regional palsy, 5–6
— distinction from movement, 284
— march of, 68–70
— — importance for localisation of lesion, 333–334
— range of, 264–267, 332–333
— relation to subsequent paralysis, 327
— sequence of, 268–273
— spread of, relation to rate of liberation, 328–329
— starting-points of, importance for localisation of lesion, 332
— suddenness of, importance for localisation of lesion, 334–335
— unilateral, at onset of epileptic paroxysms, 308–317
— *See also* Hemispasm.
Spectral illusions, relation to epileptic discharges, 141
Speech, ataxic affection of, use of term, 65
— defect of, relation to convulsions, 91, 163
— — — to loss of speech, 85
— — use of term, 451
— defects of, as affected by different pathological processes, 221
— — description of, 22, 22 *n.*
— — in cases of convulsions, 19–23
— — post-epileptiform, 450
— — *See also* Aphasia.
— dependence on one side of the brain, 39
— internal, 55 *n.*, 85–86, 87
— involuntary, 266 *n.*
— localisation of, 452 *n.*
— loss of, in case of epileptiform convulsions caused by blow, 2–3
— — classification of cases, 191
— — order of loss of movements in, 65
— — relation to defect of speech, 85
— — significance of, 73 *n.*
— nature of, 142 *n.*
— physical process of, 452
— relation to nervous discharges, 179
Spencer (Herbert), debt to, 167, 366 *n.*
— — doctrine of evolution, 38 *n.*
— — on anger, 305
— — on cases of mistakes in words, 85 *n.*
— — on classification, 190
— — on co-ordination, 108
— — on degrees of consciousness, 188
— — on detachment of nervous centres, 375
— — on discharge of nerve centres, 96
— — on evolution of nervous centres, 107, 216, 217
— — on faculty of music, 73 *n.*
— — on grey matter of brain, 108
— — on mentation, 199
— — on mind and matter, 169
— — on modes of consciousness, 61 *n.*
— — on molecular action of nerve centres, 438–439

Spencer (Herbert), on movements of the eyes, 88
— — on nature of consciousness, 188–189
— — on nervous evolution, 123, 147 *n.*
— — on nitrogenised substances, 227
— — on "Physiological Unit," 89 *n.*
— — on psychology, 41
— — on recognition, 180
— — on rhythm in consciousness, 245
— — on the faculties of the mind, 175 *n.*
— — on the seat of consciousness, 110–111, 154, 172
— — on the sense of touch, 75, 117 *n.*, 262 *n.*
— — on the statical attributes of body, 54
— — on theory of growth, 439 *n.*
— — on time in consciousness, 205
— — on variation of quantity of grey matter, 262
— — psychological teachings of, 238 *n.*
Square, case of hemiplegia, 221 *n.*
Stammering, as sequel to convulsions, 21–22
Status epilepticus, use of term, 482
Stewart (J. Purves), case of epilepsy with warning sensation of smell, 464–473
Stomach, cerebral centre for, 249
Strychnine, effect on nerve cells, 429 *n.*
Stumps, faradising, effect of, 55 *n.*
Subject consciousness, substrata of, 243, 245
Subject-object, use of term, 152 *n.*
Subjective, use of term, 310
Subjective sensations, representation of, seat of, 311
Substrata of consciousness, use of term, 289
Succession of movements, how effected, 36
— — — loss of, in unilateral convulsions, 27, 28
Suggestion, external, modification of post-epileptic automatism by, 127
"Swollen dish" appearance of eyes, in case of convulsions, 33
Sylvian artery, 9
— region, lesions of, 25–26
Symonds (J.), on sleep, 376
Symptoms, local, caused by local lesions of brain, 24–29
— method of showing relations of, 79
— relation to destruction of part of brain, 214–215
— — to seat of discharging lesions, 137
— slight, importance of, in epilepsy, 390
— *See also* Nervous Symptoms.
Syphilis in diseases of nervous system, 229
— relation to brain tumour, 346
— — to convulsions, 474
— — to optic neuritis, 395
Syphilitic disease of hemisphere, cases of, 32
Systemic movements, representation of, 248 *n.*
— sensations, 118, 241, 311

Tactual ideas, epileptic discharge of anatomical substrata of, 57
— — relation to visual ideas, 58
— impressions, 75, 117 *n.*
— movements, relation to eye, 58, 75, 88
— organs, movements of, relation to movements of eyes, 75
— — *See also* Touch, sense of.
Taine (H.), on experiments by Vulpian, 46
Taste, sensation of, as beginning of fit, 302–303
— sense of, localisation of, 409, 461
Tasting movements, in case of epilepsy, 402, 458–463
Temporo-sphenoidal lobe, disease of, case of, 464–473
Tenner (A.), on epilepsy, 220
— — experiments on brains of animals, 109
— — on experimental production of fits in rabbits, 348
Terminal, use of term, 427 *n.*
Tetanus, caused by external injury, 17
Thinking aloud, 87
Thomson (William), Archbishop of York, on method of thinking of deaf-mutes, 86
Thorne (Thorne), on masked epilepsy, 122
Thought, duplex form of, 124 *n.*
Thrombosis, as cause of nervous instability, 232, 234
Thumb, aura of, in case of epileptiform convulsions, 1–2
— specialised character of, 91, 116, 261
Time, co-ordination, 27, 272
— necessity of, for consciousness, 143, 205
Tissues, as constituents of the body, 235
Todd (R. B.), epileptic hemiplegia of, 13, 19 *n.*, 94, 142, 168, 337, 347
— — hypothesis of effects of epileptic discharges, 135–161, 318, 321
Toe, left, case of convulsion beginning from, 116
Tongue, aura of, in case of epileptiform convulsions, 3
— biting, remarks on, 14
— movement of, in thinking, 50
— right side, effect of convulsions beginning in, 19
Tonic spasm, from epileptic discharge, 272
Touch, sense of, relation to intelligence, 117 *n.*
— — Spencer on, 262 *n.*
— *See also* Tactual.
Traumatic convulsions, case of, 2–3
Trephining, in case of convulsions, 33
Trousseau (A.), on case of visceral aura, 291–292
— — on diet in epilepsy, 225
— — on epileptic insanity, 122
— — on "remembrance" in epilepsy, 298
Trunk fits, case of, 474–486
Tuke (Hack), on relation of mental diseases to epilepsy, 119
Tumour. *See* Brain, tumour of.
Tyndall (J.), on distinction of mental and physical, 41
Types, 192, 202–203

Uncinate group of fits, 467
— gyrus, left, softening in, case of, 462
Uniformity of attacks in epilepsy, 250–251
Unilateral convulsion, use of term, 257
— convulsions. *See* Convulsions, Epileptiform, Unilateral.
Universalisation of convulsion, method of, 435
Uræmia, as cause of nervous discharge, 35
Urine, passage of, in diagnosis of epilepsy, 293

Valvular disease, associated with epilepsy, 3–4
Varied uses, distinction of voluntary part, 91
Vaso-motor centre, nature of, 374 *n.*
Velocity of nervous discharges, importance of, 227
Verbalising, relation to speech, 142 *n.*
— use of term, 65
Vertigo, association with, dreamy state, 313–314, 385, 397
— as effect of epilepsy, 140
— as motor sensation, 304–305
— as precursor of epilepsy, 286
— epileptic, significance of, 48 *n.*
— nature of, 26 *n.*, 43, 193–195
— ocular symptoms in, 55 *n.*
— sensations in, 56
— use of term, 87, 309
Violence, in epilepsy, cases of, 129–134
— in epileptic insanity, 120
Virchow (Rudolf), on a blow as start of brain tumour, 346
— — on local hyperæmia, 98
Viscera, relation to cerebral centres, 46, 47, 292
Visceral aura, nature of, 292
Vision, coloured. *See* Coloured Vision.
Visual ideas, nature of, 180, 181
— — relation to tactual ideas, 58, 239 *n.*
— — substrata of, 53–57
— impressions, relation to tactual impressions, 75
— perception, defect of. *See* Recognition, Defect of.
— sensations, as effect of epilepsy, 140
"Vital," symptoms, 110, 115 *n.*
"Voices," nature of, 141 *n.*
Voisin (F.), definition of epilepsy, 100 *n.*
— — on mental states in epilepsy, 298
— — on uniformity of attacks of epilepsy, 250
Volition, nature of, 160
Voluminous mental state, 303, 385, 386
— — — use of term, 296
Voluntary, use of term, 63 *n.*, 68 *n.*, 72 *n.*, 116
— action, relation to automatic, 64
— movements, compared with automatic, 90, 261
— part, definition of, 91
Vomiting, symptomatic of foreign body in brain, 19
Vulpian (E. F. A.), experiments on brains of animals, 46, 106, 107 *n.*, 109
— — on lateral deviation of eyes, 87, 88 *n.*
— — on movements of the eyes, 62
— — on paralysis of frog, 319

Walking, use of paralysed leg in, 34
Wallerian wasting. *See* Wasting.
Warnings in epilepsy, 137, 153
— — importance for classification, 309
Wasting, descending, of fibres, 74, 150, 151, 267, 326 *n.*
Weakness, relation to paralysis, 325, 327, 337
Weber (Sir Herman), on affections of speech after fits, 450
West (Charles), in inward fits, 351
— — on diet in epilepsy, 225
Westphal (C.), on post-epileptiform reflexes, 337
Whateley, on case of Laura Bridgman, 86
Whewell (W.), on types, 192 *n.*, 202–203
Whooping cough, relation to fits, 360
Wilks (Sir Samuel), on causes of convulsions, 164 *n.*
Will. *See* entries under Volition, Voluntary.
Words, memory of, centre for, 49–53
— — loss of, 50, 65, 83–85
— place of, in thinking, 39, 40
— relation of left side of brain to, 65
— substrata of, 49, 52, 53, 181
Writing, as test of defect of speech, 20
— relation to sensori-motor processes, 85